ALTERNATIVE
MEDICINE

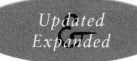

Updated &
Expanded

ALTERNATIVE MEDICINE

• the options • the claims • the evidence
• how to choose wisely

THE CHRISTIAN HANDBOOK

DÓNAL O'MATHÚNA, PHD
WALT LARIMORE, MD

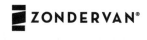

ZONDERVAN®

ZONDERVAN.com/
AUTHORTRACKER
follow your favorite authors

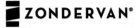

Alternative Medicine
Copyright © 2001, 2007 by Dónal O'Mathúna and Walter L. Larimore

Requests for information should be addressed to:

Zondervan, *Grand Rapids, Michigan 49530*

Library of Congress Cataloging-in-Publication Data

O'Mathúna, Dónal, 1961–.
     Alternative medicine : the Christian handbook / Dónal O'Mathúna and Walt Larimore.
  —Updated and expanded.
       p.   cm.
    Includes bibliographical references and index.
    ISBN 978-0-310-26999-1
    1. Alternative medicine—Handbooks, manuals, etc. 2. Holistic medicine—Religious aspects—
Christianity—Handbooks, manuals, etc. I. Larimore, Walter L. II. Title.
    R733.O48   2006
    610—dc22

                                                        2006024642

The website addresses recommended throughout this book are offered as a resource to you. These websites are not intended in any way to be or imply an endorsement on the part of Zondervan, nor do we vouch for their content for the life of this book.

This book contains advice and information relating to health and medicine. It is designed for your personal knowledge and to help you be a more informed consumer of medical and health services. It is not intended to be exhaustive or to replace medical advice from your physician and should be used to supplement rather than replace regular care by your physician. Readers are encouraged to consult their physicians with specific questions and concerns.

Interior design by Beth Shagene

Printed in the United States of America

11 12 13 14 • 28 27 26 25 24 23 22 21 20 19 18 17 16 15 14 13 12 11 10 9 8 7 6 5 4

FOR CHERI AND BARB—
OUR WIVES AND BEST FRIENDS,
WHO HAVE ALWAYS ENCOURAGED
AND PRAYED FOR US

CONTENTS

PART THREE
HERBAL REMEDIES, VITAMINS, AND DIETARY SUPPLEMENTS

9. Reviews of Remedies / 277

FOREWORD

DAVID STEVENS, M.D.

Have you ever noticed that the more we learn about health, the more complicated our lives become?

Scientific knowledge is increasing at a logarithmic rate. More knowledge means more options. Making choices — especially about something as important as our health — produces anxiety and stress.

Not only do we have to make a choice; we also have to evaluate the trustworthiness of each messenger and the validity of the message. What is the real motivation of the messenger? Is it to make money or a true altruistic motive? Have others verified the evidence?

Christians have yet another task. They must evaluate their choices in light of the question, "What would Jesus do?"

The explosion of health care knowledge has generated a plethora of ethical and spiritual issues. Some are obvious ethical issues, such as abortion, physician-assisted suicide, and human cloning. Other issues facing Christians are not so obvious. How would Jesus have me deal with cancer or some other life-threatening illness? Should I select my treatment based solely on how well I think it might work, or do spiritual issues impact some of those decisions? Must I always pursue *some* treatment? What

does it mean to die well? How should I prepare myself and my loved ones for my death?

You may feel there are more questions than answers. Most Christians do. As a physician who has cared for and counseled with tens of thousands of patients, I understand your confusion. You want and need a trusted expert to assist you. That is why the Christian Medical Association has joined with Zondervan to produce resources on health care issues — resources you can trust. Each resource, written by one or more carefully chosen experts who are eminently qualified to give you guidance, will provide solid scientific information in language you can understand. Most important, our authors will present and evaluate your choices from a Christian worldview. Then you can make God-honoring decisions.

The Christian Medical Association (CMA) is a *movement* of Christian doctors. The ministry was established in 1931 to help Christian health care professionals integrate their personal faith and professional practice.

Today, the Christian Medical Association helps thousands of members integrate faith and practice in hospitals and clinics, in private practices, on the mission field, and in academic institutions.

FOREWORD

Presently, over 90 percent of medical schools in the United States have a CMA student chapter that helps students from the first day of classes begin to integrate their faith and profession. Our goal is to help members become like the Great Physician, Jesus Christ.

The Christian Medical Association also holds conferences, produces resources, and develops positions on some of the tough ethical issues of our day. As the voice of Christian doctors, CMA provides testimony before Congress, submits amicus curiae briefs to the Supreme Court, provides public service announcements, and conducts national and local media interviews. We also want to fulfill an obligation to provide educational resources and other helpful information to the church.

Why this particular book? One of the most perplexing health care issues facing Christians today is how to evaluate alternative medicine in two areas:

• How can we evaluate therapies as effective, possibly helpful, or without merit?

• What alternative medicine systems contain non-Christian belief systems?

This book helps define what alternative medicine is and provides a distinctly Christian framework to evaluate each modality. In encyclopedic format, the authors evaluate dozens of alternative medicines and therapies, from reflexology to St. John's wort. The book gives you the evidence for what is helpful. When the evidence is unclear, this book gives you the facts. When a method presents physical or spiritual dangers, this book sounds the alert.

This book has been created by experts in the area of alternative medicine. The manuscript has been reviewed by a committee made up of doctors with a variety of training and experience. The result is a resource that should make its way to every Christian's reference shelf.

May you use this book to learn the facts, weigh the evidence, and make sound, God-honoring decisions.

ACKNOWLEDGMENTS

Many people have contributed to this book. We are deeply indebted to the Christian Medical Association (CMA) for their initiative in bringing us together to work on this project. Dave Stevens, M.D., and Gene Rudd, M.D., through their leadership roles in CMA, saw the need for a resource like this and have encouraged us at every stage. CMA provided a Professional Review Committee for the first edition; Gene Rudd, Al Weir, M.D., and Carol Bence, M.S., R.N., reviewed this edition. We are very grateful for their helpful comments and insightful critiques.

We are grateful to Zondervan for their support of the first edition of this book and their continued and enthusiastic support of this revised and expanded edition. Sandy Vander Zicht has been our main contact, encourager, equipper, and editor. Many others at Zondervan contributed to the final book, but we are especially thankful for the excellent editing of Jane Haradine and Dirk Buursma. We are indebted to literary agent Lee Hough at Alive Communications and attorney Ned McLeod for their valuable assistance and advice.

We especially want to acknowledge the prayers, love, support, and encouragement of our wives, Cheri O'Mathúna and Barb Larimore. We thank God daily for the privilege of being fathers to our precious children — for Dónal, Catrina, Conor, and Peter; and for Walt, Kate and Scott. We thank our families for all the things they have done and sacrificed to make it possible for us to write.

Finally, we are most grateful to our Lord and Savior, Jesus Christ, for choosing us to serve him through writing. Our deepest prayer is that this book will bring glory to God. To the extent that what we wrote is truthful and helpful, the praise and glory go to him. But if we have erred in anything, we accept sole responsibility.

Dónal O'Mathúna
Dunboyne, County Meath, Ireland

Walt Larimore
Colorado Springs, Colorado

March 2006

NOTE FROM THE AUTHORS

We have written this book together because we share two deeply held beliefs — one involving faith, the other science.

Growing up in different parts of the world has given us many different experiences (Walt grew up in Louisiana, while Dónal grew up in Ireland.) We'll use our first names occasionally in the book when referring to something only one of us has experienced. Our education and professional training also give us different perspectives (Dónal has a Ph.D. in pharmacy from The Ohio State University and an M.A. in theology from Ashland Theological Seminary; Walt is an M.D. trained at Duke University). Nevertheless, our lives have come to have a common purpose based on the relationship we each have with God. We seek to serve God and his people out of gratitude for the many blessings we have received from him.

The second common belief that motivates us is our appreciation for science. This may seem like a contradiction to those who hear about the antagonism between science and Christianity. We see science and Christianity as highly compatible. Both involve faith and evidence, usually applied to different topics. Science accumulates evidence about the natural world; scientists have faith in their beliefs that scientific laws apply to the universe and that human observation gives reliable information. Christianity provides evidence that God exists, that Jesus lived and died and rose again, and that the Bible accurately reveals God's character and will. But evidence only goes so far, and then a step of faith is needed to believe in Jesus Christ. We, along with many other respected scientists throughout history, see science as a vital tool in both understanding God's creation and learning to be wise stewards of the resources God has given us to improve people's health and lives. We disagree with those who misuse science in an attempt to deny God's existence or to validate some theory that is not only worthless but dangerous.

Several observations led us to write the first edition of this book, *Alternative Medicine: The Christian Handbook*, published in 2001. We saw patients taking herbal remedies and supplements about which very little information (good or bad) was known. People were diagnosing and treating themselves with herbs and dietary supplements without obtaining the best possible diagnoses. People were being harmed by delaying or avoiding proven medical treatment. People were enduring unnecessary suffering, risks, and even death. We met patients who were exposed to "therapies" without being told of their religious roots or spiritual implications. Faith communities were embroiled in controversy about alternative medicine, sometimes with limited or no evidence to support either side of the debate. Some claimed to have discovered God's approach to health, and some Christian media carried advertisements endorsing all sorts of unproven and potentially harmful supplements.

Most commonly, though, people had questions. What works? What is safe? Where can we get trustworthy information? Where can we find quality products? How do we pick a therapist? What is in keeping with our faith commitment?

Patients and health care professionals had few resources they could easily access for reliable information about alternative medicine. Even when information *was* available on the effectiveness and safety of therapies and remedies, the spiritual background and faith implications usually were not examined.

We put together a single resource on alternative medicine that combined the latest and most accurate information from these two important perspectives — science and an orthodox Judeo-Christian worldview. By "worldview" we mean the broad set of beliefs a person has about the way the world is, the way things really are, and the way things should be. We looked to scientific research for evidence about effectiveness and safety, and we looked to Scripture for evidence regarding spiritual issues and the implications of certain therapies for Christians.

We combed the medical literature and published reports from the United States and many other countries. We talked to conventional and alternative practitioners to find out more about the effectiveness and safety of the most common alternative therapies. To compile this information in a practical and user-friendly manner, we developed categories of treatment, tools for ranking the research that has been done, and tools for ranking the effectiveness of the therapies and remedies. We organized all this information to help you quickly find both information and our recommendations on a specific therapy or herb or dietary supplement.

Many of the issues that led to our first edition remain the same. Information on alternative medicine is more readily available today, but its reliability must be carefully evaluated. Few other resources offer a detailed evaluation of both the scientific and theological issues surrounding specific forms of alternative medicine.

As we predicted in our first edition, new studies have become available on some of the therapies and remedies we evaluated. This new and expanded edition incorporates this new evidence. To our satisfaction, most of these new studies have confirmed our initial recommendations. In a few cases, we have changed our recommendations. In addition, we added new entries for therapies and remedies that have become popular since the first edition. Some entries were removed because surveys reported they were seldom used.

Many readers report going straight to the evaluations of the therapies and remedies that interest them. That is understandable. We urge you to read Part 1, as it contains important information to help you evaluate alternative medicine in general. There we explain why scientists place such emphasis on research and clinical trials. We show how medicine without the scientific method was a free-for-all that often caused more harm than good. Part 1 gives you the tools you need to evaluate therapies and offers tips on understanding the results of various types of studies. It explains the "evidence-based" aspect of this book, an approach to evaluating all forms of drugs and therapies that is widely recognized around the world.

NOTE FROM THE AUTHORS

Christians should be concerned about much more than whether a therapy is effective. Certain therapies raise spiritual issues. Part 1 examines why people need to understand the beliefs underlying therapies. We give guidelines for evaluating therapies and therapists in light of Scripture.

Christianity is much more than a list of dos and don'ts. Our reading and study of Scripture convinces us that God wants to influence the way in which his people approach health and healing. We let you in on what we found during our study, giving you verse after verse to guide you in making your decisions and to help you answer those who would distort Scripture for their own reasons. We offer guidelines for a faith-based approach to health and healing, whether one pursues conventional medicine or alternative therapies.

Parts 2 and 3 evaluate particular therapies or remedies. Almost all the entries are arranged according to a set format; a small number of entries required a different approach or a more extensive entry. Alternative therapies are listed alphabetically in Part 2; herbal remedies, dietary supplements, and some vitamins are listed in Part 3. Each entry is as concise as possible to give you the most useful information as conveniently as possible.

We pray that this book will be a service to you. Join us in praying that God will guide you as you make decisions about your health and the health of those in your care.

Dónal O'Mathúna
Dunboyne, County Meath, Ireland

Walt Larimore
Colorado Springs, Colorado

PART ONE

EVALUATING ALTERNATIVE MEDICINE

CHAPTER 1

PURSUING ALTERNATIVE MEDICINE

Alternative medicine remains very popular. Several surveys have found that roughly one-third of adults in the United States use some form of complementary and alternative medicine.1 But what are these people using? Is what they are using safe? An accurate picture of the situation is complicated.

If you've decided to try alternative medicine, you may have had difficulty finding accurate information. Our book provides a summary of the best scientific evidence available on dozens of the most popular products and therapies. We also examine the spiritual benefits and risks from an orthodox Judeo-Christian worldview. This book may well be the only one on alternative medicine that is both evidence-based and faith-based.

Alternative medicine includes many things — some good, some bad. There is the potential for great benefit, but there is also the potential for serious harm. Before trying any remedy or therapy, give careful consideration to the whole area of alternative medicine.

First we need to define a few terms. What do we mean by "alternative medicine"? What do we mean by "evidence-based"? And what do we mean by "faith-based"? The first question we'll examine here. The two others will be our concern in each of the next two chapters.

What Is Alternative Medicine?

Many would like to replace the term "alternative medicine" with "complementary and alternative medicine" and its acronym, CAM. The term "alternative" suggests that people use these approaches instead of conventional medicine. However, surveys have found that most people combine all these approaches to medicine. In other words, alternative medicine is most typically used to complement (or supplement) standard health care. Hence, the term "complementary" is preferred by some. We will use "alternative medicine" since that term remains most popular in everyday discussions. We use it in its broadest sense to include therapies and remedies used instead of or along with conventional medicine.

What is included within alternative medicine varies considerably from one definition to another. The simplest definition, and the one we will use, is that alternative medicine includes any therapy or remedy that is not generally accepted or provided by the dominant medical establishment in a given culture. Alternative medicine has a number of general characteristics:

- **Passed over by conventional medicine,** alternative medicine includes remedies, therapies, and healing systems that conventional Western health care professionals are unlikely to provide their patients. The dominant medical establishment tends to look with disfavor (or disgust) on alternative medicine, or views its approaches as going beyond the proper domain of medicine. Sometimes, alternative medicine claims to have been pushed aside by practitioners of conventional medicine for reasons of political or financial gain.

- **Holistic approaches** to health care are commonly stressed in alternative medicine. This means different things to different practitioners, but in general they treat the body, mind, and spirit. It also means relying on noninvasive "natural" methods of healing with an emphasis on disease prevention. Although conventional medicine can be holistic, physicians usually do not stress that fact.

- **Spirituality** is frequently addressed within alternative medicine, though often in ways that are unfamiliar or alien to Christianity (and to other major religions such as Judaism and Islam). Without understanding the roots of a particular therapy, you may find yourself involved with a theology dangerously different from what the Scriptures teach or what Jesus would want his followers doing.

- **Little good-quality scientific evidence** is available to support many of alternative medicine's assertions about healing. However, as we will show, some aspects of alternative medicine have excellent scientific support yet are not utilized by many conventional Western physicians. Other therapies, with proper testing, might garner support for their claims. Without such evidence, no one, not even an expert in alternative medicine, knows for certain whether the untested, unproven alternative therapies actually have healed anyone or not. All we know is that patients relate how they were helped or cured or went into remission after using an alternative therapy.

Before you embark on any path that takes you into the world of alternative medicine, even to buy an herbal remedy suggested by a friend, we recommend that you investigate the realities of alternative medicine — the prospective benefits *as well as* the potential costs and the risks you might face. Not all stories are positive.

Hazel (in this book, the cases are real; the names and some of the details have been changed to protect patients' confidentiality) struggled for months with terrible pain in her shoulder. She avoided her physician, afraid she would be urged to take powerful painkillers with nasty side effects or to undergo surgery. So she went to a variety of alternative therapists who said they could massage or manipulate the problem away. Her shoulder would be a little better after each session but soon would hurt again.

Hazel tried all sorts of supplements and went on special diets. No improvement. She was told that the problem was with her energy and could be resolved if she had her energy "cleared." She tried Therapeutic Touch and then Reiki (see Therapeutic Touch and Reiki entries). She felt more relaxed after the sessions, but then the pain would return. Over-the-counter pain relievers helped a little, and Hazel began to wonder if she should give conventional medicine a try.

Frustrated, in constant pain, and unable to use her arm, she consulted Walt. A brief history, a physical exam, and an X-ray quickly revealed a condition called "chronic bursitis." An injection of a nonabsorbable steroid into the bursa — a common and proven conventional treatment — gave Hazel full use of her crippled shoulder within fifteen minutes. Hazel cried, realizing she had needlessly suffered chronic pain for so long while trying alternative medicine.

We don't label alternative medicine as good or bad. Our book points out the *proven* benefits and the *unproven* claims. We expose and explain the risks that many purveyors of alternative therapies appear to be concealing. We will present the background out of which various alternative therapies and remedies arose. And we will also look at what the use of alternative therapies could mean for a Christian. We have tried to anticipate your heartfelt questions and concerns so we can provide objective answers.

We have *nothing* to sell (except this book). We want you to have the best information, the best evidence, so that you can make the best and wisest decisions for your health.

In Part 2 we will discuss each of the most popular alternative therapies available today in North America. Many of these are also popular in Europe, Asia, and Australia. The entries in this section explain the origins of the therapies, give evidence of effectiveness, and list reasons for caution or concern.

Part 3 will give detailed information on popular herbal remedies, dietary supplements, and a few vitamins. We have chosen those popularly used as a form of self-help and available without much direction in health food stores, drugstores, and many supermarkets and on the Internet. Here, too, you'll be able to read our recommendations along with any cautions and concerns.

We know that some people will disagree with our conclusions. Some will reject our insistence on high-quality evidence, saying it's not available yet or can't be provided for particular therapies and remedies. Some claim research costs too much. Yet supplements are now big business, producing large profits, some of which should be put into properly testing the products to protect people using them.

Others may agree with us in general but disagree with specific recommendations. Understandably, those who practice, promote, or sell therapies and remedies will not want to see criticism of things they value or on which they base their living. We accept such disagreements and welcome discussion about our conclusions. We stand ready to change our opinions on one condition: that high-quality evidence be produced that persuades us to change our recommendation. Those familiar with our first edition will see that we have changed some recommendations, based on new evidence. But heartfelt stories or impassioned pleas or appeals based on flawed research will not persuade us to change our recommendations — nor should they persuade you.

Conventional Medicine Takes an Interest in Alternative Medicine

As more research is done, we believe that conventional medicine and alternative medicine will increasingly be used together (hence the move toward CAM). Some alternative therapists recognize the potential of a holistic approach in contemporary conventional medicine and work in tandem with medical physicians to give high-quality care. And many conventional medicine practitioners recognize that one or more alternative therapies might benefit their patients when used in tandem with surgery and pharmaceuticals.

Increasing numbers of doctors, nurses, and other health care professionals are incorporating the best of both approaches into what is called "integrative medicine."[2] Professional continuing medical education (CME) courses also are providing information on alternative medicine. In fact, some of the most popular CME courses for doctors, nurses, and phar-

macists focus specifically on alternative medicine. Pharmacies are increasingly making alternative remedies available, although natural food and health food stores, the Internet, and mail-order companies still account for most of these sales. Some areas of alternative medicine have become more popular even while sales in other areas have decreased. In 2003, overall herbal remedy sales in the United States dropped, but homeopathy sales grew by 3 percent overall and by almost 50 percent in mainstream outlets such as drugstores.[3] In addition, pharmaceutical companies have begun distributing alternative remedies and are doing some testing.

Interest Grows among Christians

Interest among Christians appears to mirror — and sometimes exceed — these general trends. Christian radio stations carry advertisements for herbal remedies and nutritional supplements even more commonly than the secular media. We have serious reservations about most of these "infomercials." Our God is a God of truth, and claims made in Christian media should be supportable and true. A Christian company should have the courage to insist that its advertisers support the accuracy of their claims. Those who declare that their therapies and remedies can treat or cure conditions should provide the sort of verifiable evidence of effectiveness and lack of harm we discuss throughout the book — we'll explain why as we go along.

Specific "Christian" alternative therapies are also promoted. One entrepreneur claimed to have figured out the recipe for manna and alleged it would protect people from all forms of illness, just as the original manna protected the Israelites in the wilderness. Another is the "Genesis 1:29 Diet," based on God's declaration, "I give you every seed-bearing plant on the face of the whole earth and every tree that has fruit with seed in it. They will be yours for food." Believers in this diet teach that people will be most healthy when eating a biblically based vegetarian diet.

Are there really "Christian therapies"? We frequently hear Christian "success" stories promoted to encourage Christian involvement in alternative medicine. Some Christians claim to have found particular ways to cure or alleviate cancer.[4] One prominent Christian author wrote about the benefits he experienced from an alternative cancer therapy available only in Europe.[5]

Highly sophisticated medical studies have been conducted on the effectiveness of prayer for healing. Results of research into the impact of spirituality and religious faith on health and healing have been published in mainstream medical journals.[6] Some Christians now claim the power of prayer is supported by scientific research with "overwhelming, undeniable results".[7] Is that really the case and does that make prayer a therapy? Both of us are firm believers in the power of prayer as described in the Bible, but we question whether scientific studies should be used to validate that belief. We will examine this issue in detail in the Prayer for Healing entry.

NIH Begins Evaluation of Alternative Medicine Treatments

In 1992, the National Institutes of Health began an evaluation of alternative medical treatments, establishing the Office of Alternative Medicine (since renamed the National Center for Complementary and Alternative Medicine, or NCCAM). Funding has increased from $2 million in 1992 to $50 million in 1999 and $123 million in 2005.[8] Prominent universities and major medical centers have received substantial grants to encourage research in and teaching of alternative medicine. Many medical schools and nursing schools have courses in alternative therapies.

Since the 1990s, a number of new publications devoted to alternative medicine have been launched. The main database for peer-reviewed medical publications (called PubMed) includes twelve such journals, and we are aware of at least four others whose primary audience is physicians and health care professionals. Well-established conventional medical journals (such as the *Journal of the American Medical Association*, *New England Journal of Medicine*, *American Family Physician,* and *Lancet*) regularly publish articles about alternative medicine.

Medical insurance and managed-care companies have started paying for some alternative therapies. Some jurisdictions now require that alternative therapies be included among the therapies covered by insurers. However, some of these trends have started to change. In 1999, basic health insurance in Switzerland was required to cover five complementary therapies, including herbal remedies, homeopathy, and traditional Chinese medicine.[9] In 2005, the Swiss government reversed its policy, claiming the alternatives did not meet requirements for efficacy or cost-effectiveness.

Alternative Medicine Is Big Business

Despite some problems with and concerns about alternative medicine, Americans are increasingly spending more and more money on alternative medicine.[10] Between 1997 and 2002, significant increases in the use of herbal remedies occurred. In 2002, 18.6 percent of Americans were using herbal remedies, *not* including vitamins and dietary supplements not of plant origin.[11] Over $4 billion is now spent annually in the United States on herbal remedies, although sales through mainstream markets dropped 7 percent in 2004.[12] No longer can it be said that alternative medicine is a small fringe market. It is a major business enterprise with all of the advantages and limitations that this brings.

Risks in Alternative Medicine

The risks with alternative medicine are real. Reliance on unproven alternative therapies can have tragic results.

Walt first became involved with Joe's care after Joe was brought to the emergency room in severe pain from a collapsed vertebra. An MRI (a diagnostic imaging test) showed cancer had spread to his brain and bones. Joe, an energetic African-American father of four, told how he had been diagnosed a few years earlier with early-stage prostate cancer and was concerned that the medical options to "cure" the cancer were invasive and fraught with significant cost and risk.

A friend took Joe to their local health food store, where the owner recommended a number of nutritional therapies and dietary supplements "proven to cure cancer" and "not known to most doctors." Joe then saw a local alternative medicine practitioner who, without even examining him, recommended only alternative therapies. The therapist told Joe that

the therapies she recommended were "being kept secret by the government."

Days passed, then weeks, and then a couple of years. Slowly Joe began to develop more symptoms. By the time I saw Joe, a young man in his forties, there would be no cure, no happy ending. I could only try to relieve his pain, his guilt and suffering, and comfort him as his wife and children, the staff, and I helplessly watched his life fade away.

The outcome most likely would have been different with conventional medical therapy. Medical literature is filled with well-documented evidence that early detection of and intervention in prostate cancer frequently results in cure. Joe probably died prematurely because he put his trust and faith in unproven alternative therapies suggested by those not trained in medical diagnosis and treatment. Although he was sincere in his belief about alternative medicine, as were the folks who recommended the unproven therapies, they were all sincerely wrong.

Unfortunately, these types of stories are not uncommon. A researcher for the British Research Council for Complementary Medicine visited twenty-nine health food stores in London asking advice about frequent, severe headaches.[13] Her fictitious symptoms were chosen so that a trained professional would easily recognize them as suggesting a brain tumor or other serious problem. The researcher was told by health food store employees that her headaches were caused by the flu, low blood sugar, tension, the weather, or using her brain too much. Forty-two different therapies were recommended, with no consistency in the advice given. At fewer than one in four of the stores was the researcher advised to see a physician.

In another study in Hawaii, a researcher visited forty health food stores stating she was gathering information on herbal remedies for her mother, whose advanced breast cancer had spread throughout her body (metastasized).[14] In 90 percent of the stores, employees recommended various products to cure cancer, even though making such a claim is against the law. The most popular remedy, recommended at almost half the stores, was shark cartilage. Later in the book we discuss the complete lack of evidence that shark cartilage cures cancer — or anything else. Of great concern is that almost one in five employees counseled *against* using conventional cancer therapies that have been proven to be effective.

Of course, we can point to many stories of how our large conventional medical system has also caused harm to patients. Alternative medicine proponents jump all over these stories and cite an endless parade of pharmaceutical horror stories — such as thalidomide given to pregnant women to treat nausea, resulting in their babies having serious birth defects, including missing or shortened arms or legs. They relate how mass inoculation against the swine flu virus resulted in serious illness, even death. They tell of people who have become overly dependent on the latest tranquilizer or sedative. They note that wonder drugs, such as Vioxx to treat arthritis pain, have been withdrawn from the market after being linked to patients' deaths — in spite of all sorts of controlled studies beforehand. They tell how people die every year from medication mistakes in hospitals and from prescription errors. And they are right. Conventional medicine is not perfect. It is a human enterprise in which practitioners are always learning and sometimes making mistakes — terrible mistakes.

What the proponents of alternative medicine rarely, if ever, reveal to those seeking advice are the failures and mistakes from their past — stories of those who believed false or inaccurate claims and suffered, even died, needlessly.

With this book, we want you to become "as wise as serpents" about the risks and benefits of conventional *and* alternative medicine. We don't want you to continue to merely ask, "What do you recommend?" or "What do you think is best?" We want you to ask the practitioners of conventional or alternative medicine, "What is the evidence that supports what you believe or recommend?" We want you to learn how to wisely gather the accurate and trustworthy information you need for the decisions you must make about your health.

Jonathan Swift, the great eighteenth-century Irish satirist, summed up our concerns beautifully: "Falsehood flies and the truth comes limping after; so that when men come to be undeceived it is too late: the jest is over and the tale has had its effect."

Proof of Effectiveness Is Missing for Many Alternative Therapies

Most people we talk to are stunned when they learn that most alternative therapies have little or no compelling clinical evidence to support their effectiveness or safety. Evidence that does exist is often ambiguous or based on seriously flawed studies. In some cases the "proof" that a therapy is effective is based on interpretations of controversial theories. For many therapies, the only evidence offered is in the form of anecdotal reports — testimony of users of the therapy.

Perhaps even worse is the way the popular media cover developments in alternative medicine. As soon as a new therapy begins to show some positive results in some people (or even in animals), reports appear promoting it as though it has already been proven to work. The fact that the reports are from those with a vested interest in the therapy, or that the positive result could just as likely be a coincidence, is virtually *never* mentioned. Instead, we see the touting of a cancer "cure" or a diabetes breakthrough, based only on preliminary evidence and supposition. And if the "cure" is subsequently disproven, there may be little if any coverage of this fact.

The story of Coenzyme Q_{10} is a good example of such a media blitz. Coenzyme Q_{10} was at one time one of the most popular dietary supplements. Physicians and researchers know that Coenzyme Q_{10} is a critical factor in generating energy in all living organisms. They also know that older people and those with a number of different ailments often have reduced levels of Coenzyme Q_{10}. Therefore, some alternative practitioners reasoned, if a person took Coenzyme Q_{10} as part of a regimen of daily nutritional supplements, it might slow or stop the aging process and the person would be assured of better health.

Soon several popular books were touting this theory as fact. Coenzyme Q_{10} became a "must have" nutritional supplement. There was even talk that it could combat or reduce the severity of AIDS, slow or reverse aging, and give people longer, better lives.

Then long-term, carefully controlled studies began to be conducted. Coenzyme Q_{10} is indeed showing some preliminary evidence of having potential in treating some illnesses. But it is not an antiaging pill or an HIV treatment. It's true that Coenzyme Q_{10} is critical for energy and that its level is reduced in certain people. But the supplement is nothing like the "fountain of youth" it was originally advertised to be. Because of the premature claims, countless consumers may have wasted millions of dollars on Coenzyme Q_{10}.

Alternative Therapies Lack Adequate Regulation

Most European countries strictly regulate the manufacture and sale of herbal and other botanical products. In Germany, the Federal Health Agency set up what became known as Commission E to evaluate the safety, efficacy, and quality of herbal products. Although the Federal Health Agency does not test herbal products, manufacturers are required to submit proof of a product's quality, safety, and effectiveness. Each product's license must be renewed every five years.

Once established, Commission E functioned independently of the Federal Health Agency. From 1978 to 1994, Commission E reviewed all available literature on the safety and efficacy of 360 herbal remedies. These technical reports were published and are now available in English.[15] In countries with such regulations, consumers are assured of the consistency and safety of what they purchase — and they have some confidence that the claims made about a substance are accurate.

Unfortunately, this is not true in the United States, as there are no such standards or regulations. Consumers not only have no guarantee of the safety or efficacy of what they purchase; in many cases they can't even be sure that the amount of the herb or other active ingredient indicated on the label is actually there. We'll discuss these issues in more detail in Parts 2 and 3, but studies have shown the following:

- **missing ingredients** where what was listed on the label was not in the container.[16]
- **contaminants** in some products, including dangerous chemicals or pharmaceuticals not listed on the label.[17]

- **differences** in the contents of the same product from different manufacturers (or even from the same manufacturer).[18]
- **prescription medications** found in "natural" remedies and supplements without being listed on the label.[19]
- **unacceptable variation** in the amounts of active ingredients in different batches of the same product.[20]

For example, the *Los Angeles Times* commissioned a study to examine St. John's wort, an herb known to be effective against some forms of mild to moderate general depression.[21] *Times* reporters purchased the ten most popular brands from several retail outlets and had the pills tested by an independent laboratory.

The results were startling. Only one had between 90 and 110 percent of what the label indicated (an acceptable standard for over-the-counter products, based on the German standards). One manufacturer's pills had only 20 percent of the amount of active ingredient claimed on the label. Two others had a third *more* than the labels claimed.

Such problems exist in the United States in large part because of the way dietary supplements are regulated. Prescription and over-the-counter drugs are heavily regulated and closely monitored. For this reason, when you pick up a prescription at the pharmacy, you can be confident you have a high-quality product in your hands. Manufacturers are required to show that these products are effective and safe and made to the highest standards before they are allowed on the market.

Not so with dietary supplements. The Food and Drug Administration (FDA) oversees the regulation of drugs, food, and dietary supplements. In the early 1990s, the FDA was concerned about the way dietary supplements were being regulated and sought to tighten its control over these products and their labeling. However, manufacturers and consumers lobbied against the new regulations in Congress. The result was passage of the Dietary Supplement Health and Education Act of 1994 (DSHEA). This legislation expanded the list of items regulated as dietary supplements and limited the FDA's role in their regulation.

Under DSHEA, the term "dietary supplement" includes dietary substances added to supplement the diet as well as vitamins, minerals, herbs, and extracts of any such ingredients. Manufacturers are not required to submit evidence of effectiveness or safety prior to marketing a dietary supplement. The burden is on the FDA to prove that a dietary supplement is unsafe before it can be taken off the market. Hence, in spite of the many reports of adverse effects from ephedra, it took from 1997 to 2004 for the FDA to succeed in banning ephedra products.[22] (By contrast, the manufacturer of a new pharmaceutical drug must prove the drug is safe and effective *before* the company is allowed to put it on the market.)

Controversy reigns over precisely what claims can be made for a dietary supplement. General health claims — "maintains a healthy heart," "helps relaxation" — are allowed. Claims cannot be made that a product prevents or treats a disease. The DSHEA also requires all statements about health claims on dietary supplements to prominently display the words, "This statement has not been evaluated by the Food and Drug Administration. This product is not intended to diagnose, treat, cure, or prevent any disease."[23]

The warning appears to have had little effect. Consumers continue to buy these products, believing manufacturer claims and ignoring the DSHEA warning. The warning actually gives the makers of these products an easy "out" — deniability.

Alternative Medicine and Ancient or Traditional Cultures

The ancient or traditional cultures with which many alternative therapies are associated have been viewed through romantic lenses, their lifestyles seen as healthier than modern, fast-paced ones. The medicines, especially the herbs, used for centuries in these cultures would, it is claimed, never have gained acceptance if they were not effective. Thus, the therapies are declared by the proponents of alternative medicine to be valid. Some champions of a product will claim that their therapies were suppressed for years by Western imperialism and Christian missionary crusades. Only now, they say, are they being rediscovered and made available in the West.

Some of the more vigorous supporters of alternative medicine blame many of the concerns about alternative medicine on Western culture. They claim that research on these therapies is lacking because of biases in the Western medical and pharmaceutical establishments. Claims are made that the pharmaceutical industry will not research herbal remedies because it cannot patent the products and hence cannot make much money from them. Conventional medicine, they claim, is concerned only with retaining power and market share.

Partisans of alternative medicine advocate giving individuals the freedom to choose whatever form of health care they want. The argument is made that people's responsibility to care for their own health should be acknowledged and promoted by giving the individual greater freedom in matters of health care. They view those seeking to regulate alternative medicine, such as the FDA and the Institute of Medicine (IOM), with suspicion.

Spiritual Therapies and Christians

The link with other cultures raises another concern, especially for Christians and others who take their religious or spiritual faith seriously. Some alternative therapies are based on practices and rituals that have long been part of pagan or spiritual traditions and other religious practices.

Spirituality is an important concept in many forms of alternative medicine. Practitioners can be devout Christians or they can believe in worldviews that are radically different from a biblically based worldview. Sometimes the same terms are used, but with meanings that are quite different. For example, prayer may be recommended by various therapists, but they may have completely different practices in mind. A valid concern is that some forms of alternative medicine may be vehicles for the promotion of religious perspectives that are opposed to Christianity. A few may actually involve occult practices.

Some alternative medicine practitioners believe they cannot help their patients without first introducing them to one or another of the ancient Eastern or New Age faith systems. This leads to potential conflict for Christians. They may hear anecdotal stories from friends about shamanism easing arthritis pain without drugs, Therapeutic Touch increasing the speed of healing after a severe burn, or Reiki easing a chronic health condition. The stories are positive. Nothing is said about the potential spiritual side of the treatments. And are these therapies safe?

For example, Therapeutic Touch seems, on the surface, to be related to the biblical laying on of hands — even though hands never actually touch the patient. Practitioners claim to have removed any religious connotations from the practice. However, the nurse who helped develop the practice is a Buddhist and has stated that the principles behind Therapeutic Touch are the three main principles of Buddhist teachings.[24] An almost identical practice based on healing energy, called "pranic healing," is found within occult traditions.

Even Christians disagree on such therapies. Some say these therapies go against biblical teaching. They warn that some may lead to involvement in the occult. But others teach that ultimately all healing comes from God. They emphasize that Jesus is called the "Great Physician." They point out that in his day, Jesus would have been considered an alternative healer. Both perspectives can't be right, can they?

A few points can be made here. One of the central tenets believed by many in the New Age movement is that all spirituality is good, that no form is any better than another.[25] This is in opposition to the Bible's message that many problems originate, either directly or indirectly, in the conflict between the spiritual forces of good and evil. Paul wrote in Ephesians 6:12, "Our struggle is not against flesh and blood, but against the rulers, against the authorities, against the powers of this dark world and against the spiritual forces of evil in the heavenly realms." (We will address these issues more fully in chapter 3.)

The "openness" advocated by many in the alternative medicine community could expose people to practices and spiritual beings whose primary purpose is to harm people and lead them away from the loving Father of the universe. Although some question the existence of evil spiritual forces, Jesus speaks repeatedly about them, and the Bible warns that "your enemy the devil prowls around like a roaring lion looking for someone to devour" (1 Peter 5:8). Before trying any therapy, carefully evaluate the background and methods used.

Categories of Therapies

We have raised a variety of issues that should be explored prior to trying alternative medicine. Each alternative therapy or remedy will not raise every issue. To help focus your attention on the type of issue to be resolved, we have developed six categories. In Parts 2 and 3, we use these categories in our evaluation of each alternative therapy or remedy. The system is not absolute, and some therapies and remedies will fit into several categories.

1. Conventional Therapies

Conventional therapies and remedies are those we associate most closely with medical physicians, hospitals, and the modern Western health care system. Conventional medicine focuses on the use of pharmaceuticals, surgery, technology, and physical devices to prevent, diagnose, treat, and cure disease. These are the therapies either practiced routinely by Western-trained physicians or taught in nearly all medical schools. Alternative medicine therapies and remedies move into this category when high-quality research accumulates to show evidence of benefit and safety, and when a growing number of conventional health care professionals recommend the therapy.

2. Complementary Therapies

Complementary therapies and remedies are those either not practiced routinely by Western-trained physicians or not taught (or incompletely taught) in most medical schools. The therapies are not primarily designed to cure illness but focus instead on promoting health and preventing illness. Many seek to bring comfort or relieve stress. Some of the more popular complementary therapies include nutrition, exercise, stress reduction, marriage and parenting classes, support groups, massage, prayer, and spirituality. Many people would say that some of these — things such as prayer or marital advice — are not therapies at all. Common sense and mounting evidence from studies show that these factors are important for healthy lifestyles and the prevention of illness. However, these factors are often included in discussions about alternative medicine, and therefore we include them in this category. Any therapy with spiritual connections we will include in our fifth category.

3. Scientifically Unproven Therapies

Scientifically unproven therapies have not gone through even the most basic testing required for scientific demonstration of effectiveness and safety. Yet these therapies need not be rejected outright if they are based on established scientific principles. An old adage that is often brought up is that "absence of evidence of an effect is not evidence of the absence of an effect."[26] While that is true, this adage actually arose in reference to adverse effects. Sometimes evidence of harm appears slowly only after many people have used the product. Many herbal remedies fall into this category.

Remedies and therapies in this category generally cannot be recommended because of the lack of evidence. But sometimes it may be appropriate to try a therapy that shows some evidence of effectiveness if there is no evidence of it causing harm and its cost is reasonable. Approach all therapies that are scientifically unproven with caution.

4. Scientifically Questionable Therapies

Scientifically questionable therapies and remedies are based on theories or principles that contradict widely held scientific beliefs and have little or no scientific evidence to back up their claims. This category includes therapies that have been proven ineffective or even harmful.

For example, we categorize homeopathy as not only unproven but scientifically questionable because of the theory on which it is based. Homeopathic remedies are made by repeatedly diluting and shaking various herbal and mineral ingredients. Homeopathic dilutions are continued, in some cases, to the point where every molecule of the original "active" ingredient has been diluted out of the solution. None of the starting material is left in the final solution, and yet homeopaths claim these have the strongest effects. This contradicts the scientific finding that the more dilute a drug's concentration, the weaker its effect on the body.

We are skeptical of scientifically questionable therapies and do not recommend them. However, we recognize that a therapy may have some usefulness via some unknown mechanism and we would examine carefully any good-quality evidence that shows such a therapy is effective *and* safe. Only then, based on that evidence, would we consider recommending using any scientifically questionable therapy.

5. Spiritual Therapies

Spiritual therapies take us into an area of alternative medicine that is highly problematic for Christians and believers of other faiths. And yet most alternative medicine books do not discuss this important aspect. For example, "energy medicine" is a general term for a collection of diverse practices based on what is called "life energy." This life energy is nonphysical and universal. True health, these practitioners say, results from a balanced flow of this energy through the body and unblocked exchange of this energy with one's environment.

Our focus here is less on the accuracy of these beliefs (which we examine in Part 2) than on the fact that they have deep spiritual and religious roots and that this is often not acknowledged by those who promote therapies based on these beliefs. These beliefs underlie a vast array of alternative therapies, including Therapeutic Touch, Reiki, reflexology, Deepak Chopra's Ayurvedic medicine, Larry Dossey's healing words, and many others.

Such therapies raise important faith issues and require theological evaluation even more than scientific analysis. That is why we assign them to their own category. Where they best belong is sometimes not clear, as certain therapies can be practiced in very different ways. For example, controlled breathing exercises can be part of a spiritual therapy such as yoga or have no spiritual connections (as with the Lamaze approach to childbirth). The important thing is to be aware of the context and know how to evaluate therapies spiritually. Christians are called to test all spirits and thereby all spiritual teaching and claims. The standard is clearly described in 1 John 4:1 – 3:

> Dear friends, do not believe every spirit, but test the spirits to see whether they are from God, because many false prophets have gone out into the world. This is how you can recognize the Spirit of God: Every spirit that acknowledges that Jesus Christ has come in the flesh is from God, but every spirit that does not acknowledge Jesus is not from God. This is the spirit of the antichrist, which you have heard is coming and even now is already in the world.

6. Quackery or Fraud

False claims, unproven products, and products known to be ineffective or harmful rob people of money, trust, and frequently their health. The sad truth is that some individuals will intentionally deceive others about a product's efficacy just to make money. That's fraud.

Almost as bad are the therapies touted by people who truly believe they are of value even though they are not. That's quackery.

In chapter 5 we will give you examples of both quackery and fraud. We also describe some warning signs you should be aware of to protect yourself from these problems.

What to Do When Considering Alternative Medicine

Many people, including physicians, are left confused and frustrated about alternative medicine. People with health-related questions don't want theological or political debates; they want relief. They don't want conflicting information; they want trustworthy guidance. They want to know the right thing to do. Christians also want to please God in their actions, base their beliefs on his Word, the Bible, and reflect his character in their decisions and actions.

When considering a treatment, we should know why we are using whatever therapies or remedies we use — or don't use. We need to know that a particular remedy is not only effective but reasonably safe. To be good stewards of our resources, we should be able to know if the label on the bottle is accurate and reliable. Others' experiences and recommendations can be an important part of any evaluation, but they are not enough.

We must also evaluate remedies from an investment, or stewardship, perspective. We are all limited in the amount of time and money available to us. We should not squander our resources. Christians especially are called to be accountable stewards of these resources. Jesus asked, "So if you have not been trustworthy in handling worldly wealth, who will trust you with true riches? And if you have not been trustworthy with someone else's property, who will give you property of your own?" (Luke 16:11).

We should all investigate the claims made about the remedies we put into or onto our bodies, the therapies we allow to be practiced on us, and the practitioners in whom we place our trust. "Do you not know that your body is a temple of the Holy Spirit, who is in you, whom you have received from God? You are not your own; you were bought at a price. Therefore honor God with your body" (1 Corinthians 6:19–20). To do this, we need to gather information that is medically reliable *and* biblically sound, weigh the options, seek sensible counsel, carefully pray, and then make as informed and as wise a decision as possible.

We cannot emphasize strongly enough that this investigation should be done whether we are pursuing conventional *or* alternative medicine. Yet with both forms of medical care, we see people trusting blindly in someone or something for no reason other than the chance happenings that led them to a certain practitioner.

This book is designed to help you make reliable decisions. The next two chapters provide you with some of the most important tools and principles you need to do this. First we will look at how medical science evaluates whether something is effective or safe (the evidence-based approach). Then we will look at how the Bible evaluates the spiritual dimensions (the faith-based approach). We apply those principles to specific therapies and remedies in the rest of the book. We'll give you the facts — fairly, evenhandedly, and as objectively as we can.

We are on your side. Our goal is to help you make wise decisions. Not only will our advice and recommendations be evidence-based and medically reliable; they will also be biblically sound.

Chapter 1: Pursuing Alternative Medicine

1. Patricia M. Barnes, Eve Powell-Griner, Kim McFann, and Richard L. Nahin, "Complementary and Alternative Medicine Use Among Adults: United States, 2002," *Advance Data from Vital and Health Statistics* 343 (May 27, 2004). *U.S. Department of Health and Human Services: www.cdc. gov/nchs/data/ad/ad343.pdf* (September 13, 2005).

2. Iris R. Bell, Opher Caspi, Gary E. R. Schwartz, Kathryn L. Grant, Tracy W. Gaudet, David Rychener, Victoria Maizes, and Andrew Weil, "Integrative medicine and systemic outcomes research: issues in the emergence of a new model for primary health care," *Archives of Internal Medicine* 162, no. 2 (January 2002): 133–40.

3. PR Newswire, "New Safe, No Worry Medicines (TM) From EuroPharma Deliver Results Without Side Effects; Homeopathy a Growing Healthcare Movement Posting 46.5% Sales Increase in 2002" (July 17, 2003). *HighBeam Research: www.highbeam.com* (September 23, 2005).

4. Anne E. Frähm with David J. Frähm, *A Cancer Battle Plan: Six Strategies for Beating Cancer from a Recovered "Hopeless Case"* (Colorado Springs, Colo.: Piñon, 1992).

5. Larry Burkett with Michael E. Taylor, *Damaged But Not Broken: A Personal Testimony of How to Deal With the Impact of Cancer* (Chicago: Moody, 1996); Larry Burkett, *Nothing to Fear: The Key to Cancer Survival* (Chicago: Moody, 2003).

6. Harold G. Koenig, Michael E. McCullough, and David B. Larson, *Handbook of Religion and Health* (Oxford: Oxford University Press, 2001).

7. Reginald Cherry, *Healing Prayer* (Nashville: Thomas Nelson, 1999), xiv.

8. NCCAM, "NCCAM Funding: Appropriations History." *National Center for Complementary and Alternative Medicine: http://nccam.nih.gov/about/appropriations/index. htm* (September 23, 2005).

9. Swissinfo, "Voters to Decide on Alternative Medicine" (September 16, 2005). *Neue Zürcher Zeitung: www.nzz. ch/2005/09/16/eng/article6088911.html* (September 23, 2005).

10. David M. Eisenberg, Roger B. Davis, Susan L. Ettner, Scott Appel, Sonja Wilkey, Maria Van Rompay, and Ronald C. Kessler, "Trends in Alternative Medicine Use in the United States," *Journal of the American Medical Association* 280, no. 18 (November 11, 1998): 1569 – 75.

11. Hilary A. Tindle, Roger B. Davis, Russell S. Phillips, and David E. Eisenberg, "Trends in Use of Complementary and Alternative Medicine by US Adults: 1997 – 2002," *Alternative Therapies in Health and Medicine* 11, no. 1 (January – February 2005): 42 – 49.

12. Mark Blumenthal, "Herb Sales Down 7.4 Percent in Mainstream Market; Garlic Is Top-Selling Herb; Herb Combinations See Increase," *HerbalGram* 66 (2005): 63.

13. A. J. Vickers, R. W. Rees, and A. Robin, "Advice Given by Health Food Shops: Is It Clinically Safe?" *Journal of the Royal College of Physicians of London* 32, no. 5 (September/October 1998): 426 – 28.

14. Carolyn Cook Gotay and Daniella Dumitriu, "Health Food Store Recommendations for Breast Cancer Patients," *Archives of Family Medicine* 9, no. 8 (August 2000): 692 – 99.

15. Mark Blumenthal, ed., *The Complete German Commission E Monographs: Therapeutic Guide to Herbal Medicines* (Austin, Tex.: American Botanical Council, 1998).

16. J. Parasrampurra, K. Schwartz, and R. Petesch, "Quality Control of Dehydroepiandrosterone Dietary Supplement Products," *Journal of the American Medical Association* 280, no. 18 (November 11, 1998): 1565.

17. Donald M. Marcus and Arthur P. Grollman, "Botanical Medicines — The Need for New Regulations," *New England Journal of Medicine* 347, no. 25 (December 19, 2002): 2073 – 76.

18. B. J. Gurley, P. Wang, and S. F. Gardner, "Ephedrine-type Alkaloid Content of Nutritional Supplements Containing *Ephedra sinica* (Ma-huang) as Determined by High Performance Liquid Chromatography," *Journal of Pharmaceutical Sciences* 87, no. 12 (December 1998): 1547 – 53.

19. Edward W. Boyer, Susan Kearney, Michael W. Shannon, Lawrence Quang, Alan Woolf, and Kathi Kemper, "Poisoning From a Dietary Supplement Administered During Hospitalization," *Pediatrics* 109, no. 3 (March 2002): 49 – 51.

20. Walter L. Larimore and Dónal P. O'Mathúna, "Quality Assessment Programs for Dietary Supplements," *Annals of Pharmacotherapy* 37, no. 6 (June 2003): 893 – 98.

21. Terence Monmaney, "Remedy's U.S. Sales Zoom, But Quality Control Lags," *Los Angeles Times* (August 31, 1998). *www.biopsychiatry.com/hypericum.html* (September 20, 1999).

22. FDA, "Sales of Supplements Containing Ephedrine Alkaloids (Ephedra) Prohibited." Last updated April 12, 2004. *U.S. Food and Drug Administration: www.fda.gov/oc/ initiatives/ephedra/february2004/* (September 26, 2005).

23. U.S. Congress, "Dietary Supplement Health and Education Act of 1994; Public Law 103-417; 103rd Congress." Approved October 25, 1994. *U.S. Food and Drug Administration: www.fda.gov/opacom/laws/dshea.html* (September 26, 2005).

24. Robert Calvert, "Dolores Krieger, Ph.D., and Her Therapeutic Touch," *Massage* 47 (January/February 1994): 56 – 60.

25. John P. Newport, *The New Age Movement and the Biblical Worldview: Conflict and Dialogue* (Grand Rapids: Eerdmans, 1998).

26. Edzard Ernst, "Absence of Evidence . . ." *FACT: Focus on Alternative and Complementary Therapies* 10, no. 3 (September 2005): 165 – 66.

EVIDENCE-BASED HEALTH AND HEALING

An evidence-based approach to health care means that recommendations and decisions are based on the results of well-conducted studies. Science values evidence over opinion. Scientific studies provide the best evidence for many (but not all) of the decisions that must be made in medicine. What distinguishes science from other branches of inquiry is the high priority placed on objective information, such as observable data and repeatable experiments.

Science has developed a method of seeking truth about the physical world that requires objective testing of ideas. Ideally, theories arise from observations, not prior beliefs and assumptions. The theories are changed or discarded if new data contradict or expand previous information. An important way of checking results is to use tests that can be repeated by others to see whether the results are consistent or just arose from chance.

Over the last few centuries, several types of studies have been developed to provide evidence for health care decisions. Each study provides important information. But each addresses a different question about the therapy or remedy. It is important to know the differences among the different types of studies when evaluating whether a study supports something's effectiveness. The National Center for Complementary and Alternative Medicine acknowledges that there is a hierarchy in the different types of evidence for therapies. The following table is adapted from the center's Five-Year Strategic Plan.[1]

Hierarchy of Evidence	Type of Research
Highest	Large randomized controlled trial
↑	Small randomized controlled trial
	Uncontrolled trials
	Observational studies
↓	Case reports
Lowest	Anecdotes

Randomized Controlled Trials

The randomized controlled trial is regarded as the "gold standard" of studies used to measure the effectiveness and safety of a therapy or remedy. Throughout the nineteenth and twentieth centuries, physicians and others saw that "controlled clinical trials" provided the best type of evidence of effectiveness and safety. The term "control group" is used when one or more groups receive something other than the treatment being tested. Sometimes the control group receives a placebo (e.g., a sugar pill), sometimes it receives the current standard treatment, and sometimes it receives nothing (to mimic normal activity). A controlled study can have more than one control group. Controlled clinical trials are designed to distinguish whether a therapy is beneficial in and of itself or works primarily by the placebo effect.

By the twentieth century, researchers realized the importance of controlling as many aspects of a trial as possible. A study of drugs being used to treat angina (pain arising due to heart problems) represented an important development.[2] The drugs were all xanthine alkaloids, the chemical group that includes caffeine. Two other xanthines, theobromine and aminophylline, had been widely used to relieve angina since 1895. By 1932, almost every cardiac patient used them. However, one physician-researcher, Harry Gold, was skeptical of their efficacy and started an experiment in which some patients received the drug and some received a lactose (or milk-sugar) pill. This was a "single-blind trial." The patients didn't know which pill they received, but the physicians evaluating them did.

After more than two years of treatments, Gold and his colleague, Nathaniel Kwit, noticed that patients were giving contradictory answers to questions about their pain levels. On closer review, they discovered that the physicians talking to patients would ask slightly different questions depending on whether the patient was receiving xanthines or the control. In effect, they asked leading questions that biased the results and introduced errors.

Gold and Kwit changed their methodology so that the physicians did not know which patients received which pill. This was the first example of a clinical trial in which neither the patients nor the physicians knew what was being given. This type of controlled study would later become known as a "double-blind study" — the patient and the physician are both "blinded" to whether the patient is receiving the active or inactive intervention.

Kwit summarized the essence of this method: "Toward the end of the study we realized that the doctor must not know what he gives, the patient must not know what he receives, and the questioner must not know what was given."[3] With this new element of control introduced, the study went on to reveal that xanthines were no more effective at relieving angina pain than a sugar pill, a finding confirmed by later studies.

Many other studies have shown that patients have an amazing ability to detect whether researchers expect to see them improve. Somehow researchers inadvertently or even subconsciously transmit their knowledge or expectations to patients. This can occur in very subtle ways, through facial expressions, body movements, or tone of voice.[4] People differ in their ability to pick up on these cues, an ability that has been demonstrated even in animals. Hence, the best research must control researchers' expectations by keeping them unaware of, or "blinded to," which treatment they are giving. That is the essence of the double-blind clinical trial. Research over the years has confirmed that the double-blind controlled study is much more likely to give accurate results than the single-blind controlled study — and both are far superior to observational studies or anecdotal reports.

Randomization Improves Accuracy of Results

The first randomized clinical trial was conducted with tuberculosis (TB) patients around the same time as Gold's research with angina patients. During the nineteenth century, TB led to one in every seven deaths. Many different remedies were touted as cures for TB; only later did researchers find they made little difference. Up until the 1940s, standard treatment for TB in one lung was to deliberately collapse that lung; if both lungs were infected, bed rest was the only treatment.[5]

Sir Austin Bradford Hill is often referred to as the "father of clinical trials" because of his influence on clinical research. Hill contracted TB during World War I and was one of the fortunate to survive. He was seriously ill for five years, making it impossible for him to achieve his dream of attending medical school. His love of medicine led him to study statistics, which he applied to medical questions as an epidemiologist. Epidemiology is the study of how frequently diseases occur in populations and the factors that contribute to increasing or decreasing that frequency.

Hill remained interested in studying TB and was a member of the British Medical Research Council when a new drug, streptomycin, was reported to be effective against TB. The council designed a clinical trial for streptomycin that incorporated Hill's expertise in statistics.[6] Researchers at that time were becoming aware that if the individuals in the control group were not very similar to those receiving the test treatment, the results could be biased.[7] For example, if by chance one group contained mostly younger people and another mostly older people, different results might be due to the age differences, not the treatment. These other factors (such as age, gender, and economic status) are known as "confounding variables." The best way to avoid such differences is to randomly assign people to the groups and use statistical methods to check whether the groups are similar in all known and relevant ways.

Today these random assignments are made based on computer-generated random allocation tables. Researchers have no way of influencing which patients end up in which group. This is best done by having someone who does not see the patients determine the group assignment and not tell the researcher until after the study is completed. Research that is not properly randomized has, on average, been found to overestimate a treatment's benefit by 41 percent.[8]

Hill's streptomycin study emphasized the importance of randomly assigning people to the study groups. In his study, one group received streptomycin injections and bed rest, and the other group received bed rest alone. The study would have been scientifically stronger if the second group had received injections containing no active drug. However, other considerations sometimes have to outweigh the scientific issues. Streptomycin was given in four intramuscular injections daily for six months. These injections are painful. To give this number of painful injections that could not benefit the patients was viewed as inappropriate. The researchers recognized that the scientific benefit was overridden by the ethical issue of avoiding needless pain and discomfort.

Obviously, the patients knew which group they were in. The researchers compensated for this by blinding the radiologists who read patients' chest X-rays and the physicians who evaluated the patients clinically. Results showed that the streptomycin group had less than half the death rate of the control group and almost double the rate of improvement. Thus, the study provided important evidence for the efficacy of an early antibiotic and gave new insights into the design of research studies.

The Powerful "Placebo Effect"

The way a patient's beliefs or the professional's bedside manner influences recovery is often called the "placebo effect." This plays an important and often beneficial role in all forms of medical and surgical care. Some medical historians have concluded that the history of medicine is mostly a history of the placebo effect. It helps to explain why, even today, people report feeling better after receiving a wide variety of treatments — even if the treatment is a sham. Randomized controlled trials identify whether a treatment works in and of itself or takes advantage of the placebo effect.

Placebos, and the placebo effect, have been defined in various ways. A placebo is any pill or injection or intervention, or part of any intervention, that produces a beneficial effect in a patient without the treatment itself having any known specific effect on the body. Maybe the patient gets better because the physician instills hope. Or the patient believes the "pill" or "shot" offers a cure, even if it doesn't.

Studies have been pointing to the role of the placebo effect for quite some time. A competent and respected New England physician, Elisha Perkins (1741 – 1799), claimed to relieve many painful ailments using metallic rods (called Perkins' tractors).[9] He claimed his metal rods worked because of the magnetic properties of the metal. He would stroke the afflicted part of a person's body and report great success. Perkins was so convinced of his tractors' effectiveness that he went to New York to cure people during a yellow fever epidemic, but he contracted the disease and died. Yet the reputation of the tractors lived on.

Another physician, John Haygarth, was skeptical of the successes Perkins had reported and devised an experiment — what we would now call a "placebo-controlled study." Haygarth made wooden tractors, painting them to look metallic — which made them the placebo, or control treatment. He then treated five patients with rheumatism, alternating between using the Perkins' metallic rods one day and his wooden rods the next. The patients who believed they were being rubbed with Perkins' rods reported the same relief with both rods.

Haygarth's experiment was a demonstration of the placebo effect. Patients improved, not because of Perkins' tractors, but because of the complex dynamics that make up the placebo effect. "The curative factors ... were the patient's and physician's imagination and faith. The physician's fame ... was an additional factor that contributed to the patient's faith: that is, the more important the physician, the more likely it was that the treatment would be effective."[10]

The placebo effect is probably the most important aspect to control in clinical trials. Studying its effect is complicated by the fact that it varies among people and procedures. It is often reported that the placebo effect can account for a third of the improvements found with any therapy. This claim is based on an influential 1955 article.[11] The author found that 35 percent was the *average* placebo effect. It can be much larger or smaller.

For example, angina was sometimes treated surgically in the 1950s. A double-blind study compared patients who received this surgery to a group who received only a skin incision (the ethics of these types of studies are seriously questioned and debated today, but that is another issue). Over half of those who received the placebo surgery reported significant improvements, approximately the same proportion as those who received the actual surgery.[12] Another study shortly after this one reported that every patient getting the placebo surgery showed significant improvements. This surgery was soon abandoned but remains an important symbol of the importance of the placebo effect.

Placebos are more effective in treating certain types of disorders. They work best with pain, nausea, phobias, depression, and anxiety.[13] Disorders related to blood pressure and bronchial airways also respond well to placebos. However, placebos do not appear to work as well in acute situations (such as a heart attack) or in degenerative diseases.

Placebos and Alternative Medicine

The conditions in which placebos work well are, for the most part, the same conditions for which alternative therapies are commonly used. Studies have shown that people pursuing alternative medicine tend to be more anxious than the general population.[14] Some commentators describe them as "the worried well" who monitor their bodies carefully and "spend more on all forms of health care, even though most are fairly healthy."[15] This heightened anxiety is relevant here because anxiety is one of the conditions most strongly affected by placebos.[16] A positive interaction between patients and health care professionals can strongly influence the placebo effect, which is why we place such importance on this interpersonal aspect of alternative therapies.

Placebo effects are much more prevalent, even today, than many health care professionals or the public may realize. Placebo effects have been observed with drugs, herbs and other botanicals, surgery, medical procedures, inactive compounds, psychotherapy, and diagnostic tests. However, the term "placebo" often carries negative connotations. Many people think of placebos as useless fakes given to trick patients into thinking they are getting something helpful when the doctor can find no reason for their symptoms. Placebos are thought to be prescribed as a pacifier for people with psychosomatic illnesses (ailments that are "just in their heads"). (The word *placebo* comes from the Latin verb that means "to please.")

But others question whether this really matters. If the patient gets better after the therapy, does it matter whether the benefit came from the therapy or the placebo effect? Those who promoted a product called "obecalp" (no longer available) didn't think so. If you spell it backwards, you'll see how it had its effect. When an herb or therapy has been shown to be ineffective, sometimes people defend its continued use on the basis that it might do some good through the placebo effect. They claim "it can't do any harm."

But if the "treatment" is costly or requires extensive training and it actually works via the placebo effect, people will be misled and their resources used unwisely.

There is also a dark side to placebos. The placebo effect is real. But so, too, is the harm that can come from placebos.

The Negative Placebo

What usually is not mentioned outside scientific circles is something called the "nocebo effect" in which a patient has a negative, or bad, reaction to a placebo. We bring this up to help you understand how unpredictable a person's response to a treatment can be.

Reviews of medical research studies have found that almost one-quarter of those being given placebos (such as sugar pills) spontaneously report adverse effects.[17] When researchers actively questioned participants, up to three-quarters of them reported at least one bothersome effect. In some studies, those taking placebos had more side effects than those taking active drugs. Most nocebo effects are relatively mild, with headaches, drowsiness, nausea, fatigue, and insomnia being common.

Many factors may explain how nocebo effects arise. Any clinic or hospital setting or past negative experiences with any drug can trigger a negative reaction. The power of suggestion is important. In one study, people with asthma were asked to inhale a spray containing only salt water (saline solution, which is harmless).[18] As expected, it caused no effect in a control group. However, when the participants were told that it contained substances that commonly cause allergic reactions, half the people developed breathing difficulties. Twelve had full-blown asthmatic attacks. When they were asked to inhale the exact same saline spray, but this time told it was an antiasthmatic drug, their asthma attacks went away.

Salt solutions, sugar pills, and nonexistent electric fields have all produced negative effects in some people. They reveal problems about the promotion of ineffective remedies. The placebo and nocebo effects point to the power of words and the importance of trust between patients and health care professionals. They also show why it can be so difficult to figure out if a therapy or remedy *really* works.

Statistics and Controlled Studies

Once the researchers have collected their data, they may find that the results in one group are somewhat different from those in another group. But the results must be carefully evaluated. If the results in the treatment group are not drastically different from those in the control group, how big must the difference be before we can be sure the therapy is useful? In other words, how do you tell which differences are significant and which are not significant?

Differences between two groups could be due to chance or they could be due to the treatment really being better. A number of complex statistical calculations are done to address these issues. Reports of studies will then state that the differences between the two groups were statistically significant or not. If they were statistically significant, there is a higher probability that the positive results were due to the treatment and not to chance. If the differences were not statistically significant, we cannot place much confidence in the effectiveness of the therapy. In those cases, it is important not to make definite statements about the treatment based on that study.

These statistical calculations are influenced by the number of people in the studies. In clinical research, the more patients enrolled, the more reliable the results. The fewer the patients, the less reliable the study and the more likely that any differences found would be due to chance. This impacts the costs of research. To be more confident of the results, studies must enroll more participants, and that means the studies will take longer and cost more to conduct.

Uncontrolled Research Studies

You should now have a good idea why uncontrolled studies are placed lower on the hierarchy of research studies. Without a control group to compare with the treatment group, we cannot be sure whether the treatment or some other factor (or combination of factors) caused whatever changes were observed. Such studies still reveal useful information. But they should not be used to claim that a treatment caused the effects seen.

As medical science began to develop in the sixteenth century, early experiments focused on careful observation. For example, a common treatment for poisonings in ancient times was the bezoar stone. Legend had it that these stones were the crystallized tears of a deer bitten by a snake (actually, they were gallstones). The legend was that when they were swallowed, they would stay in the stomach and absorb any poison taken by the person. A French surgeon, Ambroise Paré (1510 – 1590), conducted an observational experiment that would not be viewed as ethical today. Paré, better known for bringing respectability to medieval surgery at a time when it was a barber's side trade, gave a bezoar stone to a palace cook who had been condemned to death for stealing. The cook was given mercuric chloride, a common poison, and subsequently died in agony,

despite having been given the "antidote."[19] Clearly, the bezoar stone was useless.

The Natural Course of Illnesses

Observational studies are limited because a number of factors may contribute to the changes observed. One important factor is the natural course of illness and disease. Many illnesses and pains will diminish or disappear on their own. Some estimates claim that people will recover from as much as 80 percent of all illnesses regardless of what treatments they use.[20] There is much common sense behind the saying that if you have a viral upper respiratory infection, "take aspirin or acetaminophen and it'll be gone in a week; do nothing and it'll be gone in seven days." Even illnesses as serious as cancer are known to inexplicably disappear, which is known medically as "spontaneous remission." Many chronic conditions fluctuate in their severity, so if a treatment is started when the condition is at its worst, it may appear that the treatment helped when in fact the condition merely improved on its own, only to return later.

Studying the Health of Populations

Epidemiology is the study of factors affecting the health of large populations. These studies are carried out to try to find connections between health and illness and various activities, traits, and lifestyles. Technically, these are called "epidemiological studies." Although they may find an association between an illness and something else, that correlation does not necessarily show causation.

A widely reported example was an investigation into the eating habits of various Western nations. Traditional French cuisine was always rich in sauces full of ingredients that contribute to heart disease. Yet the French had a lower rate of heart disease than Americans eating meals just as rich in fat. This observation became known as the "French paradox."

Epidemiologists examined many reports from different countries trying to figure out what protected the French. Those French people who consumed wine regularly had a lower incidence of death from heart problems than Americans did with a similar diet. This led to speculation that drinking a glass of wine with dinner might somehow protect people from heart disease.[21] It sounded like scientific validation of the age-old practice of drinking wine!

The protective value of various grapes, both fermented and unfermented, due to certain active ingredients (called "antioxidants") became a topic of serious experimentation that continues to this day. However, less publicity was given to another epidemiological finding: the French have a higher incidence of death due to alcohol-related causes.[22] The French are not somehow magically protected from alcohol abuse just because their consumption of wine is both routine and ritualized at meals. Yet some Americans decided they should increase their alcohol intake based on the French experience. One commentator quipped, "Eat like the French, die like the French."

The lesson to be learned is that not all scientific studies are alike. Epidemiological studies are not randomized clinical trials. Epidemiologists survey people, asking them lots of questions about lifestyle issues, such as their diet. These studies can identify correlations: for example, that those who drink wine moderately have less heart disease. But this does not prove that heart disease is prevented by moderate wine consumption. Proof would require a controlled study in which two groups differed in no other way than one added wine to their diet and the other did

not. That sort of scientific evidence is not yet available, so controversy continues over whether people should add wine to their diet.

Case Reports

The next level of study is called a "case report." These present in detail the results of giving a certain treatment to a single patient or a small group of patients (called a "case series report"). A case report gives as complete a description as possible of all factors involved in a patient's experience. If several case reports are published for a particular treatment, especially if the patients have similar conditions, patterns may be spotted. Then someone may initiate a more controlled study to evaluate whether the suspected common factor in the case reports is truly the cause of the effect noted.

Anecdotal Evidence Is Only a Starting Point

Case reports do not provide evidence that something is effective because they are a form of anecdotal evidence. This sort of evidence consists of the stories people tell about experiencing relief or a cure after a particular therapy. We *all* tell these stories. We tell what happened when we did or took something, especially when the product, therapy, or service helped us. Sometimes, all we have is anecdotal evidence.

Anecdotal evidence alone is *not* enough to come to any valid conclusion about what caused the healing. Focusing solely on reports of positive results ignores the possibility that for some people, the therapy may do nothing or even prove dangerous. Focusing solely on negative results can result in rejection of what might actually be a new and important treatment for an illness.

With the exception of unsubstantiated opinion, anecdotal evidence is the least useful of the types of evidence available to judge the effectiveness of a therapy, whether conventional or alternative. Yet much of alternative medicine is promoted primarily on the basis of anecdotal evidence. Part of the problem is that anecdotal evidence has supported the usefulness of many of the most unlikely and bizarre treatments in the world. However, anecdotal evidence generally does not take into account the many other things going on in a patient's life that could have contributed to what happened. The purpose of the scientific method is to cut through the anecdotal information to reveal whether there is any kernel of truth hidden within.

For example, imagine a widow whose husband died two years ago. Each year, on the anniversary of his death, she becomes deeply depressed. Friends, not remembering the exact date, assume her depression is "chemical" and suggest she try an over-the-counter product advertised as being more effective and safer than any pharmaceutical.

The widow takes the product but at about the same time decides to volunteer in a church outreach program. There she meets a widower who shares many of her interests and values in life. They go to church together. They go to lunch together. They begin dating. They both discover they can love someone new. The widow thanks God for the new life that has brought her joy. Her friends start recommending the over-the-counter product to others because of the dramatic improvement in her outlook.

Their recommendations are based on their observations, which are accurate. Her depression has dramatically lifted. But their conclusion that the product *caused* the improvement is false. Her improvement is more likely due to the other changes she made in her life or to a complicated interaction among all of them.

The importance of anecdotal evidence is in suggesting that something about a treatment may be effective. Thus, if many people report being helped by a therapy, it may warrant further investigation. This is why, for example, the herbal remedy St. John's wort was and is being tested in scores of clinical trials. Anecdotal evidence overwhelmingly suggested it had value in treating mild depression. The scientific method is now confirming that what was suspected through anecdotes is actually true.

Proponents of alternative medicine often claim that centuries of using a therapy or remedy should count as valuable evidence of its efficacy. "Why else would people have kept using it?" they reason. Most scientists and physicians would agree that this does constitute valuable evidence. However, this "anecdotal" or "testimonial" evidence is of the least value when evaluating the effectiveness of any therapy.

Historical usage of a remedy is just another form of anecdotal evidence. It records *what* happened, not *why* it happened. In fact, many reasons could explain why a remedy was used for centuries. People sometimes use something because nothing else is available. Or they may use a remedy because it is intricately interlinked with their culture and religion. Or, because the illness lasts only a short time, or comes and goes in cycles, they do not realize that the relief they experience has nothing to do with the remedy.

Birth control at one time was believed to involve a woman avoiding particular sacred areas. A woman might be resting by the water of a sacred lake and feel her baby moving within her for the first time.

Because the time between sexual intercourse and first awareness of a baby growing in the womb was so long, the connection between the two was not made. Thus, birth control for that woman, and for her culture, might mean avoiding the watery area.

Most people over the age of fifty remember being told that if they were burned while cooking, they should immediately cover the burn with butter. Years later, emergency medical personnel are still trying to explain that grease not only doesn't work but might delay the healing effect of proper treatment. Cold water (not ice) has been shown by multiple well-performed clinical trials to be the best therapy to use immediately on a burn, before seeing a physician or going to an emergency care center.

Many other examples exist. The longer a culture has used a therapy, the more likely it is considered to have some value. But that value may be minimal. The positive result may be nothing more than the placebo effect enhanced by a few reports of positive experiences, repeated over and over, with the negative experiences forgotten.

The Role of Basic Scientific Research

The studies and reports we have discussed so far involve humans. Other research contributes to our understanding of human anatomy and the natural course of diseases. This is vital to understanding how to promote health and treat disease. Scientific studies of these factors are called "basic research." During the seventeenth and eighteenth centuries, developments in human anatomy and microbiology occurred that contradicted many of the assertions and theories of the Greco-Roman physician Galen (AD 131 – 200). This new information raised serious questions about whether therapies based on Galen's theories could ever be effective. Yet Galen's theories dominated Western medical practice for 1,500 years. Galen held that ingested food was continuously converted into blood in the liver. The blood, according to Galen, then permeated all the tissues of the body, passing through the heart, where it mysteriously picked up the "vital spirit" that controlled all bodily functions.

Part of the problem with Galen's theory was that it was not based on evidence — he derived it from his philosophical views. Yet because of the authority placed in Galen's conclusions, his theory was passed on from one generation to another. That began to change only when modern science developed with its insistence on evidence.

William Harvey (1578 – 1657) dissected animals and discovered that blood circulates continuously around the body, pumped by the heart. Harvey emphasized the importance of observation in medicine and was the first to use quantitative analysis. He calculated the volume of blood in the body, showing that the volume was incompatible with Galen's theories on blood.

Harvey feared what might happen to his livelihood if he published his controversial results. After he did publish, he reflected, "But now the die is cast; my hope is in the love of truth and in the integrity of intelligence."[23] Harvey's claims could be objectively demonstrated for all to see, which is an important feature of basic scientific research. Harvey's discoveries weakened the influence of Galen's theory and opened the possibility that popular remedies based on Galen's theories (such as bleeding and purging) might be ineffective.

Today, an alternative therapy or remedy will be viewed as questionable if its claims contradict a significant body of basic research findings. This in part explains why homeopathy is viewed skeptically, since it contradicts the vast amount of evidence showing that larger quantities of a drug cause stronger effects, not the opposite.

Studies and Regulation

During World War II, the need to develop reliable ways to evaluate product effectiveness was very pressing. This applied not only to drugs but also to other items important to the war effort, such as food, clothing, shelter, and vehicles.[24] From this effort came scientists trained in comparing the effectiveness of similar products using the most objective methods possible. Much of this effort is motivated by a concern for safety. Most people are surprised to learn that only a few drugs developed by pharmaceutical companies actually make it to commercial production. In a twenty-year search for antimalarial drugs alone, 300,000 chemicals were tested on animals, of which only twelve were found useful and safe enough to try with humans.[25] Fewer made it onto the market.

Further impetus for conducting controlled clinical trials came from legislative pressure. In the late 1950s, a new drug was introduced in Europe as a mild sedative. Since large doses appeared to result in little harm, it was viewed as safe and recommended for morning sickness caused by pregnancy, high blood pressure, and migraines.[26] In 1961, reports surfaced of deformities among babies born to women who had taken this drug when they were pregnant. The drug, thalidomide, was quickly taken off the market throughout the world, but not before about eight thousand children were born deformed, often with missing limbs. These deformities appeared in about

20 percent of the pregnant women who had taken thalidomide.

Thalidomide had never been approved for sale in the United States, but not because anyone suspected it could harm unborn children. Drug manufacturers were required to show that their products were safe before receiving permission from the FDA to market them in the United States. Because some animals given thalidomide suffered nerve damage (technically called "peripheral neuropathy"), the FDA kept the drug off the market. During clinical trials in the United States, thalidomide was given to some pregnant women, resulting in seventeen children being born with the characteristic deformities.

Many believed the FDA regulations averted a much larger tragedy. As a result, even stricter regulations were introduced. A bill passed by Congress in 1962 added the requirement that manufacturers submit "adequate and well-controlled experiments by experts qualified by scientific training and experience to evaluate the effectiveness of the drug involved."[27] Gradually the precise nature of these experiments was defined. Since the early 1980s, FDA approval of new drugs has effectively required the use of randomized, placebo-controlled, double-blind clinical trials.

Some Scientific Studies Are Not Well Designed

Evidence-based medicine has developed methods of reliably determining whether or not treatments work. The randomized double-blind clinical trial has made important contributions to conventional medicine's ability to determine safety and effectiveness. These methods are increasingly being applied to alternative medicine. A 2005 examination of randomized controlled trials of alternative medicine found that, in general, they are of the same quality as those conducted in conventional medicine.[28]

However, these methods are not without problems and limitations. Probably the biggest problems arise when studies are thought to be well designed when in fact they are not. Much training is needed to properly conduct clinical trials. Otherwise, inexperienced or unscrupulous researchers can publish studies with serious methodological flaws. You should be aware of some of the more common flaws.

Sometimes *claims* of scientific support are unfounded or exaggerated. Sometimes close examination of a study will show that it contains serious flaws and doesn't really support what is claimed. For example, a study reported that Therapeutic Touch relieved problematic behavioral symptoms in people with dementia.[29] Therapeutic Touch is said to work by manipulating nonphysical "life energy" and therefore requires no physical contact between therapist and patient. In this particular study, the "Therapeutic Touch" included massage of the head, neck, and shoulders. This is completely different from what is normally described as Therapeutic Touch. While the Therapeutic Touch group showed statistically significant improvements compared to the group receiving no intervention, a third group received massage only, and no differences were found between it and the Therapeutic Touch group. This study therefore supports the use of neck, head, and shoulder massage, not Therapeutic Touch, though that is not how it was reported.

Another study claimed that women receiving Therapeutic Touch had significantly reduced tension, confusion, and anxiety, and increased vigor, compared to a control group.[30] The participants were randomly assigned to the two groups, but these differed in more ways than whether or not they received Therapeutic Touch. The control group was brought into a room and completed the study questionnaires. Members of the other group were brought into a quiet room, removed their shoes, lay on a hospital bed, spent time talking to the therapist, and listened to soft music while receiving Therapeutic Touch. Any or all of these "confounding variables" could have contributed to the beneficial effects found in this study. Once again, this study does not support the effectiveness of Therapeutic Touch itself, although that is what has been claimed.

Willow bark offers another interesting case. Willow bark has been used for centuries as a natural remedy for headache and joint inflammation. During the nineteenth century, scientists found that willow bark contains an active ingredient called "salicylic acid," which does relieve pain. However, it is very irritating to the stomach. To make it less irritating, they chemically converted it to acetylsalicylic acid — what we know today as aspirin. In this way, an herb with a long tradition of anecdotal evidence led to a scientifically verifiable medication.

Some now promote the use of willow bark as a "natural alternative" to pharmaceutical aspirin. The evidence supporting the safety and effectiveness of aspirin should not be used as support for willow bark. The two are clearly not the same. Aspirin tablets contain acetylsalicylic acid and other inactive ingredients used to hold the tablets together. Willow bark contains salicylic acid plus numerous other naturally occurring chemicals. Aspirin tablets each contain the same amount of active ingredient, while the amounts of active ingredients in willow bark will vary depending on where the willow bark was obtained, when it was harvested, and how it was packaged. If the bark is used to prepare a tea, many other variables will be introduced, such as the amount used, the temperature of the water, and how long the bark was soaked. Therefore, results of studies using purified active ingredients should not be used to support the effectiveness of naturally occurring remedies.

Reviewing the Literature Is Vital

With the widespread use of clinical trials today, health care professionals have a new problem: the sheer volume of information available. There are about 20,000 to 30,000 health and medical journals publishing two million scientific articles every year.[31] If placed on top of one another, these articles would make a pillar more than 150 feet high.[32] Someone estimated that for health care professionals to remain up-to-date in their own area of practice, they need to read nineteen original articles *every day.*[33] Many of these articles report clinical trials that are not a quick read. Even with this amount of written information, only about half of the clinical studies conducted are ever published in written form, the rest being reported orally at meetings or not accepted for publication.[34]

Narrative Reviews

All this information has to be condensed and combined into a usable form for busy practitioners and interested patients. For this purpose, systematic reviews are carried out. Reviewers search for all the studies conducted on a certain therapy or drug and summarize their findings in different ways. The most common way of doing this is called a "narrative review." The reviewer, usually an expert in the field, selects the most important studies on a treatment and writes an essay on the strengths and weaknesses of each. The reviewer comes to a con-

clusion about all the evidence and its implications for clinical practice. These reviews provide concise summaries from someone familiar with the details of that research.

While narrative reviews are useful, they have an important limitation. Most reviewers are likely to have some preconceived idea about the research. This bias tends to come through in the conclusions. This is especially the case if the reviewer has done research on the therapy itself, which is probably why the person was chosen to write the review. Reviewers must be as objective as possible. Publishers now put safeguards in place to minimize this sort of bias.

A famous case of this involved the usefulness of vitamin C for treating the common cold. Linus Pauling (1901 – 1994) was a biochemist who won two Nobel prizes, one in 1954 for chemistry and the other in 1963 for peace. He reviewed the available research on vitamin C and the common cold and published two books on his findings. He concluded, from research done by others, that high doses of vitamin C would both prevent colds and, if you have a cold, decrease its severity and duration, adding, "Catching a cold and letting it run its course is a sign that you are not taking enough vitamin C."[35]

Pauling referred to thirty studies in his review but did not explain how he found these or how exhaustively he searched. He rated some studies as being of high quality and some of low quality but nowhere explained how he made those evaluations. He did not state if he "blinded" himself to the findings of the studies when evaluating their quality. The best way to review a study is to evaluate its quality without looking at its results. This method avoids judging studies that support a preconceived conclusion as being of higher quality. In Pauling's review, most studies supported his conclusion, and those that didn't he labeled "unfortunately flawed" without explaining why.

Years later, a researcher preparing to conduct another clinical trial on vitamin C and the common cold reexamined Pauling's data.[36] He searched exhaustively for all previous studies and found sixty-one. He had decided ahead of time what would constitute high quality and low quality in a study. He then covered up the results section of each study while grading how well the study was conducted. Only then did he look at their conclusions.

On a scale of 0 to 12 (with 12 being the best), only fifteen of the sixty-one studies scored 7 or more points. Based on the results of the best fifteen studies, this reviewer concluded, "Vitamin C, even in gram quantities per day, cannot prevent a cold. On the other hand, if you already have a cold, a megadose of, say, 1 g of vitamin C may slightly decrease the duration and severity of your cold (perhaps by 10%)."[37]

Systematic Reviews

This more rigorous and objective form of review is called a "systematic review." This conclusion, not Pauling's, has been consistently supported by other studies and reviews, which is why large doses of vitamin C are still not recommended by conventional medicine to prevent or cure colds.[38]

In spite of safeguards, no review can be absolutely objective since no human reviewer can be completely unbiased. Since decisions have to be made on what constitutes high and low quality, and what score counts for inclusion among the "best studies," any review will be somewhat biased. However, the more details given about how the review was conducted, the easier it is to determine how objectively it was done.

Meta-analysis

A newer method of reviewing research, called a "meta-analysis," has been developed to eliminate even more bias. This is a statistical method of combining the results of several trials that have given unclear or conflicting results. Most clinical trials with alternative therapies tend to be very small and are often poorly controlled. The theory behind the meta-analysis is that instead of running another large, expensive trial with hundreds of patients, the results of numerous small trials can be combined to give an accurate overall picture of the therapy's effectiveness.

However, a meta-analysis is only as good as the quality of the original studies. If the studies are of poor quality, then the meta-analysis will be of poor quality. All the studies combined in a meta-analysis must be very similar for the conclusion to be valid, and this is not always possible. A chain of evidence made up of weak links will not be made stronger by adding more weak links.

Unreliable "Reviews"

Unfortunately, some reports about therapies use unreliable and unobjective methods of "reviewing" therapies. Far too often, people who market alternative therapies try to promote or sell those therapies by using either media reports or poorly performed research studies. For example, reports stating "studies have found …" or "the latest evidence shows …" tell us nothing about the overall quality and significance of the research. In fact, these reports can be completely misleading, as they can pick studies that support only the conclusion the author wants to promote. It takes a lot more time and work to do a comprehensive review of the literature.

When making decisions about therapies, rely on the most systematic reviews available. We have used the principles and methods of systematic reviewing in making the recommendations given in Parts 2 and 3 of this book. A very helpful library of carefully conducted systematic reviews (including many on alternative therapies and remedies) is *The Cochrane Library*. This is available online from many public and medical libraries in versions for both health care professionals and the general public.[39]

The Limits of Scientific Testing

Scientific research has limitations. So, too, does conventional medicine. Diseases remain for which no cure is available, and symptoms for which there is no relief. Medicine cannot fix everything.

All physicians, if they practice long enough, will encounter the unexplainable: the patient who is too healthy to die yet dies at an early age; the man who has been given only a few weeks to live but years later is still doing well. Some people will do everything right as we understand healthy living and still die young. Some will do everything wrong and live to a grand old age. We don't know why.

Conventional medicine is not an exact science. It has been a long road of trial and error, of theory and testing — and change — to get where we are today. There are limitations to diagnosis and prognosis.

Every patient is different and responds somewhat differently to the same therapy. Evidence-based decisions involve an element of judgment — informed judgment.

Randomized controlled trials are the gold standard of clinical research. Even with their limitations, they provide the best evidence for discovering what works and what doesn't, what's safe and what's not. As one author concluded, "Even the sharpest critics of the way clinical trials are currently conducted, however, would not advocate that they not be done, for one simple reason: There's no better alternative."[40]

Evidence-based practice is a way for health care professionals and patients to determine which are the best therapies available. As good stewards of the "temple" God has given us, we should restrict ourselves to treatments and therapies that are reliable, safe, and effective. We would encourage our readers not to ask, "What do you think of this or that therapy?" but rather to ask, "What is the evidence supporting this or that therapy?"

Why do we suggest this? Because the therapy, if chosen, will be applied to one of the most valuable possessions on earth: "Do you not know that your body is a temple of the Holy Spirit, who is in you, whom you have received from God? You are not your own; you were bought at a price. Therefore honor God with your body" (1 Corinthians 6:19 – 20).

Chapter 2: Evidence-Based Health and Healing

1. National Center for Complementary and Alternative Medicine, *Expanding Horizons of Healthcare: Five-Year Strategic Plan 2001 – 2005. National Center for Complementary and Alternative Medicine: http://nccam.nih. gov/about/plans/fiveyear/index.htm* (August 30, 2005).

2. Harry Gold, Nathaniel T. Kwit, and Harold Otto, "The Xanthines (Theobromine and Aminophylline) in the Treatment of Cardiac Pain," *Journal of the American Medical Association* 108, no. 26 (June 1937): 2173 – 79.

3. Nathaniel T. Kwit, quoted in Arthur K. Shapiro and Elaine Shapiro, *The Powerful Placebo: From Ancient Priest to Modern Physician* (Baltimore: Johns Hopkins University Press, 1997), 142.

4. Robert Rosenthal, *Experimenter Effects in Behavioral Research* (New York: Irvington, 1976).

5. Flávio D. Fuchs, Michael J. Klag, and Paul K. Whelton, "The Classics: A Tribute to the Fiftieth Anniversary of the Randomized Clinical Trial," *Journal of Clinical Epidemiology* 53, no. 4 (April 2000): 335 – 42.

6. Medical Research Council, "Streptomycin Treatment of Pulmonary Tuberculosis," *British Medical Journal* 2 (October 1948): 769 – 82.

7. Theodore H. Greiner, Harry Gold, McKeen Cattel, Janet Travell, Hyman Bakst, Seymour H. Rinzler, Zachery H. Benjamin, Leon J. Warshaw, Audrie L. Bobb, Nathaniel T. Kwit, Walter Modell, Harold H. Rothendler, and Charles R. Messeloff, "A Method for the Evaluation of the Effects of Drugs on Cardiac Pain in Patients with Angina of Effort: A Study of Khellin (Visammin)," *American Journal of Medicine* 9 (August 1950): 143 – 55.

8. Kenneth F. Schulz, Iain Chalmers, Richard J. Hayes, and Douglas G. Altman, "Empirical Evidence of Bias: Dimensions of Methodological Quality Associated with Estimates of Treatment Effects in Controlled Trials," *Journal of the American Medical Association* 273, no. 5 (February 1995): 408 – 12.

9. Jacques M. Quen, "Elisha Perkins, Physician, Nostrum-Vendor, or Charlatan?" *Bulletin of the History of Medicine* 37 (1963): 159 – 66.

10. Shapiro and Shapiro, *Powerful Placebo*, 127.

11. Henry K. Beecher, "The Powerful Placebo," *Journal of the American Medical Association* 159, no. 17 (December 1955): 1602 – 6.

12. Leonard A. Cobb, George I. Thomas, David H. Dillard, K. Alvin Merendino, and Robert A. Bruce, "An Evaluation of Internal-Mammary-Artery Ligation by a Double-Blind Technic," *New England Journal of Medicine* 260, no. 22 (May 1959): 1115 – 18.

13. Vernon M. S. Oh, "The Placebo Effect: Can We Use It Better?" *British Medical Journal* 309 (July 1994): 69 – 70.

14. John A. Astin, "Why Patients Use Alternative Medicine: Results of a National Study," *Journal of the American Medical Association* 279, no. 19 (May 1998): 1548 – 53.

15. Paul H. Ray, "The Emerging Culture," *American Demographics* (February 1997): 7.

16. Judith A. Turner, Richard A. Deyo, John D. Loeser, Michael Von Korff, and Wilbert E. Fordyce, "The Importance of Placebo Effects in Pain Treatment and Research," *Journal of the American Medical Association* 271, no. 20 (May 1994): 1609 – 14.

17. Arthur J. Barsky, Ralph Saintfort, Malcolm P. Rogers, and Jonathan F. Borus, "Nonspecific Medication Side Effects and the Nocebo Phenomenon," *Journal of the American Medical Association* 287, no. 5 (February 2002): 622 – 27.

18. Robert A. Hahn, "The Nocebo Phenomenon: Concept, Evidence, and Implications for Public Health," *Preventive Medicine* 26, no. 5 (September/October 1997): 607 – 11.

19. Anonymous, "Charitable Chirurgion," *MD* 4 (May 1960): 188 – 93.

20. Shapiro and Shapiro, *Powerful Placebo*, 51, 134.

21. E. N. Frankel, J. Kanner, J. B. German, E. Parks, and J. E. Kinsella, "Inhibition of Oxidation of Human Low-Density Lipoprotein by Phenolic Substances in Red Wine," *Lancet* 341 (February 1993): 454 – 57.

22. Malcolm Law and Nicholas Wald, "Why Heart Disease Mortality Is Low in France: The Time Lag Explanation," *British Medical Journal* 318 (May 1999): 1471 – 76. This article sparked considerable controversy from numerous authors, whose comments are found in *British Medical Journal* 318 (May 1999): 1476 – 80; *British Medical Journal* 319 (July 1999): 255 – 56; *British Medical Journal* 320 (January 2000): 249 – 50.

23. M. E. Silverman, "William Harvey and the Discovery of the Circulation of Blood," *Clinical Cardiology* 8, no. 4 (April 1985): 244 – 46.

24. Shapiro and Shapiro, *Powerful Placebo*, 158.

25. Ibid.

26. George J. Annas and Sherman Elias, "Thalidomide and the *Titanic*: Reconstructing the Technology Tragedies of the Twentieth Century," *American Journal of Public Health* 89, no. 1 (January 1999): 98 – 101.

27. Kefauver-Harris Amendment to the Food and Drug Act (1962), quoted in Shapiro and Shapiro, *Powerful Placebo*, 172.

28. Terry P. Klassen, Ba' Pham, Margaret L. Lawson, and David Moher, "For Randomized Controlled Trials, the Quality of Reports of Complementary and Alternative Medicine Was As Good As Reports of Conventional Medicine," *Journal of Clinical Epidemiology* 58 (2005): 763 – 68.

29. Diana L. Woods, Ruth F. Craven, and Joie Whitney, "The Effect of Therapeutic Touch on Behavioral Symptoms of Persons with Dementia," *Alternative Therapies in Health and Medicine* 11, no. 1 (January/February 2005): 66 – 74.

30. Kathryn D. Lafreniere, Bulent Mutus, Sheila Cameron, Marie Tannous, Maria Giannotti, Hakam Abu-Zahra, and Ethan Laukkanen, "Effects of Therapeutic Touch on Biochemical and Mood Indicators in Women," *Journal of Alternative and Complementary Medicine* 5, no. 4 (August 1999): 367 – 70.

31. Tikki Pang, Ariel Pablos-Mendez, and Carel Usselmuiden, "From Bangkok to Mexico: Towards a Framework for Turning Knowledge Into Action to Improve Health Systems," *Bulletin of the World Health Organization* 82, no. 10 (October 2004): 720 – 22.

32. Cynthia D. Mulrow, "Rationale for Systematic Reviews," in *Systematic Reviews*, ed. Iain Chalmers and Douglas G. Altman (London: BMJ, 1995), 1.

33. Klassen et al., "For Randomized Controlled Trials," 763 – 68.

34. Kay Dickersin, Roberta Scherer, and Carol Lefebvre, "Identifying Relevant Studies for Systematic Reviews," in Chalmers and Altman, *Systematic Reviews*, 17 – 36.

35. Linus Pauling, *How to Live Longer and Feel Better* (New York: W. H. Freeman, 1986), 122; see also Linus Pauling, *Vitamin C and the Common Cold* (San Francisco: W. H. Freeman, 1970).

36. Paul Knipschild, "Some Examples of Systematic Reviews," in Chalmers and Altman, *Systematic Reviews*, 9 – 16.

37. Ibid., 11 – 12.

38. Robert M. Douglas and Harri Hemilä, "Vitamin C for Preventing and Treating the Common Cold," *PLoS Medicine* 2, no. 6 (June 2005): e168. *Public Library of Science: http://medicine.plosjournals.org/perlserv/?request=get-document&doi=10.1371/journal.pmed.0020168* (October 3, 2005).

39. *The Cochrane Library: www.cochrane.org.*

40. Rachel Nowak, "Problems in Clinical Trials Go Far Beyond Misconduct," Science 264 (June 1994): 1541.

FAITH-BASED HEALTH AND HEALING

Health is a major focus today. Many people think of physical wellness when they think about health, but the trend is toward a much broader view, a "holistic" view of health. This acknowledges the many influences on our health and healing — the physical, mental, emotional, relational, and spiritual factors. We now know that many nonphysical factors play an important role in the development of certain illnesses and in keeping us healthy.

What Does the Bible Say About Health?

The teaching of the Bible and the miracles of Jesus show that God cares for people's physical health. One of the best-known exemplars of biblical love is the Good Samaritan (Luke 10:30 – 37). He cared for the injured man holistically, including his relational and financial needs. But first the Samaritan bandaged the man's wounds, poured oil and wine on them, and took the man to a place where he could rest and recover physically.

The Bible teaches that God values our physical bodies. He considers our bodies to be temples, the dwelling place of the Holy Spirit (1 Corinthians 6:19). Paul mentions that physical training has value (1 Timothy 4:8). God is concerned about our health.

The word "health" is rarely found in English translations of the Bible. Yet the Old Testament uses a number of Hebrew terms to reflect a broad concept of "health as wholeness." Obedience to God and humility before him are frequently associated with promises of health and blessing: "Do not be wise in your own eyes; fear the LORD and shun evil. This will bring health to your body and nourishment to your bones" (Proverbs 3:7 – 8; see also Deuteronomy 30:15 – 16).

Some of the Old Testament laws reflect God's concern for the health of his people and how he expected them to use natural means to promote health. Obeying some of these laws would have promoted health in the same way that public health regulations do today. For example, the Israelites were forbidden to eat meat that we now know was more likely to carry diseases. They were to quarantine people with possible signs of infectious diseases, just as we use certain "isolation techniques" today to prevent spread of infection (Leviticus 11; 13; 14).

The clear teaching of the Old Testament is that good health depends on living one's life according to God's will. This produces *tsedeq*, which means "righteousness," or being in a right relationship with God. This leads to a long and healthy life. This multidimensional description of health is carried into the New Testament.

The underlying truth is that humans are more than merely physical beings; we are complicated persons with physical as well as emotional, relational, moral, and spiritual dimensions. The following passages show some of the ways in which holistic health is taught throughout the Bible:

- Emotions are linked to health, as in Proverbs 17:22: "A cheerful heart is good medicine, but a crushed spirit dries up the bones."
- Health is influenced by the morality of our actions: "For anyone who eats and drinks without recognizing the body of the Lord eats and drinks judgment on himself. That is why

many among you are weak and sick, and a number of you have fallen asleep" (1 Corinthians 11:29 – 30).
- Our spiritual vitality is linked to our health: "Dear friend, I pray that you may enjoy good health and that all may go well with you, even as your soul is getting along well" (3 John 2).

Health is also described in the Bible as blessedness, a significant theme in both the Old and New Testaments. The Sermon on the Mount most clearly describes this view (Matthew 5:3 – 12; Luke 6:20 – 26). The poor, the meek, the downtrodden, and the underprivileged are blessed, not rejected, by God. People can be blessed, and therefore healthy, despite undesirable circumstances. A quadriplegic can be blessed and right with God and "healthy" in the biblical sense of health. The Beatitudes describe people's overall well-being and imply that our health depends on our inner life, which God wants to nourish and promote.

The Bible teaches that health involves the restoration and strengthening of one's personal relationship with God. A healthy lifestyle includes pursuing healthy relationships (physically, emotionally, and spiritually) with family, others, and, most importantly, God himself.

However, we sometimes need to prioritize the different aspects of our health. The Bible describes situations in which physical health must be sacrificed for the promotion of spiritual health. Jesus tells us, "If your right eye causes you to sin, gouge it out and throw it away. It is better for you to lose one part of your body than for your whole body to be thrown into hell" (Matthew 5:29). Such a passage is not to be taken literally. It reflects a literary way of making a point. Christians are not called on to mutilate themselves or to neglect their physical health. In most situations, promoting physical health is compatible with promoting spiritual health. But sometimes a choice has to be made. That's what Jesus is teaching here. And in those cases, Jesus says our spiritual health should be given higher priority than physical health.

Sometimes we will have to make difficult choices not to pursue some means of promoting physical health — for the sake of our spiritual health. Jesus sums up this principle: "What good will it be for a man if he gains the whole world, yet forfeits his soul? Or what can a man give in exchange for his soul?" (Matthew 16:26).

Central to all of these ideas is the declaration that Jesus Christ came to offer ultimate health to people in the form of a life on earth that would be full and satisfying and meaningful, coupled with the promise of an eternal life that is disease-free, sin-free, and tear-free. "I have come that they may have life, and have it to the full" (John 10:10). Christians should be real examples of such contented living.

Good Health Can Become an Idol

Many of the more recent controversial developments in conventional medicine (cloning, assisted suicide, embryo research) have arisen because some believe that the purpose of life is to promote life itself — and not just *any* life, but life that is judged by human standards to be valuable or of good quality. Good health can become the most important thing in a person's life.

Our modern world makes it easy to become consumed with maintaining a very high quality of physical life for as long as possible. Cosmetic surgery, pills such as Viagra, and medical "treatments" for baldness or wrinkles become central to maintaining a certain quality of life, or "health." Each of these treatments can have a legitimate use in specific cases, but their popularity is a natural outgrowth of the idea that the purpose of life is to promote life itself.

This sort of focus can also lead people to pursue whatever spiritual, relational, or emotional factors they believe will contribute to their goals in this life. If religion and spirituality are said to help people live longer, healthier lives, they are willing to try them. Whether the beliefs are based on truth doesn't matter to someone with such a mind-set. To such individuals, the purpose of life remains rooted in the here and now, the period from birth to a painless, gentle physical death.

For many within the New Age movement, this attitude toward life is taken one step further. Health involves self-actualization. This requires getting in touch with one's intuitive side, the inner self. Various forms of meditation become important. One's own health becomes of central importance. And only the individual is able to judge what is beneficial. According to one commentator, this leads to a view that "anything that could conceivably contribute to human growth, whether scientifically verified or not, [is] admissible — and [is] admitted."[1]

Such thinking underlies the openness within New Age thought to alternative therapies. With health defined as broadly as "well-being" — and the most important test being how people feel after a therapy — almost anything could be included as "therapy." If the ultimate purpose in life is good health, then a person ought to pursue anything that might improve health.

This belief actually makes it more difficult to accept illness, limitations, aging, and death. When physical health is most important, a lack of health can be devastating — and even lead people to belittle their own value, worth, and purpose. A person's very identity can be shaken by illness. This may partially explain why people expend huge resources to keep their bodies "healthy" and demand assistance in suicide when they deem their lives to be of no further value.

What Value Should We Place on Our Health?

It is good to be healthy. We should maximize our physical, emotional, relational, and spiritual health. But they should not become ends in and of themselves. The pursuit of physical health must be balanced against other values.

Jesus proclaimed that the two greatest commandments are to love God and serve others (Matthew 22:36 – 40). Good health is a means toward these goals. Paul expressed a similar idea when he told Christians, "You were bought at a price. Therefore honor God with your body" (1 Corinthians 6:20).

In God's system, there are sometimes good reasons to sacrifice our health and even our lives. Jesus touched the lepers and other "untouchables" of his day for the greater value of their spiritual health. Doctors, nurses, and others still imitate Jesus when they take care of those with infectious diseases. Those who go on the mission field to countries where little health care is available make these same choices for themselves and their families. They are to be admired. They know that there is more to life than just physical health.

The entire law of God is summarized in both the Old and New Testaments as loving our neighbors as ourselves (Leviticus 19:18; Matthew 22:39; Galatians 5:14). This sometimes involves decisions to give the health of others a higher priority than our own health. This can range from a relatively small decision to get less sleep in order to care for someone in their illness to a major decision to move to an underprivileged country or the inner city to serve the poor.

Putting others' needs before our own is never easy. The teachings of many popular "gurus" within the alternative medicine movement make it even more difficult. Secular sociologists have pointed out that the gurus' message is very much focused on individuals and their own health.[2] This approach fits into an individualistic lifestyle, which attracts many.

God's view of a healthy lifestyle is dramatically different. It is one of significant relationships built on people's commitment to serve one another before themselves. Jesus said, "It is more blessed to give than to receive" (Acts 20:35). And even science is starting to show that this leads to better health.

Devout Faith Helps but Does Not Guarantee Good Health

Interest in the connection between faith and health has led to a relatively large number of studies investigating the link. Some religious groups, including some actively involved in alternative medicine, claim to offer complete health to their adherents. Evaluating the health of believers in those religions would provide important evidence about the truth or falsity of those religions (as has been done for the First Church of Christ, Scientist, or Christian Scientists).[3] For this reason, it is important to examine whether the Bible teaches that God promises to heal Christians.

Scientific studies seem to support the idea that religion and faith are important factors in health. Numerous studies show a positive correlation between involvement in religious practices and people's health. A large proportion of the published studies suggest that religious commitment may play a beneficial role in preventing mental and physical illness, improving how people cope with mental and physical illness, and facilitating recovery from illness.[4] The foreword to a recent book summarizing the results of hundreds of these studies put it this way: "As those of us who have labored in this field for many years have long suspected, the relationship between religion and health, on average and at the population level, is overwhelmingly positive. Now we can say, finally, that we know this to be true."[5]

This conclusion is not held by all researchers. Much still remains to be investigated with improved studies specially designed to investigate the connection between religious involvement and health status. However, a better picture of the situation has emerged over the last several years. As would be expected, things are complicated. One review, which used only high-quality studies, arrived at some general conclusions.[6]

- **Frequent church attendance** is strongly connected to increased life expectancy (by up to 25 percent).
- **Viewing oneself as religious** seems to be connected with having less heart disease, although not all studies confirmed this.
- **Prayer improves recovery** from some acute diseases, though again, only some of the evidence supports this claim (we will examine this in more detail in the Prayer for Healing entry, p. 236).
- **People who value religion** consistently showed no benefit in recovering from acute

diseases and in some cases were found to have slower recovery. Researchers have suggested that this may be due to patients' struggling over why God had "abandoned them" in their illness, an issue we address in the next section.
- **Religiosity** failed to protect people against cancer, disability, or death.
- **Benefits are greatest** when religious faith is an important part of who that person is.
- **Strong faith** not only influences a person's understanding of the meaning of life but also serves as a guide for living, motivating people to avoid risky or unhealthy behavior.[7]

A 2005 study provides a good example of the complexities of this research. Chronic stress puts people at higher risk for several diseases, including diabetes, heart disease, and cognitive disorders. A person's long-term risk correlates well with measurements of blood pressure and of a hormone called "cortisol." Higher levels of both correlate well with a higher level of chronic stress and a higher risk of disease.

When these levels were measured in university students, some interesting patterns were seen between the results and the students' levels of religiosity and spirituality.[8] Students reporting themselves as religious to any extent had lower cortisol levels after receiving stressful stimuli compared to those who said they were "not at all religious." Closer examination of the students' religiosity revealed that those with better cortisol scores prayed more frequently and rated themselves high in ability to forgive. No significant correlations were found for attendance at religious services, frequency of meditation, or use of religion to deal with stressful situations. Blood pressure measurements actually revealed conflicting results. Men who were more religious had lower blood pressure, while more religious women had higher blood pressure. This finding differs from other studies in which, in general, higher religiosity correlates with lower blood pressure.[9]

Other studies of the impact of religion on health also have not been uniformly positive. A small number of researchers found no correlation between faith and health, and in some cases they found a negative effect.

From a scientific perspective, some of these studies have significant limitations.[10] Some were poorly designed and sometimes did not take into account the difficulty in measuring such factors as people's religiosity or spirituality. Many used simple questions such as, "Do you attend church?" to measure people's religiosity.

In spite of these limitations, the studies seem to indicate that those who rarely attend religious services, or have little personal faith, are at higher risk for disease and illness, especially those connected with stress.

The general health benefits of faith are real — and the deeper and more internalized the faith, the greater the benefits. Scientific research has demonstrated that much, even if it hasn't (and probably can't) prove *why* people benefit from religious faith. That also is a matter of faith.

Christians Are Told to Expect Suffering

Although faith can improve our health, we should not assume that our lives can or will be trouble-free. In fact, the Bible tells Christians to expect suffering and not to be surprised by suffering. "For it has been granted to you on behalf of Christ not only to believe on him, but also to suffer for him" (Philippians 1:29; see also 1 Thessalonians 3:4; 1 Peter 4:12).

We are to comfort one another and encourage one another with the knowledge that our destiny is secure in the arms of the Lord, even in the face of suffering and death (1 Thessalonians 4:13 – 5:11).

Some claim illness and suffering reflect weakness in an individual's faith, but this is not borne out by the biblical record. The New Testament mentions by name a number of early church leaders, people we can assume had strong faith, who got sick. All died. Every faith healer in recorded history has gotten sick and died — some at a young age.

Can Faith Be Unhealthy?

While faith can have positive effects on health, it can also have negative effects.

Although religious beliefs are a source of comfort and support for many people, for others they are a source of stress and emotional turmoil. In one large study of hospitalized patients, the researchers looked at those who believed that

- God was punishing them;
- God had abandoned them;
- God didn't love them;
- God didn't have the power to help; or
- their church had deserted them.

People who held these beliefs had a 19 to 28 percent *higher* death rate in the two years after being discharged from a hospital.[11] This effect was statistically significant and independent of physical health, mental health, and social support.

Another potential negative effect of religion or religiosity is crippling guilt that can arise from a misunderstanding of the connection between faith and health. Sincerely religious people can come to believe that their faith will protect them from illness and suffering, a belief reinforced by pastoral professionals and others who proclaim that God will heal them if they have enough faith. Some hold that illness and suffering are a result of sin, and if they become ill, God will heal them if they have strong enough faith. When they aren't healed, they believe this means their faith is weak or they have sinned in some way. The result can be excessive guilt or anger at God, leading to a loss of faith and trust in God. This can have tragic consequences. For these reasons it is vital that we understand what the Bible actually teaches about faith and healing.

Sickness and Sin

We can say, in one sense, that all sickness has its ultimate origin in sin because human suffering stems from the fall and the sin of Adam and Eve (Genesis 2:15 – 17; Romans 1:28 – 32). But that's not the way some people think of sin causing sickness. They believe a specific sin caused a particular illness. The Bible shows that there can be a simple cause-and-effect relationship between sin and sickness. But the Bible doesn't claim that sin *always* leads to illness or that every illness has its cause in some sin. The Bible teaches that disobedience to God *can* lead to sickness that ultimately is of supernatural origin. For example, "If you do not obey the Lord your God and do not carefully follow all his commands and decrees I am giving you today, ... The Lord will plague you with diseases until he has destroyed you from the land you are entering to possess. The Lord will strike you with wasting disease, with fever and inflammation, with scorching heat and drought, with blight and mildew, which will plague you until you perish"

(Deuteronomy 28:15, 21 – 22). Several accounts are given in which an illness is sent as a punishment for specific sins (e.g., Exodus 4:11; Leviticus 26:16; Deuteronomy 32:39; Numbers 12:9 – 10; 2 Chronicles 7:13; 21:14 – 15).

Jesus himself made a strong connection between sin and sickness when he healed the man at the pool in Bethesda (John 5:1 – 15). He basically equated forgiveness with healing, although his emphasis was on the fact that only God brings about either. As Jesus bid farewell to this healed man, he made the clearest connection between sin and sickness, warning, "See, you are well again. Stop sinning or something worse may happen to you" (John 5:14). The clear implication is that if the man sinned again (possibly in some specific way well known to the man), something worse than thirty-eight years of crippling illness would befall him.

This incident may have left the disciples (and readers of John's gospel) wondering if most illnesses result from sin. John later warned that some sins lead to death and others do not (1 John 5:16). Two believers, Ananias and Sapphira, were struck dead because of a specific sin (Acts 5:1 – 11). Some Corinthian believers got ill and died because of their sin (1 Corinthians 11:27 – 34). Little wonder that some believe the Bible teaches that when people sin, bad things happen. Today when someone gets seriously ill, has a tragic accident, or is told their disease will be fatal, it is common to ask, "Why? What have I done wrong?"

However, it is neither biblical nor logical to believe that a simple one-to-one cause-and-effect relationship exists between sin and illness. God related to the ancient nation of Israel in significantly different ways than he relates to people today. Israel entered into an agreement with God in which they knew they would be blessed if they obeyed God — and swiftly punished for disobedience. God told them, "See, I set before you today life and prosperity, death and destruction" (Deuteronomy 30:15). He then told them to choose which they wanted.

The Christian church today does not have such an agreement with God. We know from experience that God does not cause people to be ill every time they sin. If he did, we would be struck by an illness or suffering every time we did anything wrong — in word, deed, or thought.

Another reason we can be confident that not all illness is sent by God as a punishment is that Jesus tells us this is not the case:

> As [Jesus] went along, he saw a man blind from birth. His disciples asked him, "Rabbi, who sinned, this man or his parents, that he was born blind?"
>
> "Neither this man nor his parents sinned," said Jesus, "but this happened so that the work of God might be displayed in his life"
>
> *John 9:1 – 3*

Jesus is very clear: we should not assume that someone's sickness occurred because the person (or the parents) sinned. The implication is that sickness and disease can arise from purely physical sources such as viruses, bacteria, cancer-causing agents, genetic factors, overeating, lack of exercise, or some environmental factor that might poison our bodies.

Many biblical accounts of healing simply state that the person was ill (2 Kings 4:18 – 37; Matthew 4:23 – 24; Acts 5:16). Sometimes illness and death were caused by others' actions, as with John the Baptist (Matthew 14:1 – 12). In another important incident, Jesus states that sometimes people suffer because they happen to be in the wrong place at the wrong time.

> Now there were some present at that time who told Jesus about the Galileans whose blood Pilate had mixed with their sacrifices. Jesus answered, "Do you think that these Galileans were worse sinners than all the other Galileans because they suffered this way? I tell you, no! But unless you repent, you too will all perish. Or those eighteen who died when the tower in Siloam fell on them — do you think they were more guilty than all the others living in Jerusalem? I tell you, no! But unless you repent, you too will all perish."
>
> *Luke 13:1 – 5*

Jesus directs his listeners to reflect on their position before God rather than trying to figure out what sin caused the suffering. The response we are encouraged to have in the face of illness or suffering is not "Why is God doing this to me?" but "What is God doing in this situation?" That question indicates a belief and trust that what a loving God allows to happen can be used for good. It is more in keeping with what Paul says in Romans 8:28: "We know that in all things God works for the good of those who love him, who have been called according to his purpose."

God's Response Isn't Always Healing

The Bible does not teach that God's response to illness is immediate physical healing. Sometimes it is healing in other realms, as exemplified by Tom's story.

Tom grew up in a small local traditional church, as had his dad and his dad's dad. Going to church every Sunday was just something that people in his hometown did.

The minister was nice, but his sermons never led Tom to consider anything beyond Sunday morning religion — such as his need for a personal relationship with God. Perhaps Tom wasn't led because the minister never had such a relationship himself. His desire was to *serve* others, not *inspire* them. The pastor and Tom never really got to know each other.

During a routine physical exam, Tom's family doctor found a lump in his prostate. Further testing confirmed that it was a potentially lethal form of cancer. Radical surgery offered the best hope of cure. The alternatives — watchful waiting, herbs and vitamins, or radiation therapy — could, according to the consultants, mean the spread of the cancer to other parts of his body. Tom was terrified.

Tom remembered a Sunday school lesson on the book of James that taught sick people to see their church elders for prayer and anointing with oil. So Tom talked with his pastor. He asked if God might cure him. To his surprise, the pastor didn't think God healed people these days. More disappointingly, the pastor didn't offer Tom anything that gave him hope.

The night before surgery, Tom slept fitfully. Waiting in the preoperative area, Tom became increasingly nervous and frightened. He wanted to call out to God; he wanted to pray — but he didn't know how.

Then he saw his family doctor, dressed in green operating room scrubs. "Tom," he said, "I know surgery can be scary. For most of us, it brings up questions about God. Every time I've ever taken patients to the OR, they've wanted to somehow talk to God and ask for his protection and healing. Would you mind if I had a little prayer with you?"

Tom was dumbfounded. Never had he seen religion like this — played out in the workplace. Object? No way!

When the doctor bowed his head, Tom reached up and grasped his hand. As the doctor prayed, Tom felt a sense of peace and something he could not remember feeling for a long time — tears running down his cheeks. Tom found himself squeezing the doctor's hand.

After the prayer, Tom dried his tears and felt somewhat embarrassed. The doctor asked if he had any questions. "Just one," replied Tom. "You won't tell anyone, will you?"

"Tell them what?" inquired the doctor. "That we prayed?"

"No. That we held hands!"

In the days following surgery, Tom's pastor stopped by his room to talk briefly. It was a nice gesture, but that was all. To Tom's surprise, his family doctor suggested that Tom begin looking at what the Bible had to say about health, prayer, and recovery. During his reading, Tom realized he did not have a personal relationship with God. His doctor suggested he read the gospel of John. Verses 12 and 13 of the first chapter hit him hard: "Yet to all who received [Jesus], to those who believed in his name, he gave the right to become children of God — children born not of natural descent, nor of human decision or a husband's will, but born of God."

Tom realized he had never had the spiritual birth described there. Tom wanted a personal relationship with God. He prayed for forgiveness and thanked God for Jesus' sacrifice on the cross that paid the penalty for his sins. He pictured Jesus standing at the door and invited him in (Revelation 3:20).

God could have healed Tom's cancer miraculously, but he chose instead to let Tom be healed through human agency. God could have appeared personally to Tom, but instead he sent a messenger — another human being. Tom was allowed to grapple with his cancer so that God could bring about the ultimate healing: spiritual restoration of Tom's relationship with God.

Part of the general healing available through Jesus Christ is the total and complete forgiveness of sin, which provides a person relief from both the penalty of sin and the guilt of sin. This forgiveness cannot be earned by keeping rules or performing rituals. Forgiveness is available as a free gift from God: "It is by grace you have been saved, through faith — and this not from yourselves, it is the gift of God — not by works, so that no one can boast" (Ephesians 2:8 – 9). We believe this is an important aspect of the connection between healing and confession described in James 5:14 – 16.

God can use disease to draw people toward himself. How we respond to disease or disorders that he causes or allows is very important to him. According to the Bible, he can use these experiences (illness and injury) to refine or purify his people: "We also rejoice in our sufferings, because we know that suffering produces perseverance; perseverance, character; and character, hope. And hope does not disappoint us, because God has poured out his love into our hearts by the Holy Spirit, whom he has given us" (Romans 5:3 – 5).

The World Is Not the Way the World Should Be

The healing experienced by Tom went deeper than his body. The Bible teaches that there is a very general way in which sickness is connected to sin. The world is not the way God intended it to be: it is a fallen world in which suffering occurs. When sin entered the world, humans changed — not only spiritually, but mentally, emotionally, and physically. With the entrance of sin, humans lost intimacy with God and became alienated from God (spiritually). This resulted in the progression from health to dis-

ease (physically), wholeness to emptiness (emotionally and psychologically), and harmony to anarchy (socially). Spiritual separation from God, physical disease, psychological dysfunction, and social disorder all find their origin in sin.

When the New Testament writers mention people being sick, they rarely associate the illness with spiritual issues. The implication is that much illness is of natural origin and exists simply because people live in a fallen world. We can even gain some hope from the knowledge that the world is not the way God wants it to be and that he promises us a better future:

> We know that the whole creation has been groaning as in the pains of childbirth right up to the present time. Not only so, but we ourselves, who have the firstfruits of the Spirit, groan inwardly as we wait eagerly for our adoption as sons, the redemption of our bodies. For in this hope we were saved. But hope that is seen is no hope at all. Who hopes for what he already has? But if we hope for what we do not yet have, we wait for it patiently.
>
> *Romans 8:22 – 25*

The Dark Side

We cannot ignore another source of illness described in the Bible. Many people today deny or scoff at the existence of a demonic realm. Yet the biblical worldview makes little sense without the inclusion of evil spiritual beings. The Bible mentions these beings repeatedly, particularly in the New Testament. Paul's thorn in the flesh that caused him illness is described as a messenger of Satan (2 Corinthians 12:7 – 10). The gospels of Matthew and Luke are especially clear that illness can have a demonic source (Matthew 4:23 – 25; 17:14 – 21; Luke 13:11).[12]

Some Christians claim that all illness has a demonic origin and that therefore all illnesses can be healed through confession of sin and prayer. They hold that since illness is from Satan and healing is from God, prayer expressed in faith *always* leads to healing. Their belief is that if people pray persistently and are not healed, they either lack faith or are infested with unconfessed sin.

However, the New Testament simply does *not* paint a picture of demonic activity causing *all* illness. Clear distinctions are made between illness of demonic origin and illness with other causes. Consider these examples:

> News about [Jesus] spread all over Syria, and people brought to him all who were ill with various diseases, those suffering severe pain, the demon-possessed, those having seizures, and the paralyzed, and he healed them.
>
> *Matthew 4:24*

> [Jesus] called his twelve disciples to him and gave them authority to drive out evil spirits and to heal every disease and sickness.
>
> *Matthew 10:1*

> Crowds gathered also from the towns around Jerusalem, bringing their sick and those tormented by evil spirits, and all of them were healed.
>
> *Acts 5:16*

The overall teaching of the Bible is that sickness can have different origins. Therefore, claims that all illnesses can be cured by casting out demons are not biblical. This has important implications for what are called "deliverance ministries," healing through casting out demons. While deliverance ministries may have a role in the church, claims that the primary focus of the church should be on delivering

Christians from demon possession must be seriously questioned.

Pentecostal scholar John Christopher Thomas notes that since only about 10 percent of the infirmities described in the New Testament are attributed to demons, "it would seem wise to avoid the temptation of assuming that in most cases an infirmity is caused by Satan and/or demons.... The current specialization in exorcisms by some in the church is misdirected at best."[13]

On the other hand, one of Satan's most effective tactics in the Western world has been to convince people that he does not exist. This means that the role of demons in illness and suffering is often completely ignored. We believe that if an illness, after careful and prayerful discernment, is deemed to be caused by demons, Christians can be confident that the power of God can bring healing. God's power is greater than any demonic power. Referring to evil spirits, John encourages the early believers, "You, dear children, are from God and have overcome them, because the one who is in you is greater than the one who is in the world" (1 John 4:4).

Failure to accept the biblical teaching on the existence and activity of Satan and his demons has another important consequence. People who do not believe in evil spiritual beings will have little concern for their own safety and well-being as they dabble in spiritual practices, including some promoted as therapies, that can be spiritually harmful.

An Uncomfortable Improvement

Mary, a secretary for the president of a large department store, began having backaches that seemed to start for no particular reason, though she realized she had poor posture when working at her computer. The backaches got worse after the man Mary thought might propose marriage broke off the relationship. She also began working a lot of overtime. Sleeping became difficult.

Mary went to a new wellness center, recommended by a woman at church who said the center had helped a relative with arthritis. Mary was advised to make some simple changes to her work area and begin taking walks outside, in sunlight, to alter her mood. Encouraged by her improvement, Mary tried a healing technique called Reiki that the center said was similar to the laying on of hands, only older. The practitioner told Mary her body had "energy blockages" that he would "unblock" by using his hands to direct energy to her. "I did feel better after the treatments, though I later realized I felt no better than after I changed my lifestyle," Mary said.

"I also had the feeling that this Reiki was some New Age practice that had nothing to do with God. When I asked the practitioner, he said if I wanted to believe that Universal Life Energy was God, I could. It would not hinder my healing."

Afraid that some Reiki practices went against Christian teachings, Mary stopped the treatments. The woman who had recommended the center held a different view, saying if Mary felt better, the treatment must be good. "After all," she said, "we know that all healing comes from God."

Not All Healing Is from God

How we pursue health and healing is very important. Our concern, as Christians, is that there are wrong ways (even evil ways) people can pursue and receive healing. We wish to make the case that heal-

ing achieved by inappropriate means is healing that is not good and, in our view, is healing that is not from God. Some people seem stunned to learn that we believe that sometimes healing can occur that is not pleasing to God.

We believe that certain alternative therapies have spiritual roots that make their use inappropriate for Christians and unwise for anyone. Any type of healing that might occur via these therapies is not worth the spiritual cost. Therefore, from a biblical perspective, some therapies are *always* wrong. Any seeking of healing, even "good healing," for the wrong reasons or with the wrong motives may be wrong.

We must point out that not all Christian theologians and health care providers agree with our view on this issue. The people of God come from different traditions and have different beliefs. They differ in their interpretation of different Bible passages and how they apply to current situations.

We therefore believe it is essential that we explain our thinking and give the biblical basis for our reasoning. The information we give in Part 2 on the origins of alternative therapies will help you understand why some Christian physicians, theologians, and pastors are so concerned about certain aspects of alternative medicine.

Illegitimate Spiritual Practices

Alternative medicine as a whole is not rooted in any particular religious tradition, but some therapies are. A number of healing rituals and traditions are part of the Wiccan religion (also called "white witchcraft"). Eastern religions often view healing as dependent on the movement of "life energy" through nonphysical channels that coincide with the physical body. Native-American religion uses herbs as part of its healing rituals. In a number of nature religions, shamans contact spirit beings or guides to get advice on how to treat and heal those under their care.

The current interest in holistic healing includes concern for spirituality, the meaning of which can be whatever the individual wants it to mean. What *is* important, this new approach says, is that a person be on *some* spiritual path. Any therapy can be pursued for its potential healing benefits. All that matters is whether it works. And if others claim it works, it's worth a try. This leads to a strong emphasis on "personal experience" being the deciding factor. As the developer of Therapeutic Touch stated, "Therapeutic Touch works.... You can do it; everyone who is willing to undertake the discipline to learn Therapeutic Touch can do it. You need only try in order to determine the truth of this statement for yourself. So, I invite you: TRY."[14]

The problem that Christians *should* have with this approach is that the Bible tells us not to engage in certain practices. Certain forms of healing are always wrong because they are accomplished via prohibited methods and have been consistently condemned by God in the Bible. Many of these practices have been incorporated into certain alternative therapies. The most complete list of prohibitions is found in Deuteronomy 18:9 – 14, although each practice is prohibited in many other passages (see also 1 Corinthians 10:18 – 21). Prohibited are divination, necromancy (channeling), mediumship, spiritualism, witchcraft, magic, and sorcery.

- **Divination** covers a variety of practices used to discover information by supernatural means (Leviticus 19:26; 2 Kings 21:6; Jeremiah 14:14). Also included as divination would be tarot cards, the reading or interpreting of omens, crystal gazing, and any technique that attempts to discern information transmitted from the spiritual realm through natural objects. Divination includes direct attempts to contact the spirit world for information, as in the use of spirit guides and shamans.

- **Astrology** is based on the same principles as divination but uses the stars to uncover hidden information. It is denounced as a waste of time in Isaiah 47:13 – 14 (see also Jeremiah 10:2).

- **Channeling, or necromancy,** has become popular within New Age circles. It involves calling up the spirits of the dead. Isaiah specifically denounces this practice, and not because it doesn't "work." Rather, necromancy, as with all these practices, displays an attitude of rebellion against God by refusing to do things his way: "When men tell you to consult mediums and spiritists, who whisper and mutter, should not a people inquire of their God? Why consult the dead on behalf of the living?" (Isaiah 8:19).

- **Mediums and spiritists** are those who possess the ability to contact the spirits of the dead (Leviticus 19:31; 20:6, 27; 1 Samuel 28; 2 Kings 21:6; 1 Chronicles 10:13 – 14).

- **Witchcraft** is the use of magical spells and charms to obtain desires through supernatural or psychic powers. God makes his views about magic very clear through Ezekiel. "I am against your magic charms with which you ensnare people like birds and I will tear them from your arms; I will set free the people that you ensnare like birds" (Ezekiel 13:20; see also 2 Kings 21:6; Acts 19:18 – 19).

- **Sorcery** is the ability to use magical spells, an ability usually obtained through contacting evil spirits. The prophet Micah brought this message from God to those in his day who dabbled in these occult practices: "I will destroy your witchcraft and you will no longer cast spells" (Micah 5:12; see also Galatians 5:20).

These practices are all condemned because they lead people away from the true God and entrap people in false ways. The use of magic and charms to influence the future reflects a lack of trust in the goodness of God to bring about what is best in a situation. Instead of trying to manipulate the future, we are called to trust in God's trustworthiness.

The Bible clearly teaches that good and evil spiritual forces exist. Many today deny or ignore this teaching. Performing spiritual acts with good intentions and getting good results does not excuse being unaware of the source of the power behind those acts. Scripture states that evil spiritual forces are powerful and dangerous and should not be dabbled with (Ephesians 6:12; 1 Peter 5:8; 1 John 4:4).

In our opinion, it is naïve and unsafe to think or teach that Satan would not use his powers to heal people, especially since healing is such an important sign of the Messiah. Satan will resort to "good deeds" to deceive people and draw them away from God. Jesus warned us, "For false Christs and false prophets will appear and perform signs and miracles to deceive even the elect — if that were possible" (Matthew 24:24; Mark 13:22).

Clearly, great discernment must be exercised before dabbling in alternative therapies with spiritual backgrounds. It is never appropriate to use therapies that involve magic, contact with spirit guides or the spirits of the dead, or any attempt to manipulate spiritual powers.

"Life Energy" or "Medical Magic"

Alternative therapies based on "life energy" use principles just like those generally attributed to magic. Although "magic" is difficult to define concisely, magical practices do have common features. Magic involves specific techniques or rituals by which people attempt to manipulate supernatural powers to meet their immediate needs.[15] Practitioners of energy medicine claim they can manipulate a supernatural force using certain techniques to bring about healing or relaxation.

- **Healing is demanded** by practitioners of magic. "There is never anything humble about the requests addressed to supernatural agents."[16] Incidentally, this leads us to have great concern about Christian healers who demand healing from God. This contrasts with the way Christians are encouraged to humbly make requests of God yet trust in his will.

- **Healing is guaranteed** when magical instructions are followed precisely, or so it is claimed. "In magic a ritual is performed and if it is correct in every detail, the desired result must follow unless countered by stronger magic."[17]

- **Present-day desires** of the individual are the focus in magic, not the long-term needs or goals of the community.

When magic doesn't work, it can still do harm. It wastes precious time, time that could have been used to seek proven, effective remedies. A cancer continues to grow. Diabetes and high blood pressure go untreated. Pain lingers.

An even bigger problem arises when magical practices do work. Long associated with occult traditions, many of these practices can lead people into all sorts of entanglements with evil spiritual beings. Kurt Koch, a Christian theologian and an authority on the occult, recounts many stories of people being healed by alternative therapies without knowing of the occult connections. One young man went to an iridologist, someone who claims to be able to diagnose and treat illnesses by examining the irises of people's eyes.[18] Soon afterward, this young man recovered completely from his illness. But then he noticed some disturbing changes. Every time he tried to enter a church, he experienced physical pain. The same thing happened whenever he tried to read a Bible or sing a Christian hymn. He rapidly became severely depressed, started abusing drugs, and eventually had a complete emotional breakdown. Certainly, not all iridologists (or alternative practitioners in general) are connected with the occult, but this particular one seems to have been. We acknowledge that this story has all the limitations of testimonials that we describe elsewhere in our book. But it fits the pattern of stories in which people inadvertently received an occult healing and paid for it with their emotional and spiritual health.

Be suspicious of any practitioner who claims he or she can accurately diagnose illnesses by "extraordinary" means or who knows things about others through some "amazing" intuition. Those powers, if real, must come from somewhere. Chances are they are supernatural powers. Great caution and discernment are necessary to ensure they are not occult powers.

Biblical Characters Condemned for Pursuing Certain Forms of Healing

The Bible recognizes the great temptation inherent in healing by evil spirits and illicit healers. The Old Testament describes an intense conflict between legitimate and illegitimate approaches to healing and spirituality. An incident involving King Ahaziah, the eighth king of Israel, clearly demonstrates this:

> Now Ahaziah had fallen through the lattice of his upper room in Samaria and injured himself. So he sent messengers, saying to them, "Go and consult Baal-Zebub, the god of Ekron, to see if I will recover from this injury."
>
> But the angel of the LORD said to Elijah the Tishbite, "Go up and meet the messengers of the king of Samaria and ask them, 'Is it because there is no God in Israel that you are going off to consult Baal-Zebub, the god of Ekron?' Therefore this is what the LORD says: 'You will not leave the bed you are lying on. You will certainly die!'" So Elijah went.
>
> *2 Kings 1:2 – 4*

In contrast, King Hezekiah of Judah became deathly ill and was told by the prophet Isaiah that he would not recover. Hezekiah responded differently, which resulted in God healing him.

> Hezekiah turned his face to the wall and prayed to the LORD, "Remember, O LORD, how I have walked before you faithfully and with wholehearted devotion and have done what is good in your eyes." And Hezekiah wept bitterly.
>
> Then the word of the LORD came to Isaiah: "Go and tell Hezekiah, 'This is what the LORD, the God of your father David, says: I have heard your prayer and seen your tears; I will add fifteen years to your life.'"
>
> *Isaiah 38:2 – 5; see also 2 Kings 20:2 – 6*

Interpretation of another incident has sparked controversy on the role of physicians. King Asa was a godly king in Judah during the early years of his reign. However, "in the thirty-ninth year of his reign Asa was afflicted with a disease in his feet. Though his disease was severe, even in his illness he did not seek help from the LORD, but only from the physicians. Then in the forty-first year of his reign Asa died and rested with his fathers" (2 Chronicles 16:12 – 13).

Some conclude from this passage that the Bible condemns using physicians and calls on people to seek healing only from God. Yet Scripture refers to physicians and their role in healing (Jeremiah 8:22; Matthew 9:12), and Luke, the author of a gospel and of Acts, was a physician (Colossians 4:14).

Even the context of the passage about Asa makes it clear that Asa's primary problem was not his use of physicians but his refusal to ask God for help. It is most likely that the physicians Asa relied on were Gentiles who practiced pagan magical healing.[19] Support for this view comes immediately after Asa's death, when his son, who succeeded him as king, is praised because he followed God and "did not consult the Baals" or carry out the idolatrous practices of Israel (2 Chronicles 17:3 – 4). Biblical examples show the need for discernment regarding where we turn for healing.

Such a decision was captured dramatically by C. S. Lewis in The Chronicles of Narnia. The series' first book, *The Magician's Nephew*, reaches its climax when Digory must decide whether to heal his mother or obey Aslan, the lion who plays the role of God. The choice is stark, especially when the Witch describes what will happen to Digory's mother. "Do you not see, Fool, that one bite of that apple would heal her? . . . Next day everyone will be saying how wonderfully she has recovered. Soon she will be quite well again. All will be well again. Your home will be happy again. You will be like other boys."[20]

Lewis skillfully raises all the usual justifications we think of when we struggle with whether to do the right thing or not. What if Digory's mother finds out he could have removed her pain and didn't? Who will ever know that he stole the apple? What has Aslan ever done to deserve obedience? Digory struggles, as we all do when something a little wrong seems able to bring about a lot of good. But Digory finds the courage to make the right choice. He chooses to trust Aslan.

A similar choice faces those who look to alternative spiritual therapies for healing. Maybe they will bring a lot of good, though there's no guarantee. Wouldn't God be pleased at the good that could come about? Not if "good" comes by illegitimate means. God has warned us that certain spiritual practices are not just harmful, but wrong. Are we going to trust him? Will we put our faith in him and his promises? If we do, we will avoid spiritual therapies that connect us with spiritual powers or beings apart from the God of the Bible.

The Gray Area of Alternative Medicine for Christians

Alternative therapies are practiced in different ways by different people. When Julie, a Christian who feels called to teach others about some alternative therapies, practices Therapeutic Touch, she prays to God and asks him to bring about healing. She honestly believes she is getting in touch with the power of God and being used by him to minister to those she treats. Yet many others trained in the same technique call on a universal life energy to bring healing. Do Christians who practice life energy therapies in the name of God avoid inappropriate spiritual connections?

Meditation can be practiced as a way to get general spiritual guidance, to become more at peace with one's inner self, to simply relax — or to contact spirit guides. Similarly, yoga can theoretically be practiced in spiritual and nonspiritual ways. Meditation and yoga are taught by both practitioners of the occult and some Christians! How are we to discern which is which? How can we know whether an alternative therapy violates the biblical commands to avoid inappropriate spiritual influences?

Some homeopaths believe they spiritually vitalize their preparations as they make them. Dana Ullman, president of the Foundation for Homeopathic Education and Research, wrote, "Homeopaths conceptualize a 'life force,' or 'vital force,' they describe as the inherent, underlying, interconnective, self-healing process of the organism. This bioenergetic force is similar to what the Chinese call 'chi,' the Japanese call 'ki,' yogis call 'prana,' Russian scientists call 'bioplasm,' and Star Wars characters call 'The Force.'"[21]

Some believe herbal remedies are effective because of the nature spirits they say dwell in them. Rosemary Gladstar, an herbalist, says she decides which herbs to use by first examining a patient; "then I pray and let the spirit of the herbs guide me."[22] What if a Christian happens to use one of these remedies? Have they spiritually "contaminated" themselves?

Look to the Bible, Not Inner Voices, for Guidance

When investigating an alternative therapy, be concerned about those that involve listening to other spirits. But what about listening to an inner guiding voice? Guidance by intuition and inner voices has become more in vogue today than guidance through reason and objective evidence. Postmodernism has contributed to this acceptance with its notion that we all create our own reality, that whatever we believe is OK.

Christians may even be attracted to these ideas because of our belief that God reveals his will to us through Scripture and the Holy Spirit. If Christians believe they are being led by the Holy Spirit to practice a certain therapy, should we question them? If during meditation or visualization someone gets a strong feeling that God is telling them that a certain practitioner can help or heal them, should we say anything more?

Again, Christians must look to the Bible for guidance. The Old Testament was clear that anyone claiming to have a message from God, that is, to be a prophet, was to be put to the test. "You may say to yourselves, 'How can we know when a message has not been spoken by the LORD?' If what a prophet proclaims in the name of the LORD does not take place or come true, that is a message the LORD has not spoken. That prophet has spoken presumptuously. Do not be afraid of him" (Deuteronomy 18:21–22).

We must evaluate claims. This is especially important when it comes to information received in an altered state of consciousness. Occult activities and healing rituals have always used a variety of ways to induce meditative states and altered states of consciousness. Through meditation, occultists claim that details concerning what to do during a healing treatment "will soon come 'intuitively' to the healer. Do not be afraid to follow your intuitive sense in this direction."[23]

Deepak Chopra, M.D., one of alternative medicine's popularizers, encourages people to "experience the effortless way that intentions can get fulfilled, bypassing the ego and the rational mind."[24] Larry Dossey, M.D., another popular author, encourages us to trust what we feel led to do even though our unconscious mind may lead us to "violate the values we hold dearest in our aware, conscious life, such as our moral and ethical codes, in order to help us."[25]

Underlying these ideas are three core beliefs that contradict clear biblical teaching:

- Personal autonomy is of supreme value.
- Humans are innately good.
- Humans are potentially or actually divine.

According to those who adopt such worldviews, meditative practices bring healing by enlightening people about their "true" nature. Transcendental Meditation (TM), versions of which underlie numerous alternative therapies, claims that "on the level of the Transcendental Consciousness we are Divine already."[26] All our problems arise, according to TM, because we don't realize this. "Although we are all 100% Divine, consciously we do not know that we are Divine."[27] Chopra similarly claims that the healthy person affirms to himself, "I know myself as the immeasurable potential of all that was, is and will be.... There is no other I than the entire universe. I am being and I am nowhere and everywhere at the same time. I am omnipresent, omniscient; I am the eternal spirit that animates everything in existence."[28]

Nothing could be further from the truth, according to the Bible. There is one God, one Creator, who is completely distinct from his creation. "For there is one God and one mediator between God and men, the man Christ Jesus" (1 Timothy 2:5).

TM misuses the Bible by claiming that God's statement about himself in Psalm 46:10 applies to all people. To quote TM's founder, Maharishi Mahesh Yogi, "Christ said, 'Be still and know that I am God.' Be still and know that you are God and when you know that you are God you will begin to live Godhood, and living Godhood there is no reason to suffer, absolutely no reason to suffer, Man is not born to suffer."[29]

Such teaching sounds attractive, as none of us want to suffer. But Maharishi's view can lead to a constant search for life without suffering. The Bible's view is completely different — and more realistic. Peter instructed us, "Dear friends, do not be surprised at the painful trial you are suffering, as though something strange were happening to you" (1 Peter 4:12). Paul taught that some things are worth suffering for: "Join with me in suffering for the gospel, by the power of God" (2 Timothy 1:8).

Humanity throughout the ages has sought insight through various meditative practices and altered states of consciousness. Scripture has consistently condemned these practices for at least three reasons:

- **The demonic realm** is sometimes encountered in these states, which is spiritually and physically dangerous for people.
- **Unreliable knowledge** is all that can be obtained in these states. The false prophets of Israel claimed to get trustworthy information through visions, trances, dreams, and

altered states of consciousness. Scripture labels the information obtained by these "prophets who wag their own tongues" as "false hopes," "delusions of their own minds," "false dreams," and "reckless lies" (Jeremiah 23:16 – 32). These ways of gaining knowledge lead to deception, not true insight. "Woe to the foolish prophets who follow their own spirit and have seen nothing!... Their visions are false and their divinations a lie" (Ezekiel 13:3 – 6).

- **Human nature** that is good and perfect, if not divine, is assumed by the worldviews depending on intuition and the inner self. A book on white magic claims that a practitioner "has to learn to do the right thing as he sees and knows it.... He must depend on himself."[30] The Bible holds that humans are not divine or perfect: "The heart is deceitful above all things and beyond cure. Who can understand it?" (Jeremiah 17:9). Dependence on the self is the root of humanity's problems.

Biblical Principles on Which to Base Decisions

Scripture gives clear principles on which we can rely when making decisions about alternative therapies with spiritual roots. Some have noted that most of the passages condemning occult practices come from the Old Testament. Most theologians teach that Christians are not bound by many of the Old Testament laws, such as those related to worshiping in God's temple. Does that mean that prohibitions of divination and magic no longer apply to Christians?

Paul makes it clear that events described in the Old Testament remain important teaching tools for Christians. "Now these things occurred as examples to keep us from setting our hearts on evil things as they did.... These things happened to them as examples and were written down as warnings for us, on whom the fulfillment of the ages has come" (1 Corinthians 10:6, 11).

We should learn from the Old Testament accounts. Occult practices are denounced in the most forceful language possible. Nowhere in the New Testament are we told that these practices are now permissible or that God has changed his perspective on them. Whenever magic and sorcery are mentioned in the New Testament, they are viewed negatively (e.g., Acts 8:9 – 24; 19:19; Revelation 9:21; 21:8; 22:15). Those magical and occult practices forbidden in the Old Testament remain forbidden. The Old Testament accounts of Israelites conducting these practices make clear their shame and detriment and remain as examples to us of things not to be practiced under any circumstances, even in the pursuit of healing.

Later in 1 Corinthians 10, Paul addresses our topic more directly. He teaches that Christians should have no involvement whatsoever in sacrifices made to idols or demons. "No, but the sacrifices of pagans are offered to demons, not to God, and I do not want you to be participants with demons. You cannot drink the cup of the Lord and the cup of demons too; you cannot have a part in both the Lord's table and the table of demons" (1 Corinthians 10:20 – 21).

Any alternative therapy involving contact with any spirit other than God is forbidden. Shamanism, Reiki, channeling, divination, and any other "therapy" that attempts to bring knowledge or healing from other spirits or spirit guides should be avoided. Let us be clear, there can be no such thing as "Christian Shamanism" or "Christian Reiki."

Paul's advice arose in response to concerns faced by the early church about meat from animals sacrificed in pagan temples. The meat would later be sold in the marketplace and eaten in people's homes. Some Christians feared that eating this meat involved them in occult activities, but others disagreed (Romans 14; 1 Corinthians 8; 10). Paul said, "Eat anything sold in the meat market without raising questions of conscience, for, 'The earth is the Lord's, and everything in it.' If some unbeliever invites you to a meal and you want to go, eat whatever is put before you without raising questions of conscience" (1 Corinthians 10:25–27).

We must remember that Paul was talking about food, not remedies and therapies. When applying these verses to alternative medicine, we must ensure that the issues of concern are analogous in all important ways. The freedom to use something would, we believe, apply only if the physical components can be separated from the underlying belief system, analogous to the way Paul separated the meat from the idolatry. Meat sacrificed in a pagan ceremony would still have nutritional value. In the same way, a therapy or remedy may be used if it has some benefit independent of any spiritual ceremony it may have been passed through. Only therapies and remedies with demonstrated benefits (and devoid of any divination, necromancy, mediumship, spiritism, witchcraft, or sorcery) should be used. The physical benefits of all remedies are then best evaluated by scientific criteria.

Acupuncture adds another degree of complication. Some people use acupuncture needles to manipulate life energy in a method more similar to a spiritual practice. However, the needles do physically impact the body and have been shown to cause physiological effects. Therefore, we believe that if the spiritual connections are avoided, acupuncture can be a legitimate option for Christians. However, as with herbal remedies, it should only be used when there is evidence to show that it is effective for the condition being treated.

The principles developed here apply differently when discussing alternative therapies that do not incorporate physical materials. Knowledge of the precise details of the therapy is needed. Alternative therapies such as shamanism and Reiki may "work" because they contact spirit guides and, therefore, according to God's Word, should not be used under any circumstances.

Other therapies, especially various meditative and consciousness-altering practices, are even more complicated. Included here would be such things as meditation, yoga, visualization, and guided imagery. These are sometimes used for relaxation, but other times they are used to get in touch with the "inner self" or some spirit being. This is sometimes viewed as a source of healing in and of itself, and other times it is seen as a means to gain insight and guidance into health-related issues. Before trying any of these types of practices, investigate them thoroughly. Find out what sort of teaching you will be exposed to. Ask others who attended exactly what the sessions involved.

Be Careful of the Impact Your Decisions May Have on Others

Christians must be concerned about more than their own freedom to choose; they must consider the impact their choices have on others and how others will interpret their actions. If a Christian uses a therapy or remedy with links to the occult, their example may cause others to follow that lead. In one of the passages about meat sacrificed to idols, Paul uses very strong language to condemn actions that lead others astray by calling the actions a "sin against Christ" (1 Corinthians 8:12).

The impact of how others view our involvement in these practices should always be taken into consideration. Our witness to the power of Christ may be damaged in the eyes of the world if we are feverishly chasing after ineffective or spiritually dangerous therapies or remedies. That is particularly tragic given everything that faith in Christ, coupled with evidence-based recommendations, has to offer.

The Power of Faith

Faith in Jesus Christ has many benefits. Fundamentally, it restores a person's relationship with God. This is spiritual healing in the ultimate sense. But Jesus did not come just to bring spiritual healing. The life he offers should impact every aspect of our lives. It allows relational, emotional, and psychological healing. Sometimes faith in Jesus also brings physical healing. To those who receive him, God promises spiritual reconciliation to become children of God, to be spiritually reborn, to be able to relate intimately with him (John 1:12 – 13; Revelation 3:20). He also promises ultimate and complete healing (physically, mentally, emotionally, relationally, and spiritually) in heaven. Healing of all our other illnesses and damage is not promised in this life, though it *will* occur in the afterlife (Revelation 21:4).

Faith in God is the beginning of a new way of living. Walking closely with God brings a life filled with "love, joy, peace, patience, kindness, goodness, faithfulness, gentleness and self-control" (Galatians 5:22 – 23). Such contentment is promised regardless of our circumstances, whether we are rich or poor, in sickness or in health. A life characterized by these features is the opposite of the high-stress, discontented rat race many find themselves in.

Adopting faith just to get the benefits will not work. The benefits are secondary to the spiritual reconciliation that Christian faith brings. The first concern should not be whether something spiritual "works." Rather, the first concern should be whether it is true and brings glory to God. Spiritual practices that arise from belief systems that deny or ignore the claims of God will not lead to true health. Strong faith in something false is like a tower built on sand. Eventually it will crumble.

A life built on the truth of Jesus Christ will unleash the true power of faith. Be alert and prayerful as you talk to others about what they offer. Remember the words of Paul:

> Live as children of light (for the fruit of the light consists in all goodness, righteousness and truth) and find out what pleases the Lord. Have nothing to do with the fruitless deeds of darkness, but rather expose them. . . .
>
> Be very careful, then, how you live — not as unwise but as wise, making the most of every opportunity, because the days are evil.
>
> *Ephesians 5:8 – 11, 15 – 16*

Chapter 3: Faith-Based Health and Healing

1. John P. Newport, *The New Age Movement and the Biblical Worldview: Conflict and Dialogue* (Grand Rapids: Eerdmans, 1998), 119.

2. Hans A. Baer, "The Work of Andrew Weil and Deepak Chopra — Two Holistic Health/New Age Gurus: A Critique of the Holistic Health/New Age Movements," *Medical Anthropology Quarterly* 17, no. 2 (June 2003): 233 – 50.

3. William Franklin Simpson, "Comparative Longevity in a College Cohort of Christian Scientists," *Journal of the American Medical Association* 262, no. 12 (September 1989): 1657 – 58; Andrew Skolnick, "Christian Scientists Claim Healing Efficacy Equal If Not Superior to That of Medicine," *Journal of the American Medical Association* 264, no. 11 (September 1990): 1379 – 81.

4. Dale A. Matthews, Michael E. McCullough, David B. Larson, Harold G. Koenig, James P. Swyers, and Mary G. Milano, "Religious Commitment and Health Status: A Review of the Research and Implications for Family Medicine," *Archives of Family Medicine* 7, no. 2 (March – April 1998): 118 – 24.

5. Jeff Levin, foreword to Harold G. Koenig, Michael E. McCullough, and David B. Larson, *Handbook of Religion and Health* (Oxford: Oxford University Press, 2001), vii.

6. Lynda H. Powell, Leila Shahabi, and Carl E. Thoresen, "Religion and Spirituality: Linkages to Physical Health," *American Psychologist* 58, no. 1 (January 2003): 36 – 52.

7. J. LeBron McBride, Gary Arthur, Robin Brooks, and Lloyd Pilkington, "The Relationship Between a Patient's Spirituality and Health Experiences," *Family Medicine* 30, no. 2 (February 1998): 122 – 26.

8. Jessica Tartaro, Linda J. Luecken, and Heather E. Gunn, "Exploring Heart and Soul: Effects of Religiosity/Spirituality and Gender on Blood Pressure and Cortisol Stress Responses," *Journal of Health Psychology* 10, no. 6 (December 2005): 753 – 66.

9. Koenig, McCullough, and Larson, *Handbook of Religion and Health*, 250 – 63.

10. Jeffrey S. Levin and Harold Y. Vanderpool, "Is Frequent Religious Attendance *Really* Conducive to Better Health? Toward an Epidemiology of Religion," *Social Science and Medicine* 24, no. 7 (1987): 589 – 600.

11. Kenneth I. Pargament, Harold G. Koenig, Nalini Tarakeshwar, and June Hahn, "Religious Struggle as a Predictor of Mortality Among Medically Ill Elderly Patients: A Two-Year Longitudinal Study," *Archives of Internal Medicine* 161, no. 15 (August 2001): 1881 – 85.

12. John Christopher Thomas, *The Devil, Disease and Deliverance: Origins of Illness in New Testament Thought* (Sheffield: Sheffield Academic Press, 1998), 63 – 64.

13. Ibid., 317.

14. Dolores Krieger, *Accepting Your Power to Heal: The Personal Practice of Therapeutic Touch* (Santa Fe, N.M.: Bear, 1993), 8.

15. Howard Clark Kee, "Magic and Messiah," in *Religion, Science, and Magic: In Concert and In Conflict*, ed. Jacob Neusner, Ernest S. Frerichs, and Paul Virgil McCracken Flesher (New York: Oxford University Press, 1989), 121 – 41.

16. Ibid., 126.

17. John Ferguson, quoted in ibid., 123.

18. Kurt E. Koch, *Occult ABC* (Grand Rapids: Kregel, 1986), 104.

19. Darrel W. Amundsen and Gary B. Ferngren, "Medicine and Religion: Pre-Christian Antiquity," in *Health/Medicine and the Faith Traditions: An Inquiry into Religion and Medicine*, ed. Martin E. Marty and Kenneth L. Vaux (Philadelphia: Fortress, 1982), 53 – 92.

20. C. S. Lewis, *The Magician's Nephew* (New York: HarperTrophy, 1955), 192 – 93.

21. Dana Ullman, *Discovering Homeopathy: Medicine for the 21st Century*, rev. ed. (Berkeley, Calif.: North Atlantic, 1991), 15.

22. Rosemary Gladstar, *Herbal Remedies for Children's Health* (Pownal, Vt.: Storey, 1999), 24.

23. Yogi Ramacharaka, *The Science of Psychic Healing* (Chicago: Yogi, 1909), 70.

24. Deepak Chopra, *Ageless Body, Timeless Mind: The Quantum Alternative to Growing Old* (New York: Harmony, 1993), 99.

25. Larry Dossey, *Healing Words: The Power of Prayer and the Practice of Medicine* (New York: HarperSanFrancisco, 1993), 61.

26. Maharishi Mahesh Yogi, *Meditations of Maharishi Mahesh Yogi* (New York: Bantam, 1968), 177.

27. Ibid., 177.

28. Deepak Chopra, *Escaping the Prison of the Mind: A Journey from Here to Here* (San Rafael, Calif.: New World Library, 1992), audiocassette.

29. Maharishi Mahesh Yogi, *Meditations*, 178.

30. Alice A. Bailey, *A Treatise On White Magic*, 6th ed. (New York: Lucis, 1963), 586.

CHAPTER 4

ALTERNATIVE MEDICINE AND CHILDREN

The growing interest in alternative medicine among adults has carried over to children and into the offices of pediatricians and family physicians. If a parent is taking echinacea, should it be given to a child with a runny nose? (Echinacea is a popular remedy for preventing colds that we consider to be scientifically unproven though apparently safe for many adults.) Is garlic oil a better eardrop than commercial products made specifically for children? What about acupuncture for children with cerebral palsy, or megavitamin or nutritional therapy for children with Attention Deficit/Hyperactivity Disorder (AD/HD)?

A national survey published in 2004 found that 87 percent of pediatricians had been asked questions about complementary and alternative medicine (CAM) by parents or children in the previous three months.[1] Two-thirds of the pediatricians in the survey believed CAM therapies could be beneficial, and one-third said they or an immediate family member had used them in the previous year. However, three-quarters were concerned about possible side effects, and another three-quarters believed CAM use could delay conventional care.

According to the Association of American Medical Colleges, in 2005, three-quarters of the nation's

125 medical schools required some kind of CAM coursework.[2] Yet fewer than 5 percent of practicing pediatricians felt very knowledgeable about CAM therapies, and most wanted more CAM information.[3] It's no wonder only about one-third of parents tell doctors they are using alternative therapies with their children.[4]

The use of CAM may even be more popular with parents for their children than for themselves. When parents were surveyed at pediatricians' offices in the United States, one-third reported using CAM with their children in the previous year.[5] The most popular therapies were infant massage, massage therapy, vitamin therapy, and herbal remedies. A survey found that CAM was used with about half of the children at a large Australian children's hospital.[6] The most commonly used remedies were multivitamins, vitamin C, and echinacea; the most common therapies were chiropractic and aromatherapy. When the same survey was conducted at a large children's hospital in Wales, 41 percent of the children were reported to have used CAM in the previous year.[7] There, the most commonly used remedies were multivitamins, herbal remedies, and dietary supplements; the most common therapies were aromatherapy and reflexology.

These surveys often use such a broad definition of alternative medicine that the numbers are inflated. The study in the United States found that by far the most popular "therapies" parents used with their children were prayer (47 percent) and exercise (19 percent).[8] These researchers did not include these in their report of overall CAM use, though other researchers have. No parents in that study had used therapies such as acupuncture, acupressure, or hypnosis with their children in the previous year, and use of other alternatives was relatively small: herbal remedies (7 percent), homeopathy (3 percent), and chiropractic (2 percent).

Why Parents Use Alternative Medicine with Children

The most common reason parents give for using CAM with healthy children is that they use CAM themselves. Parents give children herbal remedies because they believe they are cheaper and safer than conventional treatment and have little risk of side effects.

When children have chronic or incurable conditions, fear of conventional medicine's side effects becomes a bigger issue. A survey was conducted with children diagnosed with AD/HD attending an Australian outpatient clinic.[9] CAM was being, or had been, used by two-thirds of the children, who most commonly used modified diets, vitamins, and dietary supplements.

Children with cancer are commonly given CAM. Several studies in the United States between 1997 and 2003 found that between 46 and 84 percent of these children were given CAM, a huge increase from the 1980s.[10] Children with cancer most commonly used what researchers called "spiritual/mental strategies."[11] These included prayer, faith, and guided imagery. We have concerns about listing prayer and faith as "therapies," but that is how these (and many other) researchers classify them. The second most popular category was physical strategies (e.g., acupuncture or massage), followed by herbal remedies. Many children with cancer use CAM to relieve pain or chemotherapy side effects but do not report this to those providing chemotherapy.

While they or their parents may believe they are receiving the benefits of both approaches, interactions between the two can have detrimental effects. Most parents would have been shocked to hear Cora Collette Breuner tell pediatricians at the 2005 American Academy of Pediatrics meeting, "Some widely available supplements can sicken or kill kids."[12]

Evidence Is Lacking but Growing

A number of university hospital programs are now experimenting with aspects of alternative medicine for children. While much remains inconclusive at this writing, some therapies are starting to show some positive results. Many of these are ways to help children relax as they learn to cope with chronic or serious illnesses. Others represent ways to include good nutritional strategies and vitamin therapy within conventional care.

As mentioned earlier, the vast majority of pediatricians (and, we suspect, family physicians who care for children) would welcome more guidance on CAM for children. Randomized controlled trials (RCTs) provide the best evidence of effectiveness, and almost all the pediatric CAM RCTs have been published in mainstream medical journals.[13] The number of studies investigating CAM for children is increasing, but the quality of many of these has been found to be particularly poor.[14] There are signs of improvement, but still over three-quarters of all CAM trials with children mentioned nothing about adverse effects. This leaves parents and doctors without clear guidance on this crucial issue. Few systematic reviews of this research are available, but these reviews have been found to be of the same quality as those of conventional therapies.[15] Such developments are to be welcomed.

Some CAM procedures may be relatively harmless for children to try. Acupressure and acupuncture are felt by many practitioners to be generally safe for children, though their effectiveness for many children's problems remains questionable. It must be stressed that much remains unknown about whether CAM is effective or safe for children. However, some popular CAM approaches are more controversial and even raise some concerns.

Chiropractic for Children

The most common pediatric CAM therapy requiring a therapist is chiropractic. One estimate claims that the number of children being treated by chiropractors increased 50 percent between 1997 and 2000.[16] This same study found that while many adults seek chiropractic care for musculoskeletal problems, children are commonly treated by chiropractors for ear infections, allergies, asthma, colic, and bedwetting. Yet virtually no randomized controlled trials of chiropractic exist for *any* pediatric condition. One of the first such trials found it was no more beneficial than a placebo for children with asthma.[17] Those results have since been confirmed by other trials. The first high-quality randomized controlled trial of chiropractic for colic similarly found negative results.[18] Infants improved to the same degree whether they received three ten-minute chiropractic treatments or were held three times by nurses for ten minutes.

While in general chiropractic is safe, there have been rare cases of very serious problems developing shortly after children have received chiropractic manipulation.[19] The cost of such treatments must also be borne in mind, especially given the lack of high-quality evidence of benefit for chiropractic on children. We agree with the Canadian Paediatric Society, which states the following: "Open and honest discussions with families using or planning to use chiropractic for their children will, hopefully, bring about a rational use of this treatment in selected musculoskeletal conditions for which there is proof of efficacy, and enable parents to make informed choices about this form of therapy. Further, well-designed studies are needed to evaluate the chiropractic belief that musculoskeletal dysfunctions can be located and treated in children with nonmusculoskeletal conditions."[20]

Herbs for Children and the Risks

As they performed surgery on children, some doctors noticed an increase in bleeding problems.[21] Research led Kathi J. Kemper, M.D., to a connection between bleeding problems and children's use of herbal remedies. In one survey of pediatric surgery patients, the proportion of children using herbal remedies was only 4 percent, but fifteen of these children were scheduled for major surgeries, and thirteen were taking herbs known to interfere with normal blood clotting.[22]

Some herbs may lead to more serious physical harm. For example, one herbalist claims children can use "gentle herbs" such as borage and licorice "with no residual buildup or side effects" and also use "stronger" herbs such as comfrey and chaparral.[23] In Part 3, we discuss clinical evidence that these particular herbs have all caused serious side effects in adults. We believe this is strong evidence that they should never be used by children.

Even products that can safely be given to an adult might be overwhelming for a child. Children differ significantly from adults in how substances are absorbed into and distributed around the body, and then how they are broken down and excreted from the body. A child's central nervous system and immune system are still developing and may therefore be damaged by substances that would have little impact on an adult. Herbs such as buckthorn, senna, and aloe cause diarrhea, and some herbal teas and juniper oil are diuretic (increase urine production). These effects may be tolerated in an adult but quickly cause dehydration and electrolyte imbalance in children. Products also affect children differently. Some children are particularly susceptible to allergies and thus may have allergic reactions to herbs since these are plant products. When herbal remedies or dietary supplements are taken by children over extended periods of time, particular substances may accumulate in their systems.

Paul (we'll call him) was ten years old, blind, mentally retarded, and having dozens of seizures every day.[24] Paul was under the care of conventional physicians, but drugs were only moderately successful. His mother, Mary, heard from other parents about a Chinese herbal product called Diankexing. She discussed this with Paul's primary care physician and his neurologist. She had a lab analyze the product, and they concluded it was safe.

Imagine the joy and surprise when Paul's seizures dramatically diminished. Mary gradually increased Paul's dose of Diankexing until the seizures stopped completely. She then weaned her son off his conventional drugs. The seizures had not returned a couple of months later.

Mary noticed, however, that Paul was becoming increasingly tired and lethargic. Then he developed an upper respiratory tract infection. After a few days, she took him to the emergency room. He was admitted, and Mary asked the physician if she could continue giving Diankexing to Paul. He agreed. But immediately after taking a capsule, Paul developed serious breathing problems and deteriorated into a coma. Thankfully, he was taken immediately to the intensive care unit and stabilized.

Complete blood and urine analyses revealed two unusual findings. Paul's blood contained more than ten times the normal concentration of bromide, an ion from the same family as chloride and iodide. His urine contained barbiturates, a group of pharmaceutical drugs sometimes used to control seizures. However, Paul's levels were three times higher than standard therapeutic levels. Laboratory analysis revealed that the Diankexing capsules contained two types of pharmaceutical barbiturates and several salts containing bromide.

Now everything made sense. Paul's improvements had resulted from the pharmaceuticals in the capsules, not from any natural ingredients. Having discovered the source of the problems, Paul was treated for overdoses of both substances and two weeks later was released from the hospital.

Current regulations do not require the sort of product evaluation that would detect such problems. While adulterating dietary supplements with pharmaceuticals is illegal, the salts added were not illegal but were in such high concentrations that the bromide built up in Paul's system. Continuously taking bromide salts leads to a condition called "brominism" in which a person's mental status gradually deteriorates.

In this case, a concerned mother did everything she could to ensure that her child was being given something safe. In spite of all her precautions and the complete cooperation of conventional practitioners, the child was placed in serious danger. Given the current regulatory situation in the United States, no one can know for sure that something similar won't happen with any dietary supplement. This is particularly the case with products containing complex mixtures of ingredients, which are becoming increasingly popular.

Herbs and Herbalism

So far we have been concerned with the chemical aspects of herbal remedies. Herbalism is more like a religious approach to herbs and raises spiritual and pharmacological problems. Rosemary Gladstar is an herbalist who has written a number of books on herbal remedies, one for their use in children. She claims herbal remedies are safe for children, stating, "Contrary to what you may have heard or read, my experience has been that almost any herb that is safe for an adult is safe for a child so long as the size and weight of the child are accounted for and the dosage is adjusted accordingly."[25]

Gladstar's approach is simply to treat children as small adults. She describes two "rules" for calculating doses for children based on their ages and the adult dose.[26] One she calls Young's Rule, which calculates that a four-year-old should be given one-quarter the adult dose. The second she calls Cowling's Rule, which calls for a four-year-old to be given one-sixth the adult dose.

Yet Gladstar's own dosing recommendations call for a four-year-old to be given less than one-twentieth of the adult dose. Such inconsistency reveals how little is known about the correct doses of herbal remedies for children. We have little information on the dosage and effectiveness of herbal remedies in adults; we have almost none for children.

Conventional medicine has learned through tragic experience that the approach of just reducing the adult dosage can be dangerous for children. Reye's syndrome, a condition that can cause permanent disability or death, is one example. Until the 1980s, hundreds of children in the United States got this disease every year.[27] The culprit: aspirin. A link was discovered between aspirin and Reye's syndrome, leading to much publicity discouraging aspirin use for children seventeen years of age or younger. By the late 1990s, only two cases of Reye's syndrome were being reported per year. We now know that the developing body chemistry of children is very different from the body chemistry of adults. This success story should serve as a precaution against giving children any medicine without knowing how safe it is — for children.

Gladstar, the herbalist, does not refer to any controlled scientific studies to support her decisions. On the contrary, her belief in herbalism leads her to "rely on years of experience and intuition." Her view of scientific research is summed up in the following statement: "If a plant has been found safe and effective for a thousand years of human use, it may be wise to question the validity and applicability of the scientific tests now being used. There is generally some unidentified magic in the plant in the form of another chemical or an innate natural wisdom that allows the medicine, when taken as a whole, to function in a safe and beneficial manner."[28]

After examining a child, Gladstar says she will "pray and let the spirit of the herbs guide me. This, of course, is balanced with a thorough understanding of the herbs I am using, plus many years of experience."[29]

We would challenge her claim to have a balanced approach. Although she tips her hat to a scientific approach, her recommendations consistently come down on the side of her experience and the herbalist tradition. Gladstar is directly comparing the validity of science with the validity of human experience before the scientific method was developed. We have serious concerns about her approach and believe it could lead to dangerous recommendations.

Gladstar's approach also demonstrates why Christians need both spiritual and scientific discernment when investigating alternative therapies. We will elaborate more on herbalism in the Herbal Medicine and Folk Medicine entries, but it teaches that the healing power of herbs comes as much from spirits that reside throughout nature as it does from chemicals in the plants. In contrast, herbal medicine refers to the "secular" approach to herbs: the idea that they work naturally through the chemicals they contain. Taking children to an herbalist could expose them to teachings that contradict the Bible and may expose them to spiritual and physical harm if herbs are inappropriately used.

Homeopathy

Homeopathic remedies are commonly given to children. One study found that children comprised one-third of all the patients seen by homeopaths.[30] Homeopathy is often recommended for ear infections in children. Before they are three years old, most children will get at least one ear infection. While at least three-quarters of all ear infections in children go away on their own, some infections can progress to more serious conditions, most of which can be treated effectively with antibiotics.

Given the high rate of spontaneous remission of these ear infections, use of homeopathic remedies frequently appears to be successful. Some then claim that homeopathy cures ear infections. However, a 2000 review of all relevant research found "there is no published evidence to support this claim."[31] This review uncovered only two studies involving homeopathy and ear infections. Even though both studies showed positive results for the homeopathic remedies, they were neither blinded nor properly randomized. The research design therefore made it impossible to place any confidence in these results.

Since that time, we located only one additional study, a pilot study in which the authors stressed that "it is impossible to draw conclusions from a preliminary study such as this."[32] The homeopathy and placebo groups did not have significant differences in most outcomes measured, although better symptom relief was recorded by parents for the children receiving homeopathy. Overall, the evidence remains scant that homeopathy provides any benefit for children with ear infections. Similarly, results of better-designed research has found homeopathy to be no more effective than placebo in treating a variety of other conditions.[33]

Parents considering treating their children with alternative therapies should keep in mind that many alternative medicine practitioners have little conventional medical training. In Massachusetts, half of the homeopaths involved in one study had no medical training, and their training in homeopathy ranged from twenty years to *three weeks*.[34]

All practitioners should know their limitations and when to seek input from others. The Massachusetts homeopaths stated they would, on average, treat a child for three to four months before concluding that their therapies were not working. Only half of the nonphysician homeopaths would refer a two-week-old child with a fever of 101.5 degrees to a physician even though any newborn with such a high fever needs to be seen immediately by a physician.

Vaccination and Alternative Medicine

In the Massachusetts study mentioned above, less than one-third of the homeopaths recommended immunization, and almost 10 percent actively opposed immunization. In England, the most common reason given for not having children immunized is the recommendation parents receive from a homeopath.[35] A study of children attending a Canadian naturopathic clinic raised public health concerns when it found that 9 percent were unvaccinated, compared to 3 percent of the general population.[36] A survey of Canadian naturopathic students found that 13 percent would recommend full vaccination, 74 percent would recommend some vaccination, and 13 percent were unwilling to recommend any vaccination.[37]

While all vaccines carry a small risk of adverse effects, lack of immunization carries significant risks. Children in the United States who were not immunized against measles were between twenty-two and thirty-five times more likely to contract the illness than those who received the measles vaccine.[38] As more people refuse to be immunized, the health of the community can be affected negatively. During the 1970s and 1980s, concerns about alleged side effects from the pertussis vaccine led to reduced usage, resulting in a major resurgence in whooping cough (also called "pertussis"). This infection can be very serious in young children, which is why those alternative therapists who preach against established immunization programs do not have scientific support. Reluctance to recommend vaccination, or actively campaigning against it, has been found in CAM practitioners in general, which is another indirect risk of CAM, since widespread vaccination is crucial for effective protection.[39]

A broader concern raised by opposition to vaccination is what it reveals about the value therapists place on research evidence. For example, only 30 percent of chiropractors in the Boston area promote immunization, the effectiveness of which is supported by high-quality studies, while 70 percent recommend herbs and dietary supplements with little or no research support.[40] Different values will impact different decisions, but all health care professionals should make recommendations based on the best research evidence available.

Risks Are Too Great for Children

In general, we believe that alternative medicine is inappropriate for children. The potential risks are too high. Until high-quality studies show clearly that a particular alternative therapy is safe and effective for children, that therapy should be avoided. Children should never be given herbal remedies or vitamin megadoses in the belief that they are safer than pharmaceuticals. We know too little about what works and what doesn't and about the appropriate preparation and proper dosage for age and body weight to risk trying such potentially dangerous products as herbal remedies on our children. Children are not just miniature versions of adults.

If you are thinking of trying any alternative remedy with your children, first talk with their physician or primary health care provider.[41] Keep in mind that many minor illnesses play an important role in early childhood development. They challenge the body and help build the immune system we need as healthy adults. Compromise the immune system in a child, and you may have an adult with a chronic condition that could readily have been avoided by letting a child's minor illness run its natural course. Parents might limit their exploration of alternative treatments to those that do not alter the body's chemistry — such as acupressure or massage.

Chapter 4: Alternative Medicine and Children

1. Kathi J. Kemper and Karen G. O'Connor, "Pediatricians' Recommendations for Complementary and Alternative Medical (CAM) Therapies," *Ambulatory Pediatrics* 4, no. 6 (November – December 2004): 482 – 87.

2. Joann Loviglio, "Schools Opening Up to Alternative Medicine," *ABC News*, June 6, 2005. *ABC News: http://abcnews. go.com/Health/wireStory?id=823180* (October 30, 2005).

3. Kemper and O'Connor, "Pediatricians' Recommendations," 482 – 87.

4. Marilyn Elias, "Some 'Alternative' Remedies Can Harm Kids," *USA Today*, October 11, 2005. *USA Today: http:// www.usatoday.com/news/health/2005-10-11-alternative-remedies_x.htm* (October 30, 2005).

5. Deborah G. Loman, "The Use of Complementary and Alternative Health Care Practices Among Children," *Journal of Pediatric Health Care* 17, no. 2 (March/April 2003): 58 – 63.

6. Alissa Lim, Noel Cranswick, Susan Skull, and Mike South, "Survey of Complementary and Alternative Medicine Use at a Tertiary Children's Hospital," *Journal of Paediatrics and Child Health* 41, no. 8 (August 2005): 424 – 27.

7. Domenic R. Cincotta, Nigel W. Crawford, Alissa Lim, Noel E. Cranswick, Sue Skull, Mike South, and Colin V. E. Powell, "Comparison of Complementary and Alternative Medicine Use: Reasons and Motivations Between Two Tertiary Children's Hospitals," *Archives of Disease in Children* 91 (February 2006): 153 – 58.

8. Loman, "Use of Complementary and Alternative Health Care Practices," 58–63.

9. D. Sinha and D. Efron, "Complementary and Alternative Medicine Use in Children with Attention Deficit Hyperactivity Disorder," *Journal of Paediatrics and Child Health* 41, nos. 1–2 (January–February 2005): 23–26.

10. Kara M. Kelly, "Complementary and Alternative Medical Therapies for Children with Cancer," *European Journal of Cancer* 40, no. 14 (September 2004): 2041–46.

11. Dominique Martel, Jean-François Bussières, Yves Théorêt, Denis Lebel, Sandra Kish, Albert Moghrabi, and Claudine Laurier, "Use of Alternative and Complementary Therapies in Children with Cancer," *Pediatric Blood Cancer* 44, no. 7 (June 2005): 660–68.

12. Elias, "Some 'Alternative' Remedies."

13. The four journals are *American Journal of Clinical Nutrition, Pediatrics, Journal of Pediatrics,* and *Lancet.* Margaret Sampson, Kaitryn Campbell, Isola Ajiferuke, and David Moher, "Randomized Controlled Trials in Pediatric Complementary and Alternative Medicine: Where Can They Be Found?" *BMC Pediatrics* 3, no. 1 (February 14, 2003). *BioMed Central: www.biomedcentral.com/1471-2431/3/1* (October 10, 2005).

14. David Moher, Margaret Sampson, Kaitryn Campbell, William Beckner, Leah Lepage, Isabelle Gaboury, and Brian Berman, "Assessing the Quality of Reports of Randomized Trials in Pediatric Complementary and Alternative Medicine," *BMC Pediatrics* 2, no. 2 (February 27, 2002). *BioMed Central: www.biomedcentral.com/1471-2431/2/2* (October 10, 2005).

15. David Moher, Karen Soeken, Margaret Sampson, Leah Ben-Porat, and Brian Berman, "Assessing the Quality of Reports of Systematic Reviews in Pediatric Complementary and Alternative Medicine," *BMC Pediatrics* 2, no. 3 (February 27, 2002). *BioMed Central: www.biomedcentral.com/1471-2431/2/3* (October 10, 2005).

16. Anne C. C. Lee, Dawn H. Li, and Kathi J. Kemper, "Chiropractic Care for Children," *Archives of Pediatric and Adolescent Medicine* 154, no. 4 (April 2000): 401–7.

17. Jeffrey Balon, Peter D. Aker, Edward R. Crowther, Clark Danielson, P. Gerard Cox, Denise O'Shaughnessy, Corinne Walker, Charles H. Goldsmith, Reic Duku, and Malcolm R. Sears, "A Comparison of Active and Simulated Chiropractic Manipulation as Adjunctive Treatment for Childhood Asthma," *New England Journal of Medicine* 339, no. 15 (October 1998): 1013–20.

18. E. Olafsdottir, S. Forshei, G. Fluge, and T. Markestad, "Randomised Controlled Trial of Infantile Colic Treated with Chiropractic Spinal Manipulation," *Archives of Disease in Childhood* 84, no. 2 (February 2001): 138–41.

19. Michael H. Cohen and Kathi J. Kemper, "Complementary Therapies in Pediatrics: A Legal Perspective," *Pediatrics* 115, no. 3 (March 2005): 774–80.

20. Canadian Paediatric Society, "Chiropractic Care for Children: Controversies and Issues," *Paediatrics and Child Health* 7, no. 2 (2002): 85–89. *Canadian Paediatric Society: www.cps.ca/english/statements/CP/cp02-01.htm* (October 30, 2005).

21. Paula Gardiner and Kathi J. Kemper, "Herbs in Pediatric and Adolescent Medicine," *Pediatrics in Review* 21, no. 2 (February 2000): 44–57.

22. Kristin Noonan, Robert M. Arensman, and J. David Hoover, "Herbal Medication Use in the Pediatric Surgical Patient," *Journal of Pediatric Surgery* 39, no. 3 (March 2004): 500–503.

23. Rosemary Gladstar, *Herbal Remedies for Children's Health* (Pownal, Vt.: Storey, 1999), 11.

24. See Edward W. Boyer, Susan Kearney, Michael W. Shannon, Lawrence Quang, Alan Woolf, and Kathi Kemper, "Poisoning From a Dietary Supplement Administered During Hospitalization," *Pediatrics* 109, no. 3 (March 2002): 49–51.

25. Gladstar, *Herbal Remedies for Children's Health*, 10.

26. Ibid., 25–26.

27. Ermias D. Belay, Joseph S. Bresee, Robert C. Holman, Ali S. Khan, Abtin Shahriari, and Lawrence B. Schonberger, "Reye's Syndrome in the United States from 1981 through 1997," *New England Journal of Medicine* 340, no. 18 (May 1999): 1377–82.

28. Rosemary Gladstar, *Herbal Healing for Women* (New York: Fireside, 1993), 25.

29. Gladstar, *Herbal Remedies*, 24.

30. Anne C. C. Lee and Kathi J. Kemper, "Homeopathy and Naturopathy: Practice Characteristics and Pediatric Care," *Archives of Pediatric and Adolescent Medicine* 154, no. 1 (January 2000): 75 – 80.

31. E. P. Barrette, "Homeopathy for Acute and Chronic Otitis Media," *Alternative Medicine Alert* 3, no. 4 (April 2000): 37 – 40.

32. Jennifer Jacobs, David A. Springer, and Dean Crothers, "Homeopathic Treatment of Acute Otitis Media in Children: A Preliminary Randomized Placebo-Controlled Trial," *Pediatric Infectious Disease Journal* 20, no. 2 (February 2001): 177 – 83.

33. Aijing Shang, Karin Huwiler-Müntener, Linda Nartey, Peter Jüni, Stephan Dörig, Jonathan A. C. Sterne, Daniel Pewsner, and Matthias Egger, "Are the Clinical Effects of Homoeopathy Placebo Effects? Comparative Study of Placebo-Controlled Trials of Homoeopathy and Allopathy," *Lancet* 366 (August 2005): 726 – 32.

34. Lee and Kemper, "Homeopathy and Naturopathy," 75 – 80.

35. Neil Simpson, Simon Lenton, and Robina Randall, "Parental Refusal to Have Children Immunised: Extent and Reasons," *British Medical Journal* 310 (January 1995): 227.

36. Kumanan Wilson, Jason W. Busse, Amy Gilchrist, Sunita Vohra, Heather Boon, and Edward Mills, "Characteristics of Pediatric and Adolescent Patients Attending a Naturopathic College Clinic in Canada," *Pediatrics* 115, no. 3 (March 2005): 338 – 43.

37. Kumanan Wilson, Ed Mills, Heather Boon, George Tomlinson, and Paul Ritvo, "Attitudes of Naturopathic Students to Paediatric Vaccinations Amongst Canadian Naturopathic Students," *Vaccine* 22 (2004): 329 – 34.

38. Daniel R. Feikin, Dennis C. Lezotte, Richard F. Hamman, Daniel A. Salmon, Robert T. Chen, and Richard E. Hoffman, "Individual and Community Risks of Measles and Pertussis Associated with Personal Exemptions to Immunization," *Journal of the American Medical Association* 284, no. 24 (December 2000): 3145 – 50; Daniel A. Salmon, Michael Haber, Eugene J. Gangarosa, Lynelle Phillips, Natalie J. Smith, and Robert T. Chen, "Health Consequences of Religious and Philosophical Exemptions from Immunization Laws: Individual and Societal Risk of Measles," *Journal of the American Medical Association* 282, no. 1 (July 1999): 47 – 53.

39. E. Ernst, "Rise in Popularity of Complementary and Alternative Medicine: Reasons and Consequences for Vaccination," *Vaccine* 20, suppl. 1 (2001): S90 – 93.

40. Lee, Li, and Kemper, "Chiropractic Care for Children," 401 – 7.

41. Kemper and O'Connor, "Pediatricians' Recommendations," 482 – 87.

CHAPTER 5

THE GURUS: FRAUD, QUACKERY, OR WISDOM?

Many have tried alternative medicine. Some have become practitioners. A few have gained a significant following as authorities. These are the gurus of alternative medicine: those whose guidance is held by many to be authoritative. What separates the gurus from others with many of the same beliefs is their popularity. They've written a book or established a strong Internet presence and built up a following through appearances on radio and television. It's easy to believe someone who seems so honest and compassionate, whose voice is pleasant and authoritative. Their words lay out a case so compelling that many blindly follow their recommendations.

The vast majority of these writers are fervent advocates for what they believe to be the truth about healing and wellness. Most are well educated. We believe most of these gurus are sincere.

We also believe that some are sincerely wrong. Their ideas are spiritually questionable (based on biblical truth) or medically unsound (based on the best medical evidence) — or both. They are not necessarily or knowingly trying to mislead anyone. They seem to care about their followers and the public at large. They believe conventional medicine (and sometimes aspects of alternative medicine) is naive or even dangerous. They have experienced a different form of health care and developed an approach that — when you listen to their success stories — seems excellent.

We see why people are drawn to this type of person, especially if they have had a bad experience with a conventional medical practitioner. Also vulnerable are those with little hope of a cure, who have been told there is no treatment, no relief for constant pain. Desperation can drive such individuals to try anything that offers hope — a tiny miracle. "What have I got to lose?" they ask, no matter how unlikely, how expensive, how outlandish the claims.

When people are desperate, they don't care about objective evaluation of remedies. They want help. And that's when they fall prey to frauds, quacks, or those who are true believers in what is truly wrong. These terms are not easily distinguished. People don't agree on precisely how to define each one. But any discussion of alternative medicine is sure to raise one or all of these terms. Therefore, we need to discuss what they mean and how we will be using the terms.

Frauds Know They Offer Worthless Treatments

Fraud occurs when people promote a medical treatment they know is worthless. Good examples of medical fraud are a variety of electronic devices sold over the years to "treat" cancer, heart disease, arthritis, and numerous other conditions. The precise type of device and the claims vary, but what they have in common is a "box" that looks scientific. The gauges, dials, lights, and switches all work, but they don't cure anything. The more complex the box appears and the more knowledgeable the provider (or salesperson) seems to be about the device, the more confident patients become that the treatment will work. Many will leave a session feeling better. The reason: they've received the concentrated attention of a seemingly caring individual who has carefully listened to their complaints, commiserated with

their suffering, and strongly suggested that healing will take place.

Fraud can occur in almost any area of medicine. Studies of the quality of herbal remedies and dietary supplements have found products with none of the active ingredient listed on the label. That's fraud. "Natural" remedies that contain pharmaceutical drugs also indicate fraud.

When claims of a product's effectiveness are invented to mislead the customer, it's fraud. The people offering the therapy know the treatment does *not* work, yet they make up stories about people they claim have benefited. They leave out the stories of those who have been unhappy with the product, hurt by the therapy, or even killed by their wrong advice.

What Quacks Don't Know Could Harm You

Quacks differ from frauds in their motivations. While fraud is intentionally selling therapies and remedies the practitioner knows can't do what is claimed, quackery has more to do with medical incompetence. Quacks don't know the therapies and remedies they're promoting can't work. The word *quack* comes from *quacksalver*, which originally referred to untrained persons who practiced medicine. We expand that meaning to include practitioners of medical and spiritual nonsense, some of whom may have been duped by someone who knew a therapy was fraudulent.

Generally quacks are not trying to mislead anyone. Quacks are convinced their therapies work. They genuinely believe that what they are doing and recommending helps patients, and they have anecdotal evidence for support. Yet even when there's plenty of evidence that a therapy is useless, they continue to hold on to their mistaken beliefs and offer their therapies. They usually don't *want* to know about the evidence that proves their therapy is worthless.

Quacks are often inspired by the misunderstood geniuses of the past who fought against the establishment until they finally achieved some radical breakthrough. What was viewed as outlandish and impossible in their day eventually became "obvious" and routine. Many quacks see themselves as heirs to such misunderstanding and, consequently, heirs to the ultimate triumph of those historical figures. They love to quote Arthur Schopenhauer, the nineteenth-century German philosopher who said, "All truth passes through three stages. First, it is ridiculed. Second, it is violently opposed. Third, it is accepted as being self-evident." Indeed, some of today's quackery may hold grains of truth that will prove useful in tomorrow's medicine.

But most will not. We think a close examination will reveal the difference between a medical breakthrough and quackery. For example, in the 1970s, a medical professional promoted the idea that a healthy diet was determined by eating only vegetables arranged by color. He had his wife arrange vegetable platters with careful attention to green, red, and other colors according to an elaborate theory that he followed. His health was excellent, his vitality the envy of much younger men and women. For a while he lectured to employees of major corporations — divisions of IBM, General Motors, and others.

He was serious. He believed that his theory, disseminated widely enough, would improve the health of people everywhere and become part of mainstream medicine. Yet no valid evidence has demonstrated that his approach works. We are fairly certain that his claims may meet our definition of quackery (and that if he knew his claims were false, he may have been guilty of fraud).

Common Claims of Frauds and Quacks

Frauds, quacks, and some gurus are selling products and a dream — to be disease-free until a peaceful death from old age. The cost may be "only a few dollars" a month (although some products can be expensive). The claim is that you'll save money in the long run. So millions order and start using a "simple" and "natural" preparation. It's money, they reason, that would have gone to "doctoring" anyway.

Examine the claims made by promoters of alternative therapies. These are claims designed to get your attention.

A good example is a booklet distributed through the mail offering information on old remedies.[1] On the front cover were the words "Read This or Die." The back cover stated in part, "After you read this bulletin ... you probably won't die of cancer, won't die from a heart attack, won't die of a stroke, won't die of diabetes — or any common condition." The fine print promised even more: "And I'm fairly certain you'll never suffer from arthritis, osteoporosis, high blood pressure, insomnia, cataracts, glaucoma, memory loss, Alzheimer's, impotence, depression, candida, or any long-term viral disease." The brochure claimed, "Doctors have usually ignored or suppressed the truly great discoveries — for about 50 years, on average." The actual information on these "truly great discoveries" was offered via a subscription to a newsletter that promised to lead readers to the best sources for "effective treatments and cures for every major disease troubling mankind." Some of the products listed were available from only one supplier, according to the booklet. The booklet stated that although people throughout the world have found ways to stop "every killer disease and chronic illness … you just haven't been told about their solutions yet."

Another example is the controversial book *Natural Cures "They" Don't Want You to Know About* by Kevin Trudeau. The book allegedly is the most popular self-published book in history. The cover claims the book "includes the natural cures for more than 50 specific diseases." Teresa Santiago, the executive director of the New York State Consumer Protection Board, points out that "after 355 pages, Trudeau writes: 'It's important to know that people who are looking for a specific cure for a specific disease are missing the point of this book.'" If so, then why is the word "cures" all over the cover and liberally sprinkled through the first 355 pages? Santiago gives the obvious answer: "From cover to cover, this book is a fraud."[2]

Like Trudeau, other writers of such brochures, books, and websites often play up the popular, though erroneous, idea that there is a conspiracy to keep the public from learning about simple ways to become and stay healthy.

Here's an example from Trudeau's website, which claims to provide you "with information about non-drug, non-surgical and all-natural cures for virtually every disease. These are the natural cures the drug companies, the FDA, the FTC, the American Medical Association, and government agencies DO NOT want you to know about because it would cut into the profits of multinational pharmaceutical corporations."[3]

The implication is that many organizations have a financial stake in keeping you sick. The realities of the health care industry would even seem to confirm such claims. Pharmaceutical companies make money selling medicines only if you are sick. Physicians are needed only when there is sickness or injury.

In his infomercial, Trudeau claims, "It's all about money.… The drug industry does not want people to get healthy. The drug industry wants people to buy more drugs. Healthy people don't need drugs. If everyone in America was healthy, the drug industry would be out of business."[4]

Many people buy this argument without thinking about the fact that disease simply will not be eliminated from the world as we know it. The truth is that pharmaceutical companies make money only when their products are safe and effective so people can regain their health.

We have to admit, the false claims are alluring. For example, examine this claim: "There *are* all-natural cures. You'll never hear about them because the manufacturers can't tell you what they are. Diabetes, migraines, cancer, heart disease, acid reflux, Attention Deficit Disorder, depression, stress, phobias, fibromyalgia, pain of all sorts, arthritis, the list goes on. Lupus, multiple sclerosis; there are cures for multiple sclerosis."[5]

Promoters of such claims find it a lucrative way to make a lot of money. If someone is offering a cure-all, a panacea, giving a laundry list of ailments guaranteed to be cured by the same remedy, it's almost certainly deliberate fraud. If something seems too good to be true, it probably is.

For Opportunists, Timing Is Everything

Opportunists and frauds make big bucks when they persuade us to take blind leaps of faith over knowledge gaps. They take what is still unproven and hype it as the latest breakthrough. They pick up on major newspaper reports of a promising new therapy in the early stages of scientific testing and promote it as the answer to whatever ailment is currently in the media. During the months after 9/11 and the mailing of anthrax to several prominent people, websites started popping up with natural products guaranteed to protect people from anthrax. Such opportunists feed on people's fear and lack of knowledge about health threats new and old.

An ideal situation for an opportunist would be reports that an herbal remedy seems to slow tumor growth in mice. We're talking about herbs (which are unregulated) and cancer (a universal fear) and research suggesting the herbal remedy offers some hope to cancer victims. Timing is crucial. The opportunist's sales pitch would give all the positives about the initial finding and none of the negatives.

Opportunists don't mention that the initial test has not been repeated. Those "promising results" reported with such certainty may turn out to have been in error or may not be obtained in humans.

They don't say that the idea of the herb, or some component in it, providing a safe preventive for cancer is just a theory — a hope — based on preliminary findings. Careful studies are still needed, first with other animals, then with humans. Until then, no one can be sure if it really works in humans. The product is years away from enough testing to be sure it is safe — another fact ignored by opportunists.

Of all the drugs that show early encouraging signs, very few are ever approved. This is because they are found to be either dangerous or ineffective. Of those that reach human trials, less than a quarter gain approval — primarily because of adverse side effects. The whole process, from discovery to pharmacy, can take ten to twelve years. In 2001, an estimated $26 billion was spent on drug development — and only nine completely new drugs were approved (not including drugs that were modifications of earlier drugs).[6]

Opportunists don't wait. If they can market a product based on some "promising" preliminary report, they will. They give no warnings. Their failure to be open requires a "buyer beware" approach. The opportunist enlists others to sell the product. Multilevel marketing strategies spread the product rapidly. Thus the people actually selling a product like this to consumers believe what they've been told. They want you to believe it so you'll buy. But this sales force often has the telltale signs of the quack: a person with little or no training in medicine or any health care field related to what they are selling. If you place your faith in them and their remedies, and they turn out to be wrong, you have made a costly mistake — you've risked your health and thrown away your money.

Warning Signs of Quackery and Fraud

Suspect quackery? Fraud? How can you know if your suspicions are right?

What are the warning signs? We don't claim this is an original list. We have heard these warnings from many people over the years. We've modified and combined the ideas and added some of our own. The more times you answer yes to these questions as you evaluate a therapy or remedy, the greater the chance it is fraudulent or quackery.

1. **Is the product or practice promoted as a "major breakthrough," "revolutionary," "magic," or "miraculous"?** The real value of a medical therapy is rarely known until after it has been in use for many years. Only after a large segment of the population has received the therapy can a profile of the ideal patient

be known. Only after many people have used a therapy (preferably in controlled studies) can we know with some certainty whether it is truly effective and safe. It often takes years to uncover the side effects. Look at our entries on ephedra and coenzyme Q_{10}. These are remedies initially promoted as major breakthroughs that eventually were shown to be much less beneficial and, in the case of ephedra, turned out to have life-threatening side effects. With any new remedy, caution is needed.

2. **Is the promotion trying to elicit an emotional reaction from you rather than presenting clear information to help you make an informed decision about the product?** Marketing strategies play on our emotions to get us to buy a product. Promoters of questionable health products prey on the emotions of the vulnerable and the desperate. People are asked if they are tired of fad diets, then are presented with yet another. Outrageous claims scare people into thinking their water, or food additives, or the air in their homes is poisoning them. And once the ad has them feeling scared, they're ready to try anything that claims to protect them.

Guilt is another emotion that is effective in a sales pitch. Here's a quote from the booklet we mentioned that was distributed through the mail: "Let me be blunt: Cancer, heart disease, stroke, and the other major killers now fall into the category of 'diseases for dummies.'" The implication is that if you get any of these diseases, it's your own fault! If only you had bought the advertised products earlier!

3. **Is only anecdotal or testimonial evidence used to support claims of effectiveness?** Quotes from numerous satisfied customers,

even satisfied doctors and nurses, adorn websites and ads on radio and TV and in magazines and newspapers. When a celebrity endorses a product, that's meant to be evidence that the product actually works, even though the celebrity is no more qualified to speak about the product than you are.

4. **Are claims made about scientific support without specific details?** Even quacks and frauds will claim to have scientific evidence supporting their therapies, but it is important to examine the details. Watch out for the following:

- few or no references to original research studies;
- studies done by only one researcher;
- studies done at obscure, unknown institutions;
- studies reported in small or virtually unknown journals;
- studies reported decades ago;
- studies that have not been repeated; and
- funding of research by someone with a financial or professional stake in the results.

Beware of any promotional material that says, "Studies have shown ..." without giving any details about the studies.

5. **Is the information about the therapy or product being provided by a professional lacking the proper credentials?** The essence of quackery is someone without adequate training giving medical advice. Don't be misled by long lists of letters after people's names. Some of these come from very short training courses or simply joining an organization. Look for well-known credentials, such as M.D., R.N., R.D., Ph.D., not an alphabet soup of unfamiliar qualifications. Find out

if the "experts" have accredited training in a health care field specific to the problem they are treating. Someone might have a Ph.D. but no training in a relevant area of health care.

6. **Are technical words used without clear definitions?** "Energy" is one of those words. Claims that a therapy "boosts energy" can mean anything from the common idea that you feel better able to do things to Eastern ideas of promoting the flow of *chi* or *prana*. Introducing ideas from quantum physics is usually not necessary if the product really works. Information sheets should clarify, not baffle with mind-boggling gobbledygook.

7. **Would a treatment require you to abandon common sense or any well-established scientific laws or principles?** This is often subtle in quackery, blatant in fraud. For example, psychic surgery requires you to believe that a hand, without first cutting an opening, can enter the human body, perform whatever surgery is necessary to remove tumors or organs, then be withdrawn, all with no marks, no obvious place where the flesh was separated. Since it goes against everything we know about the human body, it may be fraudulent. If it actually works, then it most likely involves supernatural forces. Either way, don't get caught up in the hype.

8. **Do proponents claim that a medical system is so flawless ("airtight") that there is no need for further testing?** No area of science should be closed to further developments or revisions. The same is true of good medicine. That's part of the reason medical recommendations are always changing, whether in small or large ways. When a system remains the same for hundreds of years, chances are it has missed out learning from the experiences of those using it.

9. **Is the treatment said to be effective for a wide variety of unrelated physiological problems?** If something really does work, it usually has a limited effect — a specific action on a specific part of the body. If a treatment or product is said to cure everything, chances are it cures nothing or works as a placebo. A general relaxation response is beneficial, but that doesn't mean a specific condition is cured.

10. **Is the product a quick and easy fix for a complicated and frustrating condition?** A "favorite" is called Exercise in a Bottle — said to help people lose weight and boost athletic performance. It appeals to our desire to find easy answers and avoid the difficult lifestyle changes needed to lose weight and get fit. The idea that you can get the benefits of exercise by taking a pill is ridiculous.

11. **Does the proponent of the therapy claim to be criticized unfairly?** Some proponents of complementary and alternative medicine portray themselves as martyrs, persecuted by the government, the medical establishment, or some other organization with a stake in keeping you unaware of their breakthrough. Conspiracy theories may be brought up, such as the theory that the medical and pharmaceutical establishments are protecting their lucrative territory by keeping people sick. A physician may claim that his license to practice medicine was revoked in order to silence him. Check the facts. His license may have been revoked because of behavior that endangered the health and lives of patients. He may have been censured in the public interest, not against it.

Kevin Trudeau, author of a bestselling book on natural cures, claimed, "I have been attacked by the FTC and the FDA for making statements that are *true*."[7] His claim is not accurate. He was found guilty of making false statements. *QuackWatch* made the following observation:

> He made so many [false statements] that the FTC finally got a court order making it illegal for his [*sic*] to sell any products except publications. When challenged by the FTC, Trudeau had the opportunity to defend himself by presenting evidence that his product claims were true. Instead ... he agreed to go out of the "natural cures" business. If he had facts to back him up, do you think he would [have] agreed to stop selling products whose sales totaled hundreds of millions of dollars?[8]

12. **When challenged, do defenders attack the critic instead of responding to the challenge?** Be wary of those who attack the messenger to avoid dealing with the message. Proponents of a therapy with sufficient evidence to back up their claims do not need to attack the challenger. They respond by giving the evidence to support their claims.

13. **Do proponents claim that research will prove their therapy is effective as soon as studies are conducted?** A lack of evidence means there is no support for claims of effectiveness. In science, a lack of data never supports a conclusion.

14. **Is training to provide the therapy offered only at obscure private institutions instead of accredited professional schools?** Can anyone, with payment of a sizable tuition or fee to an unknown private school, which is the only school offering the training, become a practitioner? Does the school accept all applicants, regardless of prior education or experience?

15. **Is training in the therapy relatively short and informal?** Is the length of training only a few hours or a few days? That may be all it takes to learn how to administer the therapy. But without adequate training, therapists may not know enough to realize when they need to refer people to a trained health care professional.

16. **Is a therapy encouraged simply because it has been used for centuries in some remote place?** This might simply mean that those people had nothing else to use. If the best texts on the therapy are decades or centuries old, you'll probably find that many of the old ideas being promoted by therapists were discredited long ago. Medicine evolves as continued use uncovers side effects, fine-tunes dosage, and provides a better understanding of how the remedy works. Just think about all we have discovered about nutrition in the last few decades.

17. **Do proponents use statements that are basically true but unrelated to the therapy?** Promoters of energy-based therapies such as Therapeutic Touch and Reiki often mention the value of massage and touch. While both are valuable, these energy-based therapies are said to work through a nonphysical energy that does not require touching the patient.

18. **Do proponents blame failed tests of effectiveness on the skepticism or outright nonbelief of observers?** A physician who uses applied kinesiology stated in a training video that his therapy doesn't work well when skeptical relatives of patients are present. He recommended that practitioners allow only

"believers" in applied kinesiology to be present during their sessions. We acknowledge the role of psychological factors in healing, but an effective therapy should work whether the person believes in it or not.

19. **Do proponents claim it is too difficult for most to understand how a therapy works or that only the "enlightened" can understand?** This is often disguised in terms of someone being too rational or logical to understand how the therapy works. It's true you don't have to understand all the details of how some therapy works. You do need to understand the evidence that proves the therapy works.

20. **Does the proponent disguise the truth with vague and misleading statements?** A statement such as "this therapy has been thoroughly tested by seven leading medical research facilities" may fail to add that the tests showed the product is worthless. The "research facilities" should be legitimate, independent organizations whose findings are made available for independent review.

21. **Does the product you're considering require advance payment?** You may never receive what you bought or get your money back.

22. **Does the advertisement promise a "money-back guarantee"?** Fraudulent businesses will have closed shop and moved on before you have a chance to complain.

23. **Is the therapy available only in other countries?** Foreign countries have legitimate clinics, but they also have fraudulent ones. Some countries have very lax regulations for clinics and products and do not protect patients from harmful treatments in the way the FDA attempts to in the United States. Physicians may not be required to have the same credentials as you would expect in the United States. Before traveling, contact the local health authority where the clinic is located.

24. **Are there conflicts of interest?** Websites and people who recommend and sell products may not be as objective about the product as you would hope. You need to be as cautious about doctors and nurses selling magnets and herbs as you are about an acupuncturist selling vitamins. If practitioners tell you they have discovered a great new product and then try to sell it to you, you need a second opinion from someone who does not stand to gain financially from the sale.

25. **Is the term "natural" the main advantage of the remedy?** Do promoters claim that the product is safer because it's natural? Natural does not necessarily mean safe. Nature contains many poisons that are fatal (such as certain mushrooms) or highly irritating (think about poison ivy) or that cause allergic reactions (such as pollen or even milk, for some people). If something natural has the potential to heal, it also has the potential to hurt.

A good place to start when looking for specific information on frauds and quacks is the website run by Stephen Barrett, M.D., *QuackWatch* (*www. quackwatch.org*). Barrett is a nationally renowned consumer advocate who has published dozens of books, including *The Health Robbers: A Close Look at Quackery in America*.[9] We believe he gets close to the truth about many therapies — at least on scientific grounds. We disagree with some of his conclusions, especially on spiritual issues. But even there, when he looks at the scientific evidence related to faith and health, he is fair.

The Gurus

Alternative medicine has its "gurus," men and women whose books are scooped off the shelves. The beliefs and health systems promoted by two of these gurus are currently very popular.

Deepak Chopra, M.D.

The popular Deepak Chopra, M.D., has become one of the most prolific authors in alternative medicine. He has published at least thirty-five books, including bestselling alternative health titles such as *Creating Health*, *Quantum Healing*, *Perfect Health*, and *Ageless Body, Timeless Mind*.[10] He then moved on to promote the religious and spiritual views that underlie his approach to health.[11] More recently he has focused on topics with mass appeal — a cookbook, a book on herbs, and a book on the spiritual lessons of golf.[12]

Chopra was trained as a physician in India and in 1970 moved to the United States, where he focused on endocrinology (the study of the hormones that regulate much of the body). In 1985, he was appointed chief of staff at what is now called Boston Regional Medical Center.

After achieving much success in modern Western medicine, Chopra became disillusioned with its approach. All he did as a doctor, he has said, was write prescriptions to alleviate symptoms: "Medical training doesn't equip doctors to help patients make changes that will have a significant impact on their health."[13] He also picked up some unhealthy practices himself.

Chopra read about Transcendental Meditation (TM) and put it into practice. Within weeks he had stopped smoking and drinking whiskey. He started reading about the medicine of his native India, called Ayurveda. He returned to India to rediscover his "roots" and was soon involved with Maharishi Mahesh Yogi, the man who introduced TM to the West. Maharishi asked Chopra to start a company with him called Maharishi Ayur-Veda Products International, Inc. Together they distributed herbal remedies, teas, oils, and other Ayurvedic products (the hyphen allowed them to register "Ayur-Veda" as a trademark). Chopra resigned his hospital position to direct an Ayur-Veda health clinic in Lancaster, Massachusetts, which soon attracted the rich and famous. With all this success, Maharishi, in 1989, bestowed on Chopra the title "Dhanvantari [Lord of Immortality], the keeper of perfect health for the world."[14]

During this time, Chopra started writing books that sold widely. A charismatic and extremely persuasive speaker, he was soon on the bestsellers' lecture circuit (charging $25,000 per lecture) and appearing on television.[15]

In 1993, Chopra resigned from all involvement with the TM organization and started a clinic in California as part of Sharp Healthcare. The new clinic focused on the rich and famous, with reported charges to clients of $4,000 a week.[16] Maharishi removed all of Chopra's materials from his clinics and deleted all references to Chopra from Ayur-Veda materials.[17]

The California clinic abruptly closed in 1995 and Chopra started his own clinic close to San Diego. Now known as the Chopra Center, the plan is to franchise the approach to select locations around the world. In 2004, a large resort company announced it will open five Chopra Centers, and two others are planned for resorts in New York and London.[18] Chopra himself now focuses on writing and speaking, with occasional appearances at his resorts.

Chopra's Philosophy

Chopra provides an important example of why Christians need to critically evaluate the spiritual claims made by some within alternative medicine. A complete analysis of these claims would take up our whole book. An excellent resource on this topic, including a more detailed evaluation of Chopra's philosophy, has been written by a group of Christian physicians.[19]

Chopra's views on health and medicine appear to us to be based on his modernized version of Ayurveda and Hinduism mixed with some conventional medicine. For this reason, it is difficult to separate his views of health from his religious beliefs, so we will consider them together. He preaches that to be healthy, people first need enlightenment. Chopra states, "We all need to be healed in the highest sense by making ourselves perfect in mind, body and spirit. The first step is to realize that this is even possible. To create health you need a new kind of knowledge based on a deeper concept of life. Although our package of skin and bones looks very convincing, it is a mask, an illusion, disguising our true self which has no limitations."[20]

Chopra's approach is that we need to realize we are both infinite and all-powerful. In his words: "The truth is: I am here, but I am also everywhere else. That you are there, but you are also here because here is there, and there is everywhere, and everywhere is nowhere, specifically."[21] And again: "We all have the power to make reality."[22] Once we come to believe these things, according to Chopra, we can create the health we so deeply desire. For Chopra, mind has complete control over matter. "People can become happy simply by realizing that the source of change is inside themselves. The responsibility for all illness and all cure resides within us."[23]

We get ill, Chopra claims, when our mind and our consciousness are not aligned with what he calls the Universal Consciousness. "Sickness, disease is a self-correcting signal to realign the patterns that structure the whole."[24] In other words, we get sick when our thoughts distract us from the way things really are.

Chopra believes that the Universal Consciousness is all-powerful, all-knowing, perfect, and good. According to Chopra, we, too, are like this: perfect and all-knowing. If we are sick, it is because we don't believe what Chopra believes. If we did believe it, we would be aligned with the Universal Consciousness. We would be healthy if we believed that our true nature is one of perfection and complete goodness. Health will arise, he says, when we can affirm, "I know myself as the immeasurable potential of all that was, is and will be.... There is no other I than the entire universe. I am being and I am nowhere and everywhere at the same time. I am omnipresent, omniscient; I am the eternal spirit that animates everything in existence."[25] In other words, Chopra claims each of us is God.

Chopra says that to come to believe this about ourselves involves meditation and a return to Hinduism. Meditation is how we reestablish contact with our inner self, which is more closely aligned with the Universal Consciousness. Chopra disagrees with the Western view that meditation is just a mental activity. He says that "meditation is a spiritual practice."[26]

We agree with this point on meditation being a spiritual practice. This is why we are very concerned about the type of meditation someone promotes. For Chopra, meditation allows people to "settle down to a silent state of awareness, beyond thought, to the experiential level of total unity with the universe. You experience the fact that you are part of the larger wholeness."[27] Assuming that the Universal Consciousness is loving and cares for us, we will sense guidance and direction when meditating. "You will tap into the cosmic mind, the voice that whispers to you non-verbally in the silent spaces between your thoughts. This is your inner intelligence and it is the ultimate and supreme genius that mirrors the wisdom of the universe. Trust this inner wisdom and all your dreams will come true."[28]

Part of what makes Chopra's system so attractive is his declaration that our dreams for health, wealth, and happiness are legitimate. In fact, our purpose in life is to be satisfied. He declares that when we live according to his Seven Spiritual Laws, "we experience the ecstasy and exultation of our own spirit, which is the ultimate goal of all goals."[29] To help people attain this goal, Chopra developed a special treatment for his clinics, called the "Pizzichilli treatment."[30] This involves two technicians massaging and bathing a naked patient in warm sesame oil for two hours. We find it hard to determine whether this practice is therapy or self-indulgence!

Meditation is central to Chopra's approach to health, but he also recommends other products and practices. Ayurvedic remedies are herbal but given to stimulate and balance life energy (or *prana*), which we describe in more detail in the entry Energy Medicine. "In Ayurvedic terms, they [herbal remedies] stimulate the intelligence of the body, which is the ultimate and supreme genius mirroring the wisdom of the universe."[31] More traditional Ayurvedic approaches place importance on detoxification, personality typing, pulse diagnosis, adequate rest and exercise, and attention to relationships.

Deepak Chopra's immense popularity points to the high value many Americans place on personal comfort and pleasure. His system offers the universe — literally. Only the rich and famous can afford many aspects of his approach to health and healing. Yet their enthusiasm for his services makes the whole system more attractive to the masses. An editorial accompanying a *Newsweek* article on Chopra is worth reading. In it, Wendy Kaminer points out that "gurus" like Chopra "always confirm our essential godliness. They lead by flattery.... Gurus often tell us exactly what we want to hear."[32]

In reality, the spiritual aspects of Chopra's approach to health contradict biblical teaching. The Bible teaches that humans are not "little gods," and we are not, by nature, extensions of the Big God. We are created beings, loved by the Creator of the world in which we live. The Bible's spiritual laws conflict drastically with Chopra's spiritual laws. Both cannot be right.

The Bible teaches that we humans are fallen human beings, creatures created by the one true Creator. Romans 3:23 states that "all have sinned and fall short of the glory of God." Yes, we are extremely valuable to God and have great potential. The psalmist gave thanks for how God made humanity. "You made him a little lower than the heavenly beings and crowned him with glory and honor. You made him ruler over the works of your hands; you put everything under his feet" (Psalm 8:5 – 6). But our potential is not realized by listening to our inner selves and having our selfish dreams fulfilled. We need to listen to the voice of God, which comes through his Word and his Holy Spirit. This message is not as attractive to rebellious humans as a Pizzichilli massage. Nor is it an easy path to pursue. But it is true.

As Kaminer points out in her *Newsweek* editorial, Chopra and his fellow gurus ask very little. "The spiritual peace and enlightenment offered by pop gurus doesn't require a lifetime of discipline. It requires only that you suspend your critical judgment, attend their lectures and workshops and buy their books."[33]

While this low-cost, high-pleasure system may be more appealing, we question its long-term value and its spiritual veracity. Chopra's approach is sprinkled with enough good information about diet, sleep, and relationships that applying his ideas will bring some improvements to those who have not cared for their health. However, when we are faced with serious illness and disease, his system appears to have little to offer. When pressed for scientific support for his remedies and therapies, Chopra admits, "I am not at all attached to the scientific worldview at the moment. I see myself as a bum on the street who has a lot of fun writing."[34] However, he doesn't forget to include his "M.D." on his books and continues to speak to an apparently adoring and growing choir of people around the world committed to consumerism and postmodernism.

Chopra is like many other alternative medicine gurus. His teaching must be rejected for the scientific and spiritual reasons we describe throughout our book. Chopra seems to truly believe in his methods, theories, and spiritual path. He believes that utilizing Ayurveda and his other practices will result in the best possible health. He has achieved fame and, presumably, a significant degree of wealth from promoting his ideas. However, the discerning Christian seeking wellness needs to recognize that popularity, fame, and financial success do not prove that the possessor has an inside track on healthy living. Nor do they indicate a right relationship with God.

Larry Dossey, M.D.

Chopra is not alone as a doctor-writer who has discovered "new answers." Others offer an approach with a seemingly Christian subtext. Larry Dossey is a physician who has come to public prominence through his books on prayer and healing: *Healing Words*, *Prayer Is Good Medicine*, and *Be Careful What You Pray For ... You Just Might Get It*.[35] Raised in a fundamentalist Christian home in Texas, he drifted away from his religious upbringing into agnosticism.[36] However, as a physician, he was confronted by the way many of his patients relied on prayer. He undertook a spiritual journey that brought him into contact with Eastern religions. Here he claimed to find the universal aspects of all religions and has come to believe that all world religions lead people in basically the same direction.

Dossey's Views on Health, Prayer, and God

Dossey proposes a view called "nonlocal medicine."[37] According to this belief, each person does not have an individual mind confined to his or her own brain. Instead, Dossey believes that the minds of everyone are joined in one Universal Consciousness. This means that each person, through prayer or another distance method, such as telepathy, clairvoyance, or voodoo, can affect the mind of another. Dossey admits his view is not supported by scientific evidence, but this is because these anomalous, nonlocal events "seem to have no possibility, even in principle, of being explained in the local, physicalistic, reductionistic framework" of current science and medicine.[38]

For Dossey, then, "prayerfulness" is more important than "prayer." By prayerfulness he means "a sense of simply being attuned or aligned with 'something higher.' Prayer tends to follow instructions laid down by the great religious traditions; prayerfulness does not. It is a feeling of unity with the All, rather than with specific leaders, traditions, or holy books."[39] In many ways, Dossey understands the problems Christians sometimes have when they pray. He says we sometimes arrive at God's doorstep with a laundry list of expectations rather than with the humble attitude God calls on us to express. In *Healing Words*, Dossey observes, "Intercessory prayer has a tendency to ask for definite outcomes, to structure the future, to 'tell God what to do,' such as taking the cancer away. Prayerfulness, on the other hand, is accepting without being passive, is grateful without giving up. It is more willing to stand in the mystery, to tolerate ambiguity and the unknown. It honors the rightness of whatever happens, even cancer."[40]

While Dossey's emphasis on the attitude for prayer seems on the surface to be biblically sound, his last sentence reveals where his theology differs from orthodox Christianity. Dossey acknowledges that his view of prayer is "far different" from the "old biblically based views of prayer" where requests were offered to a God distinct from humans.[41] He claims the biblical view of prayer arises from a worldview that "is now antiquated and incomplete" and constitutes a "uniquely 'pathological mythology.'" He seems to have rejected belief in a personal God whose loving will determines the outcome of prayer.

In Dossey's view, a Cosmic Consciousness directs all things. Interestingly, Dossey refers to this Consciousness as loving, trustworthy, caring, benevolent, wise, and something with which we can communicate. All these are personal attributes, yet Dossey never seems to admit this. Nor does he give us any reasons for accepting his description of Consciousness. Instead, we are left to take it on faith that the universe is loving, that cancer, for example, must be right.

In contrast, we see the biblical explanation as much more satisfying and reasonable. The Bible teaches that the universe (cosmos) is not loving, wise, and benevolent. The universe is not the way it should be, but one day it "will be liberated from its bondage to decay and brought into the glorious freedom of the children of God. We know that the whole creation has been groaning as in the pains of childbirth right up to the present time" (Romans 8:21 – 22). Cancer, pain, and suffering are not right; they are the tragic consequences of living in a fallen world. We should not go along with Dossey's advice to "honor the rightness of whatever happens, even cancer."[42] We can grieve the loss, suffering, and death that disease brings, decry the existence of such suffering, express our pain, and turn to the loving Creator of this world for comfort. He did not make the world to be this way, and he promises in his Word to one day restore it to how it ought to be. Because of this, God says we can have confidence that he will help and comfort us while we grapple with illness, disability, or death.

Dossey ultimately seems to hold that prayer is a form of language or energy. It is a way that minds have of interacting with one another. He refuses to believe that a personal God is needed to determine what outcomes will arise. The words need only be spoken, or the thoughts expressed, for us to get the desired outcomes.

We might want to have this type of powerful prayer that always works, but it raises the ominous possibility that our thoughts might also harm people. According to Dossey, even an inadvertent "God damn it!" thus becomes a dangerous weapon. This is the focus of Dossey's book on harmful prayer.[43] As such, he admits that his view of prayer has become a magical one. All those negative thoughts of others, or things we mumble under our breath, become expressions of the Cosmic Mind that impact the people against whom they are directed.

Dossey is to be admired for tackling such a controversial and difficult topic. Yet his conclusion is, to us, completely unsatisfactory and unscriptural.

Given his belief in prayer as something like an energy, independent of our will or the will of God, he is forced to conclude that these negative thoughts do "hit" others. He uses stories about voodoo hexing as illustrations of this effect. Just as he refuses to accept the role of a personal God in bringing about good, he does not accept a role for evil spiritual beings in bringing about harm.

We therefore ask why people do not die when people maliciously or inadvertently tell them to "drop dead." Dossey's answer is that humans "have evolved forms of protection against the negative thoughts of others — a kind of 'spiritual immune system' that is analogous to our immune system against infections."[44] As with most of Dossey's assertions, he has no evidence to back up his claims. He has to invent new propositions to resolve problems in his original theory. That is a clear sign of a theory in trouble, of one that doesn't match reality. We can take comfort in the fact that our thoughts are not all-powerful.

However, Dossey raises good points about the impact of our attitudes toward others. People can often sense the negative attitudes and feelings we harbor toward them, which could be potentially harmful to them. This is not because of some energy that emanates from our mind to the Cosmic Mind and into the other person's mind. We harm them because these thoughts can lead to actions. "For out of the heart come evil thoughts, murder, adultery, sexual immorality, theft, false testimony, slander" (Matthew 15:19).

At the very least, thinking negatively about others distracts us from focusing on how we might love and serve them. "Let us consider how we may spur one another on toward love and good deeds" (Hebrews 10:24). Paul encourages us, "Whatever is true, whatever is noble, whatever is right, whatever is pure, whatever is lovely, whatever is admirable — if anything is excellent or praiseworthy — think about such things" (Philippians 4:8).

Our thoughts and words are filtered through the mind of God. David prayed, "Search me, O God, and know my heart; test me and know my anxious thoughts" (Psalm 139:23; cf. Hebrews 4:12). God hears our requests but does not automatically act on them in the way we feel is best. He determines what is most loving, most just, most needed in a situation to accomplish *his* purpose for humankind. God sees the totality of the other options, not just the limited view we have. This is why we cannot predict the outcome of our prayers like we can the effects of an injection or X-ray. We examine the whole area of controlled research on prayer in the Prayer for Healing entry (pp. 236 – 45).

Dossey's books on prayer have done much to stimulate discussion, research, and interest in prayer for healing. As such, his contributions are welcome. However, Christians cannot welcome his ideas with open arms. His beliefs about prayer, as he himself admits, are based on completely different views of reality, people, and God. His description of prayerfulness is quite insightful but not accurate in the light of biblical truth. Dossey's proposals suffer from a number of ironic twists. While rejecting the God of the Bible, he wants to hold on to a "god" who has many of the attributes of God, but not those aspects that Dossey does not want to accept. He fails to provide evidence for why we should accept those bits of Christianity he wants to hold on to. Nor does he show why we should accept the eclectic nature of his view of prayer. Christians who choose to be exposed to his teachings should read his books with a critical eye, realizing he makes some good points but that his message is fundamentally at odds with the message of the Bible.

Other Health Gurus

There are numerous other gurus who write and speak widely on alternative medicine, wellness, and spiritual healing. Some are more like Chopra, using some good medical common sense to promote a form of spirituality that is usually alien to Christian spirituality. They often endorse a variety of other products that prove to be financially rewarding for them. Others are more like Dossey, who use their medical credentials to speak on spiritual issues. They take well-established Christian concepts and redefine them.

Some are well known in evangelical Christian circles, such as Lorraine Day, M.D., the Rev. George Malkmus, and Jordan Rubin. However, these Christians have been listed among *QuackWatch*'s "promoters of questionable methods."[45] According to this website, all of them have "been involved in some way with the promotion or administration of questionable health products and/or services." Even though they hold sincere beliefs, and we agree with many of their spiritual views, their books contain at least some medically unreliable information.

For example, Lorraine Day's website contains much valid information on the benefits of a healthy diet. But she goes too far when she claims that drugs can't cure disease. She herself seems to have had an amazing recovery from cancer. But that doesn't mean that she knows what cured her — or that what she thinks cured her will cure anyone else. In every case, Christians should evaluate all that is being said in light of biblical revelation and sound medical research.

Writers who adhere to an approach to healing far different from that with a biblical base must be questioned in the same manner in which we question proponents of other therapies and herbal remedies.

In some instances, their work should be avoided because it requires the acceptance of religious ideas and values in opposition to those of orthodox Christianity. In other instances, they may be orthodox Christians who have fallen into the realm of medical uncertainty, fraud, or quackery.

Common Sense Is Key

The health-related advice of the gurus must be evaluated medically and scientifically. Although science has flaws and limitations and has led to mistakes, the scientific method remains the best way to figure out whether something works. While scientists are never completely unbiased, they look to data and empirical evidence as the bottom line in discovering truth. Promotion of health-related products on any other basis must remain questionable.

The spiritual teachings of the health gurus must be evaluated spiritually. Reflect on the following passages and how they apply to your reading about health. We believe they call on us to actively engage our minds and to think critically and biblically whenever our reading addresses spiritual issues. And, of course, we should also pray as we read on these issues.

> Let no one deceive you with empty words, for because of such things God's wrath comes on those who are disobedient. Therefore do not be partners with them.
>
> For you were once darkness, but now you are light in the Lord. Live as children of light (for the fruit of the light consists in all goodness, righteousness and truth) and find out what pleases the Lord. Have nothing to do with the fruitless deeds of darkness, but rather expose them. For it is shameful even to mention what the disobedient do in secret. But everything

exposed by the light becomes visible, for it is light that makes everything visible.

Ephesians 5:6 – 14a

See to it that no one takes you captive through hollow and deceptive philosophy, which depends on human tradition and the basic principles of this world rather than on Christ.

For in Christ all the fullness of the Deity lives in bodily form, and you have been given fullness in Christ, who is the head over every power and authority.

Colossians 2:8 – 10

Timothy, guard what has been entrusted to your care. Turn away from godless chatter and the opposing ideas of what is falsely called knowledge, which some have professed and in so doing have wandered from the faith.

1 Timothy 6:20 – 21

Chapter 5: The Gurus: Fraud, Quackery, or Wisdom?

1. David G. Williams, *Read This or Die* (Rockville, Md.: Mountain Home, n.d.).

2. Michael Gormley, "Agency: 'Natural Cures' Guy Selling Names" *ABC News,* October 27, 2005. *ABC News: http://abcnews.go.com/Health/wireStory?id=1257608* (October 30, 2005).

3. Natural Cures, "Natural Cures, Alternative Medicine," 2005. *NaturalCures.com: www.naturalcures.com* (October 30, 2005).

4. Stephen Barrett, "Analysis of Kevin Trudeau's 'Natural Cures' Infomercial (2004)." Posted February 2, 2005. *Infomercial Watch: www.infomercialwatch.org/tran/trudeau.shtml* (October 30, 2005).

5. Ibid.

6. Jason S. Bardi, "The Other Side of Drug Discovery, Part 1," *News and Views* 2, no. 14 (April 22, 2002). *Scripps Research Institute: www.scripps.edu/newsandviews/e_20020422/drug.html* (October 17, 2005).

7. Barrett, "Analysis of Kevin Trudeau's 'Natural Cures' Infomercial."

8. Ibid.

9. Stephen Barrett and William T. Jarvis, eds., *The Health Robbers: A Close Look at Quackery in America* (Buffalo, N.Y.: Prometheus, 1993).

10. Deepak Chopra, *Creating Health: Beyond Prevention, Toward Perfection* (Boston: Houghton Mifflin, 1985); *Quantum Healing: Exploring the Frontiers of Mind/Body Medicine* (New York: Bantam, 1989); *Perfect Health: The Complete Mind/Body Guide* (New York: Harmony, 1990); *Ageless Body, Timeless Mind: The Quantum Alternative to Growing Old* (New York: Harmony, 1993).

11. Deepak Chopra, *Everyday Immortality: A Concise Course in Spiritual Transformation* (New York: Harmony, 1999); *How to Know God: The Soul's Journey into the Mystery of Mysteries* (New York: Harmony, 2000).

12. Deepak Chopra, David Simon, and Leanne Backer, *The Chopra Center Cookbook* (Hoboken, N.J.: John Wiley & Sons, 2003); Deepak Chopra and David Simon, *The Chopra Center Herbal Handbook: Forty Natural Prescriptions for Perfect Health* (New York: Three Rivers, 2000); Deepak Chopra, *Golf for Enlightenment: The Seven Lessons for the Game of Life* (New York: Harmony, 2003).

13. Deepak Chopra, quoted in *Current Biography Yearbook,* ed. Judith Graham (New York: H. W. Wilson, 1995), 91 – 96.

14. Andrew A. Skolnick, "Maharishi Ayur-Veda: Guru's Marketing Scheme Promises the World Eternal 'Perfect Health,'" *Journal of the American Medical Association* 266, no. 13 (October 1991): 1741 – 50.

15. See John Leland and Carla Power, "Deepak's Instant Karma," *Newsweek* (October 20, 1997): 52 – 58.

16. Elise Pettus, "The Mind-Body Problems," *New York* (August 14, 1995): 28 – 31, 95.

17. Ibid., 31.

18. Conor Dougherty, "Spiritual-Healing Guru Deepak Chopra's Carlsbad, Calif., Firm Plans Growth," *San Diego Union-Tribune Knight Ridder* (January 17, 2004). *HighBeam Research: www.highbeam.com* (October 17, 2005).

19. Paul Reisser, Robert Belarde, and Dale Mabe, *Examining Alternative Medicine* (Downers Grove, Ill.: InterVarsity, 2001).

20. Deepak Chopra, *Journey Into Healing: Awakening the Wisdom Within You* (New York: Random House Audio, 1995), audiocassette.

21. Deepak Chopra, *Escaping the Prison of the Mind: A Journey from Here to Here* (San Rafael, Calif.: New World Library, 1992), audiocassette.

22. Chopra, *Journey Into Healing*.

23. Deepak Chopra, *Creating Health*, rev. ed. (New York: Random House Audio, 1995), audiocassette.

24. D. Scott Rogo, "The Healing Reality: An Interview with Deepak Chopra, M.D.," in *New Techniques of Inner Healing* (New York: Paragon, 1992), 158.

25. Chopra, *Escaping the Prison*.

26. Chopra, *Ageless Body, Timeless Mind*, 167.

27. Rogo, "Healing Reality," 161.

28. Chopra, *Journey Into Healing*.

29. Deepak Chopra, *The Seven Spiritual Laws of Success: A Practical Guide to the Fulfillment of Your Dreams* (San Rafael, Calif.: Amber-Allen, 1994), 93.

30. Pettus, "Mind-Body Problems," 30.

31. Rogo, "Healing Reality," 162.

32. Wendy Kaminer, "Why We Love Gurus," *Newsweek* (October 20, 1997): 60.

33. Ibid.

34. Zina Moukheiber, "Lord of Immortality," *Forbes* 153, no. 8 (April 11, 1994): 132.

35. Larry Dossey, *Healing Words: The Power of Prayer and the Practice of Medicine* (New York: HarperSanFrancisco, 1993); *Prayer Is Good Medicine: How to Reap the Healing Benefits of Prayer* (New York: HarperSanFrancisco, 1996); *Be Careful What You Pray For ... You Just Might Get It: What We Can Do About the Unintentional Effects of Our Thoughts, Prayers, and Wishes* (New York: HarperSanFrancisco, 1997).

36. Dossey, *Healing Words*, preface.

37. Larry Dossey, *Reinventing Medicine: Beyond Mind-Body to a New Era of Healing* (New York: HarperSanFrancisco, 2000).

38. Dossey, *Healing Words*, 44.

39. Ibid., 24.

40. Ibid., 24.

41. Ibid., 7.

42. Ibid., 24.

43. Dossey, *Be Careful What You Pray For*.

44. Ibid., 8.

45. Stephen Barrett, "Promoters of Questionable Methods." *QuackWatch: www.quackwatch.org/11Ind/index.html* (October 30, 2005).

CHAPTER 6

HEALTHY LIFESTYLES

At the beginning of the twentieth century, physicians faced the challenge of trying to treat numerous diseases that had no known cures. Influenza took the lives of millions. Pneumonia, diarrhea, chicken pox, measles, and scarlet fever were deadly threats to children. Heart disease guaranteed that many men would not see their fiftieth birthday.

At the beginning of the twenty-first century, one of the biggest challenges facing society is the problem of symptoms in search of a disease. Companies making pharmaceutical drugs and those making herbal remedies are getting rich from products made to elevate mood, relax tense nerves, fight sleep disorders, and improve sexual performance. Fatigue, lethargy, and a sense of spiritual emptiness are as likely to underlie many people's sense of unwellness as any physical disease.

Take Mike, for example. A master chef in New York, he worked at least sixty hours a week for the owner of an upscale Manhattan restaurant. He loved the work, but it was strenuous. Mike's body ached from the constant handling of large pots and pans in the commercial kitchen. He ate properly when he ate but often skipped meals because he was too busy. He always skipped breakfast just to get a few more minutes in bed.

Mike knew he needed a change. So when he was recruited to be the private chef for a wealthy family, he left the restaurant. He was soon eating better, getting enough rest, and taking long walks every afternoon. His achiness and fatigue diminished drastically but did not disappear.

Friends suggested an array of vitamins and herbal supplements. They were all natural, "safe," his friends told him, available in any health food store. Mike thought they might help. But he decided to see his doctor first and get an expert's opinion. The physician praised Mike's lifestyle changes but recognized that Mike's symptoms were a concern. He was right. Extensive testing revealed that Mike was in the early stages of multiple sclerosis.

That early diagnosis probably prolonged Mike's life. Multiple sclerosis is much easier to treat in its early stages. Mike's increase in exercise, improved diet, and regular rest strengthened him for the long fight to come. There's a good chance he will lead a rich, full life, with the disease progressing slowly enough to be little more than a tolerable burden to which he can adapt. To Mike's surprise, his physician suggested he take some of the nutritional supplements recommended by his friends.

Had Mike tried to be his own physician, treating himself first with the nutritional supplements, his multiple sclerosis might have progressed untreated to the point where it could no longer be dismissed as mild fatigue, and the potential for his future likely would have been far bleaker.

Busyness and Stress Contribute to Illness

Mike found a specific cause for his symptoms. Many others do not. They end up with a vague collection of symptoms that seem to defy explanation.

One contributing factor is busyness. We spend more hours on the job, either by choice or by necessity. Some work two jobs in order to meet their expenses. Working longer hours leads to a series of complications. Few working couples get adequate rest during the week. To do *something* different from the regular workday, we rob a half hour, an hour, or

even more from our sleep time to watch television, play on the computer, or spend more time with our children (sometimes keeping them awake too long as well).

Most people are sleep-deprived, a fact reflected in highway accident statistics. Some researchers warn that people who work long hours and then fail to get enough sleep once they get home could be putting their lives at risk. Law enforcement agencies increasingly warn that overtired drivers falling asleep at the wheel may be as great a problem as drunk driving. One study carried out in Australia suggested that the effects of sleep loss could be similar or even worse than the effects of drinking too much alcohol.[1]

Family interaction, once an essential and enjoyable aspect of every day, is increasingly seen as an intrusion into other activities now viewed as more important. The shared breakfast or evening meal is now a weekly event at best. Job requirements for parents and teenagers, extracurricular school activities, sports, exercise, music, and so on, all mean that most families rarely spend more than a few minutes a day together, and those few minutes are often filled with tension. The push is to get ready for the next event, not be together as a family.

Christians active in their churches add a list of other activities to their schedule. An appropriate focus on our spiritual health and that of our loved ones commits us to activities that can further isolate family members from one another. Church services, Bible studies, youth programs, weekend retreats, and service to the needy can result in even less time with loved ones who also need our spiritual support and encouragement. All these are important, but we need balance.

Some adults add to their stress by combining too many unrelated activities. There was a time when parents would attend their children's athletic events, school plays, and Christmas pageants with nothing more on their minds than enjoying the diversion and encouraging their children. Today it is difficult to go to such an activity without seeing adults using cell phones, PDAs, and other electronic devices. Soccer, baseball, and football practice fields often have parents using laptop computers in their cars or in the bleachers. They glance up from time to time, waving vaguely in the direction of their sons or daughters, trying to give the impression they are watching, yet fooling no one, especially not their children.

Our point is not that any of these activities are wrong. Nor are we saying that being busy is wrong. The Gospels record that Jesus had a very busy schedule during his public ministry. Paul covered many hundreds of miles in his missionary journeys, preached often, discipled many, and allowed the burdens of many people to weigh heavily on his heart (2 Corinthians 11:28 – 29). Christian servants throughout history have led active lives and done much to further the kingdom of God.

But there is something wrong when the first thing everyone comments on these days is how busy and stressed out they are. The problem is not our busyness, but how we balance our activities with times of empowerment. The problem has less to do with what we're doing and more to do with the mind-set with which we approach our activities. If we don't get this right, the consequences can be serious.

Overactivity can lead directly to health problems. Excessive busyness also negatively impacts our significant relationships: with God, with our spouses, with our children, and with those few really close friends we all need. This lack of critical interaction with others can affect our health. Doctors know that a loving touch combined with leisure time spent with a loved one usually reduces stress, lowers blood pressure, and can have a positive effect on the immune system. If you are a parent who has held a sick child when he or she awakens frightened, feverish, and confused, you have experienced the slower heart rate and more relaxed breathing that come from the simple act of being enveloped in love. The child is still sick, but the symptoms seem to ease as your child falls asleep in your arms.

The Negative Effect of a Sense of Isolation

Isolation also has a negative impact. Many of us are isolated from family members, living in different cities, different states, and even different countries. We've lost the old-fashioned connection with neighbors. The isolation from neighbors started innocently enough with the proliferation of televisions that took people off their porches and stoops. Then the Walkman-type device appeared and it became acceptable to walk down the street wearing earphones. Now look at how far things have come with iPods and 3G cell phones allowing people to enjoy music, surf the Internet, or check email while on the move. Gone is the social nicety of acknowledging a passerby. What used to be rude has become acceptable.

We have gradually abandoned other forms of casual conversation. When was the last time you shared a salesclerk's joy at her daughter being accepted into college or her son making her a grandmother? When did you last extend your sympathies to another supermarket regular who just lost a spouse? When did you last see anyone offering commiseration and an old family home remedy to a cold-sufferer wandering the aisles of the neighborhood pharmacy?

These were the familiar strangers of daily life, the momentary interactions providing a respite from troubles, a sense of community, an awareness that, if ever so briefly, we all matter in someone else's life. For some elderly living alone, this tenuous community can be the incentive to get out of bed each day and go for a walk. This sense of community is the reason some people mourned the demise of the old five-and-dime with its lunch counter where they would mourn the passing of a loved one. The longtime waitresses and the men and women who stopped in for coffee and doughnuts all became a family of sorts. They shared casual conversation. And everyone felt as though they mattered.

The shopping mall food court has become a substitute for some, certainly for our youth. But it requires a car or bus to get to the mall. It's not part of a casual stroll through the neighborhood. Coffee shops also are filling this void to a degree. Unfortunately, they're creating an environment that partially perpetuates the trend they could have countered. Many have added rental computer terminals with Internet access so patrons have the illusion of community while focusing solely on the screen, oblivious to anyone nearby.

The Internet itself is said to offer a form of friendship — a virtual community. We can instantly write messages and keep up personal contact through chat rooms and email, but all without face-to-face contact. You cannot see a smile or a tear. You cannot get a hug or hold a hand, share a kiss or walk together in silence. Real interaction is missing. The sense of community and caring that can reduce blood pressure, slow the pulse rate, and trigger what has been called the "relaxation response" is gone.

Participation in a real community can lead to a longer life, regardless of other factors such as diet and exercise. In 1983, a study of the residents of Alameda County, California, showed that people who eat right and exercise regularly, yet are basically loners, frequently have shorter life spans than those

who may not take such good care of their bodies yet feel they are needed, wanted, and loved as part of a community.[2] We may instinctively sense this but let the popular culture lull us into an increasingly isolated way of living and working.

How the Invasion of the Computer Affects Health

There is yet another challenge to our physical and emotional health, namely, the widespread use of the computer. In just a few years, the Internet went from being a link among colleges, universities, and government agencies, all engaged in research, to a significant tool of business, interpersonal communication, entertainment, and relaxation. Individuals who have escaped the computer on the job (a rapidly diminishing number) typically have one at home for Internet access and email.

For some workers, a free personal computer for home use is a perk of their job. Ostensibly, employer-provided computers upgrade the technical skills of employees and their families. Practically, these computers seductively enter the home, and work hours are extended into what was once leisure time.

Computers not only further our isolation from one another but also create health problems. Some are placed on desks never meant to hold them. Keyboards and mouse pads are often in the wrong position for proper use, resulting in the pain and disability of carpal tunnel syndrome — now the most common workplace disability in America. We are also likely to resort to poor posture in an effort to compensate for the bad angle of the keyboard and, in many instances, the monitor, increasing the risk of low back pain, shoulder and neck pain, headaches, and other similar discomforts.

Adding to our problems is room lighting produced by either standard tungsten or fluorescent bulbs. We are deprived of full-spectrum light, the type found outdoors at noon. Such light stimulates our body's production of a natural tranquilizer and mood-elevating brain hormones. When you spend your day indoors, staring at a computer screen, without any sunlight, you may feel depressed for seemingly no reason. You are likely to feel emotionally uplifted if you take at least a brisk fifteen- to twenty-minute walk outdoors.

Computer use has also altered our eating habits in much the same way that early television use changed mealtime. The newness of television led many families to make TV-watching the focus of their lives. The dinner hour was shared with television news programs. Since many sets were placed in the living room or family room, dinners were moved to be near the sets. Family members, eating dinner from plates set on TV trays, abandoned conversation in favor of watching TV.

Soon normal preparation of food was considered a time-consuming nuisance and the TV dinner — a frozen meal of meat, vegetable, potato, and dessert — entered the home. The nutritional quality was questionable, but the convenience was undeniable.

Fast-food restaurants and takeouts are offering another time-saver that has had a negative impact on the diet. Between 1978 and 1995, people in the United States more than tripled the percent of calories they got from fast foods and almost doubled the percent they got at restaurants in general.[3] Restaurants may serve healthy food, but what people order has more fat, sodium, refined sugars, and calories than what people cook at home. Diets with nutritious meals are sabotaged by overindulgence in caffeinated beverages and snack foods — pastries, chips, and ice cream. Sugar and caffeine are stimulants that enable people to work longer hours than are healthy, increasing the risk of heart disease, hypoglycemia, diabetes, and obesity.

We could go on and on about the way modern lifestyles contribute to unhealthy habits. Frequent flyers on airplanes know they might experience headaches from dehydration. Driving to more places increases our risk of being in an accident simply because our way of life puts us on the roads more. "Weekend warriors" — sedentary workers active in sports on weekends — know their muscles will ache on Monday. The late-night movie watcher expects to be tired the next morning.

Physicians are seeing the common complaints linked to these lifestyle changes. Patients say they are tired. Many have headaches or chronic back pain. Depression is frequently mentioned, and many admit their relationships are strained. Many visit doctors asking for a sleeping pill or an antidepressant. Others seek a stimulant. Still others want a tranquilizer. Some worry that they might have chronic fatigue and immune dysfunction syndrome, fibromyalgia, or the early stages of heart disease or cancer. If a doctor asks about their spiritual life, they smile a bit sheepishly and say that Sunday is often their only day of rest — unless their children have a baseball game, a soccer game, a . . .

Do You Need a Remedy or a Lifestyle Change?

Perhaps you see yourself in this situation. You probably have seen it in friends and coworkers. You wonder what you can do. You may have heard that some have found relief from a particular pharmaceutical, an herbal supplement, acupuncture, or some other form of health care. What you may not have heard is that all of these therapies, conventional and alternative, may be helping people avoid their true need while, in some cases, putting them at further risk. These remedies may bring relief for the moment, but something more fundamental may need to change. The person may have a real medical problem that is being ignored. The lifestyle may even be compounding existing medical problems.

Before we look at how to analyze your lifestyle to determine whether anything is adversely affecting your health, consider the following principles.

First Do No Harm

Perhaps the classic story of the man who ignored medical advice is that of runner and author James Fixx. The author came from a family of men with a history of heart disease that killed them when they were in their early forties. All had been overweight and underexercised, so Fixx decided to be the exception.

Fixx changed his diet and began running. At first he could pass only a couple of houses before becoming so winded he'd have to slow to a walk. After a while he could run from one end of his suburban street to the other before pausing to catch his breath. Then he went around the block. Over time, his distances increased and his weight decreased. He became fit and trim. He began writing bestselling books showing others how they could do what he did.

He also stopped seeking medical advice, even though, because of his genetic heritage, he remained at high risk for heart problems. Mild chest discomfort while running did lead him back to his doctor, who recommended tests to determine whether he needed medicine, surgery, or both to treat his heart problem. His prognosis, with treatment, was excellent.

Instead of keeping the appointment, Fixx decided to run out the pain. Most athletes experience a certain amount of discomfort in the early stages of exertion. Then their bodies begin producing beta-endorphins, natural painkillers that allow them to continue their activity without further problems. Long-distance runners know that once they get "through the pain" and "into the zone," they'll feel better and be able to continue for a few more miles. This phenomenon is called "the runner's high."

Beta-endorphins are a natural reaction to discomfort. They are not some naturally produced medication that can heal what is wrong with the body. If anything, they mask the seriousness of a symptom.

Fixx apparently believed that his natural beta-endorphins could deal with his chest pain and continued running. His body was found by the side of the road. He died, like other men in his family, in his forties from a heart attack. The sad part of the story is that if Fixx had combined his admirable new lifestyle with a medically appropriate program designed specifically for his damaged heart, his life might have been dramatically prolonged.

Rule Out Any Medical Problems

What does all this mean for you? Before you embark on any lifestyle changes, especially any alternative therapies or remedies, see a doctor to rule out any medical problems, whether you have any symptoms or not. Early diagnosis and proper treatment can mean the difference between life and death. In this initial medical review, you should do the following:

- **Have a physical exam** to learn if you have any health problems that must be addressed in conventional ways.

- **Examine your lifestyle** to determine how it might be creating or contributing to any "symptoms" or ailments.
- **Inform your physician** (one you can trust) of your entire lifestyle — exercise, diet, and unusual stress factors (divorce, loss of a loved one, loss of a job, a new marriage or child, a move to a new house).
- **Ask your physician** to review all prescription medications as well as the vitamins, dietary supplements, herbal products, and over-the-counter medications you take.
- **Talk with your pharmacist** about possible interactions between the medications and nutritional supplements you take, even any infrequently taken over-the-counter products.

Take the "Four Wheels" Assessment

Examining your lifestyle may be just as important for your health and sense of well-being as having a periodic exam by a physician. Lack of rest, lack of adequate daylight exercise, a faulty diet, concerns about your job, and pressures from family and friends and even church may all have a negative effect on your health.

Walt has developed a number of assessment tools that allow you to evaluate your physical, emotional, relational, and spiritual health in less than thirty minutes. Different tools for adults, teenagers, and children are available in his book *God's Design for the Highly Healthy Person* and via the Internet at no cost.[4]

Take the Lifestyle Exam

Another evaluation to consider as you plan for making lifestyle changes involves asking yourself the following questions. There are no right or wrong answers. These questions are meant to focus your awareness on issues that may be influencing your stress level and affecting your health. Some may not apply to you; others could be key.

1. What is the average time you spend walking outdoors during daylight hours each day? Include going to and from a parking lot or public transportation pickup point if the distance is at least a half mile. Include lunchtime activity, though not if you regularly pause at store windows or go in and out of shops to briefly check merchandise. The ideal is at least a twenty-minute, uninterrupted walk each day during daylight hours.

2. Do you regularly take the stairs at work? If you are on an upper floor of your building, do you walk up at least one flight of stairs? You might walk a flight and then catch the elevator or take the elevator to a floor just below your own. You might also walk up one flight from your office, then catch the elevator to go down to the lobby. However you do it, walking up at least one flight of steps enhances your cardio-vascular system.

3. What type of lighting do you have at work and at home? Is it bright or subdued? Do you have full-spectrum bulbs or traditional fluorescent or incandescent lights? If the latter, arrange to replace them with full-spectrum bulbs or add a light to your desk that will use such bulbs.

4. Can you open windows where you work, or do you work in a building that is sealed and recycles air? Sealed buildings, even with cleaned, recycled air, can pose health problems that don't occur in buildings with fresh air.

5. How many hours a week do you spend watching television? How long do you use a computer

in any manner — from working to surfing the Internet to using a DVD drive to enjoy a movie?

6. Do you live alone or in an emotionally unsatisfying relationship?

7. Do you feel loved and needed by a spouse, other family members, friends, or coworkers?

8. Do you enjoy activities with others? These might include religious services and programs, such as Bible study as well as social clubs and athletic leagues. Do you participate regularly or just occasionally?

9. How many times a week do you eat convenience foods? Include meals in fast-food restaurants, snack foods, and prepackaged meals.

10. How many times a week do you eat fresh fruits and vegetables?

11. When you go out to lunch in a restaurant or coffee shop, do you focus on sandwiches and fries, or do you order salads and lunch specials that include a vegetable and lean meat, poultry, or fish?

12. Are you in a caretaker position for a loved one with a chronic illness such as Alzheimer's?

13. Do you have financial concerns you worry you cannot handle?

14. Do you work in a job requiring extensive overtime?

15. Do you work more than one job, either full- or part-time?

16. Do you regularly attend a religious service where you feel a part of the congregation?

17. Do you participate in spiritual activities with others, such as Bible study, prayer groups, or food programs?

18. Have you recently relocated, changed your job (or retired), had an illness, or lost a loved one?

19. How much restful sleep do you get on an average night?

20. How many mornings a week do you awaken feeling tired?

21. Do you drink plenty of fluids every day, or do you regularly feel thirsty, as though you have cotton balls in your mouth?

22. Do you keep putting off activities that give you pleasure because you feel you should use that time in some other "useful" way?

23. Do you have any personal space at home or at work? This is an area that might have flowers or pictures, personal mementos or special collectibles, handicrafts from children — items that can make you smile, remind you of loved ones, help you relax.

24. How often do you have a quiet time with the Lord, and how often do you take time to read the Bible and pray — alone?

25. Do you feel overly obligated to others? Do you feel you should say no more often but cannot bring yourself to do it?

26. Do you serve others in a regular way? This is important among friends and family and those we don't know. When you do serve others, are you grateful for the opportunity or resentful?

27. Are you your own harshest critic, or do you have a healthy appreciation for the unique and special person you are in God's eyes?

28. Do you see the role God has for you in life and the gifts and talents he has given you that bring purpose to your life?

29. When you spend time with your spouse or children, are you happy to be with them or worried about your busy schedule? What would they say?

30. Do you have a friend who knows your loftiest dreams and your deepest fears? Do you know

what they are? Does anyone know what character issue God is working on in your life at the moment? Do you know?

Did you recognize other areas that are negatively impacting your physical, spiritual, and emotional well-being? Consider how you can modify your lifestyle to improve your quality of life. If you're tired, how can you get more sleep? If you're overweight, how can you modify your diet and get more exercise? For most people, a change in lifestyle alone will result in at least some improvement in their health.

Maybe the first step you need to take is a risky one. Do you have anyone you could talk to about the issues raised by these questions? If not, we believe you would benefit immensely from using these questions to help you get to know someone better. If you are married, your spouse would be an ideal person. If you are involved in a church or small group, someone there might be a good candidate. There can be great benefits from having a friend of the same gender with whom you can talk about these sorts of issues. We know that asking someone to talk about personal issues can raise feelings of uncertainty or embarrassment. But once you do, you may find that they have had similar questions or concerns about their health. Use our questions as a rough guideline to start talking about these issues. As your friendship develops, you may find you want to start to exercise together, or support one another as you improve your diet, or pray together, or study the Bible, or just get out and have some relaxing fun

together. The important thing is to start to address the unhealthy habits these questions may reveal and make the healthy lifestyle choices you may have been neglecting.

If you also need some form of aggressive medical treatment, don't make the mistake James Fixx and others have made. For anyone with a medical problem, lifestyle changes must be a part of proper treatment, as prescribed by a doctor.

What the Alternatives Can Offer

You've seen your doctor, who finds no medical problems. You've changed your diet — cut down on fats and added more vegetables and fruits, more whole grains. You now walk four times a week. And you've become actively involved in a good church, gaining a few friends you see regularly.

But you wonder if there's more you can do, should do. Alternative medicine seems to have so much to offer. You hear about the megadoses of vitamins and herbal remedies that people are taking to prevent a laundry list of ailments, and the "therapist" who helped a man with back pain. Are these for real? Should you try some of them?

In the next chapter we explain how you can get answers to these questions and get the most out of the information on specific therapies and remedies detailed in the rest of the book.

Chapter 6: Healthy Lifestyles

1. BBC, "Lack of Sleep 'Risks Lives,'" *BBC News*, September 19, 2000. *BBC News: http://news.bbc.co.uk/hi/english/health/newsid_930000/930615.stm* (October 30, 2005).

2. Lisa F. Berkman and Lester Breslow, *Health and Ways of Living: The Alameda County Study* (New York: Oxford University Press, 1983).

3. Bonnie Liebman and David Schardt, "Diet and Health: Ten Megatrends," *Nutrition Action Health Letter* 28, no. 1 (January/February 2001): 4 – 12.

4. Walt Larimore, *God's Design for the Highly Healthy Person* (Grand Rapids: Zondervan, 2005). *DrWalt.com: www.drwalt.com/PDF/hlthpers.pdf* (for adults); *www.drwalt.com/PDF/Assessteenhealth.pdf* (for teens); *www.drwalt.com/PDF/Assesschildhealth.pdf* (for children).

PART TWO

ALTERNATIVE THERAPIES

HOW TO USE THE REST OF THIS BOOK

To help you make better choices, the alternative therapies, herbal remedies, dietary supplements, and vitamins listed alphabetically in these next two parts of the book are presented as concisely as possible.

The entry for each therapy or remedy describes the origins of its use (What It Is) and the claims that are made: what some people claim it is useful for and how it is said to work (Claims).

The scientific information for each therapy or remedy is then presented (Study Findings). We summarize the results of all sorts of studies. Some studies support the claims made about each therapy, some contradict the claims, and others give evidence about possible harms. In describing the sorts of studies available on a remedy or therapy, we used a scale

of positive (✓) and negative (✗) symbols to indicate the overall strength of the evidence.

The same evidence scale is used to discuss what is known about possible or actual harmful effects of the therapies or remedies (Cautions). Contrary to the false claim that everything "natural" is safe, you will see that therapies and remedies can be dangerous — physically, mentally, or spiritually.

We conclude each entry with our overall recommendations about the therapy or remedy (Recommendations) and then categorize each remedy (Treatment Categories). Here we use a second easy-to-understand scale that shows not how effective or harmful a product may be but how confident we are either that a remedy is potentially effective (☺) or that it potentially has no benefit or may even be harmful (☹). For example, one symbol means we have some confidence that the remedy is effective; four symbols means we are very confident the remedy is potentially beneficial. We include a third symbol to alert readers to a need to monitor for serious adverse effects (⊘). Even if a therapy or remedy is effective, it may have serious side effects. This symbol will warn you if this is the case. One final symbol addresses spiritual concerns (☞). An effective therapy may still raise spiritual concerns. If so, this symbol will call this to your attention. We conclude each entry with a list of additional material we recommend should you want to study the therapy or remedy in more detail (Further Reading).

How We Rated the Evidence

Evidence Rating Scale

If you're having problems with your car, you could turn to lots of different people and places for help. You could come to us and ask our opinion. You should be warned, though, that we rarely do anything under the hood beyond checking the oil! You would be better served going to a car mechanic. But even then, different mechanics could make recommendations based on different evidence. One might tell you that the last dozen cars he has seen needed new spark plugs; therefore, that's what he recommends for your car. Another might take a quick look under the hood and tell you what she thinks the problem is. A third might run a number of tests and explain to you what the results indicated. Whose advice would you take?

Not all evidence is the same. The instruments used by the mechanic are not 100 percent foolproof,

and the results must be correctly interpreted. But they will tend to give more reliable evidence than a guess or a one-solution-fits-all approach.

The same situation exists regarding the evidence used to make decisions about therapies and remedies — whether conventional or alternative. There is not a *conventional* way to evaluate medicine and drugs and a different *alternative* way to evaluate alternative therapies and herbal remedies. Conventional, standard, alternative, new, and old therapies all need to be evaluated through the same evidentiary lens. If *any* therapy has evidence that it is harmful, you have the right to know that. If *any* therapy has no or little evidence that it is helpful or harmful, you have the right to know that. You have the right to know *all* the options available to you — as well as the cost, risks, and benefits of each — *and* the evidence supporting or refuting each.

This standard was summed up in a 2002 report issued by the White House Commission on Complementary and Alternative Medicine Policy, a body composed almost completely of advocates and practitioners of complementary and alternative medicine (CAM). It stated, "The Commission's position is that the same high standards of quality, rigor, and ethics must be met in both CAM and conventional medical research, research training, publication of research results in scientific and medical journals, presentations at research conferences, and review of products and devices."[1]

Modern health care practice is based on what is known as evidence-based practice. The underlying premise of this approach is that health care decisions should be based on the best evidence available. Health care professionals and researchers agree that a hierarchy exists among the types of evidence available for decision-making. The following table is adapted from the United States National Center for Complementary and Alternative Medicine.[2]

Hierarchy of Evidence	Type of Research
Highest	Large randomized controlled trial
↑	Small randomized controlled trial
	Uncontrolled trials
	Observational studies
↓	Case reports
Lowest	Anecdotes

The higher the research falls on the scale, the more confident we can be that decisions based on that evidence will lead to reliable and safe outcomes.

When none of the higher levels of research are available for a therapy, we must be more tentative in our recommendations and expectations. Alternative medicine is often recommended on the basis of other people's reports and testimonies (anecdotes). Unfortunately, this is the least reliable form of evidence that something works or is safe.

Evidence should be accurate and appropriate. Unfortunately, that's not always the case. For example, let's say dozens of randomized controlled trials support the use of a particular therapy for heart disease. That evidence should not be used to support the use of that therapy for treating an entirely different ailment.

In the Study Findings and the Cautions sections of Parts 2 and 3, we mention many studies. We developed one scale to use here so you can quickly gauge how high or low those studies fall on the hierarchy of evidence. If the evidence being discussed shows a therapy has benefit, we rated the *evidence* using a score of one to four ✓ symbols. The number of symbols was assigned according to the following criteria based on the amount of evidence and the type of evidence supporting the therapy.

Symbol	Type of Evidence
✓✓✓✓	Multiple high-quality randomized controlled trials demonstrate the efficacy and safety of this therapy.
✓✓✓	At least one randomized controlled trial or multiple nonrandomized trials support the efficacy and safety of this therapy.
✓✓	Nonrandomized series or numerous case reports in the peer-reviewed medical literature support the efficacy and safety of this therapy.
✓	Anecdotal evidence exists to support the efficacy and safety of this therapy.

Evidence against Using Therapies

Studies can also provide evidence that a therapy or remedy should not be used for a particular condition. Those results could be evidence either of a lack of effectiveness or of harmful effects. To represent these sorts of studies, we developed a similar scale of one to four ✗ symbols. If the studies showed either no benefit, the potential for harm, or actual harm, we rated the *evidence* (not the potential for harm) using the following criteria:

Symbol	Type of Evidence
✗✗✗✗	Multiple high-quality randomized controlled trials demonstrate the lack of benefit or the significant potential for harm with this therapy.
✗✗✗	At least one randomized controlled trial or multiple nonrandomized trials support the lack of benefit or the significant potential for harm with this therapy.
✗✗	Nonrandomized series or numerous case reports in the peer-reviewed medical literature support the lack of benefit or the significant potential for harm with this therapy.
✗	Anecdotal evidence exists to support the lack of benefit or the significant potential for harm with this therapy.

Overall Recommendation Scale

As more research has been conducted on alternative medicine, studies have sometimes produced conflicting evidence. A particular therapy can have some studies supporting its effectiveness or safety and other studies finding no benefits or pointing to some potential for harm. This is why evaluations of therapies and remedies should be as comprehensive as possible. Sometimes a news report will point out that a high-quality study found that a remedy was effective. However, before deciding whether this remedy should be recommended, the results of other studies should be examined. If this is the first study of this remedy, caution is needed until the results are confirmed. If other studies have been published, all the results should be taken into account before coming to an overall conclusion.

We compiled the results of all the studies we located into a single guide. This rating scale is our "best estimate" of the physical benefit of a remedy (☺ to ☺☺☺☺). We also give a confidence rating for therapies that are of no benefit or potentially harmful (☹ to ☹☹☹☹) for particular conditions. When a therapy or remedy is commonly used for a number of indications, we have developed separate recommendations. All of these are presented under the Treatment Categories section.

Overall Recommendation	Criteria
☺☺☺☺	75% – 100% confidence that the therapy is potentially beneficial (the potential benefits outweigh the risks)
☺☺☺	50% – 74% confidence that the therapy is potentially beneficial
☺☺	25% – 49% confidence that the therapy is potentially beneficial
☺	0% – 24% confidence that the therapy is potentially beneficial
☹	0% – 24% confidence that the therapy is of no benefit or potentially harmful (the risks outweigh the potential benefits)
☹☹	25% – 49% confidence that the therapy is of no benefit or potentially harmful
☹☹☹	50% – 74% confidence that the therapy is of no benefit or potentially harmful
☹☹☹☹	75% – 100% confidence that the therapy is of no benefit or potentially harmful

One of the new features in this expanded edition is another scale of one to four ⊘ symbols. If a therapy or remedy raises concerns about serious adverse effects, these symbols are placed in the Treatment Categories section (Risk of Serious Side Effects). Even if evidence supports the effectiveness of a therapy or remedy, the risk of serious adverse effects may make its use unwarranted. If an entry has any of these symbols, read the Cautions section carefully.

Another new feature is an additional recommendation scale on spiritual concerns. Readers of the first edition expressed concern that our recommendations were unclear regarding therapies that raised spiritual questions and concerns. The first edition's recommendation scale only took scientific evidence into account. To make our spiritual evaluations more explicit, we have made two changes to this expanded edition. The first change is that the category of therapies called Energy Medicine in the first edition is now called Spiritual Therapies. These were explained in more detail in chapter 3. The second change is that when a therapy is included in the Spiritual Therapies category, a level of overall spiritual concern is assigned using the following scale. The greater the number of ☝ symbols, the greater our concern about the spiritual implications of the therapy.

Overall Spiritual Concern Level	Criteria
👎	We have some concerns about the therapy's spiritual roots or the way some practitioners use it. Once these are kept in mind, the practice may be helpful.
👎👎	The therapy developed within a spiritual worldview that conflicts with Christianity but can be divorced from those beliefs. Caution should be exercised in choosing a therapist.
👎👎👎	The therapy has significant spiritual connections and is most frequently practiced within a worldview in conflict with Christian beliefs. It should only be used under mature guidance.
👎👎👎👎	The therapy involves spiritual practices that are in direct conflict with biblical teaching. We cannot see any justification for Christians to use this therapy.

Underlying our concern here is a belief that effectiveness alone does not justify the use of any treatment. The search for cures and treatments must be influenced by the importance of upholding ethical principles and values. When these are not upheld, we end up with the situations that underlie many of today's bioethical controversies. For example, therapies that kill human embryos or practices that intentionally kill patients should not be accepted, no matter how beneficial they are.

When someone is sick or dying, he or she is tempted to try any therapy or remedy, alternative or conventional, looking for a cure. Such thinking should not be accepted by Christians for reasons we discussed in chapter 3. With alternative medicine, an unbiblical spiritual practice should not be accepted as a therapy even if it is effective. People of faith should seek to do all things to the glory of God,

and that includes being willing to forgo therapies that are spiritually inappropriate.

The Implications of Current Regulations

The alternative medicine scene today is a huge business. So is conventional medicine. However, doctors, nurses, nutritionists, hospitals, pharmacies, pharmaceutical companies, and most other aspects of conventional medicine are heavily regulated and scrutinized. These safeguards protect patients from many, but not all, harms. They go a long way toward ensuring that most health care professionals are adequately trained and most products are of good quality.

The same cannot be said of complementary and alternative medicine (CAM). The White House Commission mentioned earlier noted that regulation of CAM was highly variable and in some areas nonexistent. The report stated that it was premature to recommend or reimburse for CAM therapies and remedies because most have not been shown to be effective or safe. Some sort of regulation is needed, with the report recommending, "Decisions on regulating the use of and reimbursement for CAM therapies should be based on published evidence of safety (including toxicity, side effects, and adverse interactions), clinical efficacy, general effectiveness, and cost-effectiveness and cost-benefit analyses rather than on traditional use, anecdotal reports, consumer interest, and market demand."[3]

Yet in spite of these recommendations, great variability exists in the quality and nature of the products and services available within alternative medicine. This means that all of the recommendations made in this book must be qualified. Even if we report that the evidence favors using a particular remedy, care must be taken in picking a high-quality brand. Even if we report that the evidence favors using a particular therapy, care must be taken in picking a therapist.

Many of these problems arise because of the way alternative medicine is regulated in the United States. Until effective oversight and regulation are in place, additional caution must be exercised in deciding which brand of remedy to use and which therapist to see. Learning as much as possible about the therapies and remedies is the first step in making wise decisions. The following guidelines should provide additional help when choosing a product or therapist.

Picking a Brand

Since 1994, dietary supplements, vitamins, and herbal remedies have been regulated in the United States under the Dietary Supplement Health and Education Act (DSHEA). They are not subject to the strict regulations that govern over-the-counter drugs and prescription medications. Studies show that dietary supplements sold in the United States are frequently of poor quality.[4]

Currently, the only guidance for product quality comes from independent agencies. For example, products that claim to be produced to the United States Pharmacopeia (USP) standards of quality, purity, and potency (and carry the USP symbol on their label) are supposed to be laboratory tested and theoretically should be of higher quality — but may not be — than products not meeting this standard. The United States Pharmacopeia is an independent pharmacy organization, not a government agency. A commercial company doing something similar makes its conclusions available to anyone subscrib-

ing to its website (*www.consumerlab.com*). This company has tested hundreds of products in three ways: (1) to be sure the product contains what the label claims, (2) to be sure the product has no contaminants, and (3) to be sure the product is actually absorbable by the human body.

Recognize the dangers and use caution. Even if studies are available to show that a substance is effective and safe, different brands will be of different quality. If you decide to use a particular substance, first try to find a brand that has been certified by an independent testing laboratory (such as USP or consumerlab.com) or another country's regulatory agency. If neither is available, try to find a brand that seems to work well for you and stay with that brand.

Picking a Therapist

In addition to knowing about a therapy, you must exercise discernment when choosing a practitioner to provide the therapy. The same therapy can be practiced in different ways. For example, a Christian chiropractor could treat you holistically, in a biblical sense, based on the best scientific evidence available for your condition, including referring you to a conventional physician when needed. Another chiropractor may claim to be able to treat all of your ailments, manipulate your aura, introduce you to Eastern meditation, and try to sell you dietary supplements. Both are practicing what they call "holistic health care," but their approaches are different, and what their patients receive is very different.

Part of the problem arises because training programs within much of alternative medicine vary. For example, an acupuncturist could be a physician with much medical knowledge who has taken a short course in acupuncture, or someone who has trained for years under an experienced traditional acupuncturist, or someone with no health care training who has attended a few weekend sessions on acupuncture. Some of the more esoteric therapies (such as Reiki, shamanism, and herbalism) are even more variable.

Another complication arises when practitioners mix different therapies. You may think you are receiving only a massage when in fact the practitioner is mixing massage with Therapeutic Touch and color therapy.

Because of these differences in practitioners' training and approach, it is important to investigate each practitioner before agreeing to receive therapy. Ask questions of the practitioner and staff. Ask for references. Seek the advice of others. Take your time.

Consider carefully not only the therapy but also the character and worldview of those offering the treatment. Medical literature now gives health care providers guidance on discussing issues of spirituality with patients. One such tool uses the mnemonic SPIRIT to remind physicians of the types of questions they might ask patients.[5] You could use the same types of questions to gather information on a therapist's spiritual views.

S for spiritual belief system. Ask therapists to describe their belief system.

P for personal spirituality. Ask what they believe personally and how important spirituality is to them.

I for integration into a spiritual community. Ask if they are involved in a spiritual group, formally or informally.

R for rituals and restrictions. Ask if they include any spiritual rituals in their

therapies, or if their beliefs restrict them from offering certain therapies.

I for implications for medical care. Most important, ask how their spiritual beliefs impact the care and therapies they offer.

T for terminal care (probably the least relevant here). Ask about how their beliefs impact the care they offer when patients reach the end of their lives.

In Walt's book *God's Design for the Highly Healthy Person*, he suggests ways of interviewing your physician about spiritual issues.[6] You can use some or all of these same questions with an alternative therapist. Asking these questions in an interview style might not be comfortable or even appropriate. You may instead want to look for opportunities to raise these sorts of questions informally during a visit. You might phrase the questions in ways to find out how "pushy" the therapist might be about the spiritual dimensions of the therapy (if they exist). Taking such a "spiritual history" on a therapist will alert you to potential conflicts — before they become an issue. It can help you avoid those therapists who want to draw you away from your faith and convert you to their religious beliefs. Remember, attractive remedies may sometimes be nothing more than lures to draw people into deception. The following are examples of the types of questions to ask.

1. Are you willing to consider my spiritual preferences as you care for me?
2. Are you open to discussing the religious or spiritual implications of my health care?
3. Are you willing to work with my spiritual mentors (pastor, priest, rabbi, elder) and other members of my health care team (family, friends, mentor, support group) in providing me with the best possible health care?

4. Are you willing to pray with me — or for me — if I feel the need for prayer?

5. What does spirituality mean to you? How much is religion (and God) a source of strength and comfort for you?

6. Have you ever had an experience that convinced you that God or a higher power exists?

7. How strongly religious or spiritually oriented do you consider yourself to be?

8. Do you pray? If so, how frequently?

9. Do you attend religious worship times? If so, how often do you generally attend?

Unfortunately, we know that some therapists (not all) are not honest with patients about their therapies. Possibly some are deceived themselves about the nature of what they are doing. Others are being deceptive. We have been contacted by people receiving therapies about which they have felt uneasy. When they asked the therapists about possible spiritual aspects to the therapies, they were assured there were none. Yet books and websites describing these therapies make it clear they are spiritual, sometimes even linked with the occult. Great caution is needed when investigating unfamiliar therapies, especially those that claim to involve any sort of nonphysical energy.

As you investigate a therapist, bathe your investigation in prayer. Seek out the counsel of mature believers, especially those familiar with occult, New Age, and other spiritual practices. Search for information on the practices and schools of therapy. If you are not convinced of the importance of doing this, reflect on the following Scriptures:

> The Spirit clearly says that in later times some will abandon the faith and follow deceiving spirits and things taught by demons.
>
> *1 Timothy 4:1*

> For the time will come when men will not put up with sound doctrine. Instead, to suit their own desires, they will gather around them a great number of teachers to say what their itching ears want to hear. They will turn their ears away from the truth and turn aside to myths.
>
> *2 Timothy 4:3 – 4*

Chapter 7: How to Use the Rest of This Book

1. White House Commission on Complementary and Alternative Medicine Policy, *Final Report March 2002*, 40. *White House Commission on Complementary and Alternative Medicine Policy: www.whccamp.hhs.gov/finalreport. html* (March 28, 2002). We do not agree with all of the report's recommendations. For a more complete evaluation of the report, see Dónal P. O'Mathúna, *Alternative Medicine: A Response to the White House Commission on Complementary and Alternative Medicine Policy* (2002). *Christian Medical Association: www.cmdahome.org/index. cgi?BISKIT=2639447799&CONTEXT=art&art=2180* (August 31, 2005).

2. National Center for Complementary and Alternative Medicine, *Expanding Horizons of Healthcare: Five-Year Strategic Plan 2001 – 2005. National Center for Complementary and Alternative Medicine: http://nccam.nih. gov/about/plans/fiveyear/index.htm* (August 30, 2005).

3. White House Commission on Complementary and Alternative Medicine Policy, *Final Report March 2002*, 47 – 48.

4. Walter L. Larimore and Dónal P. O'Mathúna, "Quality Assessment Programs for Dietary Supplements," *Annals of Pharmacotherapy* 37, no. 6 (June 2003): 893 – 98.

5. Todd A. Maugans, "The SPIRITual History," *Archives of Family Medicine* 5 (January 1996): 11 – 16.

6. Walt Larimore, *God's Design for the Highly Healthy Person* (Grand Rapids: Zondervan, 2005), 250 – 51.

CHAPTER 8

REVIEWS
OF THERAPIES

See chapter 7 for a complete explanation of how we rated the evidence to arrive at our recommendations. Keep in mind that we rated the *evidence*, not the benefit, based on the types of research conducted, the amount of research, and the methods used by the researchers. We detail the research on effectiveness of a therapy and the research that provides a warning that a therapy is of no benefit or could even be harmful.

In the listings of specific uses for the therapies, we rank not the effectiveness of a therapy but our *confidence* that a specific therapy is *potentially* beneficial. We use the ☺ symbol for those therapies that are potentially beneficial and the ☹ symbol for a therapy that is potentially harmful. The more confident we are that a therapy is potentially beneficial (or potentially harmful) based on the research, the more symbols, from one to four. Physical side effects are highlighted with the ⊘ symbol and spiritual concerns with the ☝ symbol, again from one to four.

ACUPRESSURE

What It Is

Acupressure involves applying pressure to specific points (acupoints) on the body using fingers, hands, elbows, or knees. Pressure can be applied by therapists or patients themselves, or by elasticized bands that press a stud onto the person's skin. Acupressure developed within traditional Chinese medicine (TCM). (See the Traditional Chinese Medicine entry to understand how acupressure is believed to work.) Central to its development is the notion of *chi* (pronounced CHEE), a nonphysical life energy central to good health in TCM. When its flow has been interrupted, pressure on the appropriate "acupoints" is believed to relieve energy blockages. An acupoint is the precise location on the skin on which pressure (or a needle) is believed to bring about a biological effect. There are some two thousand acupoints said to be interconnected. Acupressure (and acupuncture) practitioners work with acupoints to balance energy flow and restore health.

Acupressure led to the development of a Japanese form of massage called Shiatsu (which literally means "finger pressure"). Unlike typical massage, shiatsu massage is carried out to balance the flow of *chi* by applying pressure at various acupoints using practitioners' fingers, thumbs, elbows, knees, or feet.

Claims

Acupressure is most commonly believed to reduce nausea and vomiting when pressure is applied to an acupoint called P6 or Inner Gate, located between the tendons on the forearm, three fingers' width from the first wrist crease. Some companies market a do-it-yourself acupressure device with small metal or wooden balls positioned on a strap in such a way that when the device is strapped around the wrist, a ball will press on P6. These are sold in stores catering to boaters, air travelers, and others who suffer from motion sickness. They are also being investigated to prevent nausea and vomiting caused by chemotherapy or anesthesia.

Another acupoint between the thumb and index finger (called Meeting of the Valleys) is believed to help digestion. Acupressure is also believed to relieve pain, particularly headaches, back pain, and migraines.

Some claim acupressure can treat and cure just about every illness and disease. An advertisement by a "Dr. J. V. Cerney" for a book called *Acupuncture Without Needles* claims acupressure "can rub away pain . . . gently massage away chronic illness . . . restore vigor and youthfulness." Once you buy the book, you can unlock "the mystery of your body's 'magic buttons' for safe, fast relief of almost any pain or ailment." The ad contains several pages of testimonials from satisfied customers relieved of everything from migraines to asthma to impotence. People are identified only by their first names, making it impossible to check whether they even exist. The ad ends with a list of more than eighty ailments acupressure is claimed to instantly relieve. An ad for another book on acupressure claimed it could reverse the aging process.

Study Findings

Research on acupressure has focused primarily on the relief of headaches, nausea, and vomiting. A 2004 Cochrane systematic review found several studies using P6 acupressure to prevent postoperative nausea and vomiting. Overall, acupressure was effective, and in some of the studies it was found to be as effective as conventional pharmaceuticals (✓✓✓). Several studies used wristbands to apply pressure to the P6 acupoint to relieve morning sickness. However, one systematic review of these studies found that, overall, the evidence was unclear when the size and quality of these studies were taken into account (✓✓). In addition, research on the most severe form of morning sickness, hyperemesis gravidarum, has found no evidence of benefit from acupressure (✗✗✗).

Studies (✓✓) using acupressure for headaches had mixed results. Based on the results of case studies, acupressure for smoking cessation was found to be better than just advice. Overall, though, there is no clear evidence (✓✓) that acupressure is effective for smoking cessation.

Objective studies have not demonstrated the existence of the acupoint and meridian system. Though there are charts mapping this invisible system, they are only guides. Traditional Chinese medicine teaches that acupoints vary from person to person. Western scientists question the validity of the entire concept.

Conventional medicine recognizes that acupressure works for some people some of the time, especially for preventing nausea and vomiting and to some extent for relieving headaches. The question is whether acupressure is sometimes effective because it relieves energy blockage (as traditional Chinese medicine teaches), because of some poorly understood but scientifically verifiable mechanism, or because of the placebo effect.

Cautions

Although most treatments are gentle and acupressure is without serious side effects, some types of acupressure are applied with enough pressure to cause minor aches and pains that continue for hours after the procedure has been completed. More care is needed with some forms of Shiatsu massage, especially when practitioners use their elbows or feet.

Of greater concern is the belief system that can accompany these therapies. Belief in the concept of life energy and its manipulation is fundamental to Eastern religions. Certain acupressure teachers expose practitioners to these ideas and may want to convert patients to their beliefs. Some practitioners call on spiritual powers to assist in diagnosis and treatment, exposing patients to occult concepts and powers. People receiving Shiatsu massage sometimes report getting cold or flu symptoms. These are viewed by practitioners as evidence of a "healing crisis," believed to be caused as *chi* is unblocked. This appears highly speculative and should raise concerns about possible spiritual implications. For these reasons, Christians must use careful discernment when choosing a practitioner for any of these therapies with Eastern roots.

Recommendations

Readily available acupressure wristbands have had positive results in several trials for preventing nausea and vomiting. Patients who do acupressure on themselves may also be able to get some relief from certain forms of headaches. Such self-administered acupressure also avoids exposure to the Eastern religious beliefs underlying *chi*.

Therapists can give acupressure treatments that last as long as an hour and continue over several weeks. This affords ample opportunity to expose clients to the religious ideas underlying *chi* therapies. Research has not revealed much additional benefit when acupressure is carried out by therapists. Great care should be taken to ensure therapists do not call on inappropriate spiritual forces during treatment. Or choose a conventional therapist — a physical therapist or physician — who could teach you to perform acupressure on yourself.

Treatment Categories

Complementary

To treat nausea and vomiting	☺☺☺☺
To relieve headaches	☺☺
To treat morning sickness	☺
To help with smoking cessation	☹☹

Scientifically Unproven

For any other indication

Spiritual

In the hands of some practitioners ☞

Further Reading

Cassileth, Barrie R. *The Alternative Medicine Handbook.* New York: W. W. Norton, 1998, 209 – 12.

Jewell, D., and G. Young. "Interventions for Nausea and Vomiting in Early Pregnancy." *The Cochrane Database of Systematic Reviews* 2003, no. 4.

Lee, A., and M. L. Done. "Stimulation of the Wrist Acupuncture Point P6 for Preventing Postoperative Nausea and Vomiting." *The Cochrane Database of Systematic Reviews* 2004, no. 3.

ACUPUNCTURE

What It Is

Acupuncture is a therapy, like acupressure, that evolved within traditional Chinese medicine. Traditionally, acupuncture is used in combination with other therapies. Fine needles are inserted into the skin just far enough so they don't fall out — a procedure that usually is painless. Both acupuncture and acupressure are based on the idea of the body having an invisible life energy force known as *chi* (pronounced CHEE) that is said to travel through invisible pathways known as meridians. The proper flow of *chi* helps all parts of the body adjust to various stresses, keeping the organs in balance (see the Traditional Chinese Medicine entry for more details).

Alteration or blockage of the normal flow of *chi* leads to imbalances in the body that can cause disease. Traditional Chinese medicine practitioners believe acupuncture restores the proper flow of *chi*.

The earliest surviving Chinese medical texts show 365 acupoints; contemporary charts show as many as 2,000. Each point is on a meridian that affects particular organs.

Originally, a single needle was inserted at each acupoint believed to be appropriate for restoring proper flow of *chi* based on the patient's symptoms. Today, many needles are inserted.

Small variations are sometimes used. The needles can be twirled after insertion into the skin to increase stimulation. Electroacupuncture sends tiny electric charges through the needles for added stimulation. Laser acupuncture uses lasers instead of needles. In a more traditional variation called "moxibustion,"

the ends of the needles protruding from the skin are heated with burning cones of the herb mugwort. The needles are not allowed to get hot enough to burn the patient. Mugwort leaves are known to have an antibiotic effect. However, in moxibustion, mugwort is believed to help restore the flow of *chi*, whether the cone is burned to heat acupuncture needles or the leaves are used alone.

Modern interest in acupuncture was sparked during President Richard Nixon's visit to China in 1972. A reporter on the trip underwent emergency surgery for acute appendicitis and later received acupuncture for pain. News accounts led to widespread interest in acupuncture.

But the news stories led to a misconception: that for centuries acupuncture was the standard anesthetic for surgery in China. Until recently, traditional Chinese medicine rarely used surgery. Acupuncture use as an anesthetic in the operating room is almost always in conjunction with traditional forms of anesthesia. The combination is believed to *reduce* the amount of conventional anesthetic needed, not eliminate the need.

Western medical scientists, not convinced of the existence of *chi* or meridians, have developed alternative theories about how acupuncture might work. One theory is that the needles release naturally occurring hormones called "endorphins" that regulate pain perception. Endorphin release reduces pain during childbirth. Athletes commonly experience the effect of endorphins when they run long distances. If acupuncture needles stimulate the release of these hormones, pain will be reduced.

Another theory is based on the observation that pain in one area of the body can be reduced when another area is irritated. Still other scientists say that acupuncture merely causes a placebo effect.

Claims

Acupuncture is most commonly believed to reduce pain, both acute pain, as with surgery, and chronic pain. Anecdotal accounts report the use of acupuncture to control asthma, reduce nausea and vomiting, reduce weight, treat chronic sinus and allergy symptoms, and help people give up addictive behaviors, such as cigarette smoking.

Study Findings

In November 1997, a panel at the National Institutes of Health (NIH) released a review of research on acupuncture. Of the more than two thousand studies, few were determined to be high-quality clinical studies. Although the popular press generally reported the panel's findings as positive, the report actually concluded there was little evidence to support most of the claims. Good-quality evidence (✓✓✓✓) on the effectiveness of acupuncture was found for the reduction of nausea and vomiting after chemotherapy or surgery and for relief of dental pain. Numerous studies (✗✗✗) have shown that acupuncture alone is not effective in controlling asthma or reducing weight. Studies (✗✗✗) also showed it was not effective in helping people to stop smoking. Studies with drug addiction have had mixed results, but a large recent study with more than six hundred cocaine-addicted participants found ear acupuncture no more effective than placebo (✗✗✗).

Another report released by the British Medical Association in June 2000 came to almost identical conclusions but reported new evidence concerning effectiveness of acupuncture with chronic pain. A number of controlled studies have been conducted for treating low back pain, but the results have been variable. A 2003 Cochrane review concluded that there was insufficient evidence to make any recommendations about acupuncture for *acute* low back pain (✗✗✗).

However, for *chronic* low back pain, acupuncture is more effective than no treatment or a sham treatment (✓✓✓✓). When combined with other therapies, additional benefits may arise, but these are small effects. Studies on recurrent headaches and migraines (✓✓✓) have shown some improvements but with inconsistent results. Given the great variability in the origins of and responses to pain, some people's pain responds well to acupuncture while others' pain does not.

For the many other uses of acupuncture, there is even less evidence of benefit.

Cautions

Acupuncture should not be used in the hope of curing an illness. It should not be used instead of proven effective therapies. However, it may relieve some symptoms and perceptions of illness. While infrequent, infections have developed from the use of nonsterile acupuncture needles. In a couple of cases (✗), death resulted from needles puncturing a patient's lung.

Recommendations

Despite its limited effectiveness, acupuncture's low cost and relative safety can make it a viable option for some conditions, such as pain relief after dental procedures and the reduction of nausea and vomiting after chemotherapy or surgery.

Use great caution when choosing a therapist. Verify that the therapist has had adequate training. Acupuncturists who are physicians may have had little training in acupuncture. Those who adhere to acupuncture's roots in traditional Chinese medicine and religion may try to convert patients to their Eastern worldview. Others may call on spiritual powers to assist in treatments, thus exposing people to occult influences.

Treatment Categories

Complementary

To treat nausea and vomiting after chemotherapy or surgery	☺☺☺
To relieve dental pain	☺☺☺
To relieve headaches	☺
To treat chronic back pain	☺
To treat acute back pain	☹☹

Scientifically Unproven

To treat asthma	☹☹☹☹
To help with weight reduction	☹☹☹☹
To help with smoking cessation	☹☹☹☹
To treat addictions	☹☹☹☹

Scientifically Questionable

For any other indication

Spiritual

In the hands of some practitioners 👎👎

Further Reading

British Medical Association. *Acupuncture: Efficacy, Safety and Practice*. Amsterdam: Harwood Academic, 2000.

National Institutes of Health, Consensus Development on Acupuncture. "Acupuncture." *Journal of the American Medical Association* 280, no. 17 (November 1998): 1518–24.

APPLIED KINESIOLOGY

What It Is

"Applied kinesiology" began in 1964 when chiropractor George Goodheart noted that weakness in certain muscles could be corrected by massaging seemingly unrelated muscles. (Applied kinesiology must be distinguished from the discipline known as kinesiology, or biomechanics, which is the scientific study of movement.) Goodheart's work was initially based on research done about twenty years earlier concerning the evaluation of disability by a series of noninvasive muscle tests. Goodheart's work went much further, developing the idea that muscle dysfunction could be used to identify specific problems with glands and organs.

Within the theory of applied kinesiology, overall health is seen as involving a complex interaction among structural, chemical, and mental components, all requiring many different therapies. For example, the structural health of the body is maintained by conventional dentistry as well as chiropractic and acupuncture. Chemical health is promoted through the use of herbal remedies, homeopathy, and conventional medicine. And mental health is achieved through relaxation, energy medicine, and Bach flower remedies. The treatments recommended by applied kinesiologists may involve any combination of those listed here or other alternative therapies.

According to applied kinesiology, the various muscle groups are connected to the body's vital organs and systems through interconnected "energy circuits" similar in concept to the meridians found in traditional Chinese medicine. To diagnose a problem, the strength of large muscles is tested. For example, patients are asked to hold their arms out straight. Practitioners place their fingers on patients' arms and apply firm but gentle pressure. If a patient resists this pressure and the resistance feels normal to the practitioner, the systems related to the arm muscles are considered normal. If a muscle feels weak or sags under pressure, that's the sign of a problem. Further tests are carried out on other muscles to pinpoint the problem. Muscle weakness is said to be caused by life energy imbalances, physical problems, dietary deficiencies, and allergies.

Making this topic even more confusing, one estimate claims there are more than fifty types of applied kinesiology systems — including Neural Organization Technique, Contact Reflex Analysis, Health Kinesiology, Neuro Emotional Technique, Jaffe-Mellor Technique, Nambudripad's Allergy Elimination Technique, Whole System HealthScan, Thought Field Therapy, the Dawson Program (also called "vibrational kinesiology"), and Body Talk.

Claims

Practitioners claim to be able to diagnose and treat most ailments, in particular chronic problems such as asthma related to allergies and environmental toxicity. To test for allergies, muscle strength is tested in the usual way. Then a solution of a food, chemical, bacteria, etc., is placed on the patient's stomach, lips, or tongue, and the same muscle is retested. Alternatively, a vial containing the solution is held by the patient. If the muscle seems as strong when retested, the patient is not allergic to the substance. If the muscle is weaker, the patient is said to have an allergy to the substance. This type of muscle testing is also used to detect deficiencies in nutrients, vitamins, or minerals.

Study Findings

There is no compelling scientific evidence that applied kinesiology works for diagnosing or treating any health problem. While many testimonials of successful diagnoses are reported (✓✓), controlled studies consistently find no supportive evidence (✗✗✗). One review found twenty published research reports on applied kinesiology, but none of the studies fulfilled even the basic requirements for a controlled study (✗✗). A small number of randomized double-blind studies have been carried out with applied kinesiology (✗✗✗). One study involved seven German patients with known anaphylactic reactions to wasp stings. Four applied kinesiology therapists tested each patient with twenty vials, ten containing wasp venom and ten placebos. None of the patients, therapists, or evaluating researchers knew what was in each vial. Applied kinesiology gave the correct result 51.9 percent of the time. This is the same rate as random guessing or coin tossing. The only therapist to get the correct result more than half the time was the one with almost no experience. In contrast, all patients tested positive for wasp venom allergy with two conventional allergy tests.

Applied kinesiology is not a true science. Not all practitioners apply the ideas in the same way. In controlled studies, different practitioners reach different diagnoses for the same patients (✗✗✗). Outcomes vary depending on the amount of pressure applied, the angle at which pressure is exerted, and whether the patient or the practitioner exerts pressure first.

Practitioners have tried to develop instruments to standardize the muscle-testing method, but without success. Even if such instruments were developed, additional time would be needed for testing to develop consistent replicated standards of diagnosis and treatment.

Cautions

While applied kinesiology may cause little harm, it could lead someone to postpone pursuing more conventional and effective diagnosis and treatment. Decisions based on unreliable testing methods may lead to extended suffering.

Caution should be exercised concerning the beliefs accompanying this practice. Practitioners who are strong advocates of life energy ideas may try to draw people into the New Age worldview. This is particularly the case with Touch for Health, an offshoot of applied kinesiology developed by John Thie, a chiropractor and colleague of Dr. Goodheart. This popularized version, which has been significantly influenced by New Age beliefs, focuses on the need to balance "energy" in the body.

Recommendations

There is little or no reliable evidence that applied kinesiology does anything more than provide reassurance to those who have not been able to find relief through conventional medicine. As such, when it offers comfort, it probably works through a complicated placebo effect. The specific treatments involved could waste valuable time and money. Given this and the close connections between some of its many variants and New Age ideology, there seems to be no valid reason for Christians to use this practice.

Treatment Categories

Scientifically Questionable

For any indication ☹☹☹☹

Spiritual

In the hands of some practitioners 👎👎

Quackery or Fraud

In the hands of some practitioners

Risk of Serious Side Effects

When effective care is postponed ⊘

Further Reading

Barrett, Stephen. "Applied Kinesiology: Muscle-Testing for 'Allergies' and 'Nutrient Deficiencies.'" *QuackWatch: www.quackwatch.org/01QuackeryRelatedTopics/Tests/ak.html.* Accessed October 30, 2005.

Lüdtke, R., B. Kunz, N. Seeber, and J. Ring. "Test-Retest-Reliability and Validity of the Kinesiology Muscle Test." *Complementary Therapies in Medicine* 9 (2001): 141–45.

Teuber, Suzanne S., and Cristina Porch-Curren. "Unproved Diagnostic and Therapeutic Approaches to Food Allergy and Intolerance." *Current Opinion in Allergy and Clinical Immunology* 3, no. 3 (June 2003): 217–21.

AROMATHERAPY

What It Is

The concept behind aromatherapy dates back thousands of years. Everyone knows the experience of encountering the aroma of a favorite food as it is being cooked for dinner, only to suddenly become hungry. We instantly remember the last time we ate that particular meal and the pleasure we experienced. We are anxious to repeat those feelings and look forward to when the food will be ready.

A woman wears a special perfume only when she plans an intimate rendezvous with her husband. The moment he becomes aware of the scent, he is aroused, anticipating the physical pleasure of his beloved.

Then there are the aromas of special places — the mix of hay, manure, and sweat we knew from a time spent happily caring for a horse on a grandparent's farm; the rose garden in which we played as children; the salty air of the seashore we visited on our honeymoon. Perfume companies experiment with scents to find ways to sell fragrances that will revive personal aromatic pleasures of long ago.

The universal way an aroma can affect people seems to be acknowledged in the Bible. Exodus 29:18 describes the aroma of sacrificial offerings: "Then burn the entire ram on the altar. It is a burnt offering to the LORD, a pleasing aroma, an offering made to the LORD by fire."

Aromatherapy is the systematic use of volatile oils to improve a person's well-being. Plants contain many constituents, including compounds that are not water soluble. These can be extracted from the plants using other oils (such as castor oil or olive oil), by pressing on the plants, or by distilling the oil. Many of the oils produced in this manner have pleasant aromas. They are then diluted with other oils, such as sunflower oil or sweet almond oil, and the resulting mix is usually massaged into the skin by an aromatherapist.

A variation of this practice involves heating oils to give a room a pleasant scent. Oils may also be added to baths.

Claims

Aromatherapy adds a relaxing element to a lingering bath or a massage. Rooms with aromatic scents are believed to create a calmer atmosphere and relieve stress. For these reasons, aromatherapy is used by some as an adjunct to analgesics for people with a variety of painful conditions.

Various specific claims are made for particular aromatherapy oils, much like the claims for herbal remedies. Each oil contains compounds particular to the plant from which it was obtained. For example, eucalyptus oil is said to treat infections. Rose oil is used to regulate menstruation. And lavender oil is said to promote the healing of burns and wounds as well as having a calming effect.

Study Findings

Oils have been used medicinally for centuries, but little research has been done on their effects. Certainly, smells can elicit memories and emotions that can influence people's thoughts and feelings (✓✓✓✓). Most people can relate to feeling at ease (or uncomfortable) walking into a room with an aroma associated with a pleasant (or disturbing) memory.

Aromatherapy accompanied by a massage and involving an interaction with a caring provider does bring short-term relief from stress and anxiety (✓✓✓). However, a controlled study found that depression was relieved as much by a massage as by aromatherapy (✗✗✗). Research done with cancer patients found little additional benefit in reducing anxiety or improving overall well-being from aromatherapy compared to regular massage (✗✗✗), though both were better than no intervention (✓✓✓). A recent high-quality randomized controlled trial found aromatherapy no more effective than placebo in improving cancer patients' quality of life (✗✗✗).

A small number of preliminary studies have found that people experience some relief from pain during aromatherapy (✓✓). Oils used in these studies came from herbs with pain-relieving or anti-inflammatory reputations, such as chamomile, marigold, and willow.

Claims that certain oils can cure or prevent illnesses or diseases have little evidence to support them (✗✗✗). One study examined whether aromatherapy reduced nausea and vomiting in patients after surgery. Pads were soaked in peppermint oil, rubbing alcohol, or salt water. Patients requested antiemetic drugs much less frequently when given the aromatic pads, though no odor was any better than another. Researchers concluded that the benefits were due not to the specific aroma but to the way patients focused on their breathing while inhaling the vapors. A placebo response seems as plausible.

Someone who is seriously ill is likely to feel better after aromatherapy, but such feelings do not indicate that the illness itself has been improved. Most claims made for aromatherapy have not been tested, and research into therapeutic aromatherapy (or aromatology) is only beginning. Early results have shown that certain aromas influence brain activity of areas affecting sexual arousal or appetite (✔✔). Whether this will lead to products that, for example, help people attempting to diet remains to be seen.

Cautions

When used as recommended, aromatherapy oils are generally safe and soothing for most people. However, these are plant products and some people may be allergic to them.

Other potential hazards may arise because these oils are very concentrated. They should never be taken internally. Some ingredients are absorbed through the skin during proper use, so large amounts could lead to potentially troublesome side effects. A number of oils (particularly from pennyroyal, parsley seed, and juniper) have reputations for causing abortions and thus should not be used during pregnancy. Children should be massaged with only small quantities of oils that have already been well diluted.

Recommendations

Aromatherapy provides a pleasant (though not always inexpensive) means of relaxing. No evidence supports claims that the oils prevent or cure any illnesses. As with all forms of natural products, care should be taken to use reputable brands. Higher price tags do not necessarily mean higher quality. Some products have been adulterated with cheaper, synthetic oils. Aromatherapy oils are highly concentrated extracts of plants that can cause problems if taken internally. The oils should be kept out of the reach of young children.

Treatment Categories

Complementary
To promote relaxation and
   relieve stress or anxiety   ☺☺☺
To treat pain   ☺☺
To improve quality of life
   in cancer patients   ☺

Scientifically Unproven
For most specific healing uses

Scientifically Questionable
To treat or prevent diseases   ☹☹☹

Quackery or Fraud
In the hands of some practitioners

Further Reading

Anderson, Lynn A., and Jeffrey B. Gross. "Aromatherapy with Peppermint, Isopropyl Alcohol, or Placebo Is Equally Effective in Relieving Postoperative Nausea." *Journal of PeriAnesthesia Nursing* 19, no. 1 (February 2004): 29–35.

Cooke, Brian, and Edzard Ernst. "Aromatherapy: A Systematic Review." *British Journal of General Practice* 50 (June 2000): 493–96.

AYURVEDIC MEDICINE

What It Is

Ayurveda is the traditional medicine of India. The word means "knowledge of life" and thus refers to a whole approach to living, incorporating medical, philosophical, and religious beliefs. Those parts of Ayurveda that deal with one's health are difficult to separate from the religious components.

The central belief of Ayurveda is that health involves balance among physical, mental, emotional, relational, spiritual, and environmental elements. If we don't look too closely at what this means, it seems compatible with contemporary Western medical thought and Christian beliefs. A more careful examination reveals otherwise.

In its traditional form, Ayurvedic medicine teaches that life is sustained by the nonphysical life energy called *prana*. Health exists when the body has a balanced flow of *prana*, a concept very similar to the *chi* of traditional Chinese medicine. When the flow of *prana* is blocked or out of balance, people get ill, age, and die.

Energy balance, Ayurvedic practitioners believe, is not just internal. Such balance is also needed among people and their environments, a concept they say is based on a belief in the unity and interconnectedness of the universe.

According to Ayurveda, at conception each person is given a unique combination of what are called the three *doshas* — *vata*, *pitta*, and *kapha*. Since no two people have the same *dosha* combination, a practitioner must do an individualized typing and diagnosis to ensure the proper *dosha* balance for the patient. The diagnosis is made by examining the tongue, breathing patterns, and the pulse in ways that are believed to reveal information about *prana*. Prescriptions for restoring energy balance are also individualized.

Given that Ayurvedic medicine is actually a worldview, the practices recommended to balance *prana* and the *doshas* encompass every dimension of life. Meditation (of the Transcendental Meditation variety in the West) is viewed as essential for reducing stress and inducing altered states of consciousness. These changes are said to allow people to attain insight into their health and spirituality.

Ayurvedic practitioners use numerous products and practices to improve people's health. These include diet, exercise, meditation, massage, controlled breathing, *rasayanas* (herbal supplements), gemstones, *panchakarmas* (purification procedures), and *yagyas* (religious ceremonies to solicit the aid of Hindu deities).

Removal of toxins from the body is also important in Ayurvedic medicine. Negative thoughts, foods, and habits lead to the accumulation of *ama*, a negative form of energy. Purification practices include bloodletting with leaches, vomiting, laxatives, sinus cleansing, and enemas.

Deepak Chopra is the best-known proponent of Ayurvedic medicine in the United States (see p. 96). Chopra's version of Ayurveda includes the Pizzichilli treatment, in which two "technicians" massage and bathe a naked patient who reclines in a warm sesame oil bath for two hours. Formerly reserved for "the pleasure of the kings," this treatment is viewed as more appealing to Western customers than purging and bloodletting.

Claims

Ayurvedic medicine is a holistic approach to health and life. In its traditional setting, practitioners advise people on their diet, exercise, health, work, choice of spouse, sex life, personal habits, and religious beliefs. It emphasizes prevention of disease but also claims to be able to cure any and every disease. While increasing numbers of Westerners turn to Ayurvedic medicine, many Ayurvedic practitioners in India are increasingly adding conventional therapies to their practices.

Study Findings

No studies have examined Ayurvedic medicine as a complete medical system. The lifestyle changes recommended as part of Ayurveda's holistic approach to health may be beneficial if they are based on sound dietary, stress-reduction, and relational principles. No rigorous scientific evidence supports the claim that Ayurvedic remedies can cure serious diseases. This point is apparently acknowledged in India, where 75 percent of the preparations recommended by Ayurvedic practitioners were modern pharmaceutical drugs.

Some studies have been carried out on a few Ayurvedic herbs. Ancient Ayurvedic medical texts recommend 700 different herbs as medicinal. Many thousands of Ayurvedic preparations are recommended that have never been scientifically investigated (✗✗). Researchers in India note interest in more than 10,000 plant species, but fewer than 200 have been examined in any way. Case studies on a few Ayurvedic herbal remedies report some efficacy (✓✓). The quality of the studies done to date has been very poor. For example, a search for studies on Ayurvedic herbs used to treat diabetes found 1,311 articles. Among these, only 22 were clinical studies, and only one was of high quality. This review suggested that six preparations (including fenugreek) warranted further study in treating diabetes.

Cautions

Certain aspects of Ayurvedic medicine may be beneficial for disease prevention and promotion of a healthy lifestyle. Much of Ayurveda remains unproven, and some elements, such as the purification methods, may have serious side effects for some patients. In pursuing Ayurvedic medicine exclusively, people with serious illnesses may neglect more effective treatments.

Ayurvedic remedies have quality and authenticity problems. Authorities in India question whether commercial Ayurvedic preparations even conform to ancient Ayurvedic texts. The chair of the advisory board on Ayurvedic medicine to the Ministry of Health in India stated in the British journal *Lancet*, "The majority of Ayurvedic formulations on the market are either spurious, adulterated, or misbranded."

Confirmation of this claim came in 2004 in research carried out by Robert Saper and colleagues. They examined Ayurvedic herbal products manufactured in Asia and purchased in Boston-area stores. Fourteen of the seventy products (20 percent) contained levels of lead, mercury, or arsenic that exceeded maximum regulatory standards. The researchers warned that Ayurvedic practitioners often attribute therapeutic roles to mercury and lead. They claimed that perhaps 35 to 40 percent of Ayurvedic medicines contain at least one heavy metal. The authors recommended mandatory testing of these products because of the risk of heavy metal toxicity faced by users.

Other studies have had similar findings. In 2004, the Centers for Disease Control and Prevention (CDC) reported lead poisoning among adults in five states associated with Ayurvedic medications or remedies. And Health Canada in 2005 warned consumers not to use certain Ayurvedic products that contain high levels of lead, mercury, and/or arsenic. The agency notes that such products are not authorized for sale in Canada but warns consumers that they can be obtained outside Canada and over the Internet.

Also of concern is the intimate association between Ayurvedic medicine and Hinduism, along with its New Age variations, including the Transcendental Meditation movement. The holistic approach of Ayurvedic medicine means that practitioners are interested in all aspects of a patient's life, including religious beliefs, and will often suggest changes in those beliefs. While someone can obtain surgery or a drug from a physician without any questions about their belief system, this is not possible with an Ayurvedic practitioner.

Recommendations

Certain aspects of the Ayurvedic system are beneficial (such as some of its dietary and relaxation advice) and can be practiced without involving oneself in the philosophy of Ayurvedic medicine. The system should not be pursued to the neglect of conventional medicine, especially for serious illnesses. As an overall medical system and way of life, Ayurvedic medicine is so intertwined with Hinduism that Christians would find many conflicting beliefs.

Treatment Categories

Complementary
Certain aspects only ☺☺

Scientifically Unproven
Some herbs for diabetes ☺
Most herbs and other aspects ☹☹

Spiritual
Many Hindu practices 👎👎👎

Quackery or Fraud
In the hands of some practitioners

Further Reading

Kumar, Sanjay. "Indian Herbal Remedies Come Under Attack." *Lancet* 351 (April 1998): 1190.

Lalonde, Nathalie. "Some Ayurvedic Medicinal Products Contain High Levels of Heavy Metals." *Health Canada: www.hc-sc.gc.ca/ahc-asc/media/advisories-avis/2006/2006_46_e.html*. Accessed August 1, 2006.

Padma, T. V. "Ayurveda." *Nature* 436 (July 2005): 486.

Saper, Robert B., Stefanos N. Kales, Janet Paquin, Michael J. Burns, David M. Eisenberg, Roger B. Davis, and Russell S. Phillips. "Heavy Metal Content of Ayurvedic Herbal Medicine Products." *Journal of the American Medical Association* 292 (2004): 2868–73.

Shekelle, Paul G., Mary Hardy, Sally C. Morton, Ian Coulter, Swamy Venuturupalli, Joya Favreau, and Lara K. Hilton. "Are Ayurvedic Herbs for Diabetes Effective?" *Journal of Family Practice* 54, no. 10 (October 2005): 876–86.

BIOFEEDBACK

What It Is

One of the simplest ways to understand biofeedback is to think about how you drive a car, especially a stick shift. You probably don't even notice all the things you do. You certainly don't have to tell your foot when to move from the accelerator to the brake.

Now think back to when you were learning to drive. Did you watch the speedometer to know when to shift gears? Listen to the sound of the engine? Look down when you moved the gearshift lever from one position to another?

You learned to drive with the help of feedback from the various dials and sounds in your car. You learned to process the input automatically. You no longer need to consciously think about these things.

Biofeedback offers you the same sort of help as you learn to "operate" your body. Think of your body for a moment. You have been working under intense pressure. Your nerves are on edge. Your back aches. Your neck aches. You have a headache. You want to relax, but your mind is so focused on your work and how bad you feel, relaxing is impossible.

Enter the biofeedback machine. A variety of devices can be attached to your body by a biofeedback therapist. The machine might measure the electrical activity of your muscles, the temperature of your skin, or the dampness of your skin. An indicator tells you how tense you are. This might be a sound that rises or lowers in pitch, a dial with a needle that moves, or some other auditory or visual device. It can be as simple as a handheld thermometer that displays how your skin's temperature changes as you focus on warming your hand.

Just as you used to watch your car's speedometer or listen to the engine, you now watch or listen to the biofeedback machine. Just as you learned to drive a car, you can learn to control your skin temperature, heart rate, brain wave patterns, and many other functions once thought to be beyond conscious control.

You use biofeedback to help you learn how to relax your muscles. No matter what the device, it is only a short-term aid. People learn to consciously make the desired changes in their bodies without needing a machine to tell them how well they are doing.

Claims

The most common use for biofeedback is in learning to relax and reduce or eliminate pain. For example, when you are anxious, a number of physiological changes occur that are measurable — tensed muscles, colder hands, and raised heart rate and blood pressure. Biofeedback instruments show you the progress you are making as you learn to consciously alter these factors. Biofeedback also is reported to help relieve migraine and tension headaches and to help control incontinence and hypertension.

Study Findings

Numerous studies (✓✓✓) have shown that biofeedback can help people gain control over bodily functions they could not previously control. It helps people learn to reduce blood pressure and relieve tension and anxiety. Studies (✓✓✓✓) support the use of biofeedback to restore continence, especially with children. Biofeedback has become conventional therapy for incontinent children, though most study participants have been girls.

Controlled studies (✓✓✓✓) have shown that for tension headaches, biofeedback is about as effective as relaxation training alone. Results with migraine and hand-temperature biofeedback have been less encouraging, although some studies (✓✓✓) show it can be as effective in preventing migraines as relaxation training alone or the use of the drug propranolol (a conventional drug used for migraines). One study compared propranolol use with a biofeedback-assisted breathing technique and relaxation. After six months of use, two-thirds of both groups had significant improvements. One year after stopping the interventions, migraines had begun to reoccur in almost 50 percent of those taking propranolol but in only 10 percent of the biofeedback group.

Back pain occurs because of a complex variety of problems, and as such, the success of biofeedback has not been consistent (✓✓✓). This is to be expected. For some people, learning to relax works best with approaches that combine several techniques, such as biofeedback, hypnosis, and progressive muscle relaxation. Its effectiveness varies with different physiological conditions. For some people, it does not appear to work at all.

In some instances, such as heart disease, biofeedback is used to reduce one or more elements, such as blood pressure, that put you at risk. However, whether this actually impacts your chances of developing heart disease (or the severity of the problem if it develops) remains less clear.

Cautions

Biofeedback instruments have not been reported to cause any harm, nor do they have side effects. Those already using conventional medicine to control a condition (such as high blood pressure) should consult their physicians before trying biofeedback — or any other alternative therapy — so that appropriate adjustments in conventional therapies can be made, if necessary. Do not stop medications or make other significant changes before starting biofeedback.

According to *QuackWatch*, some health care providers are using "electrodiagnostic" devices and calling them "biofeedback" devices to obtain insurance reimbursement. These practitioners say this "bio" or "electrical feedback" helps them select the treatment they will prescribe, and many falsely claim they can determine the cause of any disease by detecting an "energy imbalance." Some even claim they can tell whether a disease, such as cancer or AIDS, is *not* present. There is no evidence to support these uses, and there is a good chance they are fraudulent.

Recommendations

Biofeedback is an approach that has been shown to work for some people, allowing them to consciously control their symptoms and thus reduce or eliminate medications or other therapies. Those with chronic pain who have had little relief from other therapies may find it worth trying, though they must understand it doesn't work for everyone.

As a method of relaxation, biofeedback is devoid of the need to alter one's consciousness or adopt any particular beliefs. As such, it is an alternative that is becoming more and more conventional.

Treatment Categories

Conventional
To treat incontinence in children ☺☺☺☺

Complementary
To reduce blood pressure ☺☺☺☺

To relieve tension and anxiety ☺☺☺☺

To treat tension or
migraine headaches ☺☺☺☺

To relieve back pain ☺☺

Scientifically Unproven
For most other indications or to cure any illness

Quackery or Fraud
In the hands of some practitioners, especially those using "biofeedback" or "electrodiagnostic" devices to diagnose nonexistent health problems, select inappropriate treatment, and defraud insurance companies

Further Reading

Barrett, Stephen. "Quack 'Electrodiagnostic' Devices." *QuackWatch: www.quackwatch.org/ 01QuackeryRelatedTopics/electro.html*. Accessed October 30, 2005.

Kaushika, Reshma, Rajeev M. Kaushika, Sukhdev K. Mahajana, and Vemreddi Rajeshb. "Biofeedback-Assisted Diaphragmatic Breathing and Systematic Relaxation Versus Propranolol in Long-Term Prophylaxis of Migraine." *Complementary Therapies in Medicine* 13, no. 3 (September 2005): 165 – 74.

Yagci, Sezgin, Yusuf Kibar, Ozan Akay, Selim Kilic, Fikret Erdemir, Faysal Gok, and Murat Dayanc. "The Effect of Biofeedback Treatment on Voiding and Urodynamic Parameters in Children with Voiding Dysfunction." *Journal of Urology* 174, no. 5 (November 2005): 1994 – 97.

BREATHING TECHNIQUES

What They Are

"Okay, everyone. Take a deep breath and off we go!" These are common instructions before starting something that may cause you more than a little anxiety. But maybe there's more to this than an old wives' tale. Traditional Chinese medicine, martial arts, and yoga teach the importance of breathing for good heath and function. The yoga breathing technique is called *pranayama*. Deep, even, and steady breaths are made using the diaphragm, not the chest, while sitting in a relaxed yoga position.

Within Eastern approaches, breathing is not just important for moving air in and out of the body. It is believed that proper breathing facilitates the flow of life energy (the *prana* in *pranayama*) through the person.

In Western contexts, many parents are familiar with the breathing techniques taught to expectant mothers to help them during labor. Another group of breathing techniques is known as deep diaphragmatic breathing. Deep breathing is also taught in relaxation and pain control techniques. Changes in both the rate and depth of breathing are connected with levels of arousal and anxiety. Hence, when someone is panicking, it is common to encourage them to take a few deep breaths. Given the role played by stress in modern life, and its exacerbation of some chronic illnesses, many people have turned to deep breathing to promote relaxation. When complementary and alternative medicine usage in the United States was studied in 2002, the results reported that deep breathing techniques were the fifth most popular therapy. Almost 12 percent of the population had used one of these techniques in the previous year.

Another breathing technique has gained widespread interest since being featured in a 1998 BBC television program. Called the Buteyko breathing technique, it was developed in Russia to help people with asthma. It is a complicated technique that requires five two-hour training sessions. Proponents believe asthma is caused by hyperventilation (breathing too quickly) and hypocapnia (excessive reduction of carbon dioxide levels). People are taught to breathe more slowly and shallowly. This is done twice a day and whenever asthmatic symptoms arise. Users tape their mouths closed at night to prevent mouth breathing while sleeping. They are also to avoid stress, exercise exertion, oversleeping, processed foods, and food additives. Use of asthma inhalers is permitted, but only if the breathing techniques do not bring relief.

Claims

Breathing techniques were widely used in treating asthma until several decades ago. Some of the methods used then were so extreme they worsened the asthmatic symptoms and were largely abandoned. More moderate breathing techniques became popular again in the 1980s along with other relaxation techniques. Proponents of the Buteyko technique claim that over 90 percent of 100,000 Russian asthmatic patients who learned the technique no longer use any medications. A similar success rate is claimed for 8,000 asthma patients in Australia.

The other main use of deep breathing is to relieve anxiety. Deep, steady breathing is said to directly trigger the relaxation response. Various breathing techniques are also used to reduce pain or anxiety by distracting people's attention from the source of pain or anxiety. Deep breathing has also been used to help people trying to stop smoking and to relieve migraine headaches.

Study Findings

A 2004 Cochrane review of breathing techniques used for asthma found seven small studies. In contrast with the dramatic claims made for the Buteyko technique, two small controlled studies found modest benefits (✓✓✓). A larger and longer study published after the Cochrane review involved ninety patients for six months. Patients were randomly assigned to either the Buteyko technique, a modified yoga breathing technique, or placebo. Those using the Buteyko technique had significantly improved asthma symptoms and reduced inhaler usage compared to the two other groups (✓✓✓). The patients' lung function was not changed in any group. Major drawbacks with the Buteyko approach were the length of time for training and the need to diligently practice the technique.

Two studies have examined the use of yoga breathing in asthma. One found no statistically significant differences between the yoga and placebo groups. The other found that both yoga and physical therapy led to significant improvements in patients' symptoms compared to placebo (✓✓✓).

However, only the physical therapy group showed improvements in patients' lung function. Four other small studies using various deep breathing techniques had mixed results. The authors of the Cochrane review concluded that encouraging trends have been found for symptom management (✓✓✓) but not for changes in the underlying lung disease.

Dental anxiety is one other area where deep breathing has been tested. Anxiety over visiting dentists affects almost one-third of Americans. Apart from its impact on patients, it leads to many canceled appointments, delayed procedures, and avoidance of dental care. Breathing techniques could be learned quickly and used while patients wait to see their dentists. A small number of studies with dental patients found that anxiety was reduced by deep breathing (✓✓✓). One controlled study with fifty children found it particularly effective (✓✓✓). However, a 2003 controlled study found no differences among a group practicing deep breathing, a group using distraction by focusing on their feet, or a placebo group (✗✗✗). Studies of deep breathing before surgery have had mixed results. A large 2003 randomized study found no differences between patients taught deep breathing exercises before cardiac surgery and those not taught (✗✗✗).

Other uses of deep breathing techniques have been studied very little. For example, one randomized controlled study compared the treatment of migraines with the conventional drug propranolol against a deep breathing technique with biofeedback and a muscle relaxation technique. Both approaches led to similar improvements in two-thirds of each group after six months. One year after stopping the interventions, migraines had begun to reoccur in almost 50 percent of those taking propranolol but in only 10 percent of the deep breathing group (✓✓✓). Deep breathing helped smokers who had stopped smoking the previous day. The craving of cigarettes, anxiety, and other withdrawal symptoms were significantly improved by the breathing technique compared to placebo (✓✓✓). People suffering from panic attacks have similarly responded better to deep breathing than to placebo (✓✓✓). Deep breathing is apparently effective in relieving anxiety of different origins. Despite the popularity of breathing techniques taught to expectant mothers, no controlled studies were found on their effectiveness during labor and delivery.

Cautions

Deep breathing techniques are easy to learn and without serious complications. Overly aggressive breathing should be avoided, as this can lead to hyperventilation, which could increase anxiety and breathing problems. Yoga is fundamentally a spiritual practice, although it has allegedly been secularized in the West. Some practitioners still use it to introduce people to Eastern religious beliefs. Given that other breathing techniques are available without yoga's worldview, those should be used instead.

Recommendations

Deep breathing techniques can be effective in reducing anxiety and helping people relax, including in some stressful dental and medical settings, although results have not been consistently positive. As a complementary strategy in the management of asthma, deep breathing appears to be a helpful adjunct to conventional therapy.

Treatment Categories

Complementary

For those with asthma, to relieve
symptoms and reduce inhaler usage ☺☺☺☺

To reduce anxiety of different origins ☺☺☺

To manage migraines ☺☺

Scientifically Unproven

To cure asthma ☹☹☹☹

Spiritual

When yoga breathing is taught by some 👎👎👎

Further Reading

Cooper, S., J. Oborne, S. Newton, V. Harrison, J. Thompson Coon, S. Lewis, and A. Tattersfield. "Effect of Two Breathing Exercises (Buteyko and Pranayama) in Asthma: A Randomised Controlled Trial." *Thorax* 58 (2003): 674–79.

Holloway, E., and F. S. F. Ram. "Breathing Exercises for Asthma." *The Cochrane Database of Systematic Reviews* 2004, no. 1.

CHELATION THERAPY

What It Is

The concept behind chelation therapy has made it one of the most talked about forms of alternative medicine for an aging population. As far back as 1948, chelation therapy was in regular use by physicians in the U.S. Navy to treat lead poisoning. A chemical, most commonly ethylene diamine tetraacetic acid (EDTA), is injected into the bloodstream. The EDTA molecules act like claws (the Greek word for "claw" is *chele*), engulfing other molecules. The injected substance traps the lead and other minerals, such as calcium, magnesium, and iron, and removes them from the body by way of the kidneys.

EDTA is also used as a cleaning agent to remove calcium that can build up and clog boilers and pipes. "Atherosclerosis" is the medical term for the buildup of thick, hard plaque in blood vessels that can eventually cut off blood circulation and lead to certain forms of heart disease. Calcium is involved in plaque buildup. In the late 1950s, Dr. Norman Clarke Sr., from Detroit's Providence Hospital, theorized that EDTA chelation could treat heart conditions.

Today EDTA is used as an alternative therapy for atherosclerosis. Half a million people in the United States undergo chelation therapy every year, according to estimates. Almost 10 percent of Canadians who underwent cardiac catheterization had previously tried chelation therapy. However, chelation therapy is not recommended by the Food and Drug Administration, Federal Trade Commission, National Institutes of Health, National Research Council, American Medical Association, Centers for Disease Control and Prevention, American Heart Association, American College of Physicians, American Academy of Family Physicians, American Society for Clinical Pharmacology Therapeutics, American College of Cardiology, and American Osteopathic Association.

Claims

Intravenous EDTA chelation therapy is primarily used today to treat coronary artery disease and peripheral arterial disease. Chelation therapists claim that people with high calcium blood levels have an increased risk of developing atherosclerosis and that EDTA removes calcium from plaque and cleans out a person's arteries. Therapy is said to be an economical, effective alternative to coronary bypass surgery and angioplasty, and effective for cleaning blocked arteries in the legs. However, some chelation therapists also claim the therapy can treat thyroid disorders, multiple sclerosis, cancer, Alzheimer's disease, and many other disorders. Adequate explanations for how it might act in treating these other disorders have not been proposed.

A variation of intravenous EDTA chelation therapy is called "oral chelation." Various substances are taken by mouth to allegedly reduce serum cholesterol and to treat problems such as toxicity from heavy metal (nickel, mercury, etc.). Among the suggested substances used for oral chelation have been vitamin C, zinc, garlic, and certain amino acids.

Study Findings

Oral chelation therapy is based only on anecdotal reports (✓). The few well-designed studies that have evaluated the claims of intravenous chelation therapy for atherosclerotic diseases have, without exception, found no evidence that chelation worked (✗✗✗).

When intravenous EDTA was first used for lead poisoning in the 1950s, patients who also had angina reported relief from their symptoms (✓). Angina is chest pain that results from inadequate blood supply to the heart muscle, often due to clogged coronary arteries. In the years following the introduction of EDTA,

many reports (✓✓) were published claiming that chelation therapy helped people with coronary heart disease. However, these reports involved small groups of patients, and no controls were used that could help determine if improvements were due to the EDTA.

A 1990 controlled study (✓✓), with only ten people, reported benefits from chelation, which led to a number of larger, controlled studies. All of these, including a large randomized study, have found neither short-term nor long-term benefits from the therapy (✗✗✗✗). A 1997 review of the best of these studies (✗✗✗) concluded that use of chelation therapy for atherosclerosis "should now be considered obsolete." Another concluded chelation therapy "must be regarded as ethically unsound practice." A 2002 double-blind, randomized study with eighty-four heart disease patients found no objective or subjective benefits in patients receiving EDTA chelation therapy compared to intravenous saline solutions (✗✗✗).

Not only has chelation therapy been shown to be ineffective, but the proposed rationale for how it might work has been shown to be scientifically implausible. One month of chelation therapy could remove no more than 1 percent of all the calcium in plaque. As quickly as it would be removed, more calcium would be released from bone to replace it. Plus, calcium makes up only a tiny fraction of what is in plaque. Cholesterol and fibrous tissue are much more abundant, and there is no reason to believe that these are removed by EDTA. Claims are now being made that EDTA works by removing metal ions involved in oxidation that can damage blood vessels and contribute to plaque buildup.

These research results contrast with the many stories reporting great benefits from chelation therapy. Chelation therapists usually advise patients to quit smoking, lose weight, improve their diet, begin exercising, and take vitamins. Patients may be benefiting from either (1) the caring attention given them by practitioners and their staff to cope with their symptoms or (2) the recommended changes that lead to a healthier lifestyle. In 2003, the National Institutes of Health launched a five-year high-quality study of chelation therapy in more than 2,300 patients. More than twenty times larger than previous studies, this research should provide the most conclusive evidence yet about whether chelation therapy has any benefit — or not.

Cautions

Chelation therapy has potentially serious side effects. Dangerously low levels of blood calcium can result (blood calcium is more easily removed than calcium in plaque). These low levels could lead to tetany (muscle spasms). Severe kidney damage and even death have resulted from using EDTA in lead poisoning. These risks are justified only because of the serious dangers of heavy metal poisoning. The American Heart Association and various physician organizations have reported many negative effects from the therapy and are against its use for atherosclerosis. Proponents say that some of the dangers have come from the amount of EDTA used, and that reducing the amount of EDTA reduces the risks. Intravenous infusions take three to four hours, usually requiring forty or more treatments over a couple of months. Some therapists then recommend ongoing monthly treatment to prevent recurrence. Chelation therapy is very expensive, costing between $3,000 and $10,000. This type of therapy — we believe for the right reasons — is virtually never covered by medical insurance.

Recommendations

Intravenous chelation therapy should only be used in cases of heavy metal poisoning where objective tests validate the presence of toxic levels of specific metals. The risks of other uses of intravenous chelation or any use of oral chelation are not warranted in light of the lack of evidence for effectiveness. Evidence against its effectiveness in heart disease is so clear, its continued use raises serious ethical questions. The therapy is very expensive and can be very lucrative for providers.

Treatment Categories

Conventional
To treat heavy metal poisoning ☺☺☺☺

Scientifically Questionable
For any other indication, particularly coronary heart disease, angina, and peripheral vascular disease ☹☹☹☹

Quackery or Fraud
In the hands of many practitioners

Risk of Serious Side Effects
- Direct toxic effects ⊘⊘⊘
- Avoiding effective care ⊘⊘

Further Reading

Ernst, E. "Chelation Therapy for Peripheral Arterial Occlusive Disease." *Circulation* 96 (1997): 1031 – 33.

Knudtson, Merril L., D. George Wyse, P. Diane Galbraith, Rollin Brant, Kathy Hildebrand, Diana Paterson, Deborah Richardson, Connie Burkart, and Ellen Burgess. "Chelation Therapy for Ischemic Heart Disease: A Randomized Controlled Trial." *Journal of the American Medical Association* 287, no. 4 (January 2002): 481 – 86.

Villarruz, M. V., A. Dans, and F. Tan. "Chelation Therapy for Atherosclerotic Cardiovascular Disease." *The Cochrane Database of Systematic Reviews* 2002, no. 4.

CHIROPRACTIC

What It Is

Daniel David Palmer was a self-taught healer at a time — the 1890s — when science had yet to have a serious impact on medicine. The country doctor rode his horse and buggy from home to home, giving patients more loving comfort than meaningful treatment. Patent medicine remained popular, most of it so filled with alcohol that heavy users could forget their discomfort as long as there was another dose in the bottle. Bayer, the German pharmaceutical company, was just starting to market two products that would become well known in the twentieth century: one was aspirin, and the other was heroin!

Palmer was a grocery store owner who had learned magnetic healing and mysticism. He also had the good sense to distrust much of contemporary medicine and was determined to find a way to heal others without using drugs. Spinal manipulation for the treatment of illness had been used in one form or another for centuries. Palmer developed a series of manipulative procedures that he believed would bring health to muscles, nerves, and organs that had gotten out of alignment. He named these procedures using the Greek words *cheirios* and *prakticos*, which translate to "done by hand," or "manipulation." Palmer called his method "chiropractic." Chiropractors are recognized by the D.C. after their name, which stands for Doctor of Chiropractic.

The start of chiropractic goes back to deaf janitor Harvey Lillard in Davenport, Iowa. Lillard was said to have been in good health until one day, when he was doing heavy labor, he felt something go wrong with his back. He was instantly deaf and remained that way for the next seventeen years until he encountered Palmer.

Lillard, so the story goes, had a lump on his back that Palmer determined to be a displaced vertebra. He applied pressure according to his carefully conceived theory, and the vertebra slipped back into place. Immediately the janitor could hear.

The frequent retelling of this story has left many details very sketchy. It is uncertain how the janitor became a patient of Palmer (he was not a doctor). Nor is it clear why he would allow the grocery store owner to manipulate his spine. What matters is that this story became the basis for Palmer's theories, theories he claimed were proven, at least to himself, when a second patient's heart condition was eased through similar manipulation. His techniques are now called the Palmer Method of chiropractic.

The history of chiropractic is filled with divisiveness over what problems it relieves best and precisely how manipulations bring relief. Today the Palmer concept stresses that alignment of the spine assures good health. Misalignments, called "subluxations," interfere with the body's natural ability to heal itself and thus need to be corrected by spinal manipulation.

Palmer used the term "subluxation" in a metaphysical way. In his view, subluxations interfered with the flow through the body of Innate Intelligence (or spark of life or spirit). This energy was therefore a form of life energy, as used in Eastern medical systems. His son, Bartlett Joshua Palmer, claimed that subluxations were the cause of all disease. This led to a split between those loyal to both Palmers and chiropractors who sought a scientific basis for chiropractic. In the view of those seeking scientific explanations, subluxations are displaced vertebrae that somehow disrupt the flow of nerve impulses through the spine. These somehow cause pain and physical illness. However, the nature, location, and very existence of subluxations remain disputed, even by chiropractors.

Chiropractors typically use X-rays and their hands to determine where manipulation is needed. One form of manipulation is done quickly, using hand thrusts involving different amounts of force. The manipulation causes adjustments that usually are accompanied by a distinctive cracking noise. Another form of manipulation involves slower, gentler movements. With both, relief may be immediate, may require a number of visits, or may come after an initial period of increased discomfort.

Claims

The claims made for chiropractic vary, depending on which approach a therapist uses. Some chiropractors treat only those conditions appropriate to their training. They strive to support clinical decisions with rigorous chiropractic studies that have revealed clear benefits. Other chiropractors claim they can cure almost any disease and seek to practice as the equivalent of primary care physicians. These chiropractors point out that their training involves significant numbers of science-based courses, which they claim gives them extensive medical knowledge.

Many chiropractors also function in the capacity of naturopaths — practitioners who resist the use of medicinal drugs and surgery and emphasize nutrition and natural approaches to healing. Critics of those taking this approach point out that after one hundred years their scope of practice is not defined clearly or on a scientific basis. One such critic, Wil-

liam T. Jarvis, has said that those chiropractors who distance themselves from conventional medicine fail to contribute "to the worldwide body of knowledge shared by the health sciences."

Study Findings

Hundreds of studies have been conducted, leading to more than fifty reviews of the chiropractic research. Unfortunately, many of the earlier studies had significant methodological flaws that make it difficult to use their results.

Back pain is a leading cause of pain and disability and contributes hugely to health care costs and employees missing work. Chiropractic is most frequently sought for low back pain. More than fifty randomized controlled trials of chiropractic for low back pain have been conducted. A 2003 review of this evidence found that chiropractic was superior to control therapies and therapies known to be ineffective (✓✓✓). Chiropractic was found to be no more or no less effective than more conventional interventions such as general practitioner care, physical therapy, use of painkillers, or bed rest (✓✓✓). Similar results were obtained, whether the low back pain was acute or chronic.

However, several studies have found that while outcomes are similar, patient satisfaction is higher with chiropractic than with conventional back care (✓✓). An interesting 2005 study found preliminary evidence that improved satisfaction itself may contribute to better relief from low back pain, at least in the short term.

Another common practice in chiropractic is manipulation of the cervical spine. This is carried out to relieve neck and shoulder pain, but also headaches and migraines. Supportive evidence for treating headaches is much less convincing, with about half the studies finding benefit and half not (✓✓). A 2005 review of chiropractic manipulation for acute neck pain found only one randomized study, and that had no placebo group (✓✓).

There is no compelling medical evidence (✗✗✗) that chiropractic is effective for other conditions such as asthma, allergies, or painful menstrual periods. Reports (✗✗) are similar for cancer. We have not seen any evidence that convinces us that chiropractic is appropriate for children.

Cautions

Chiropractic manipulation is not without side effects. Manipulations of the lower spine are relatively safe, but cervical manipulation around the neck is controversial. Some neck arteries are particularly prone to injury when the head and neck are suddenly rotated in unusual ways. Such injuries can trigger stroke and are sometimes fatal. Some are concerned that cervical manipulation may randomly, though rarely, cause such serious injuries. Dozens of case reports have been published identifying a connection between cervical spine manipulation and stroke (✗✗). Surveys have revealed hundreds of unreported cases of suspected connections, but this is not high-quality evidence of a connection (✗✗). The lack of any consistent pattern has led to much debate over whether the injury is caused by manipulation or just happens to occur around the same time. The risk, though very low, is serious, which is even more problematic given the lack of studies supporting neck manipulation (✗✗).

In general, chiropractic is relatively low in risk, although about 12 percent of patients reported mild adverse effects. While this risk is not very high if the treatment is effective, it becomes highly problematic if manipulation is done for conditions for which it has not been shown to be beneficial. This is a particular problem with certain chiropractors who place less weight on the best scientific evidence available and more weight on Palmer's metaphysical roots.

Given such variation among chiropractors, Jarvis recommends avoiding those who

- appear overconfident or cultist in their zeal for chiropractic care;
- disparage regular medicine as jealously antichiropractic;
- criticize prescription drugs or surgery in an ideological manner;
- attack immunization, fluoridation, pasteurization, or other public health practices;
- X-ray all of their patients or routinely use full-spine X-rays; or
- use scare tactics, such as claiming that the failure to undergo chiropractic care could lead to serious problems in the future.

Obviously, care should be taken in choosing one's chiropractor.

Recommendations

Chiropractors differ in their scientific foundations and spiritual beliefs. Some openly promote New Age and shamanistic approaches to health and healing and disdain well-supported vaccinations and promote sales of unsupported remedies (see pp. 83–84). Other chiropractors take a scientific approach to their profession and practice according to evidence-based guidelines. The Christian Chiropractic Association is to be highly commended for separating New Age beliefs and practices from the scientifically based aspects of chiropractic.

Chiropractic can be a legitimate intervention, bringing welcome relief for specific muscular and skeletal conditions. Although many chiropractors claim it is also more cost-effective than conventional medicine, economic studies have found the opposite. Individual visits to chiropractors cost less, but usually more visits are recommended, and treatment is often continued for longer periods. A *New England Journal of Medicine* study found that different treatment approaches for back pain were equally effective. However, primary care physicians offered the least expensive regimen, with chiropractic care being the most expensive option, costing even more than orthopedic surgery.

Treatment Categories

Conventional

To relieve acute and chronic
low back pain ☺☺☺☺
To treat some other
musculoskeletal conditions ☺☺☺

Complementary

To relieve headaches and migraines ☺☺
To relieve neck and shoulder pain ☹

Scientifically Unproven

To treat medical diseases
or as preventive medicine ☹☹☹☹

Spiritual

In the hands of some practitioners 👎👎

Quackery or Fraud

In the hands of some practitioners

Further Reading

Cherkin, Daniel C., Karen J. Sherman, Richard A. Deyo, and Paul G. Shekelle. "A Review of the Evidence for the Effectiveness, Safety, and Cost of Acupuncture, Massage Therapy, and Spinal Manipulation for Back Pain." *Annals of Internal Medicine* 138, no. 11 (June 2003): 898 – 906.

Haldeman, Scott, Frank J. Kohlbeck, and Marion McGregor. "Stroke, Cerebral Artery Dissection, and Cervical Spine Manipulation Therapy." *Journal of Neurology* 249, no. 8 (August 2002): 1098 – 104.

Haneline, Michael T. "Chiropractic Manipulation and Acute Neck Pain: A Review of the Evidence." *Journal of Manipulative and Physiological Therapeutics* 28, no. 7 (September 2005): 520 – 25.

Jarvis, William T. "Why Chiropractic Is Controversial." *ChiroBase: www.chirobase.org/01General/ controversy.html*. Accessed November 1, 2005.

CHRISTIAN THERAPIES

Some alternative therapies are promoted as being particularly in line with biblical teaching. A diet may be said to follow biblical guidelines, or a remedy may be promoted by a company run by Christians. This is what we mean by "Christian therapies." We do not include prayer or faith healing within this category. We examine prayer later in this part of the book and discussed faith in chapter 3.

These therapies are usually promoted by well-meaning Christians who seek to give God the glory for everything they do. It is hard to criticize a man or woman with a passion for the things of God. They are so certain, so joyous, we start thinking that all of their pronouncements must be solidly based in Scripture.

Yet the truth is that the person of passion is also human. When celebrating our Lord, he or she can sometimes go too far in ascribing to God that which is of man or nature. Such is sometimes the case with what are called "Christian therapies."

Our point is *not* to attack any particular Christian therapy or remedy. Our point is to give a broad overview of concerns we have with promoting certain therapies as "Christian" or "biblical." We as Christians are blessed with God's biblical guidance and the direction of the Holy Spirit. We are blessed with many therapies, and the Bible and the Holy Spirit can guide us as we select the ones to pursue. But we should be very cautious about labeling any therapy as "Christian."

The problem comes when someone who is alive with the Spirit, who has a passion for the Lord, enters the health field and offers health advice (whether sound or ill-founded), claiming the same authority as the Word of God. Sometimes the therapy appears to be a soundly reasoned program for a healthy lifestyle or promotes well-established methods of healing or treatment. Other times the therapies, based on faulty views of the Bible, are recommended or even "preached" by sincere Christians who have little or no medical background and no evidence to support them. Although these men and women may be sincere, they may be sincerely wrong.

Christian therapies are frequently based on personal experience. They were often discovered when someone greatly benefited from the therapy — someone experienced healing or improved health. Widespread promotion of the therapies sometimes begins with members of the clergy, lay theologians of note, or others with ready access to the media, especially Christian radio or television.

Rarely can anyone question whether a healing occurred. It often seems clear that God's hand was involved in the healing. Yet the confusion is in the details. No one can say with certainty what caused the original healing. But you'd never know that from the way the therapy is promoted. It is presented as God's answer to human ailments.

These Christian therapies are said to be biblically justified. Some fit into the theology of the particular denomination to which their proponents belong. They sound good. Unfortunately, some are not medically sound, and others are even medically dangerous. Other remedies have an important role in health and healing, but this role is expanded well beyond what is scientifically supported. We ordered an audiotape advertised as containing the Bible's recipe for healthy living. The tape presented some helpful information about the importance of vitamins, made many speculative claims about dietary supplements, and never once mentioned the Bible. The advertisement appeared to us to be no more than a marketing ploy to entice Christians into buying the company's products.

Christians are, and should be, concerned about their health. We want our book to help Christians choose alternative therapies wisely. We also believe that God sometimes grants a miracle of healing. When a Christian experiences healing, either directly from God or through a therapy, he or she may become convinced that others can be healed. Some start to reflect on exactly what they did immediately prior to the healing. Had they just changed their diet? Had they just started praying a little differently? Had they just taken a dietary supplement? Had they started attending a new church?

Motivated by a desire to help others, they search for those crucial steps that led to their healing. They hear others' experiences and develop a list of additional factors needed for healing. Soon they have formulated a new Christian therapy. Their experience, and the successes of others who have tried it, is the only proof they need that this new therapy really works. Besides, their intentions are only to share God's blessings, and the therapies are so "gentle" they couldn't harm anyone. Why should anyone be concerned?

Well, *we* are concerned — and we think *you* should be also. It is one thing to rejoice with someone whose health has been renewed; it is quite another to promote as a therapy whatever seemed to contribute to that healing. Good intentions are not enough when making recommendations that affect people's health. Labeling the therapy as "Christian" or "God's own" or "biblically supported" raises a host of other concerns.

What we suggest, in every case, is caution and wisdom. Let's examine one such therapy that goes by a variety of names.

Christian Vegetarianism

Some Christian vegetarians (or vegans) suggest that the story of the Garden of Eden teaches that Adam and Eve were meant to eat only food that grows in the ground. The most cited verse is Genesis 1:29: "Then God said, 'I give you every seed-bearing plant on the face of the whole earth and every tree that has fruit with seed in it. They will be yours for food.'"

Some scholars believe this verse can be correctly interpreted to mean that humanity, at least in the Garden of Eden, was designed to be vegetarian. From this belief stem several diet plans that are circulating in the church today, going by names such as the "Hallelujah Diet," "God's Original [or Optimal] Diet," "God's Ideal Diet," and the "Genesis 1:29 Diet." Their promoters claim that God still intends for people to eat only plant-based food.

Even if we were to agree that humans were designed by God to be vegetarians, this does not necessarily mean we are to continue to be vegetarians. This passage also tells us that Adam and Eve were naked until they sinned. Should Christians therefore be nudists? Adam and Eve lived in a garden, and Adam spent his time naming the other creatures. Is this how all humans should spend their days? Clearly, those who insist that Genesis 1:29 teaches that God wants people to be vegetarians are not interpreting this passage consistently.

More important, a significant amount of other biblical teaching contradicts the interpretation that Christians should be vegetarians. In Genesis 4 we learn that Abel was a keeper of livestock. Jabal is described as "the father of those who live in tents and raise livestock" (Genesis 4:20). It is reasonable to infer that these herdsmen would have used some products from their animals as nourishment.

When Noah enters the ark, God tells him to take both clean and unclean animals (Genesis 7:2). This distinction makes sense only if some were eaten and others were not. We admit that the evidence is not conclusive that humans ate meat before the flood. However, the passages just reviewed show that we cannot rule out the possibility that some humans did eat meat.

After the flood, God declared, "Everything that lives and moves will be food for you. Just as I gave you the green plants, I now give you everything. But you must not eat meat that has its lifeblood still in it" (Genesis 9:3 – 4). All may be eaten, except if it contains blood. In Genesis 18, Abraham served his angelic guests butter, milk, and meat. They ate meat and other cooked food, washing it all down with milk — an animal product.

Later, although being deceptive, Jacob prepared venison to obtain his father, Isaac's, blessing. Without moral qualms, Isaac ate the cooked meat (Genesis 27:25). In Exodus 16, God sent quail, a bird, to the Israelites to feed them. In God's law, he lists clean and unclean animals and says of the clean animals, "Of all the animals that live on land, these are the ones you may eat" (Leviticus 11:2).

God even taught the Israelites how to cook lamb: "Do not eat the meat raw or cooked in water, but roast it over the fire — head, legs and inner parts" (Exodus 12:9; see also Leviticus 6:24 – 26). If God's intention was that humans never eat meat, it seems strange that he provided such painstaking details about which meats the Israelites should eat, which they shouldn't, and how to cook them.

Throughout the Bible, we see references to the eating of meat and animal products without any condemnation (1 Kings 4:22 – 23; Nehemiah 13:16; Proverbs 27:27; Luke 15:29). Turning to the New Testament, we are told that John the Baptist ate more than plants: "His food was locusts and wild honey" (Matthew 3:4). Paul declares, "Eat anything sold in the meat market without raising questions of conscience" (1 Corinthians 10:25). Scripture states that Christians can even eat meat that has been sacrificed to idols!

Jesus himself ate more than plants (e.g., fish) and gave such foods to those he loved. One example is the well-known story of the loaves and the fish (Matthew 15:32 – 38). Another is the time after Jesus' resurrection when he appeared to the disciples and asked, " 'Do you have anything here to eat?' They gave him a piece of broiled fish, and he took it and ate it in their presence" (Luke 24:41 – 43). Later, they all met on the beach. "Jesus said to them, 'Come and have breakfast.' … Jesus came, took the bread and gave it to them, and did the same with the fish" (John 21:12 – 13). Why would Jesus give his apostles fish to eat if he wanted everyone to be vegetarian?

The eating of clean and unclean animals was controversial during the early years of Christianity. Jewish Christians wanted to remain faithful to their traditional laws but weren't sure if Gentile Christians should also be required to abstain from unclean foods. Peter received a vision of a large sheet. "It contained all kinds of four-footed animals, as well as reptiles of the earth and birds of the air. Then a voice told him, 'Get up, Peter. Kill and eat' " (Acts 10:12 – 13). Many of the animals were unclean, and when Peter pointed this out, he was told, three times, "Do not call anything impure that God has made clean" (Acts 10:15).

The controversy continued for a while. After much discussion, the apostles sent a letter to the Gentile believers telling them "to abstain from food sacrificed to idols, from blood, from the meat of strangled animals and from sexual immorality" (Acts 15:29). This would have been the perfect opportunity to tell the Gentiles not to eat meat, but we find no prohibition.

In Romans 14, Paul attacked the issue of eating meat by explaining that questions about diet (and which day to worship on) were "disputable matters" — in other words, there is no clear teaching from the Lord, and Christians can operate in these areas as led by the Holy Spirit. Paul, it seems to us, is teaching that no food, in and of itself, is unclean for Christians. He also teaches that one's choice of food has to be kept in perspective: "For the kingdom of God is not a matter of eating and drinking, but of righteousness, peace and joy in the Holy Spirit, because anyone who serves Christ in this way is pleasing to God and approved by men" (Romans 14:17 – 18).

Elsewhere, Paul tells Timothy to reject teachers who, among other things, call on people "to abstain from certain foods, which God created to be received with thanksgiving by those who believe and who know the truth. For everything God created is good, and nothing is to be rejected if it is received with thanksgiving, because it is consecrated by the word of God and prayer" (1 Timothy 4:3 – 5). Could Paul have been predicting teachers such as those who claim God does not want people to eat meat or cooked foods?

Paul calls on Christians not to submit to those who declare, "Do not handle! Do not taste! Do not touch!" (Colossians 2:21). He goes on to point out that "such regulations indeed have an appearance of wisdom, with their self-imposed worship, their false humility and their harsh treatment of the body, but they lack any value in restraining sensual indulgence" (Colossians 2:23).

We see this borne out in people's lives. If we accept that those who lived prior to the flood were strict vegetarians, this was no advantage for their overall spiritual health. They still became completely wicked so that "the LORD was grieved that he had made man on the earth, and his heart was filled with pain" (Genesis 6:6). The result was the flood, from which only Noah and his family were saved.

Jesus explained to his followers that true righteousness has essentially nothing to do with what one puts in one's mouth. He taught that food does not defile us. "What goes into a man's mouth does not make him 'unclean,' but what comes out of his mouth, that is what makes him 'unclean.' … Don't you see that whatever enters the mouth goes into the stomach and then out of the body? But the things that come out of the mouth come from the heart, and these make a man 'unclean'" (Matthew 15:11, 17 – 18; see also Mark 7:1 – 23).

Should people today, for health reasons, not eat those animals listed in Scripture as unclean? The two of us do not agree on that issue. Walt believes it is still a good health practice to reduce the consumption of or avoid these unclean animals; Dónal does not.

However, our preferences in this "disputable matter" are exactly that — our preferences. We would never teach either position as doctrine. Further, in accordance with Romans 14:19, we would make every effort to ensure our differences do not cause conflict or become a stumbling block for others. Jesus commanded his disciples to "eat what is set before you" (Luke 10:8). In teaching about eating meat and drinking wine, Paul says, "Whatever you believe about these things keep between yourself and God" (Romans 14:22).

The problem with teaching that all Christians should be vegetarians is not with what Christians eat and don't eat. The problem is that it easily leads people to an external focus on factors that are not what the Bible declares as most important in life. Jesus commanded us, "Do not worry about your life, what you will eat or drink; or about your body, what you will wear. Is not life more important than food, and the body more important than clothes?" (Matthew 6:25). It is too easy to become consumed with eating the perfect foods and drinking the perfect beverages. Instead, we should "seek first his kingdom and his righteousness, and all these things will be given to [us] as well" (Matthew 6:33).

The teaching of the Bible seems clear to us that humans are not commanded to abstain from meat. Vegetarianism should not be promoted as required for Christians, either on its own or as part of a therapy. At the same time, we must point out that the typical Western diet is too high in animal products and saturated fat, too low in fruits and vegetables and fiber, and too high in processed food. Medical studies are virtually unanimous in agreeing that this type of diet causes and worsens a variety of diseases.

People would be wise to eat a more plant-rich diet — and likely would be healthier. Yet a purely plant-based diet is not taught in Scripture and has some potential for harm. One of the vitamins essential for health — vitamin B_{12} — is lacking in *all* vegetarian diets (although vitamin B_{12} supplements are now available). In the past, vitamin B_{12} could be obtained only by eating at least some meat, as was almost certainly a part of the diet of Jesus and his disciples.

One version of the "Genesis 1:29 Diet," called the "Hallelujah Diet," exemplifies some of the concerns we have about many Christian alternative therapies. The Hallelujah Diet is a very popular Christian diet. The fervor of passionate Christians who feel they experienced a healing because of this Christian therapy is understandable. Their actions are based on faith and must be respected but are still open to critique.

In 1976, the Rev. George H. Malkmus stopped eating meat, processed food, and cooked food after being diagnosed with colon cancer at the age of forty-two. He had watched his mother die an agonizing death from colon cancer while undergoing conventional chemotherapy. He chose a different route. He claims that just about every sickness and illness can be prevented or cured if people "change from the world's diet of dead food to God's Diet of living food." He originally recommended a diet of only raw fruits and vegetables but later changed this to allow up to 15 percent cooked foods. He also recommends exercise, a relationship with Jesus Christ, and two dietary supplements — vitamin B_{12} and BarleyGreen, a powder made from barley grass (*Hordeum distichon*).

BarleyGreen is believed by Malkmus (and Dr. Lorraine Day, another cancer survivor who promotes Christian therapies) to stimulate the immune system and help rebuild the tissues of the body. The product has had a controversial history due in part to the multilevel marketing companies distributing it. In 1988, the FDA ordered its distributor to stop claiming it was effective against various diseases. Whereas there is some evidence that barley grain or flour may reduce total cholesterol when added to the diet, no studies support the use of BarleyGreen to treat any specific ailment.

We are concerned about anyone who puts the imprimatur of God on his or her advice, who puts a "thus sayeth the Lord ..." on any health advice without having indisputable biblical backing for the claim. It is a bold statement to claim that one's advice is directly from God or that one's therapy is God's ordained diet or remedy. At stake is God's credibility in the eyes of others, both those within the church and those outside the church.

However, the Rev. Malkmus goes even further. He stated on his website (referenced at the end of this entry) that he wants people, especially Christians, to believe that "truly, WE DON'T HAVE TO BE SICK! That disease and sickness are self-inflicted!" [emphasis his]. He claimed that the solution to all our health problems is simple: stop eating animal products and cooked food. "We see well over 90% of all physical problems just disappear in six months or less." If such claims are true, the Rev. Malkmus should produce data to back them up.

In his January 25, 2001, newsletter, he replied to a request for evidence to support his claims: "What you are seeking, for all intents and purposes, does not exist! It has been a great frustration to me through the years that practically no scientific research has been done to support or disprove RAW vegetarianism." All he can provide is anecdotal evidence. Without scientific support, some recommendations may be valid and others may not. We see this with the Hallelujah Diet. Some of it is sensible dietary advice, but overall it is not well balanced and could lead to some deficiencies.

The Word of God does not give a clear statement of doctrine on many issues. What we get in such cases are biblical principles to apply to an issue. While we can still develop clear biblical positions on some issues not addressed in the Bible, we must remain tentative on other issues. Most Christian therapies appear to us to be in the latter category. They are not based on clear teaching in God's Word but on interpretations that should be held tentatively because sometimes those opinions are wrong.

When scientific misinformation and confusion are promoted as part of a "Christian" therapy, Christianity can be further discredited. Most proponents usually are not deliberately trying to mislead anyone. But many often have no medical training or experience. They are acting on a dramatic personal experience and what we feel is an incomplete understanding of Scripture. In addition, Christians facing serious health problems who aren't aware of all the facts and who neglect effective treatment for their condition may actually be harmed by these therapies.

Christian Therapies and the Bible

Some Christians promote a therapy after finding one or more verses in the Bible that appear to support their perspective. Some proponents of herbal medicine claim the Bible specifically teaches that people should use herbs as medicine. They usually use the King James Version (KJV), and we will soon see why. The following examples come from a handout distributed by a visitor promoting herbal remedies at one of our churches:

- "And to every beast of the earth, and to every fowl of the air, and to everything that creepeth upon the earth, wherein there is life, I have given every green herb for meat; and it was so" (Genesis 1:30 KJV).
- "He causeth the grass to grow for the cattle, and herb for the service of man: that he may bring forth food out of the earth" (Psalm 104:14 KJV).

• "And by the river upon the bank thereof, on this side and on that side, shall grow all trees for meat, . . . and the fruit thereof shall be for meat, and the leaf thereof for medicine" (Ezekiel 47:12 KJV).

Those who use these verses to promote herbal medicine seem to forget one of the primary principles of biblical interpretation: seek first to understand what the text meant to the original writer and audience. Two Hebrew words are translated "herb" in the King James Version, and both mean "green plants" or "grass." Psalm 104:14 even states the purpose of the "herbs": to serve as food. Just as grass feeds cattle, "herbs" or green plants feed humans (see Psalm 37:2). This is poetry. English poetry uses rhyme. Hebrew poetry repeats the same thought in two ways.

When the King James Version was translated, the English word "herb" had a broader meaning than it does today. To take our modern usage of this word as a medicinal remedy and read that meaning back into an English translation of the Bible is inappropriate. Our belief is confirmed in more recent translations that replace the KJV "herb" with "green plants" or something similar. To us, these verses have no bearing on whether Christians should or shouldn't use herbal remedies or any other forms of medicine.

Ezekiel 47:12 does teach, however, that trees can have leaves that bring healing. This interpretation has been noted throughout history without any disagreement. However, this verse gives no help in determining which herbs bring healing and which are poisonous. It makes no statement on whether herbs or pharmaceutical drugs are preferable. In fact, it is questionable whether this verse has anything to do with the trees that grow on earth today. It falls within a section of the book of Ezekiel that contains prophecies about the kingdom of God. Many schol-

ars hold that this kingdom is yet to come, especially given the middle section of the verse, left out of the promotional literature we have seen. The following is the complete verse in the New International Version: "Fruit trees of all kinds will grow on both banks of the river. Their leaves will not wither, nor will their fruit fail. Every month they will bear, because the water from the sanctuary flows to them. Their fruit will serve for food and their leaves for healing" (Ezekiel 47:12). Leaving out the middle of the verse veils the fact that these clearly are not typical trees. These trees bear fruit every month, have leaves that never wither, and are nourished by water from the sanctuary. Such trees do not grow in the world as we know it today. This makes the applicability of this verse to today's herbal remedies very questionable.

When investigating any claim that something is a Christian therapy, basic principles of biblical interpretation should be utilized. Before accepting any "Christian teaching," carefully compare it with what the Bible actually states. Try to discern the plain meaning of the text in its most recent scholarly translations. If verses are cited, read them in your own Bible. Read the passages surrounding these verses to ensure that the interpretation fits the context.

Detailed examination of claims may require learning about how the Bible should be translated and interpreted, a study that will bear a wealth of fruit for your spiritual vitality. It may well protect you from going astray from the clear teaching of the Bible. This type of study was commended by Luke when he wrote in Acts 17:11, "Now the Bereans were of more noble character than the Thessalonians, for they received the message with great eagerness and examined the Scriptures every day to see if what Paul said was true." Such study led many of these men and women to believe the Christian message.

Many accept Christian therapies as based on biblical doctrine and medical fact. Sometimes they are not. Some even use their teachings, which we believe to be unbiblical, to judge others in the body of Christ. Worse yet, churches have been divided over these "false" teachings — which is, we suspect, exactly what Satan desires.

God, in his Word, urges us to carefully evaluate all that we are told: "Be very careful, then, how you live — not as unwise but as wise, making the most of every opportunity, because the days are evil. Therefore do not be foolish, but understand what the Lord's will is" (Ephesians 5:15 – 17).

Attacks on Conventional Medicine

Some promoters of Christian therapies attack conventional medicine with great ferocity. Lorraine Day, M.D., promotes an all-natural diet and 10-step program to health. Her website details how she recovered from breast cancer after refusing to use conventional chemotherapy and surgery. Instead, she prayed, claimed the healing promises of the Bible, and ate "the original diet God gave in the Garden of Eden." She chose to depend on God "rather than depend on human medical knowledge which is nothing more than drugs." Throughout her website and videos, she claims that conventional medicine is based on errors, that it harms people, and that it doesn't work. She urges people not to use conventional medicine. The Rev. Malkmus similarly discredits and discourages pharmaceuticals and doctors in a Web article titled "Drugs: A Killer of Mankind."

We readily admit that too many pharmaceuticals are used in the United States and that some doctors fail to practice good medicine. Many people are harmed from adverse effects of pharmaceuticals and mistakes by doctors. Some health care professionals are greedy and more interested in profits than patients. But a lot of good is done by conventional medicine. We all benefit from different aspects of modern medicine. The way to respond to problems in conventional medicine is not to reject the whole field; it is to fix the problems.

Dr. Day claims in her videotape that "sugar is as addictive as cocaine" and "paralyzes the immune system for four hours" after ingestion. She claims that "osteoporosis is not caused by lack of calcium" and that milk can make osteoporosis worse. She lists many health problems she believes are caused by common foods and drugs. According to a critical review of her claims on *QuackWatch*, "She speaks eloquently and from the heart, but her tapes contain hundreds of factual errors and far-fetched claims."

Dr. Day believes a huge conspiracy exists to keep people sick. This conspiracy includes the human creation of the AIDS virus to dramatically reduce the world's population, the use of TV to brainwash people, vaccination and fluoridation to harm people, and many other methods utilized to control people. When responding to an article in the *AARP Bulletin* that criticized her approach, she claimed the American Association of Retired Persons (AARP) was receiving $30 million to $300 million per month from the drug industry. She pulled her numbers out of thin air and then claimed the AARP had "a multi-million dollar arrangement with the drug companies," and this was why they were critical of her.

The Rev. Malkmus claims that the biblical teaching on physicians is summed up in Mark 5:25 – 26: "And a woman was there who had been subject to bleeding for twelve years. She had suffered a great deal under the care of many doctors and had spent all she had, yet instead of getting better she grew worse." The Rev. Malkmus, like Dr. Day, maintains that conventional medicine is dominated by false ideas and motivated by financial incentives.

The Rev. Malkmus goes even further in using the Bible to discredit the use of pharmaceuticals. He claims that the Bible's teaching on drugs is summed up in Revelation 18. This passage describes the overthrow of Babylon, which was the epitome of evil, and the way God will judge Babylon because of its negative impact on the world: "By your magic spell all the nations were led astray" (18:23). The Greek word here for "magic spell" ("sorcery" in other translations) is *pharmakeia*. This is the word from which we get "pharmacy" in English. Lorraine Day comes to a similar conclusion when she writes on her website, "In fact the English word pharmacy comes from the Greek word *pharmakeia*. *Pharmakeia* means sorceries and witchcraft. That's what drugs are — sorceries and witchcraft because they only treat symptoms while the underlying disease or condition continues to get worse."

The Greek word *pharmakeia* did originally mean a drug (usually a poison). But long before the New Testament was written, the word came to mean "magical material" (sometimes including drugs) that was used for purposes of hate. The word *pharmakeia* and those closely related to it are used only five times in the Bible (Galatians 5:20; Revelation 9:21; 18:23; 21:8; 22:15). The best translation in all these instances is "sorcery" or "sorcerer," as all major Bible translations render them. Virtually all theologians who have published on this topic indicate that there is no good interpretive reason to believe that this verse denounces the use of medicinal agents. That the Bible does not view medicine in general negatively is clear from numerous passages that speak positively of the use of available medicinal agents:

From the sole of your foot to the top of your head
    there is no soundness —
only wounds and welts
    and open sores,
not cleansed or bandaged
    or soothed with oil.

Isaiah 1:6

Babylon will suddenly fall and be broken.
    Wail over her!
Get balm for her pain;
    perhaps she can be healed.

Jeremiah 51:8; see also 8:22; 46:11

[The Good Samaritan] went to him and bandaged his wounds, pouring on oil and wine.

Luke 10:34

Is any one of you sick? He should call the elders of the church to pray over him and anoint him with oil in the name of the Lord.

James 5:14

Most of the scriptural references to physicians say nothing negative (see Jeremiah 8:22; Matthew 9:12; Luke 4:23), and Luke, who wrote both a gospel and the book of Acts, was a physician (Colossians 4:14). Although certainly some modern therapies can cause harm, and all can be overused, many modern therapies do much good. What is needed is appropriate use of effective and safe therapies for those conditions for which they are indicated. Some drugs do have serious side effects and risks. In those cases, a difficult risk-benefit analysis must be done by patients and their doctors to discern the best course of action.

We are concerned that a complete dismissal of conventional medicine and modern pharmaceuticals can and will lead to much harm. A variety of groups and sects, some claiming to be Christian, refuse to allow even children to be treated by conventional medicine, leading Seth Asser and Rita Swan to claim that children are dying unnecessarily in the United States. They found 140 cases between 1975 and 1995 in which a child died without medical treatment from conditions for which conventional medicine had a greater than 90 percent survival rate. In all these cases, the parents refused to use conventional medicine because of the teachings of the religious groups to which they belonged.

• Recommendations

There are numerous ways in which people can and should change common dietary practices. Many people could benefit from eating a healthier, more balanced, and more natural diet, with fewer processed foods. But doing so does not necessitate becoming a vegetarian. Nor does it require abandoning the cooking of all foods. Christianity should bring new freedom to God's people. The life of Jesus fulfilled the Old Testament rituals and ceremonial laws so that now Christians are free. "It is for freedom that Christ has set us free. Stand firm, then, and do not let yourselves be burdened again by a yoke of slavery" (Galatians 5:1). The slavery mentioned here is to arbitrary laws and dogma regarding foods and other practices.

We must be careful how we exercise our freedom. In the context of dealing with the eating of meat, Paul says, " 'Everything is permissible' — but not everything is beneficial. 'Everything is permissible' — but not everything is constructive" (1 Corinthians 10:23). We believe the Bible clearly teaches that Christians have the freedom to eat meat but not to overindulge in it. We should eat a healthy, balanced diet so that we can enjoy good health in this life and thereby glorify God and serve others.

Our primary concern here is not with the particulars of any Christian therapy. Christians are free to be vegetarians if they so choose. Our concern is with the way some Christian therapies are presented as being "God's diet" or "God's supplement" yet are based on inaccurate or incomplete scientific evidence and biblical claims arrived at by questionable methods of interpretation.

We are also concerned, and believe you should be too, when an alternative therapy advocate exhibits grandiosity ("I know more than any doctor knows"), makes messianic claims ("There will be no more illness when you follow my teachings"), or generates unrealistic fears ("All drugs are so dangerous that it pays to risk one's life to avoid them").

Christians who use these approaches appear to be absolutely certain that they are correct and completely biblical. In effect, they believe they know more than most theologians (whom they often label as "Pharisees") and medical experts (whom they often label as "frauds"). Paul told the Corinthians that when someone was speaking out in God's name (as a prophet), "the others should weigh carefully what is said" (1 Corinthians 14:29). Christian therapies should be submitted to such an examination. When a therapy fails the test of biblical reliability or does not have scientific support, we feel obligated to disagree theologically or scientifically.

As in all areas of health, what is needed is balance. Christian therapies may bring some benefits. Those that include a vegetarian diet probably will bring benefits to those who previously ate inappropriately. In *God's Way to Ultimate Health*, the Rev. Malkmus claims, "All we have to do to be well is eat and live according to the way God intended!" By this he means adhere to his diet. We respectfully disagree. Diet may contribute to illnesses, but there are many other causes. The situation is often very complicated. We cannot realistically avoid all sickness and disease.

If you decide to use any of these therapies, do so with joy, wisdom, and understanding. Do not do so dogmatically. Use them if they are based on reliable evidence, not because someone claims God has ordained this approach — an idea we don't find taught in the Bible. And do not blindly follow the teaching against conventional medicine and pharmaceuticals. We also believe it is very important to pray diligently in the midst of illness (see the Prayer for Healing entry).

● Further Reading

Asser, Seth M., and Rita Swan. "Child Fatalities from Religion-Motivated Medical Neglect." *Pediatrics* 101, no. 4 (April 1998): 625 – 29.

Day, Lorraine. *Diseases Just Don't Happen.* Thousand Palms, Calif.: Rockford Press, 1998. Videotape and various articles. *www.drday.com.* Accessed October 26, 2005.

Donaldson, Michael S. "Metabolic Vitamin B_{12} Status on a Mostly Raw Vegan Diet with Follow-up Using Tablets, Nutritional Yeast, or Probiotic Supplements." *Annals of Nutrition and Metabolism* 44, nos. 5 – 6 (December 2000): 229 – 34.

Jacobson, Michael. *The Word on Health: A Biblical and Medical Overview of How to Care for Your Body.* Chicago: Moody Press, 2000.

Malkmus, George H. *God's Way to Ultimate Health.* Eidson, Tenn.: Hallelujah Acres, 1995.

Malkmus, George H. *Why Christians Get Sick.* Shippensburg, Penn.: Treasure House, 1995. Various articles. *www.hacres.com.* Accessed March 23, 2001, and October 26, 2005.

Willett, Walter C. "Convergence of Philosophy and Science: The Third International Congress on Vegetarian Nutrition." *American Journal of Clinical Nutrition* 70, suppl. 3 (September 1999): S434 – S438.

Yamauchi, Edwin M. "Magic in the Biblical World." *Tyndale Bulletin* 34 (1983): 169 – 200. (For more on the Greek word *pharmakeia.*)

COLONICS

● What They Are

Enemas (irrigation of the colon) are used medically to relieve constipation and to clear the bowels prior to colon surgeries or procedures. Colonic hydrotherapy (colonics or colonic irrigation) is usually practiced outside of conventional medicine. Colon therapy in one form or another is actually many centuries old. Even in the early 1900s, the American Medical Association criticized colonic irrigation (also called "detoxification") when used to allegedly remove toxins and enhance health.

Since ancient Egypt, different theories have arisen tracing the origins of all human disease to feces. Those who advocate colonic hydrotherapy offer one of two theories on why patients should utilize it. The first theory, which has its roots in Darwin's concept of evolution, considers colonic hydrotherapy necessary to counter what is known as "ptosis." This term simply means that an organ has moved downward from its usual position. According to this theory, as humans evolved from four-legged to two-legged animals, gravity in the standing position pulled the abdominal cavity in a different direction. This pressure, so the theory contends, produced a drop, or ptosis, in the intestines that caused stress bands that narrowed the intestines, slowing passage of the contents. Treatment includes massage to help move bowel contents along and colonic irrigation to loosen the contents.

The second and related theory, championed by French physician Charles-Jacques Bouchard (1837 – 1915), is "autointoxication." Just when microorganisms were being identified as the cause of some diseases (leading to the germ theory of disease), Bouchard proposed that slower movement of waste through the colon would give microorganisms time to decompose that material. That would lead to the production of toxins, which could then be absorbed back into the body, causing disease and illness. This reabsorption leads to the body poisoning itself, which is what Bouchard and others called "autointoxication."

The most famous practitioner of colon therapy was Dr. John Harvey Kellogg of Battle Creek, Michigan, better known for his breakfast cereals. Dr. Kellogg practiced in the early twentieth century, and by 1920, colon therapy had become quite popular. The doctor was convinced that by using colonic therapy, he had saved almost 40,000 sufferers of gastrointestinal illness from surgery. He claimed that only twenty of his patients had to undergo the knife.

Colonics are performed by inserting a soft tube into the rectum. Gravity or a pump then gently pushes the liquid in and out of the colon. Up to 50 liters can be run in and out of the bowel this way. FDA-approved colonic machines usually come with filters to remove bacteria from the infusion liquid.

Claims

Colonics have been said to treat or cure arthritis, fatigue, depression, anxiety, headache, seizures, alcoholism, allergies, asthma, colitis, hypertension, parasites, skin disorders, fevers, and ulcerative colitis. They are also used to "detoxify" the body and generally improve health.

Although enemas are not true colonics, they can be included here. Enemas empty only the end of the colon. They have a legitimate role in health care, but some use them in the belief that they rid the body of toxins. Mineral oil enemas, called "lavages," have been used because they seem like the ideal way to eliminate feces while lubricating the colon.

Study Findings

Unfortunately, there are no well-performed, controlled medical studies to support or refute this type of therapy. Further, the FDA classifies colonic irrigation systems as Class III devices that can only be marketed for medically indicated colon cleansing (such as before certain radiologic examinations). No system has been approved for "routine" colon cleansing to promote general well-being. Some doctors believe that patients who feel better after colonics are responding to a placebo effect induced by their belief that colonics are helpful.

Cautions

Reports show (✗✗) that colonic irrigation has been associated with at least one outbreak of amoebiasis (an infection caused by a tiny one-celled organism called an "amoeba" that can be spread by the use of improperly cleaned colonic equipment contaminated with fecal material). Other types of colon infections have been caused by colonics. Three cases of colonic tubes puncturing patients' colons have been reported recently, requiring emergency treatment to prevent systemic infections — those that spread throughout a patient's body (✗✗). Two deaths associated with coffee enemas have also been reported (✗✗). Some doctors worry that colonics might change the normal bacteria in the colon, but this has never been reported. Other unproven concerns include the loss of intestinal muscle tone and normal defecation reflex, water intoxication, and electrolyte disturbances. People with any intestinal problem or illness should consult a physician before undergoing colonics.

Recommendations

We could find no studies to prove or disprove that colonics enhance health. No medical evidence supports the use of colonics other than for constipation and pre- or postoperative reasons. Adverse effects appear to be relatively infrequent. Yet when there is no evidence that something is effective, any risk is too large to take. We are also concerned that those who promote colonics do not place enough importance on having evidence to support their recommendations. There is no scientific basis for using or recommending colonics for general health.

Treatment Categories

Conventional

To treat severe constipation
(under medical care)   ☺☺☺☺

To prepare people for certain
surgeries   ☺☺☺☺

Scientifically Questionable

To use in detoxification
or other indications   ☹☹☹☹

Quackery or Fraud

In the hands of some practitioners

Further Reading

Handley, Doug V., Nick A. Rieger, and David J. Rodda. "Rectal Perforation from Colonic Irrigation Administered by Alternative Practitioners." *Medical Journal of Australia* 181, no. 10 (November 2004): 575 – 76.

Jarvis, William T. "Colonic Irrigation." *National Council Against Health Fraud: www.ncahf.org/articles/c-d/ colonic.html.* Accessed November 1, 2005.

Sullivan-Fowler, Micaela. "Doubtful Theories, Drastic Therapies: Autointoxication and Faddism in the Late Nineteenth and Early Twentieth Centuries." *Journal of the History of Medicine and Allied Sciences* 50 (July 1995): 364 – 90.

CRANIOSACRAL THERAPY

What It Is

Craniosacral therapy was popularized in the 1970s by osteopathic physician John Upledger. He adapted the older approach of W. G. Sutherland called "cranial osteopathy." Although arising out of an osteopathic approach, craniosacral therapy is not typically viewed as part of conventional osteopathic medicine.

Cranial osteopathy, on which craniosacral therapy is based, evolved from two controversial ideas. The first is the belief that the bones of the cranium (the part of the skull surrounding the brain) can be moved relative to one another. This is true with babies because movement of the bones is necessary for vaginal birth. However, these bones are naturally fused during childhood, or at least held in place by very dense connective tissue. They are no longer movable to any significant degree in older children, teenagers, or adults.

The second disputed proposal deals with cerebrospinal fluid and the idea of cranial rhythmic impulse (CRI). Cerebrospinal fluid brings nutrients and protection to the brain and the spine. Cranial osteopaths claim they can detect pulsation in this fluid using their hands. No instruments are available to objectively measure CRI. Therapists claim they can restore CRI to normal by using gentle pressure that does not manipulate or massage but stimulates inherent "potential" and releases tension and memories. Exactly what is meant here varies among therapists.

Craniosacral therapy focuses on the soft tissues (various membranes and connective tissues) around the skull and spine, while cranial osteopathy focuses on the bones. The goal of both therapies is the same: restoration of an even, rhythmic CRI in the cerebrospinal fluid. Therapy is believed to improve the function of the central nervous system, the immune system, and other systems. Craniosacral therapists apply a gentle and subtle pressure to the head and sacrum (base of the spine) to manipulate the membranes said to control CRI.

Claims

The CRI is believed to influence the connective tissues that surround all the major organs and muscles of the body. Craniosacral therapy is used primarily to relieve chronic aches and pains throughout the body, but especially muscle problems and arthritis. It is also believed to relieve stress, lift depression, correct learning disabilities, and assist in a patient's recovery from brain and head injuries, as well as stroke and meningitis. Therapists claim to be especially successful with children because their cranial bones are not yet fused. Some claim that head injuries occur in the womb and during birth so that all babies should have a craniosacral checkup soon after birth. This, they claim, will help prevent such conditions as autism, cerebral palsy, dyslexia, and learning difficulties.

Study Findings

There are many anecdotal reports (✔✔) of dramatic recoveries from chronic, persistent problems, especially through the Upledger Institute in Florida. However, a 1999 review of research literature found very few studies of the therapy and none of sufficient quality to recommend its use (✗✗✗). It remains controversial to claim that the bones of the cranium can be moved in adults. At least five controlled studies have found that craniosacral therapists did not agree on their CRI measurements or on the effects of one another's manipulations (✗✗✗✗). The most recent of these had two therapists simultaneously measure a patient's CRI, one at the cranium and the other at the sacrum. Completely different values were obtained in all cases, even though the theory predicts the values should be the same.

Cautions

Craniosacral therapy appears to be very gentle, much more so than cranial osteopathy. There appears to be little danger from craniosacral therapy so long as serious problems are not missed if conventional care is avoided or postponed. Great caution should be exercised by anyone attempting to manipulate a child's growing bones. Cranial osteopathy is offered by osteopathic physicians, but craniosacral therapy can be offered by anyone who has completed a course in the therapy. CRI practitioners may have little or no medical training and are not qualified to diagnose medical problems.

Some craniosacral therapists now claim that the therapy works by manipulating "life energy" rather than bones or fluid. Thus, people should be alert to therapists wanting to expose patients to New Age thinking and practices.

Recommendations

There is no evidence that craniosacral therapy does anything more than help people relax. Many experts claim that simply lying down will produce greater changes in the pressure of the cerebrospinal fluid than any manipulation of the bones or membranes of the head.

Treatment Categories

Scientifically Questionable
For any indication ☹☹☹☹

Spiritual
In the hands of some practitioners 👎👎

Quackery or Fraud
In the hands of some practitioners

Further Reading

Green, C., C. W. Martin, K. Bassett, and A. Kazanjian. "A Systematic Review of Craniosacral Therapy: Biological Plausibility, Assessment Reliability and Clinical Effectiveness." *Complementary Therapies in Medicine* 7, no. 4 (December 1999): 201 – 7.

Hehir, Brid. "Head Cases: An Examination of Craniosacral Therapy." *RCM Midwives Journal* 6, no. 1 (January 2003): 38 – 40.

Moran, Robert W., and Peter Gibbons. "Intraexaminer and Interexaminer Reliability for Palpation of the Cranial Rhythmic Impulse at the Head and Sacrum." *Journal of Manipulative and Physiological Therapeutics* 24, no. 3 (March – April 2001): 183 – 90.

DIET AND NUTRITION

● What They Are

Why discuss diet and nutrition in a book on alternative medicine when conventional medicine has always recognized them as important?

Many surveys reporting on the popularity of alternative medicine include nutrition as an alternative therapy, sometimes with emphasis on dietary supplements to provide critical nutrients. In our opinion, the majority of studies reveal that the nutrients everyone needs are best obtained through a healthy, balanced diet, though there are exceptions. Certain illnesses make it necessary for some people to take specific nutritional supplements.

With increased attention on dietary supplements, some people might ignore good eating habits, trusting instead in supplements to meet their needs. Others may already be eating a healthy diet, getting everything they need, but add supplements since everyone else seems to be taking them. Or, for example, news reports that antioxidants in vegetables have health benefits might prompt some to begin taking dietary supplements containing these antioxidants rather than doing what would be cheaper and better: eating more vegetables. Dietary supplements are of inconsistent quality, so you are more able to assure yourself the nutrition your body needs by eating a proper diet.

The following information gives principles to keep in mind as you plan and cook meals. We will not focus here on specific dietary supplements. The most popular of these are considered in Part 3.

Guidelines for a Healthy Diet

A healthy diet is a balanced diet containing complex carbohydrates (grains, fruits, and vegetables), oils, milk, and protein. In 2005, the old familiar USDA Food Guide Pyramid underwent a major overhaul and is now called MyPyramid. The old guidelines stipulated that a balanced diet consisted of 50 to 60 percent "good" or complex carbohydrates, 20 to 25 percent "good" fat, and 20 to 25 percent protein. The new guidelines take into greater account individual

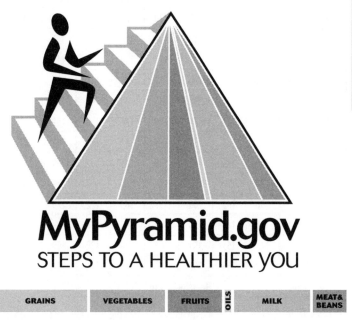

| GRAINS | VEGETABLES | FRUITS | OILS | MILK | MEAT & BEANS |

Graphic courtesy of the United States Department of Agriculture

167

variability and people's differing needs. The pyramid itself does not give specific amounts of each food category but points to relative proportions. It includes helpful ways to figure out specifically how much of the different food groups people should be eating based on their current weight, age, and activity level. And it emphasizes the importance of exercise and physical activity. By accessing MyPyramid through the Internet (*www.MyPyramid.gov*), you can get customized personal recommendations on the daily calorie needs for each family member based on the 2005 dietary guidelines.

Aim to have your weight in the range of what is normal. Being overweight or obese has negative effects on your health no matter what percentage comes from carbohydrates, oils, or protein. Your normal range will vary depending on your gender, age, height, and other relevant factors. It's easy to think that ideal weight is based on the appearance of professional athletes or underweight models. That's usually not the case. The most recent research points to determining ideal body weight by measuring body mass index (BMI). A BMI of 19 to 25 is considered an ideal body weight. Table 1 shows how to figure out your BMI.

Table 1:

BMI	18	19	20	21	22	23	24	25	26	27	28	29	30	31	32
Height	Body Weight (pounds)														
4'10"	86	91	96	100	105	110	115	119	124	129	134	138	143	148	153
4'11"	89	94	99	104	109	114	119	124	128	133	138	143	148	153	158
5'0"	92	97	102	107	112	118	123	128	133	138	143	148	153	158	163
5'1"	95	100	106	111	116	122	127	132	137	143	148	153	158	164	169
5'2"	98	104	109	115	120	126	131	136	142	147	153	158	164	169	175
5'3"	102	107	113	118	124	130	135	141	146	152	158	163	169	175	180
5'4"	105	110	116	122	128	134	140	145	151	157	163	169	174	180	186
5'5"	108	114	120	126	132	138	144	150	156	162	168	174	180	186	192
5'6"	112	118	124	130	136	142	148	155	161	167	173	179	186	192	198
5'7"	115	121	127	134	140	146	153	159	166	172	178	185	191	198	204
5'8"	118	125	131	138	144	151	158	164	171	177	184	190	197	203	210
5'9"	122	128	135	142	149	155	162	169	176	182	189	196	203	209	216
5'10"	126	132	139	146	153	160	167	174	181	188	195	202	209	216	222
5'11"	129	136	143	150	157	165	172	179	186	193	200	208	215	222	229
6'0"	132	140	147	154	162	169	177	184	191	199	206	213	221	228	235
6'1"	136	144	151	159	166	174	182	189	197	204	212	219	227	235	242
6'2"	141	148	155	163	171	179	186	194	202	210	218	225	233	241	249
Underweight	Healthy Weight						Overweight					Obese			

Find your height in the left-hand column and look across the row until you find the number closest to your weight. The number at the top of that column gives your BMI.

How much and when you eat can be as important as what you eat. If you eat more calories than you use in daily activities, you will gain weight. If you want to lose weight, you need to use more calories than you take in. Based on your current age, weight, and activity level, figure out how many calories you need to eat each day to either maintain your weight or move gradually toward your ideal weight range. You can estimate your calorie needs a few different ways, with Table 2 giving one example.

Table 2: Calculating Calorie Needs (from *www.MyPyramid.gov*)

Age (years)	Calorie Range	
	Sedentary (only typical daily activities)	Active (walking for at least one hour daily)
Toddlers		
2 – 3	1,000 ➡	1,400
Females		
4 – 8	1,200 ➡	1,800
9 – 13	1,600 ➡	2,200
14 – 18	1,800 ➡	2,400
19 – 30	2,000 ➡	2,400
31 – 50	1,800 ➡	2,200
51+	1,600 ➡	2,200
Males		
4 – 8	1,400 ➡	2,000
9 – 13	1,800 ➡	2,600
14 – 18	2,200 ➡	3,200
19 – 30	2,400 ➡	3,000
31 – 50	2,200 ➡	3,000
51+	2,000 ➡	2,800

Another rough way to calculate your calorie needs is to multiply your weight in pounds by 15 if you are moderately active or by 13 if you are relatively inactive. More precise estimates can be calculated. One is available on the *Consumer Reports* website (*www.consumerreports.org/cro/health-fitness/top-diets-how-many-calories-do-you-need-605/index.htm*). Once you know how many calories you should consume each day, *www.MyPyramid.gov* gives tables showing you how to divide up the portions of each food category. A part of those tables is reproduced in Table 3. For example, if you should consume 2,000 calories per day, you will obtain this from the food in that column (that is, 2 cups of fruit, 2.5 cups of vegetables, and so forth). These can be consumed in any combination during the day.

Table 3: Calculating Daily Food Portions

Calorie Level	1,600	2,000	2,400	2,800	3,200
Fruits	1.5 cups	2 cups	2 cups	2.5 cups	2.5 cups
Vegetables	2 cups	2.5 cups	3 cups	3.5 cups	4 cups
Grains*	5 oz-eq	6 oz-eq	8 oz-eq	10 oz-eq	10 oz-eq
Meat and Beans[†]	4 oz-eq	5.5 oz-eq	6.5 oz-eq	7 oz-eq	7 oz-eq
Milk[‡]	3 cups	3 cups	3 cups	3 cups	3 cups
Oils[§]	5 tsp	6 tsp	7 tsp	8 tsp	11 tsp
Discretion	132 calories	267 calories	362 calories	426 calories	648 calories

*1 ounce-equivalent of Grains is 1 slice of bread or 1 cup of cereal or ½ cup of cooked rice, cereal, or pasta.

[†] 1 ounce-equivalent of Meat and Beans is 1 ounce of meat, poultry, fish, or 1 egg, ¼ cup of cooked dry beans, or ½ ounce of nuts or seeds.

[‡] 1 cup of milk or yogurt is the equivalent of 1½ ounces of natural cheese or 2 ounces of processed cheese. Group does not include milk products with little calcium such as butter, cream, and cream cheese. Milk should be low-fat or fat-free.

[§] Oils include only those from plants and fish that are liquid at room temperature.

The Recommended Food Groups

Grains

The most widely eaten grains are wheat, rice, oats, cornmeal, and barley. This group includes all the foods made from these grains, including bread, pasta, cereals, tortillas, oatmeal, and grits. Grains are composed primarily of carbohydrates, a ready source of energy. But not all carbohydrates are equally nutritious. The group includes complex carbohydrates (such as those found in whole grains) and simple sugars. While bread and cereal are important, easy, and inexpensive foods, the huge popularity of low-carbohydrate diets points to a problem. A huge increase in the consumption of processed grains and simple sugars correlates well with the growth of the obesity epidemic in Western nations. The new Food Pyramid recommends that at least half of all grains should be whole grains.

Grains are an important food because of the many nutrients they contain. In addition to carbohydrates, grains contain fiber that is important for a healthy digestive system. They also contain some proteins, vitamins, and minerals. Stone-ground whole-grain bread is vastly more nutritious than highly processed (white) bread or even enriched white bread because the processing removes many nutrients and fiber. Grains are also valuable because of what they lack. Foods made from grains tend to be relatively low in fat.

However, most fast foods and bakery-produced breadlike foods, such as donuts, pastries, and sweets, have a high fat content and high calorie count and should be kept to a minimum. They represent "bad" carbohydrates, as do most simple sugars, or "sweets." Consumption of soft drinks, another source of large amounts of simple sugars, should be reduced to a minimum.

Vegetables and fruits

Many recent studies have documented the extensive health benefits of eating several servings a day of fruits and vegetables. They have been the primary source of nutrition throughout most of human history and remain so for most of the world's population. Plant foods contain nutritious complex ("good") carbohydrates, are high in fiber and low in fat, and are healthy sources of other substances (called "phytochemicals") that include vitamins, antioxidants, and other plant products. Phytochemicals have health-promoting benefits and have been shown to act as antioxidants, stimulate the immune system, lower cholesterol, improve many hormone levels, and assist the body's detoxification systems. While in some cases we know which individual phytochemical has which specific effect, the mixture of compounds found in natural foods seems to work better than the individual components taken as supplements.

Fruits make a great snack, and many are best eaten unpeeled, after thorough washing, as the skins are high in fiber. Most vegetables are best eaten uncooked, or lightly steamed, as prolonged cooking destroys some of the nutrients. However, some vegetables seem to have improved health benefits when cooked. Tomatoes are one example.

Milk

Low-fat or nonfat milk products are believed by many, but not all, experts to be an important primary source of nutrients and vitamins, especially calcium. Some people are allergic to milk or cannot digest it easily, so they will need to have other sources of these nutrients. Milk products contain vitamins A, C, and E, some of the B vitamins, and minerals such as calcium and magnesium. They also contain proteins, carbohydrates, and in some cases fats. The group includes milk, cheese, yogurt, sour cream, cottage cheese, and many other products. The new *MyPyramid.gov* guidelines recommend only those milk products that contain calcium, including milk, yogurt, and cheese.

The Old Testament frequently describes the Promised Land as "a land flowing with milk and honey" (Exodus 3:8). The abundance of milk was often used as a metaphor for God's provision (Isaiah 55:1; see also Deuteronomy 32:14; Proverbs 27:27; Isaiah 7:22). However, the milk of today is not necessarily the milk of the Bible. Most milk is now homogenized and pasteurized, which has led to debate over the benefits of processed milk. Processing prevents the transmission of many infections and makes it possible to reduce the fat content, but it also can damage some nutrients. Because of these concerns, some avoid all milk products, claiming the Bible prohibits all animal foods. We discuss in more detail under Christian Therapies why we disagree with this position. It is difficult to reconcile with the way Abraham and the angels ate curds (a delicacy somewhat like cheese or butter) and drank milk (Genesis 18:8), the way milk was recognized as important for healthy teeth (Genesis 49:12), and the way Israelites kept milk available to drink (Judges 4:19).

Milk products can contain significant amounts of saturated fat, so no-fat or low-fat milk products are preferable for those age two or older. Low-fat milk has about 1 percent fat, compared to 3 percent fat in whole milk. Because of hormones and antibiotics given to cows in commercial dairy operations, some turn to "organic" dairy products to avoid this type of exposure. Others use goat or soy milk, trying to gain the benefits of the protein without the possible detriments of commercial cow milk.

Meat and beans

The foods in this group, including meat, poultry, fish, and beans, contain significant amounts of protein and numerous vitamins and nutrients. Meat varies in the type and proportion of saturated (or "bad") fat it contains. Expensive cuts of beef contain about 20 percent saturated fat, whereas up to half of some types of lowest-priced ground beef can consist of fat. Animal fat tends to be primarily saturated fat, which is not as healthy as the unsaturated fat found to a greater extent in plants and fish.

The Bible seems to indicate that meat was eaten only on occasion, except by the rich who could afford to eat it regularly (Genesis 18:6 – 8; 27:3 – 4; 1 Samuel 2:13 – 15). Fish was an important part of the diet during the time of Jesus. The Old Testament law was very specific about which meat was clean or unclean (Leviticus 11; Deuteronomy 14). These laws demonstrate that vegetarianism is not obligatory for Christians, although some may choose such a diet. We give our reasons for this position in our entry on Christian Therapies.

Vegetarians who avoid meat and dairy products must be careful to obtain sufficient protein elsewhere and supplement their diet with certain nutrients and vitamins, especially vitamin B_{12}. Sufficient protein can also be obtained relatively easily from dried beans, nuts, and soy protein, which also are sources of other important nutrients, such as vitamins and antioxidants.

Oils

The oil group is barely visible in the new Food Pyramid. Oils and fats contain more than twice as many calories per gram as protein or carbohydrates, which is part of the reason we need less of them. Oils and fats are very similar chemically, but as with carbohydrates, there are good and bad types. Including only oils in the new Food Pyramid indicates that the bad fats should be avoided or limited. Yet the proportion of fat in the average American diet increased steadily during the twentieth century, at times approaching 50 percent.

The bad fats to avoid are saturated fats, hydrogenated fats, trans-fatty acids (TFAs), and cholesterol.

Foods high in these fats include any milk product that does not say it is nonfat, fatty meats, hydrogenated or partially hydrogenated vegetable oils (which convert them to solids), egg yolks, most margarines, most baked goods, and many fast foods. As of January 2006, food labels in the United States must indicate (under Ingredients) whether hydrogenated fats, partially hydrogenated fats, or trans-fats are in the food.

The "good" oils come primarily from plants and fish. They include the omega-9 fatty acids (contained in olive oil) and the omega-3 fatty acids (contained in the oils of cold-water fish such as cod, salmon, halibut, and swordfish, and in virtually all types of nuts). Good oils are found in canola, corn, olive, soybean, and sunflower oil and in avocados. These oils have many health benefits, and a diet deficient in them is actually associated with some poor health outcomes.

What is called the "Mediterranean Diet" is very low in the "bad" fats and has up to 25 percent "good" fat — especially olive oil. The healthiest of the olive oils appears to be "cold-pressed, extra-virgin" olive oil, which can be used instead of butter (some call it "Italian butter") and in salad dressings. However, cooking has to be done with "regular" olive oil, as the regular olive oil has a higher smoke point than extra-virgin olive oil.

For most people living in developed countries, the types of foods in the diet and the way they are prepared must change. Fried food has more fat than the same food cooked any other way. Cook with olive oil instead of butter. Instead of flavoring dishes with cream sauces or butter, use herbs and spices. When cooking with eggs, don't use the yolks. Remove the skin and fat from poultry. Reduce overall fat consumption and replace unhealthy fats with healthy oils (such as olive and canola) and omega-3 fatty acid – containing foods (such as fish). Eat less.

Water

A vital part of the diet — water — is not found anywhere on the Food Pyramid. At birth, the body is three-fourths water. This decreases as we age, but water remains the single most abundant substance in our bodies. We need water to transport nutrients around the body and remove wastes. Water plays a central role in regulating body temperature. Most chemical reactions that allow life to continue occur within a liquid environment. Water is one of the starting materials required for some reactions our cells carry out, including breaking down all of the major food groups.

To provide the body with enough water, it is commonly said that most healthy adults need to drink at least eight to ten eight-ounce glasses of water a day. Some experts recommend this rule: take your weight in pounds, divide it in half, and drink that many ounces of water every day. Many teach that water is best taken as pure water, and not in drinks such as tea or coffee. However, there is very little data to support any of these common recommendations. In fact, the prestigious Institute of Medicine's Food and Nutrition Board says that eight glasses of water isn't necessary because most people get plenty of fluid from their food. For example, many fruits and vegetables are 80 to 90 percent water. The Institute tells us that "when our body warns us through thirst that it's time to drink something — then drink up."

Most parts of the United States have a plentiful supply of clean, safe water. In other parts of the world, people live or die depending on whether their water supply is maintained. In biblical times, an abundant supply of drinking water was another reminder of God's loving provision. Jesus used the importance of water for physical life as a metaphor for the spiritual life he offered: "Jesus stood and said in a loud voice, 'If anyone is thirsty, let him come to me and drink. Whoever believes in me, as the Scripture has said, streams of living water will flow from within him.' By this he meant the Spirit, whom those who believed in him were later to receive" (John 7:37–39; see also 4:10–14).

The rise in purchases of bottled water has prompted a number of city water departments and various researchers to check the quality of tap water against the quality of the bottled mineral and spring water available at a much higher cost. In most instances, the quality of the tap water was higher — especially water purified using an ionization process as opposed to a filtration process. In fact, some studies have shown that as much as 50 percent of the bottled water samples tested had excessive amounts of viruses, bacteria, or other impurities. Water from a "natural spring" does not guarantee quality. There are health food purists who say the only water to drink is steam distilled. Certainly a safe alternative, but in most large cities, steam-distilled water is, in our opinion, a needless expense.

Water is so readily available for most of us that we are not content with "just" water. We have become used to beverages with taste — with caffeine or sugar to keep us going. Sugar is a source of needless calories, and caffeine, a diuretic, is said by some to cause the body to eliminate fluids, while other experts say this is not true for those who drink caffeine on a daily basis. So the debate continues. The "pro-water" experts argue the caffeine of coffee or tea works against the body's need to remain hydrated. They declare that the ensuing dehydration can lead to much more than just being thirsty. It can cause headaches and intestinal problems and even be a factor in more serious illnesses. They believe most people would benefit from increasing their intake of pure water and decreasing their intake of other beverages. We find the recommendations of the Institute of Medicine the most compelling — when you feel thirsty, drink water. Making water your beverage of choice at and between meals is likely to be a very healthful activity.

When you are ill, it is especially important to drink lots of water. That's one of the reasons so many people in a hospital are hooked up to an IV bag. Remember to also adjust your water intake based on weather and your activity level. Those exercising in warm weather should drink two to four extra glasses of water in the hour before exercising, a glass of water every thirty minutes during exercise (if practical), and afterward, three glasses of water for every pound of weight lost during exercise (mostly water lost through sweating). That's a lot of water, but it has been shown to improve exercise performance and may also lead to a stronger overall feeling of well-being.

Study Findings

Collectively, in studies conducted in the United States and in the United Kingdom, cardiovascular diseases, cancer, and diabetes have been shown to account for over 60 percent of all deaths. Globally, cardiovascular diseases cause about one-third of all deaths, with three-quarters of those occurring in developing countries. These diseases come with a huge cost in terms of suffering, pain, and resources. A large quantity of research has shown that these three diseases have the same three major risk factors: smoking, obesity, and physical inactivity. While several strategies to reduce smoking have been put into effect and are having some success, strategies to improve people's dietary and exercise habits are lagging behind. In 2004, the American Cancer Society, the American Diabetes Association, and the American Heart Association announced they would work together to draw attention to the importance of diet and activity for health.

ALTERNATIVE THERAPIES

The connection between the above chronic diseases and diet is supported by many epidemiological studies (✓✓). These large surveys are designed to measure different factors that might give clues about what lifestyle factors impact people's health. Winston Craig, a professor of nutrition, reported that out of 156 of these types of studies (✓✓), 82 percent found that increased fruit and vegetable consumption was connected to protection against a wide variety of cancers. Those who ate the most fruits and vegetables had roughly half the risk of getting cancer, especially those cancers that involve epithelial cells found in the lung, cervix, stomach, and colon.

Similar types of effects have been found in relation to cardiovascular disease and diabetes. A 1999 study (✓✓) found that men and women who ate five to six servings of fruits and vegetables per day had a 31 percent lower risk of stroke compared to those who ate one serving per day. A survey of more than 40,000 women asked whether they ate certain foods at least once a week. Twenty-three of these foods (such as apples, dried beans, baked fish, high-fiber cereal, low-fat milk) were included on the Food Pyramid. The women who ate the most of these foods (14 or more out of 23) had a 30 percent lower death rate than the group with the lowest scores (0–8), a statistically significant difference.

In another epidemiological study (✓✓), women who daily ate food from only two of the recommended food groups had a 40 percent higher risk of death than women who daily ate from five different food groups. In another study, men with healthier diets had a 13 percent lower risk of death.

Unfortunately, randomized controlled trials of dietary changes have not produced the positive results researchers had hoped to achieve (✗✗✗). For example, one group of patients was assigned a high-fiber diet after having surgery to remove colorectal polyps. Another similar group of patients was given a brochure on healthy eating. Over the subsequent years, no differences in the polyp recurrence rates were found between the two groups. Another similar controlled study added either 13.5 grams or 2 grams of wheat-bran fiber to patients' daily diet. After three years, the two groups' polyp recurrence rates were not statistically different.

While the results of such studies are disappointing, they do not necessarily lessen the importance of diet in the development of colorectal cancer (or for health in general). For one thing, these sorts of chronic diseases can take years to develop and therefore an intervention may take many years to make a significant difference. Most of the studies have been relatively short-lasting. More important, researching the health effects of dietary intervention is frustrated by its complexities. Benefits noticed in an epidemiological study may have more to do with general lifestyle than any one food. For example, people who eat more fruit might be different in some other ways that combine to improve their health. Mary Serdula, a physician-researcher at the Centers for Disease Control and Prevention, has shown that studies demonstrating health benefits from eating more fruits and vegetables also found that those who ate more of these foods tended to exercise more, and those who ate fewer tended to exercise less, smoke more, and drink more heavily.

The dietary recommendations given in the new Food Pyramid and discussed above are widely accepted by different professional organizations. In spite of the importance of diet for overall health, many people do not follow the recommended dietary guidelines. Professor Craig referred to one survey that found that the average American eats only one and one-half servings of vegetables and less than one serving of fruit per day. On the day the survey was taken, almost half the people said they had eaten no fruit. Only about one-third of Americans eat the recommended servings of grains, and only one-quarter consume the recommended number of dairy products.

Modern research is confirming the age-old wisdom underlying the saying, "An apple a day keeps the doctor away." In spite of both ancient wisdom and modern research, unhealthy eating habits are proving to be hard to break. Part of the problem may be that people need to improve their diet to *prevent* illness. Changes need to be made when people still feel healthy. Illness can provide strong motivation to change, but by the time symptoms are felt, it may be too late for dietary changes to make a difference. Or is it? This leads us to examine claims that dietary changes may cure diseases.

Diets as Cures

Evidence for claims that certain diets cure people of serious illnesses, such as cancer, is weak or nonexistent (✗✗✗). One such popular strategy is the Gerson Diet Therapy. This approach forms the basis of many Christian vegetarian diets. For example, Dr. Lorraine Day's website promotes the sale of many books on the Gerson Diet. Macrobiotics is very similar, incorporating aspects of traditional Chinese medicine. Other diets said to treat diseases are a group of metabolic therapies, each named for its creator: Kelley, Manner, Contreras, or Gonzalez.

Like many who claim vegetarian diets cure diseases, Dr. Max Gerson said his health improved dramatically after he changed his diet. Plagued with migraine headaches, he noticed that what he ate affected the severity and frequency of his headaches. We now know that diet directly impacts migraines because of its effects on a natural hormone called "serotonin." Conventional treatment of migraines includes elimination of certain foods.

Dr. Gerson believed that if diet relieved his migraines, it could cure other diseases. He developed a special diet for tuberculosis and then one for cancer. His ideas were not widely accepted, and he moved to Mexico to found the Gerson Clinic. He believed that cancer is caused primarily by changes in dietary patterns as countries become more developed and more affluent. People, he believed, simultaneously poison themselves with the chemicals found in foods grown using pesticides and artificial fertilizers and starve themselves of vital nutrients and vitamins by eating processed and poorly prepared food.

The Gerson Diet uses freshly prepared vegetable juices made by pressing organically grown products. Until 1989, raw liver juice was also used, but this concept was abandoned after numerous patients suffered serious adverse reactions to contaminants in the juice. The diet recommends consuming about twenty pounds of fruits and vegetables daily by drinking a glass of freshly prepared juice every hour. Supplements are added to aid digestion or replenish vitamins. Castor oil is taken to cleanse the system, and coffee enemas are used to relieve cancer pain. In addition, counseling, group therapy, and family support are strongly encouraged.

There is no question that a change in diet can help many people feel better (✓✓✓), especially given how unhealthy many people's diets are these days. Diet is important in the *prevention* of cancer (✓✓), but *curing* cancer through diet is a different matter. The main evidence cited for the Gerson Diet is anecdotal (✓). Gerson's books provide even weaker evidence, because, as he admits, he picked the best examples. What about all those people for whom his diet was not effective?

Much publicity has centered on a 1995 study (✔✔) published by Gar Hildenbrand from the Gerson Research Center. This found that melanoma patients lived longer on the Gerson Diet than those treated with conventional therapies. However, the study was not a randomized controlled trial but rather interviews with many Gerson Clinic patients. Many former patients could not be located for the study, which could have considerably skewed the results in favor of the therapy. But even with the information reported, no one could tell whether the diet caused any of the reported benefits. The researchers noted that the patients used many other conventional and alternative therapies. While at the Gerson Clinic, patients received psychological interventions and family support and achieved a sense of control from mastering the diet. Any improvements that occurred may have had as much to do with these factors as with the diet. The researchers stated in their report, "These cases are not held out by us as evidence that here is a 'cure' for cancer, but rather that some patients can get well." Yet a "cure" is exactly what many claim of the Gerson Diet and its many variants: that changing your diet will cure cancer and many other diseases. The evidence simply does not support that conclusion.

● Cautions

Remember the proper role of diet and nutrition. Although we are discovering that a healthy, balanced diet can play a role in preventing certain illnesses, a healthy diet does not guarantee good health. People develop serious illnesses for a variety of reasons. While we should do what we can to remain healthy, we cannot prevent all illness. Be wary of anyone claiming to guarantee perfect health through dietary changes alone. We must also be cautious about claims that a particular diet can cure serious diseases. Some dietary changes can be difficult to tolerate, especially when people are weakened from a serious illness or conventional treatments such as surgery or chemotherapy. Using diet alone to treat a serious illness may result in people avoiding effective treatments.

However, some diseases are caused by factors in the diet and can be treated by dietary changes. In some parts of the world, many diseases are caused by dietary deficiencies. In the Western world, most diet-related diseases are due to people's reactions to certain components in the diet. An important example of the latter involves milk products. Some people become less able to tolerate milk as they get older because of a particular type of sugar in milk called "lactose." This requires an enzyme called "lactase" to digest it properly. People whose ancestors came from northern and western Europe continue to produce lactase as they get older and usually have no problem with milk products. But people of any other ethnic origin tend to produce less lactase as they age. This gives rise to a condition called "lactose intolerance," which leads to various intestinal problems and pain whenever milk is consumed. This condition is easily treated by reducing (or eliminating) milk products in the diet or by taking supplements of lactase. These are now readily available (one example is Lactaid), to be taken whenever milk products are consumed.

Milk can also be the source of other problems. Milk is one of the most common sources of food allergies, best treated by avoiding milk products altogether. A more serious problem, called "galactosemia," occurs in a small number of newborn babies. The heel-prick blood test is done on all newborns to check for the presence of this genetic condition (and others). When lactose is digested, another sugar is produced called "galactose." If the enzyme needed to break this down is not present, galactose builds up in the blood and can lead to brain damage. A baby with this condition must avoid all milk sugar.

If you suspect that an illness is linked to food, get advice from a professional trained in nutrition. Be aware that anyone can call himself or herself a nutritionist. There is no generally accepted standard for training or certifying nutritionists. In most cases, a registered dietitian should be consulted. Registered dietitians are nationally certified.

Recommendations

A balanced diet that meets the recommendations of the new food guidelines at *www.MyPyramid.gov* can go a long way toward maintaining good health and reducing the risk of several diseases. More and more research is finding that we can make significant improvements in our health, and our long-term outlook, by adhering to these guidelines.

Most people are not successful in completely overhauling their diet in one swipe. Plan instead to make small, consistent steps toward your goal. To achieve maximum benefits, you must balance dietary changes with appropriate exercise and physical activity. Studies have found that even small dietary changes lead to some health improvements. Remember that these lifestyle changes are primarily beneficial in the prevention of disease, not its treatment.

Treatment Categories

Conventional

To reduce the risk of cardiovascular
diseases, cancer, and diabetes   ☺☺☺☺

Complementary

To reduce the risk of many
other chronic diseases   ☺☺☺☺
To improve general well-being   ☺☺☺☺

Scientifically Unproven

To cure diseases

Quackery or Fraud

Certain "miracle" foods and diets

Further Reading

Craig, Winston J. "Phytochemicals: Guardians of Our Health." *Journal of the American Dietetic Association* 97, suppl. 2 (1997): S199 – S204.

Gerson, Max. *A Cancer Therapy: Results of Fifty Cases and the Cure of Advanced Cancer by Diet Therapy.* 5th ed. Bonita, Calif.: Gerson Institute, 1990.

Hildenbrand, Gar, L. Christeene Hildenbrand, Karen Bradford, and Shirley W. Cavin. "Five-Year Survival Rates of Melanoma Patients Treated by Diet Therapy After the Manner of Gerson." *Alternative Therapies in Health and Medicine* 1, no. 4 (September 1995): 29 – 37.

Jacobson, Michael. *The Word on Health: A Biblical and Medical Overview of How to Care for Your Body and Mind.* Chicago: Moody Press, 2000.

Lampe, Johanna W. "Health Effects of Vegetables and Fruit, Assessing Mechanisms of Action in Human Experimental Studies." *American Journal of Clinical Nutrition* 70, suppl. (1999): S475 – S490.

Reddy, Srinath K., and Martijn B. Katan. "Diet, Nutrition and the Prevention of Hypertension and Cardiovascular Diseases." *Public Health Nutrition* 7, no. 1A (February 2004): 167 – 86.

Renehan, Andrew G., and Anthony Howell. "Preventing Cancer, Cardiovascular Disease, and Diabetes." *Lancet* 365 (April 2005): 1449 – 51.

DIETS AND DIETING

• What They Are

Dieting could be viewed as a national pastime (or obsession). Look at any magazine rack and you'll see the latest diet guaranteed to melt away the pounds as you sit and watch. "Lose weight while you sleep," calls the enticing ad.

In spite of all the "guaranteed" diets, the number of Americans who are overweight is growing. More than half of all adults in the United States and about a quarter of all children are overweight (body mass index [BMI] between 25 and 30; see table on p. 168). About one in three adults is obese (BMI greater than 30). In Europe, between 10 and 20 percent of the populations of various countries are obese. The rate of increase in obesity and overweight is similar in both the United States and Europe. The World Health Organization has declared obesity an "escalating epidemic" and "one of the greatest neglected public health problems of our time."

Obesity is spreading even as we learn more about the dangers of being overweight. Many chronic illnesses are caused by or made worse by being overweight. Obesity puts people at higher risk for diabetes, high blood pressure, heart disease, gallbladder disease, stroke, and some cancers. Out of an average group of one hundred obese adults, eighty will have at least one of the following: diabetes, high cholesterol levels, high blood pressure, coronary heart disease, gallbladder disease, or osteoarthritis; twenty will have at least two of these problems. Over a quarter of a million Americans die every year because of obesity, making it the second leading cause of preventable death in the United States (only smok-ing causes more). Yet three-fourths of those who are seriously overweight are not concerned about how their weight could impact their health.

In response to this problem, a $35 billion dieting industry has sprung up in the United States. More than $1 billion is spent annually in retail outlets on dietary supplements for weight loss. Of those who are trying to lose weight, a survey by Mary Serdula, M.D., found that only 20 percent were following the only well-established recommendations: eating fewer calories and engaging in two and a half hours of physical activity per week. Also of concern is a finding that in the United States almost one in three women of *normal* weight is trying to lose weight.

Because of the difficulty of making lifestyle changes and the frustration of failed diets, dieting pills have become increasingly popular. The best-known pharmaceutical weight-loss medication of the last two decades was the combination called Fen-Phen (fenfluramine taken with phentermine). Prescriptions for these drugs soared from 60,000 in 1992 to 18 million in 1996 even though the two drugs were never approved for use together. Tragically, reports of women developing valvular heart disease while taking the combination led to the "Fen" part of "Fen-Phen" being withdrawn by the manufacturer in 1997, along with a similar drug sold as Redux. At the end of 2000, the FDA called for withdrawal of phenylpropanolamine (PPA), another drug present in over-the-counter diet pills as well as cold remedies, because of the increased risk of hemorrhagic stroke (bleeding in the brain).

The vacuum created by these withdrawals has been filled by numerous herbal remedies and dietary supplements. More than fifty individual herbs and dietary supplements are marketed as weight-loss products. Many of these are formulated into complicated mixtures, such as Metabolife 356. This mixture of eighteen herbs, including ephedra, was literally cooked up in a man's kitchen for his ailing father. In spite of having no published controlled trials to support its effectiveness or safety, it was the most popular weight-loss dietary supplement until ephedra was banned in 2004 because of its adverse effects.

The most popular herbs and dietary supplements used for weight loss were recently reviewed by Dr. Robert Saper and colleagues. They found enough evidence to discourage use of ephedra and ephedra-caffeine mixtures because of adverse effects (✗✗✗). Findings like these provided evidence that led to ephedra's April 2004 ban in the United States. Chitosan, guar gum, and spirulina (or blue-green algae) have been ineffective in a number of controlled trials (✗✗✗). Dr. Saper and colleagues' review found insufficient evidence (and in some cases no controlled studies) to support the use of chromium, conjugated linoleic acid, ginseng, green tea, hydroxycitric acid, L-carnitine, psyllium, pyruvate, or St. John's wort for weight loss (✗✗✗). On the basis of available evidence, the use of any dietary supplement for weight loss cannot be recommended. Some of these are reviewed in more detail in Part 3.

In addition to diet pills, fad diets come and go every year. Many fall into the area of alternative therapies in that they often contain some grain of truth and hence work for some people. But then they are mass-marketed to help everyone lose weight. Some diets are said to be biblical; most are said to be scientifically based; all are "guaranteed" to work.

But do they? Will you shed all those pounds in so many weeks? If you do, will you stay at your lower weight? Are there any precautions to be aware of before embarking on these diets?

The following chart gives a brief overview of some of the most popular diets and approaches to losing weight, with a summary of what the available evidence suggests at this point.

Diet	Description	Claims	Evidence	Benefits	Cautions
Atkins Diet	The best-known low-carbohydrate, high-protein diet, *Dr. Atkins' New Diet Revolution*, is an updated version of his 1972 book. In the first two weeks, carbohydrates make up 5 percent of calorie intake, with unrestricted amounts of high-protein and high-fat foods. After two weeks some complex carbohydrates are allowed, but never more than 20 grams/day.	Cutting down on carbohydrates is said to reduce blood sugar levels and decrease insulin production. Less insulin forces our bodies to burn rather than store fat.	Insulin production is much more complicated. People who are overweight produce too much insulin, but not necessarily because of dietary carbohydrates. In controlled trials published after 2003, greater weight loss was found compared to low-calorie diets up to six months. After twelve months, weight loss was similar. (✓✓✓)	Eliminating carbohydrates will reduce overall calorie intake. Proteins and fats are digested more slowly, meaning people feel full longer.	Adherence to this diet is low. Large amounts of protein contain much fat. This may lead to unhealthy blood lipid levels, though studies have not found this yet. Long-term studies are needed. Diet contains little fiber, which may lead to intestinal problems. Many nutrients are lacking, requiring supplements. Bad breath results from excess fats being broken down to ketones.

ALTERNATIVE THERAPIES

Diet	Description	Claims	Evidence	Benefits	Cautions
Blood-Type Diet	People of different blood types should choose different diets.	Blood types reflect different evolutionary ancestry. For example, type O means your ancestors were Stone Age hunters, so you need lots of meat and intense exercise but few grains and dairy products.	No convincing or reputable evidence supports blood types being related to evolutionary ancestry or diet. People in the same family can have different blood types. (✗ ✗ ✗)	Some recommendations may be healthy. Type O people may start exercising more. Type A people are advised to cut down on meat, and this may be helpful.	Some recommendations may be unhealthy. Type O elimination of grains and dairy products will reduce vitamin and nutrient intake. Type A people are told to reduce exercise, which will not help.
Cabbage Soup Diet	A soup made from cabbage, onions, peppers, tomatoes, and celery is eaten exclusively for one week. A short break is taken, and then you restart with soup alone.	This diet drastically reduces your calorie intake and you lose weight.	It works to reduce weight rapidly, although much of this may be water loss. However, there is no evidence that people keep this weight off. (✗ ✗)	This diet can produce short-term, nonsustained weight loss.	Many essential nutrients and vitamins are lacking. This diet can cause serious problems if maintained for long periods and can lead to rebound weight gain
Candida Diet	The goal is to eliminate all sources of yeast (such as bread and beer) and sugar (sweets and fruit) from the diet.	Tiredness, allergies, and recurrent yeast infections are evidence of a yeast (*Candida albicans*) infection throughout the body. The claim is that yeast needs to be starved of all sugar and other yeasts need to be eliminated from the diet.	Candida is found in many healthy women. A small percent have recurrent yeast infections that are difficult to treat. There is no convincing medical evidence that eliminating certain foods cures these infections. (✗ ✗ ✗ ✗)	Because so many foods are eliminated, people should lose weight.	Following this diet strictly will lead to deficiencies in many vitamins and nutrients.
Fasting	The goal is to completely abstain from any food, usually for a specific length of time. Water is usually consumed.	Fasting can be done to lose weight, to "detoxify" the body, or for religious reasons. The biblical rationale for fasting is to allow focused attention for prayer (Matthew 6:16 – 18; Acts 13:2; 14:23) and to empathize with the poor (Isaiah 58), not to earn God's favor.	Obviously, eliminating all calories will lead to weight loss. (✓ ✓)	Weight can be lost, but for the first few days this is usually water loss.	Most Americans can easily afford to fast from time to time without any negative effects. However, extended use will lead to weakness (Psalm 109:24) and nutritional deficiencies and may contribute to the development of eating disorders.

Diet	Description	Claims	Evidence	Benefits	Cautions
Food-Combining Diet	This diet claims we need to eat foods by category. Fruit should be eaten alone in the morning. Carbohydrates should be eaten with vegetables but never with fat or protein, etc.	Health problems are caused by eating foods in the wrong combination. If mixed wrongly, our digestive enzymes are confused and the wrong enzymes produced. The food sits in the intestines, rots, and poisons us.	Few foods contain only one food group. Our digestive enzymes select the correct food and don't get "confused." (✓)	The diet can lead to more fruit and vegetable intake and a move toward smaller quantities.	This diet is highly structured and may lead some to an "all or nothing" approach. It may have some benefits, but do not neglect all mixed foods (especially dairy products).
GI Diet	Based on eating foods with a low glycemic index (GI) and avoiding those with a high GI. See discussion below under "Control blood sugar."	Foods that cause rapid increases in blood sugar lead to rapid rises in insulin and storage of energy as fat, followed by a sharp drop in blood sugar and hunger. These foods have a high GI value.	GI has been studied in diabetes much longer than for weight loss. Mechanism seems reasonable. Few controlled studies as yet for weight loss. Some studies question the connection between GI and feeling full. (✓✓)	Low GI foods may address the blood sugar peaks and valleys. Foods approved include many fruits and vegetables. The GI Diet allows food from each food group.	Eating lots of low GI foods can still provide too many calories. Some high GI foods (potatoes, carrots, watermelon) are still healthy. Diets based on GI are new and have not received long-term study.
Jenny Craig	This diet is a complete commercial food program based on 28-day preset menus that come in vacuum-sealed packages. It includes a weekly consultation with a former participant on diet and exercise.	Meals have been prepared according to USDA dietary guidelines to give 1,200 – 1,500 calories/day.	This is a balanced approach with all food groups included. No controlled studies have been published. (✓✓)	The diet is balanced (though possibly low in fiber), and calorie reduction should bring about weight loss.	The prepackaged approach to meals does not teach how to shop and prepare one's own meals. The program may be restrictive, and costs may be prohibitive, especially if a several-month contract is required.
Macrobiotics	Meals are composed of whole grains (50 to 60 percent), vegetables (25 to 30 percent), beans or soybean products (5 to 10 percent), with some nuts, seeds, miso soup, and herbal teas. Meat or seafood is allowed once a week	*Macrobiotics* literally means "way of long life" and is a quasi-religious approach to diet. Foods are chosen based on *yin* and *yang*, pulse diagnosis, and life energy beliefs.	There is no evidence that a macrobiotic diet cures cancer and other diseases as claimed. Weight loss occurs from calorie reduction. (✓✓) (👎👎)	Adherents will benefit from increasing plant products in the diet and reducing calories.	Nutrient deficiencies occur. Using macrobiotics to cure cancer may lead to neglect of effective treatments. People are at risk of great spiritual harm from Eastern religious teachings.

ALTERNATIVE THERAPIES

Diet	Description	Claims	Evidence	Benefits	Cautions
"Mayo Clinic" Diet	This diet is unrelated to the famous Mayo Clinic. Eat half a grapefruit at every meal, other specific foods at every meal, and eight glasses of water and one glass of skim milk or tomato juice a day. Do this for twelve days; then eat freely for two days.	Grapefruit is said to act as a fat burner. The combination of foods is said to promote fat burning.	There is no evidence to support the diet, and no evidence that grapefruit has any special dieting properties. (✓)	The plan is low on calories and high on vegetables and salads. The water is beneficial.	The diet contains quite a large amount of meat, which can contain significant amounts of fat and can be hard on the kidneys. It is low in calcium and quickly gets boring.
Ornish Diet	This is a vegetarian diet aiming to reduce fat to less than 10 percent of calories. As much unprocessed, fiber-rich foods as desired can be eaten in small meals throughout the day.	This is a balanced vegetarian approach to eating healthy. The program includes exercise, stress reduction, and group support but can get into New Age ideas. Caffeine, sugar, alcohol, and salt are restricted.	The Ornish Diet was developed to combat heart disease. It has small controlled studies to support its effectiveness. (✓✓✓) (☞)	This program incorporates all of the aspects of recommended nutrition guidelines except for fats, but may be very difficult to follow.	Lack of fat makes this diet very bland and requires much self-discipline. Diet is low in vitamins E, B_{12} and D, and calcium and zinc. High fiber content may cause gastrointestinal problems.
Pritikin Program	This is a very low-fat diet allowing unrestricted amounts of vegetables, fruits, whole grains, and other low-fat foods. Up to 3.5 ounces of low-fat meat, poultry, or fish is allowed per day.	This is a balanced approach to eating healthy. It also emphasizes exercise and patient education.	The Pritikin Program was developed to combat heart disease. It has some controlled studies to support its effectiveness. (✓✓✓)	This program incorporates all of the aspects of recommended nutrition guidelines. Fat intake and calorie intake are reduced.	While more balanced than the Ornish Diet, this diet can still be bland. It is low in vitamins E, B_{12} and D, and calcium, iron, and zinc. High fiber content may cause gastrointestinal problems.
Slim Fast	In this diet, breakfast and lunch are replaced by prepackaged drinks and bars. It leaves one meal to prepare using balanced nutrition guidelines.	This diet works on the principle of using a highly structured approach to dieting. Slim Fast products are nutritious.	Several controlled studies have shown short-term effectiveness. The drop-out rate is high when continued beyond a year. This diet ranked as the second-best weight-loss strategy by *Consumer Reports*. (✓✓✓)	A balanced diet is consumed. Short-term weight loss occurs through calorie reduction.	The drinks and bars can get monotonous and can also be costly compared to other foods.

DIETS AND DIETING

Diet	Description	Claims	Evidence	Benefits	Cautions
South Beach	Phase one eliminates carbohydrates and encourages high-protein foods that are high in good fats; phase two stays high-protein but reduces fat and encourages high-fiber vegetables.	This diet claims to work by eliminating foods that cause an insulin surge that promotes hunger.	Reduced carbo-hydrates will reduce calories. High protein will leave people feeling full. This diet has been studied in only two trials lasting only three months. (✓✓✓)	This diet has the short-term advantages of the Atkins Diet and the long-term advantages of the Zone Diet.	High protein intake may be tough on the kidneys.
Sugar Busters!	The goal is to eliminate white flour and all refined sugar from the diet. Lean meats high in protein are encouraged. Some carbohydrates are allowed, especially high-fiber vegetables.	This diet is based on eliminating refined carbohydrates to prevent the insulin surge that occurs after eating sugars.	There are no controlled studies available for this diet. (✓✓)	Eliminating these sugars will reduce calorie intake. Fat intake is controlled and usually reduced.	This diet eliminates some grains and fruits, so fiber level and vitamins need to be monitored. Adherence rates can be quite low.
Volumetrics	This approach is based on research by Barbara Rolls, Ph.D., into low-energy-density foods. It emphasizes low-calorie, high-bulk foods with high water content: fruits, vegetables, whole grains, soups, lean meats.	Low-energy-density foods give people the sense they are filled after consuming fewer calories. Weight is lost through calorie reduction and increased physical activity.	This diet is based on sound principles that have been studied. The diet itself has not been researched in controlled studies, which is its only shortcoming. (✓✓✓)	This diet reduces calorie intake while allowing much variety. It follows balanced diet guidelines.	Initial high-fiber intake may cause some intestinal discomfort. The diet may be low in vitamin E.
Weight Watchers	All foods are assigned "points," with 1 point being roughly 50 calories. Individual targets are set based on current weight.	This approach is based on reducing calories and eating a balanced diet. Encourages exercise and weekly support groups.	This was rated the best diet by *Consumer Reports* for the most supportive evidence and best adherence rates. (✓✓✓✓)	The balanced approach should lead to calorie reduction and long-term success.	Weekly fee for support group ($13) may be costly for some people.
Zone Diet	The goal is to lower daily intake of carbohydrates and replace them with protein and fat.	This diet claims that the perfect balance is 40-30-30, carbohydrate-protein-fat. Very detailed planning is required.	Some controlled studies have been done, but not all show the diet is effective. Long-term adherence is better than with other, less balanced diets. It was ranked as the third-best weight-loss strategy by *Consumer Reports*. (✓✓✓✓)	The balanced approach should lead to calorie reduction.	This diet requires incredible attention to detail in order to follow exactly and can be boring.

Study Findings

Almost every diet brings initial success. The pounds start coming off. You feel better. But after a few weeks or months, there's a night out. You splurge. There's cake at a birthday party. You smell your favorite food. At first, it's just a nibble. You deserve a reward. Then it's a "day off." Before you know it, the weight is coming back. You give up. The diet didn't work.

Almost all diets, weight-loss programs, and diet pills have a very high relapse rate. Studies show that few diets work well over long periods of time for most users. One of the few studies with long-term follow-up found that 95 percent of those who lost more than thirty pounds regained that weight within five years. In another study of people who had lost eleven or more pounds, 52 percent had kept the weight off a year later, but only 11 percent still kept it off five years later. This type of "yo-yo" dieting has been shown to be particularly harmful.

The news is not all bad, though. *Consumer Reports* surveyed more than 30,000 people in 2002 about weight loss. Nearly a quarter of those who had tried to lose weight lost 10 percent of their starting weight and kept it off for at least a year. Almost half of them kept it off for five years. The strategies used by these successful weight losers were compared with those of the people who didn't lose any weight. Two clear findings emerged. You must increase exercise and physical activity. And no one diet works for everyone (or even for most people). Eighty-three percent of those who kept their excess weight off for five years did not follow any established program. They figured out for themselves how they could make the necessary lifestyle changes. We will give you the general principles that have been demonstrated to work. But then you need to figure out how you can incorporate those into your lifestyle on a long-term basis — even if it means the initial weight loss is slow but steady.

Another study to figure out what worked best surveyed people who had previously lost weight. The results are summarized in the following table. Kayman and colleagues wanted to see if there were significant differences between those who remained at a lower weight (called Successful Maintainers) and those who regained lost weight (called Unsuccessful Relapsers). The results speak for themselves. More than one hundred women were interviewed and asked to list all weight-loss methods they had used.

Weight-Loss Method	Percent of Successful Maintainers Using It	Percent of Unsuccessful Relapsers Using It
At least 30 minutes exercise, 3 times per week	90	34
Devised personal eating plan	73	39
Attended Weight Watchers	76	36
Attended other program/group	10	43
Followed doctor's orders	20	34
Took pills or shots	3	47
Fasted	3	11
Underwent hypnosis	0	9
Followed book or magazine diet	10	25
Total number of different methods used by those in each group	28	121

The Successful Maintainers used a small number of well-established and highly recommended approaches: exercise, a personal eating plan, and a support group. Those who regained weight used a large number of different approaches and, to a smaller extent, followed the three well-established strategies. One of the more dramatic differences was that diet pills and shots were used by almost half of the Unsuccessful Relapsers, in contrast to only 3 percent of the Successful Maintainers.

Lifestyle changes and moderation are key. Another controlled study, published by Dansinger in 2005, found that after one year people lost similar amounts of weight using Weight Watchers or the Atkins, Ornish, or Zone diets. However, only about half of those on the more extreme Atkins and Ornish diets completed the study, while two-thirds of those on the Zone Diet or attending Weight Watchers finished the program.

The science behind weight loss is not complicated (at least not until we get into how we motivate ourselves to make the necessary changes). Calories measure energy. Energy enters the body in food; it leaves (primarily) through physical activity. The difference between energy in and energy out is seen in body weight. More energy in than out: you gain weight. More energy out than in: you lose weight. The rest follows on from this. To lose weight, you need to reduce intake (food calories) and increase output (physical activity). How doesn't seem to matter. That's where you do what works for you. If you love red meat, a vegetarian diet is going to be hard. If you hate red meat, Atkins is going to be hard for you. If your knees hurt, don't try to run. If you love the outdoors, find ways to get out there more. Maybe you've always wanted a dog and getting one would give you the motivation to get out for a walk every night. Maybe you've wanted to get to know your neighbors. Find out what activities they enjoy and see if they would do them with you. Be creative. Think about how you are going to make changes that are healthy and as enjoyable as possible.

But it's not all going to be easy. Look at where you can make big calorie savings. Having less cereal at breakfast will not be as beneficial as cutting out the donut you have with coffee. If you have several sodas every day, cut back on them. Rather than supersizing your burger and fries, order the regular size or have a salad. Every time you resist the urge to have extra calories, take note of that. Congratulate yourself. And next time, remember that you can resist the urge.

The only proven approach to losing weight and keeping it off involves combining the following strategies into a plan that works for you.

- **Reduce the number of calories and eat a balanced diet.** Under the Diet and Nutrition entry, we gave you some ways to calculate how many calories you need to maintain your current weight. If you want to lose weight, take in fewer calories. Set reasonable goals. If you consume 4,000 calories a day, aiming to get to 1,500 overnight might be too aggressive. Figure out attainable steps on the way to your target. Remember also that your body needs fewer calories when it weighs less (estimated to be about ten calories less per day for every pound lost).
- **Increase physical activity.** Two and a half hours of moderate exercise per week is believed by some to be most effective. However, *any* increase in activity will help. Take the stairs instead of the elevator. Park farther away from where you're going. Walk the dog or the kids. Ride a stationary bike or walk on a treadmill while watching the evening news or your favorite TV show. Mow your grass — with a push lawn mower!
- **Have social support.** When someone is trying to lose weight, others can encourage and help

with the necessary changes. In the study by Kayman mentioned above, one-third of those who relapsed said they had no one helping or supporting them. Support and encouragement are practical ways to love others during what can be a very difficult time. "And let us consider how we may spur one another on toward love and good deeds. Let us not give up meeting together, as some are in the habit of doing, but let us encourage one another — and all the more as you see the Day approaching" (Hebrews 10:24 – 25). This may be one of the reasons group weight-loss programs such as Weight Watchers seem to be more successful than "going it alone." Christian weight-loss programs (e.g., Weigh Down Workshop, First Place, and God's Weigh), which incorporate biblical resources and Christian insight, may prove to be successful; however, we are not aware of any published scientific studies that have evaluated these programs.

- **Fill up on low-energy-density foods.** Feeling full reminds us that we've had enough to eat. Of course, we have to listen to our stomachs and tell our mouths to stop eating. Foods differ in the number of calories contained in the same amount of space. That means your plate and your stomach can be equally full but contain very different numbers of calories. This idea is the basis of eating foods low in "energy density," a strategy that underlies the Volumetrics diet but is actually part of many other successful diets. Low-energy-density foods contain lots of water and fiber and are low in fat. Chicken-noodle soup, for example, will leave you feeling fuller than the same amount of chicken and noodles, just because of the added water. Strangely, drinking the extra water doesn't have the same effect — it needs to be cooked into the meal. Other foods low in energy density include water-rich fruits and vegetables, whole grains, and lean meats. As we saw in the Diet and Nutrition entry, these foods are good for us for other reasons too.

- **Control blood sugar.** Athletes drink special drinks containing sugars that quickly get into the bloodstream. That releases insulin, which is needed to bring the sugar into cells to give the athlete an energy boost. However, if you are not in the middle of a marathon, that same insulin release will lower your blood sugar and leave you feeling hungry. So you reach for another soda or donut or candy. And on the cycle goes. Carbohydrates are now being assigned a glycemic index (GI) value to capture this concept. Pure sugar has a GI of 100; 70 or above is considered high; 55 – 69 is medium; 54 or below is low. White bread, refined flour, white rice, and other simple carbohydrates have a high GI. Many complex carbohydrates (fruits, vegetables, whole grains, and beans) have a low GI. Low GI carbohydrates increase blood sugar and insulin more slowly and allow people to feel full longer and, as a result, eat fewer calories. While the approach seems reasonable, there are some anomalies. Some plant foods (potatoes, carrots, and watermelon) have a high GI, while chocolate fudge cake has a GI of 39. The connection between GI and feeling full is not firmly established (potatoes have a GI of 101, but they are excellent for leaving people feeling full). In addition, GI does not take into account the quantity of food eaten. A newer index called Glycemic Load incorporates the GI and grams of food but is not widely used yet. Overall,

GI is another important factor in evaluating the food in the diet, but it should not be used in isolation from the other established dieting principles or viewed as the answer to everyone's struggle with diet.

- **Measure your portions.** *Consumer Reports* evaluated popular diets in their June 2005 issue. They ranked the diets according to their adherence to well-established nutrition guidelines and their success rates in controlled clinical trials. An additional strategy found in the most successful approaches was measuring food portions. If you know people who have done Weight Watchers, you will know how all foods are assigned point values. These points correlate with calories. You are allowed a certain number of points per day, and you keep track of how you spend your points. If you want a donut, that's fine — but that might use up half your points for the day! All that measuring and counting apparently makes a difference. It was part of other successful approaches. Of course, there also needs to be a commitment to stick with rules. Fudging on amounts or points won't fool the scales.

All of these strategies, taken together, have the best chance of helping someone make the lifestyle changes necessary to not only lose weight but keep it off. But you have to find an approach that works for you.

Remember that you must be able to live with the changes you make for the rest of your life. Be realistic. Drastic diets and diet pills have not produced consistent, long-term results. Start with a plan that works. Design your own plan based on the above well-established principles.

Cautions

Almost all the popular diets involve consuming fewer calories and can lead to initial weight loss. However, drastically reducing calorie intake can cause metabolic problems as your body uses up stored energy. Losing weight actually makes it harder for many people to lose more weight. With less food available, the body's metabolic rate is lowered, meaning your same activity level requires fewer calories. If your brain senses that your body is entering "starvation mode," it will often increase how much fat is stored (sort of long-range planning).

The diets that emphasize one food or food type can easily lead to a deficiency of essential nutrients and vitamins. For example, a vegetarian diet can lead to deficiencies in vitamin B_{12}, calcium, iron, and other nutrients, although all of these are readily available as supplements. Good fats and low GI carbohydrates are important to give us a longer-lasting sense of having had enough to eat. Apart from being bland, low-fat diets lead to people being hungry sooner, putting them at higher risk of snacking too much or on the wrong foods. The best strategy is a balanced diet to ensure adequate amounts of all needed nutrients and vitamins. This is especially important with children and teenagers during these important growing periods.

With the constant attention to dieting, children often get wrong impressions about their own weight. Eighty-one percent of ten-year-olds reported they were afraid of "being fat." Some already have a problem with their weight. To some extent our society has generated a self-fulfilling prophecy. In a different study, teenage girls who reported using dieting agents and being concerned about dieting were more likely to gain weight and become obese after their teenage years.

Ineffective diets and dieting agents will lead to disappointment, but they can also make weight problems worse. People who go on diets and give up often regain even more weight. Then the cycle repeats itself. A new diet hits the media; a new product goes on the market. Another try; another failure.

When considering a diet, ask the following questions. The more times you answer yes, the greater the chance that the diet is more of a fad than a reliable strategy for healthy eating.

- Does the diet require eating a very small number of foods or focus exclusively on one food group?
- Does the diet focus on the *type* of food you eat rather than on the amount of food and making lifestyle changes necessary for healthy eating?
- Are common foods rejected because people are said to be allergic to them or because they allegedly contain toxins?
- Is losing weight said to be easy or automatic or "guaranteed"?
- Is weight loss of more than a few pounds a week promised?
- Is weight loss promised without any increase in activity (or even promised while you sleep)?
- Would you consider it unreasonable to ask the rest of your family to make the changes required by this diet?
- Are other products and supplements being sold as part of the diet?
- Does the diet ignore the fact that a calorie is a calorie, no matter what food group it comes from?
- Does the diet exclude all tasty foods that appeal to you?

Recommendations

Almost any diet will work at first, giving you short-term improvement, if it reduces your calorie intake. Long-term improvements are much more important and harder to achieve. Successful weight loss can be difficult, but the benefits are well worth the investment. The sense of accomplishment from having tackled a difficult issue and had success can flow over into all areas of your life.

Christians should be especially motivated to keep their weight within healthy limits. Food is part of God's creation, to be received with gratitude and shared with others (1 Timothy 4:3 – 5). Food is one of God's general provisions through which we can experience his loving care for us. Eating food can be a pleasant experience. Meals provide important times for building relationships among family and friends, socializing, and serving others.

But like all good things, food can be abused. Overeating harms the body and can shorten the time we have been given on this earth to glorify God and serve others. People become overweight for many reasons, some of which are beyond their control. However, we cannot ignore the fact that overeating stems from small decisions to eat when we shouldn't. In that way, some decisions to eat must be viewed as sinful. The Bible views gluttony as immoral and links it with drunkenness. "Do not join those who drink too much wine or gorge themselves on meat, for drunkards and gluttons become poor, and drowsiness clothes them in rags" (Proverbs 23:20 – 21; see also Deuteronomy 21:20).

In condemning any sinful behavior, we must be quick to remember that "all have sinned and fall short of the glory of God" (Romans 3:23). Gluttony is just one of many ways we demonstrate our selfishness and rebellion. Instead of Jesus Christ being Lord of their lives, for some "their god is their stomach" (Philippians 3:19). This leads people into slavery to their appetites and neglect of others' needs.

We in the developed world have become so rich we are dying from eating too much. Millions of others are dying from hunger. To paraphrase 1 John 3:17, how does the love of God abide in those who have most of the world's food and close their hearts against those who are hungry? Galatians 5 lists the sins of the flesh and the fruit of the Spirit. Among the sins is a Greek word translated "orgies" (v. 21), which actually describes wild parties involving drunkenness, fornication, and overeating. In contrast is "self-control" (v. 23), which involves keeping all our sensual appetites in check. The consequences of overindulging in alcohol or not keeping our sexual appetites under control are clearly visible. Christians are well known for condemning those practices. We should be as concerned about our eating habits and allow the Holy Spirit to free us from the misuse of food.

The fact that God is concerned about our weight should be a source of hope. God is with us in our attempts to get this area of our lives under control. We should approach weight loss as we would any other area of character change, with prayer, fellowship, and guidance from other Christians. We should avoid legalistic approaches or making ourselves (or others) feel guilty.

Christ came to bring us freedom, not put us under bondage. But this does not give us license to do whatever we feel like doing. "Do not offer the parts of your body to sin, as instruments of wickedness, but rather offer yourselves to God, as those who have been brought from death to life; and offer the parts of your body to him as instruments of righteousness. For sin shall not be your master, because you are not under law, but under grace" (Romans 6:13 – 14).

We need to show grace to ourselves and others who struggle with weight issues.

The best overall approach to losing weight is based on low-tech, old-fashioned principles: eat fewer calories, eat healthier foods, become more active, enlist the support of others, and depend on the Lord for the help we need in this area. Make the physical, mental, and spiritual changes that can help you eat a healthier diet. Keep in mind the following:

- **You are embarking on a challenging activity.** Don't expect it to be easy, and don't be surprised that some days will be harder than others.
- **Focus on changes** that reduce "bad" fats, "bad" carbohydrates, and overall calories, especially by increasing consumption of "good" sources of protein and oils and "good" or complex carbohydrates, such as stone-ground whole grains and fruits and vegetables.
- **Make changes that you can envision becoming part of your new lifestyle** (such as adding a fruit to your breakfast) as opposed to strategies you know cannot last long (such as eating cabbage soup every day).
- **Move your body more.** Every activity uses up calories (walk over to talk to someone rather than using the phone). Find an exercise that you like and someone you like to do it with. Being accountable to another person helps:

> As iron sharpens iron, so one man sharpens another.
>
> *Proverbs 27:17*

> If one falls down, his friend can help him up. But pity the man who falls and has no one to help him up!
>
> *Ecclesiastes 4:10*

- **Set reasonable goals** and take small steps in that direction rather than trying to take giant leaps. You might replace one of your daily cans of pop with sparkling water rather than quitting soda all at once. Some things you might want to eliminate altogether.
- **Enjoy the food you can eat** and give thanks for having it, as opposed to focusing on what you've chosen not to eat.
- **If you slip up, don't give up.** Admit what you did, show yourself some grace, and set a new goal.
- **Find a way to keep yourself accountable,** one that allows you to see your progress (such as a food journal, "coach," or support group).
- **Enlist the help, support, and prayers** of your spouse, family, and church members. The changes you are making should be healthy for everyone, and you will benefit from their support.
- **Change your thinking** from "I'm going on a diet" to "I'm going to improve my eating habits" or "I'm going to take better care of my body."
- **Eat breakfast every day.** Have a nutritious lunch. Keep dinner the smallest meal of the day and try to eat it as early in the evening as possible. Some call this the "royal" nutrition plan: eat breakfast like a king, lunch like a queen, and dinner like a pauper.
- **Increase the amount of water you drink** every day.

Further Reading

Dansinger, Michael L., Joi A. Gleason, John L. Griffith, Harry P. Selker, and Ernst J. Schaefer. "Comparison of the Atkins, Ornish, Weight Watchers, and Zone Diets for Weight Loss and Heart Disease Risk Reduction: A Randomized Trial." *Journal of the American Medical Association* 293, no. 1 (January 2005): 43 – 53.

Kayman, Susan, William Bruvold, and Judith S. Stern. "Maintenance and Relapse after Weight Loss in Women: Behavioral Aspects." *American Journal of Clinical Nutrition* 52 (1990): 800 – 807.

Pierre, Colleen. "Is There Wisdom in Those Wacky Diets?" *Prevention* 52, no. 6 (June 2000): 142 – 47, 208 – 11.

"Rating the Diets from Atkins™ to Dr. Sears Zone." *Consumer Reports* 70, no. 6 (June 2005): 18 – 22.

Saper, Robert B., David M. Eisenberg, and Russell S. Phillips. "Common Dietary Supplements for Weight Loss." *American Family Physician* 70, no. 9 (November 2004): 1731 – 38.

Serdula, Mary K., Ali H. Mokdad, David F. Williamson, Deborah A. Galuska, James M. Mendlein, and Gregory W. Heath. "Prevalence of Attempting Weight Loss and Strategies for Controlling Weight." *Journal of the American Medical Association* 282, no. 14 (October 1999): 1353 – 58.

ENERGY MEDICINE

● What It Is

Energy medicine is a branch of alternative medicine that contains numerous therapies from many parts of the world. Each is based on the existence of a non-physical energy pervading the universe, though the nature of the energy, the form of the therapies, and the way healing is believed to take place vary from culture to culture.

Energy medicine has traditionally been a part of Eastern medicine, little utilized or discussed in the United States until the 1970s. Then, with the opening of relations with China, the news media introduced the Western world to images of surgery being conducted with acupuncture appearing to be the only anesthetic. Acupuncture was heralded as a long-proven surgical anesthetic even though surgery itself was a skill very new to Chinese medicine, in contrast to its long history of use in the West. Reporters wrote glowing stories without carefully checking information that would have revealed that, in at least some cases, the acupuncture was used to *reduce* the amount of anesthetic required, not replace it. The reporters ignored the other supposed "miracle" of Chinese medicine: doctors who claimed they performed surgical procedures on patients while the patients read aloud from the Little Red Book — *The Sayings of Chairman Mao* — to keep from feeling any pain.

The interest in everything Chinese was reinforced in 1977 with the release of the George Lucas movie *Star Wars*. With this came the idea of "the Force," a mystical, invisible energy or spirituality. The Force was both good and evil, the two being kept in balance, although at odds, with either side able to triumph. Jedi knights embraced both sides, pulled in one direction, then the other. The Force did not allow for death. Instead, though your body was lost, you became one with the Force — stronger and able to communicate with the living when necessary.

The film quickly developed a cult following. Soon the concept of the Force was being used in sermons and popular theological discussions. Some people started to refer to the Force as a reality, not the creation of a writer's imagination. Newspapers reported religious groups evolving around the idea, and though they were short-lived, the "truth" of the film as interpreted by them lingered.

That generation has now grown to adulthood, and if you look at many who have sought one form of energy medicine or another, they are within that age group. It is presumed that though they are older, wiser, and have long since moved beyond talking about the Force, they remain intrigued by the possibilities inherent in the philosophies of different energy medicines.

Because energy medicine permeates so many different cultures, the names used for the energy vary from culture to culture. The energy is called *chi* (sometimes spelled *qi*) in traditional Chinese medicine, *prana* in Indian Ayurvedic medicine, *ki* in Japanese practices, and a variety of other names in Western history, such as "orgone" and "bioenergy." "Biofield" is a new term chosen by the National Center for Complementary and Alternative Medicine in the United States.

Although the details vary, this energy is believed to pervade the universe but takes on in each person a particular form called the "human energy field" (HEF). According to these theories, the HEF, or human aura, contains a number of layers, each with energy of differing frequencies. The energy is transformed between layers, and eventually into the physical body, via structures called *chakras*. These are shaped like a whirlpool, with seven major ones located around the spine and head. Illness is believed to begin with disturbances of the energy field that are eventually transferred to the physical or emotional realm. In energy medicine, the HEF must be treated first. According to practitioners, once the HEF is balanced and energy flows properly, true healing can occur.

Western Historical Development

Franz Anton Mesmer (1734 – 1815) claimed that health is dependent on "animal magnetism." He used magnets in his healing sessions but later claimed he only needed his hands, engaging in the practice we today call hypnosis. His approach is the source of the contemporary term "mesmerized." Throughout the nineteenth and twentieth centuries, claims were made that the HEF had been detected and identified as a form of electromagnetic radiation (of which light, heat, and infrared radiation are familiar examples).

Wilhelm Reich (1897 – 1957), a psychiatrist and colleague of Freud's, also claimed to identify the HEF. He called his energy "orgone," saying it was a universal life energy that he could generate with devices he sold, called "orgone boxes." In a scandal around the time of his death, one of the orgone boxes, allegedly made to his specifications, was taken apart and examined. The box contained little more than a lightbulb activated when the box was plugged in. Whether Reich or a follower or someone else was perpetrating such a scam is unknown. The orgone

box fell into disfavor with even those who followed Reich's theories, and manufacture was stopped. Reich had claimed he could use his orgone to heal and even produce living cells from inanimate matter. These claims were never independently verified.

In the early 1900s, Walter J. Kilner, a London physician, invented a special screen filled with a dye made from coal tar that he said allowed people to see one another's auras. Goggles based on these screens are still sold. When you look through these screens, people do have a colored aura. However, scientists have shown that this is caused by the dye used, which allows only blue and red light to pass through. Since these regions of the light spectrum do not exactly overlap, they give the impression of separate auras around a person. It is a little like the effect of looking at a 1950s 3-D comic book. Without the special glasses needed to see the picture in three dimensions, the illustrations are merely a series of slightly separated lines of different colors.

"Proof" of the life energy field was again claimed by Semyon and Valentina Kirlian in the 1960s. These Russian researchers, working with concepts first developed in the 1890s, claimed to be able to photograph energy fields. What are now known as Kirlian photographs allegedly capture images of life energy, also called "bioplasma." These images show auras and streams of light coming out from people's hands or plant leaves. The intensity, shape, and color of these shapes are said to provide valuable information on the health of the person or organism.

Problems arise when these admittedly dramatic Kirlian photographs are investigated by independent scientists. The images have a physical explanation. Variations in factors such as the moisture level of the object photographed, the pressure exerted on the photographic film, the length of exposure, and the type of film used result in changes to the color, shape, size, and intensity of the resulting image. To be a diagnostic aid, images taken under the same conditions should have consistent, reproducible results. This does not occur.

Additionally, Kirlian auras have been recorded for such things as pennies, paper clips, and water droplets, none of which is said to have a life energy field. The auras that show up in Kirlian photographs are clearly not a feature limited to living organisms.

In spite of all this evidence, proponents of energy medicine still claim that Kirlian photography provides objective evidence of the existence of the HEF. Some proponents of life energy therapies will admit there is no objective evidence for the existence of life energy or the HEF. Their belief becomes a faith issue that has no basis in demonstrable fact.

In contrast, electromagnetic radiation can be detected in, and does emanate from, the human body. Many conventional diagnostic techniques make use of these effects, such as EEGs and EKGs. However, these are not what energy medicine means by its HEF. Electromagnetic energies can be detected, generated, and studied objectively, while such studies have never been done with the HEF.

The Human Energy Field

Since the HEF cannot be detected objectively, meditation becomes an important aspect of energy medicine. During meditation, practitioners are believed to reach a higher level of awareness that allows them to sense the HEF. Some claim that within this state they actually see the HEF and receive guidance for the healing. The guidance may be intuitive, along the lines of what Dr. Edward Bach believed when developing his Bach flower therapy, or it may be directly from spirit guides who provide information to practitioners, as with Reiki.

Many practitioners of energy medicine say that the HEF is divided into seven layers, or bodies. Each layer deals with different aspects of the person, some having more to do with physical, emotional, mental, or spiritual issues. The healing that a practitioner will suggest may have as much to do with emotional or spiritual issues as it does with the physical symptoms someone may be experiencing.

• Study Findings

While instruments may not be able to detect the HEF, it is still possible to design studies to test whether people can reliably detect the HEF, whatever it might be. During the 1970s, a well-known English psychic healer, Matthew Manning, claimed to be able to see human auras even if he was separated from the subject by a closed door. A test was devised by researchers and accepted by Manning. He would stand on one side of a closed door and would guess whether a person was standing up against the other side of the door. He believed he could detect the presence of an aura and could tell if the person moved away from the door because the aura would fade as the person walked away.

If you or I took such a test and had to guess whether a person was behind the door, random chance would determine that we would make the right guess about half the time. Someone who really could see the aura should have a far higher success rate. When the Manning experiment was done (✗✗), he gave the correct answer just half the time. His success rate was no better than that of someone guessing or flipping a coin.

In a more recent test, ten people who claimed to be able to see human auras were given a chance to prove their abilities. Among the subjects were five individuals who earned some of their living as professional psychic healers. Four identical screens were placed in a room with volunteers who took turns standing behind one or another of them. The people being tested believed they could detect each volunteer's aura and determine which screen he or she was behind. The results: 185 correct answers out of 720 attempts.

As a control, ten other people who made no claim to any special abilities and who had no experience with the HEF were tested in exactly the same way (✖✖✖). Again, out of 720 attempts, 196 were correct, a little better than those who were certain they could detect auras. The two best individual scores among all the people tested were 50 percent and 40 percent correct. These were achieved by two of the ten people in the control group, who claimed no ability to detect auras.

The test of Therapeutic Touch practitioners with Emily Rosa, a fourth-grader, also counts as evidence against people's ability to detect the HEF. This study (✖✖) received much publicity after it was published in the April 1, 1998, *Journal of the American Medical Association*. Twenty-one Therapeutic Touch practitioners sat behind a screen with Emily on the other side. They put both their hands through the screen, palms open and facing up. They claimed they would be able to detect Emily's aura if she held one of her hands above one of theirs. They got the answer correct 44 percent of the time, which is again about what would be expected by chance.

Another study tested the claim of an energy medicine practitioner to diagnose infertility in women. The practitioner claimed he could determine which women were infertile by accessing only their energy fields. He examined thirty-seven women in the study and answered four questions related to physical abnormalities that would lead to infertility. The healer scored no better than chance on any of the four questions.

Cautions

While scientific evidence does not support the existence of an HEF or the effectiveness of many of energy medicine's therapies, there are still concerns. Energy medicine practitioners often do not separate spiritual from physical healing, and therefore spiritual practices are completely intertwined with the healing efforts of most of these practitioners. Therapies used in energy medicine often cannot be separated from the philosophical and religious beliefs underlying the practices. These practitioners will claim to rebalance one's aura by involving spiritual forces that they claim are poorly understood. While they may believe these are impersonal energies being used for good purposes, there is no way to know if this is the case.

In our opinion, people who subject themselves to energy medicine are exposing themselves to real spiritual forces over which they may have little control. This creates a serious problem for Christians who are told in 1 John 4:1 to "test the spirits to see whether they are from God, because many false prophets have gone out into the world." We should have no involvement with spiritual beings or forces other than those who clearly proclaim Jesus Christ as Lord and Savior.

While most concerns with the different energy medicine therapies are primarily spiritual, some specific therapies can have other adverse physiological and psychological effects. These are noted where appropriate in the discussions of the individual therapies.

Recommendations

Energy medicine is based on ideas and beliefs that are rooted in Eastern religions and esoteric Western philosophy. These beliefs are often in direct conflict with Christian teaching. The practices may expose people to spiritual beings and forces that are not of God.

In general, Christians should completely avoid energy medicine. However, some therapies that have arisen within these belief systems include a physical component. Acupuncture is an example. We believe a therapy such as acupuncture can be separated from the energy medicine philosophy. Medical doctors and others, including some Christians, use this sort of therapy along with conventional medicine and reject the philosophy of its Eastern origins. In cases where clear evidence demonstrates that these therapies are effective, they may be worth considering. However, you should remain alert to the possibility that you may hear some different religious ideas from some practitioners.

Most therapies based on energy medicine do not involve physical contact, although sometimes it is used in addition to energy manipulation. Therapeutic Touch and Reiki are examples. These therapies are so completely intertwined with energy manipulating approaches that they should not be used by Christians under any circumstances. Practitioners who offer these therapies to patients should make the religious roots of the therapies very clear.

Treatment Categories

Scientifically Questionable
For any indication ☹☹☹☹

Spiritual
Almost always 👎👎👎👎

Quackery or Fraud
In the hands of some practitioners

Further Reading

Albrecht, Mark, and Brooks Alexander. "The Sellout of Science." *Spiritual Counterfeits Project Journal* 2, no. 1 (August 1978): 18 – 28.

Fish, Sharon. "Therapeutic Touch: Healing Science or Mystical Midwife?" *Christian Research Journal* 12 (1995): 28 – 38.

Tart, C. T., and J. Palmer. "Some Psi Experiments with Matthew Manning." *Journal of the Society for Psychical Research* 50 (January 1979): 224 – 28.

FOLK MEDICINE

What It Is

"Folk medicine" is one of the terms used to describe the body of health-related information traditionally held as part of a culture or community. Other names are "traditional medicine" and "home remedies." The information is usually learned by observation and trial-and-error. It is then passed on by word of mouth and by being demonstrated to an apprentice. Plants indigenous to where the community lives will become part of that culture's folk medicine as the herbal remedies most commonly used.

Folk medicine can include natural and supernatural aspects and emphasize one dimension over the other. Faith healing can be part of folk medicine when the culture's religious beliefs are called on to promote health. This can include special prayers or rituals for healing or the use of certain items such as holy water or relics of saints. Visiting certain shrines or taking part in pilgrimages can be part of folk medicine. Charms may also be worn to provide protection or good luck. Voodoo and psychedelic plants may become part of folk medicine as it seeks to use the spirit world to influence health in this life.

Claims

Folk medicine is an approach to health care that includes claims about how to prevent and treat the common ailments of the culture. It involves poultices for treating wounds, herbal remedies for various illnesses, rituals for protection from illnesses and spirits, and many other recommendations to improve health and prevent or treat illnesses. Various foods and drinks are recommended within folk medicine, such as an apple a day to keep the doctor away, or chicken noodle soup for the common cold.

Study Findings

One of the characteristics of folk medicine is that it hasn't been subjected to controlled trials. In some cases, if a particular practice or remedy is tested, it is shown to have had some benefit or to have worked via the placebo effect.

Cautions

Folk medicine can include good advice that has withstood the passage of time. Some advice was only passed on because it did prove to be beneficial. But some advice is more like old wives' tales. Effective, safe medical care should not be avoided in favor of unproven home remedies and folk cures.

Another caution must also be expressed regarding the spiritual aspects of folk medicine. Sickness and death have always drawn people to ask questions about whether or not God exists. They trigger many questions on spiritual topics and have led to various answers. Many of these traditions get incorporated into the teachings of folk medicine. Christians should be particularly cautious that the answers offered by folk medicine are in keeping with biblical teaching.

● Recommendations

Folk medicine includes many remedies and practices. Some truth will exist within these practices. But often some of the beliefs will have simply been passed down from generation to generation. Little or no evidence may support their use. Some herbal remedies are showing themselves to be effective, and some folk practices are being supported by research results. We discuss these in the individual entries in Parts 2 and 3. We support the clinical testing of apparently safe folk remedies to see if they are effective or truly safe. In general, though, few reasons support the pursuit of unproven folk medicine remedies given the other well-tested approaches available to many in the developed world today.

● Treatment Categories

Complementary
Some approaches   ☺☺

Scientifically Unproven
Most approaches by definition   ☹☹

Spiritual
Some approaches   👎👎👎👎

Quackery or Fraud
In the hands of some practitioners, especially some well-meaning participants

● Further Reading

Hufford, David J. "Cultural Diversity, Folk Medicine, and Alternative Medicine." *Alternative Therapies in Health and Medicine* 3, no. 4 (July 1997): 78–80.

Logan, Patrick. *Irish Folk Medicine*. Belfast: Appletree, 1981.

HERBAL MEDICINE

What It Is

For thousands of years people have gone into the woods and selected plants they have learned have healing or soothing qualities. They make extracts, infusions, or poultices, or eat the plant alone or in a soup or stew. The plants used vary around the world depending on what grows locally. Some of these plants have been analyzed scientifically and sometimes found to contain a component that does, indeed, have medical utility. For example, when Native Americans made a tea from willow bark, they were actually getting a form of the chemical that we today call aspirin. Thus, rather than risk taking the chemical equivalent of an herb (along with binders, coloring, and other additives), why not go back to the herbs themselves?

A "back to nature" approach seems good, but it's not that straightforward. An estimated 1,400 different species are used to make the almost 30,000 herbal products available in the United States. While overall sales and sales of single-herb products have dropped a little since the early 2000s, sales of multiherb mixtures have increased. Only a small fraction of all these remedies have been scientifically tested in humans using controlled studies. Most ancient groups of indigenous people whose medical practices are well documented used a lot fewer remedies. In addition, there is no consistency in how the herbs are selected and used. One practitioner of herbal medicine might use one part of a plant, while a different practitioner uses a different part. Sometimes the plant material is dried and powdered; others insist the fresh plant must be used. Some use the powder to make capsules; others say it's best to use the powder to make a tea.

The active ingredients are sometimes removed from the plant material by extraction, a process similar to brewing coffee from coffee grounds. The liquid is usually water, although alcohol or steam can also be used. An alcohol extract is called a "tincture." Herbal remedies are sometimes given as injections in Europe, but this is rare in the United States. How the remedy is made and which plant part is used influence what the final preparation contains and what its potential uses may be, even though the same basic herb has been used to make the preparation.

Claims

Herbal medicine is growing in popularity. David Eisenberg and colleagues at Harvard Medical School have conducted the most frequently cited surveys of complementary and alternative medicine usage in the United States. The surveys were conducted in 1990, 1997, and 2002. The 2002 survey was published in 2004 and 2005, making it the most current data at the time we wrote this book. We refer to it several times throughout the book as the 2002 CDC Survey (carried out by the Centers for Disease Control and Prevention) and list it under Further Reading under the name Barnes.

Herbal remedy usage in the United States increased over the three surveys from 2.5 to 12.1 and then to 18.9 percent. In the 2002 survey, one-quarter of the population reported having used herbal remedies at some point. The most commonly used herbs were echinacea, ginseng, ginkgo, garlic, glucosamine, and St. John's wort. According to the journal *HerbalGram*, sales through retail outlets have increased from $25 million in 1991 to a peak of $430 million in 1999 and were at $258 million in 2004. Examined by retail sales, the bestselling herbal remedies were garlic, echinacea, saw palmetto, ginkgo, soy, and cranberry. The *Nutrition Business Journal* publishes information on sales of herbs to manufacturers. These figures give a broader indication of herb popularity since they take into account products that sell through other outlets (e.g., the Internet) and those that end up in multiherb mixtures, drinks, and other products. According to their reports, the bestselling herbs in 2004 were noni, green tea, garlic, echinacea, saw palmetto, and ginkgo.

People use herbal remedies for many different reasons. *Prevention* magazine conducted a survey in 1999 of herbal and other dietary supplement usage by adults in the United States. The most common reasons people gave for using herbal remedies were to ensure good health (75 percent), improve energy (61 percent), prevent or treat colds and flu (58 percent), improve memory (43 percent), ease depression (35 percent), and prevent or treat serious illness (29 percent). The survey also reported the reasons people prefer herbs over prescription medications: prefer natural products (43 percent), fewer side effects (21 percent), more effective (14 percent), allows self-treatment (11 percent), less expensive (8 percent), and more gentle or mild (6 percent).

Many people believe that because herbal remedies are natural, they are less harmful than pharmaceutical drugs. A survey released by the National Consumers League in 2002 found that 86 percent of Americans believed that if a product was labeled "natural," this meant it was safe. There is some truth to this, because in general, herbal remedies are milder and less concentrated. However, herbs are not harmless. Under the individual entries for herbs, we will point out that virtually all herbal remedies can have adverse effects. People have overdosed on popular herbs such as ephedra, leading to serious problems and even death. Some herbs, such as pennyroyal and chaparral, cause more harm than good, leading us to conclude they should never be used. Many herbal products also cause interactions with drugs, other supplements, or even foods. Natural is not necessarily safe. As renowned botanical and herbal expert James Duke, Ph.D., wrote, "There are probably safe, medicinal, toxic, and lethal doses for all chemicals, natural and synthetic" (see *www.ars-grin.gov/duke/syllabus/module15.htm*). And herb remedies contain natural chemicals.

Study Findings

Studies of herbal remedies vary widely in quality, as will be seen with the specific herbs in Part 3. Herbal medicine relies primarily on traditional usage, sometimes ignoring the fact that different indigenous people have used the same herb in radically different ways. Basically, many assume that if an herb has been used for a long time, it must be somewhat effective. That assumption is not necessarily valid.

The recent interest in herbal medicine is leading to more clinical trials, but the focus is on a small number of herbs that show promise, leaving the majority of preparations untested. Research in Europe is usually done on standardized products that often differ from products available in the United States. In addition, some promoters of herbal medicine argue that when a traditional herbal remedy is found to be ineffective in testing, the problem is with the test. They argue that if an herb was tested in the way they use it, the results would be quite different. Since such tests often have not been conducted, it is impossible to argue with their logic.

Some claim that conventional medicine is incompatible with herbal medicine. However, it should be remembered that more than one-quarter of the pharmaceutical drugs on the market today were originally isolated from plant material; over half came from natural sources when you include microorganisms and animals. Throughout the rise of conventional medicine, departments of pharmacognosy were in major schools of pharmacy. Here, herbs and other natural products were examined for potential therapeutic benefits. Their approach was to isolate the active ingredients because of difficulties preparing herbal remedies of consistent quality.

When willow bark was shown to relieve pain, or foxglove to help with congestive heart failure, preparations that would deliver consistent doses were sought. However, plants vary widely in how much active ingredient they produce. The particular variety of plant, where it is grown, the weather during growth, when it is collected, how the collected plant is treated and stored, and many other factors influence the contents of the plant. Foxglove *(Digitalis purpurea)* was found to contain drugs that have a powerful effect on the heart, but many of them were also toxic. Plants closely related to foxglove were examined for similar drugs, leading to the discovery of digoxin. Very precise doses of digoxin must be used for it to be effective without causing toxicity. To ensure that each dose contained the same amount of digoxin, the active chemical was isolated and prepared in pure form, thus removing the need to use the crude herb.

More recently, an extract of the Pacific yew tree (*Taxus brevifolia*) was found to have anticancer properties. However, the tree is an environmentally protected species and one of the slowest-growing trees in the world. To test the potential treatment in just one patient would take six one-hundred-year-old trees. To resolve this problem, researchers identified the active ingredient and how to make it from a compound found in much larger quantities in an easily cultivated species of yew (*Taxus baccata*). This gave them sufficient quantities to confirm that they had a powerful new anticancer drug called "taxol." Subsequently, chemists have developed ways to make taxol without using any plant material. Taxol has gone on to become a very useful drug in treating certain cancers, especially ovarian and breast cancers.

Once the active ingredients are identified, their amounts must be standardized so that people get the same dose each time they take the herb. The first step toward this goal is to prepare the herbal remedy in what is called a "standardized formulation" in which a specific amount of one active ingredient is contained in a dose. For example, the Australian Standard of tea tree oil contains at least 30 percent terpinene-4-ol (an active ingredient) and no more than 15 percent 1,8-cineole (a skin irritant). Australian regulators hold manufacturers to this standard to ensure high-quality, safe products. However, standardized products are more expensive, and regulation is required to enforce them. In the United States, no such regulation exists. Therefore, huge variation is found in the amount of active ingredient in products sold in the United States.

There is growing evidence to support this concern. ConsumerLab.com is an independent company that tests herbs, vitamins, and supplements sold in the United States against generally accepted testing standards. Initial tests have shown that many products contain levels of key ingredients that are lower — and in some cases *much* lower — than the package claims. In testing preparations from different companies, for example, the laboratory found that 63 percent of saw palmetto preparations did not contain the amount of active ingredient listed on the label. The lab reported similar findings with 46 percent of glucosamine-chondroitin products, 100 percent of chondroitin products, 23 percent of ginkgo products, and 15 percent of vitamin C products. You can find out which products did pass muster by subscribing to the lab's website (*www.consumerlab.com*). The company continues to release new tests nearly every month.

In 1995, *Consumer Reports* studied a number of ginseng products. The different product labels listed the amount of ginseng as anywhere from 100 mg to 700 mg of ginseng per capsule. Chemical tests of the capsules found very different amounts of ginsenosides, the chemicals believed to be the active ingredients in ginseng. (Note: With some herbs, we know what causes change in humans. Willow bark contains salicylic acid, the key ingredient in aspirin and the reason a willow bark tea will reduce or stop some pain. We do not know the specific ingredient or ingredients in ginseng that affect humans, though we suspect it is the ginsenosides.) An even bigger problem found by *Consumer Reports* was that the capsules with larger amounts of ginsenoside were not labeled as having more ginseng. In fact, there was no correlation between the labels and what was actually found in the capsules.

This type of variation in products from different manufacturers is one reason some products are less effective than others. They don't contain enough of the active ingredient. *Consumer Reports*, in May 2000, published a massive survey of 46,806 of their readers that in part measured how people subjectively perceived the effectiveness of various therapies. More than three-quarters of the survey respondents reported some, little, or no help from a number of popular herbal products that medical studies have demonstrated to be effective.

These high levels of dissatisfaction were disturbing, but not unexpected, for those aware of the great variability in these products. Possibly, the products simply did not work for the patients who tried them. For those products with evidence to support their effectiveness, poor satisfaction could be due to poor product quality.

Another problem with unregulated herbal remedies has been contamination. More than one hundred cases of severe kidney damage have occurred in Belgium because *Stephania tetrandra* was mistakenly replaced by *Aristolochia fangchi* in a Chinese herbal remedy. Of those women whose kidneys were removed because they were so badly damaged, more than half had developed cancer in the surrounding tissues. *Aristolochia* species are known to contain compounds that are poisonous to the kidneys and cause cancer. This tragedy probably was due to a simple mistake: the Chinese names of the two unrelated species are almost identical.

Other problems are more suggestive of deliberate actions. Synthetic drugs are regularly found in herbal remedies. In chapter 4, we told you about Paul, a ten-year-old boy whose mother gave him an herbal remedy to relieve his seizures (see p. 80). The remedy worked but later almost killed him because it contained pharmaceutical drugs and other compounds that weren't listed on the label (and shouldn't have been in the product at all). We'll give other examples below.

Regulation of herbal remedies and dietary supplements is needed. Consumers expect the highest quality in health products. But until changes are made, consumers cannot be assured that the herbal remedies (or vitamins and supplements) they buy contain what is listed on the label. When buying herbal remedies in the United States, you must adopt a buyer beware attitude.

• Cautions

How, then, are you going to find reliable information about herbal remedies? In chapter 1, we described studies that revealed problems with the information people receive in health food stores. Many people turn to the Internet for information on complementary and alternative medicine — 43.3 million per year in the United States according to one estimate. Many herbal remedies are marketed and purchased on the Internet. According to Morris and Avorn's 2003 study, the herbal information people find there is not very reliable. They used the five most popular search engines to research the eight bestselling herbs. Using the first page of search results, they carefully examined the information found on those websites. The results were disturbing but not really surprising.

Three-quarters of the websites offering information on herbs also sold herbal remedies or were directly linked to a seller. Only 12 percent of those websites had any references to studies to support the claims they made. Apart from whether their claims could be supported, more than three-quarters of these websites made claims about improving health that they should not legally make in the United States, and half made illegal claims about the products curing diseases. More than half omitted the required statement that their claims had not been evaluated by the FDA. Many sites did not include well-known information about the adverse effects of certain herbs. In other words, most of the popular websites offering information on herbal remedies present inaccurate, incomplete, and unreferenced information that frequently violates the United States law as set down by the 1994 Dietary Supplement Health and Education Act.

Caution is also needed because some herbal remedies can have adverse effects. For example, proponents claimed ephedra helps people lose weight and improves athletic performance. In 2001, ephedra products made up 0.8 percent of all sales of dietary supplements in the United States, yet they accounted for 64 percent of all herb-related adverse events reported to poison control centers. Ephedra products have been linked to several deaths and yet were very difficult to remove from the United States market. The FDA was finally able to ban their sale in April 2004.

Cases of deliberate adulteration of herbal remedies have been reported. Relatively inexpensive pharmaceutical drugs such as aspirin, antihistamines, barbiturates, and steroids have been found in herbal remedies in what would appear to be attempts to make the herbal remedies seem effective. A study in the Middle East by M. J. Bogusz and colleagues found that over 30 percent of 247 herbal remedies were contaminated in some way. Of these, eight contained pharmaceutical drugs, including valium-like drugs in herbal sedatives and ibuprofen in herbal capsules for rheumatism. Another study examined seventy Ayurvedic herbal remedies manufactured in India and Pakistan and purchased in the Boston area. A 2004 publication by Dr. Robert Saper and colleagues found that 20 percent of the products contained lead, mercury, and/or arsenic. When taken according to the labels' recommendations, all would have resulted in heavy metal intakes above regulatory standards — some of them three times the recommended reference doses.

Another area of concern is how herbal remedies interact with other herbs and drugs. Many herbs and drugs are eliminated from the body by the liver. If the liver is tied up metabolizing components of herbal remedies, less of the drug will be eliminated and may even reach toxic levels. Other herbs (e.g., St. John's wort) stimulate the liver to more actively eliminate other drugs, leading to those drugs being less effective. That's why it is important to let all your health care providers, conventional and alternative, physicians and pharmacists, know about *all* the medicines and remedies you are taking, including drugs, over-the-counter products, herbs, vitamins, and dietary supplements.

Very little is known about the long-term effects of taking herbal remedies. Most traditional uses of herbs involve short-term use for a specific condition, although practitioners in one country sometimes follow guidelines not used in others. For example, many practitioners of herbal medicine in Europe say that their experience requires that ginseng not be used for more than two weeks at a time. Yet in the United States, practitioners seem to feel comfortable recommending its use as an energy booster for months or years. Current use of herbal remedies and dietary supplements is often for conditions, such as mild depression, general anxiety, antiaging, and as energy boosters, for which the remedies may be taken for years. There is no information on how the body will tolerate this extended use.

Given the general lack of information on the toxic effects of many herbs, some general guidelines can be proposed. Women who are pregnant or who are sexually active and thus might become pregnant should be extremely cautious about using any herbal remedy. The same is true for nursing mothers. Very little is known about how herbal remedies affect the unborn and children, but their potential for causing them harm is even higher than for adults. We know very little about the amounts that can be considered safe doses for an adult. We know almost nothing about what is safe for the unborn and the newborn. Because of this lack of knowledge, babies and children should not be given herbal remedies unless they have been clearly proven safe and effective.

Adults taking herbal remedies should limit their use to only short periods of time unless long-term studies have been done (which is beginning to be

the case for a few herbs and supplements). Never assume that just because something is natural, it is safe. The opposite might be true. Take only reasonable amounts of any herbal remedy. If things don't improve relatively quickly, see your physician and report what you've been taking. Don't fall into the trap of assuming that if a small amount helps a little, a large amount will help a lot. This is not the case with pharmaceutical drugs, and it's not the case with herbal remedies.

Only use standardized preparations bought at reliable stores. The United States Pharmacopeia (USP) is a volunteer organization of pharmaceutical experts that evaluates the standards by which any drug or herbal remedy has been manufactured. Look for its stamp of approval as a way of determining which products at least say that they are made according to high standards. They will theoretically be the safest, though that does not mean that the manufacturer's claim for its effectiveness, or the actual amount in the bottle, will be accurate. Consider subscribing to *www.consumerlab.com* to see if the brand you're considering has been tested by this independent company. And when you find a reliable brand, don't shop around for a different brand that's cheaper. You may be better off sticking with a brand that is giving you the results you want rather than trying to save a few dollars.

Further Caution with Herbalism

All of what we have discussed so far applies to "herbal medicine," where herbal remedies are used in ways similar to how prescription drugs are used. Another term sometimes used in these discussions is "herbalism." This term usually arises within a pantheistic worldview that sees herbal remedies as an essential part of humanity's oneness with nature, not as chemicals that have certain physical effects on the body. Herbal remedies are believed by these practitioners to be one of the ways Mother Earth, or the Universal Consciousness, cares for humanity. For example, David Hoffman, a well-known herbalist, writes, "The Earth is not a physico-chemical mechanism but a living entity with the equivalent of senses, intelligence, memory and the capacity to act." In other words, the Earth is a living, personal being. For many of these practitioners, she is also the object of their worship.

Herbalism varies among cultures, but the common view is that herbs are believed to balance or strengthen a person's vital force or life energy. Herbs are chosen by how they are believed to rebalance a person's vital force or trigger natural healing mechanisms. In this way, the same herbs may be used in completely different ways in different cultures, or even with different patients within the same community.

Herbalism is a religious or magical approach to herbs. One form of magic uses the similarity of objects to allegedly cause desired effects. Thus, herbs that grow with shapes similar to parts of the human body gain magical reputations for healing those body parts. For example, mandrakes have fleshy, forked roots that resemble the lower parts of the human body and have been used since biblical times to promote fertility. Jacob's wife Leah collected mandrakes to use in this way (Genesis 30:14–17). This passage demonstrates the futility of herbalism's approach, although the main teaching is that fertility is a gift from God. Having given away her mandrakes to Rachel, Jacob's other wife, Leah then becomes pregnant. Meanwhile, Rachel uses the mandrakes and remains barren for the time being.

Since the approach is clearly at odds with Christian worship of the one true God, Christians should not use herbal remedies within this context. If you seek out an expert in herbal remedies, make sure you are not exposing yourself to those who practice herbalism.

• Recommendations

Plants have been the source of people's drugs for most of human history. Given the diversity of God's creation, it is unlikely we have discovered all the potential blessings contained in the plant kingdom. In fact, one of the tragedies of the rapid destruction of the rain forests is that we may be losing indigenous plants capable of curing some of our most devastating diseases, including certain forms of cancer.

Traditionally, the herbal market has been portrayed as an unorganized group of mom-and-pop operations trying to fight against the big, bad pharmaceutical giants. No longer is this the case. Herbal remedies are a multibillion-dollar market, with all the problems that accompany this type of giant enterprise. Common sense and careful investigation are needed before wandering into a field as dangerous as any shark-infested waters.

Additionally, some herbal remedies, such as the Bach flower remedies, are believed to work because they have been "spiritually vitalized." Others make use of herbal remedies within the context of a sort of religious practice called "herbalism." A number of hallucinogenic herbs and other preparations are used in witchcraft and shamanism to access the spirit world. In all these contexts, herbal remedies are tools to promote occult activities and should be avoided. In these situations it is very important to have discernment about those manufacturing and promoting these preparations.

Treatment Categories

Conventional

A growing number of specific herbs for specific indications — discussed under each herb's entry

Complementary

A small but growing number of herbal products for specific indications

Scientifically Unproven

Many herbal remedies

Scientifically Questionable

Many herbal products

Spiritual

Many of the same herbs when used within herbalism or as Bach flower remedies

Quackery or Fraud

In the hands of some practitioners

Further Reading

Barnes, Patricia M., Eve Powell-Griner, Kim McFann, and Richard L. Nahin. "Complementary and Alternative Medicine Use Among Adults: United States, 2002." *Advance Data from Vital and Health Statistics* no. 343 (May 27, 2004). *U.S. Department of Health and Human Services: www.cdc.gov/nchs/data/ad/ad343.pdf.* Accessed September 13, 2005. Referred to as "2002 CDC Survey."

Blumenthal, M., J. Gruenwald, T. Hall, C. Riggins, and R. Rister. *German Commission E Monographs: Medicinal Plants for Human Use.* Austin, Tex.: American Botanical Council, 1998.

Blumenthal, Mark. "Herb Sales Down 7.4 Percent in Mainstream Market; Garlic Is Top-Selling Herb; Herb Combinations See Increase." *HerbalGram* 66 (2005): 63.

Bogusz, M. J., M. al Tufail, and H. Hassan. "How Natural Are 'Natural Herbal Remedies'? A Saudi Perspective." *Adverse Drug Reactions and Toxicological Reviews* 21, no. 4 (2002): 219 – 29.

Fetrow, Charles W., and Juan R. Avila. *Professional's Handbook of Complementary and Alternative Medicine.* Springhouse, Penn.: Springhouse, 2001.

Foster, Steven, and Varro E. Tyler. *Tyler's Honest Herbal: A Sensible Guide to the Use of Herbs and Related Remedies.* 4th ed. London: Haworth Press, 1999.

Hoffman, David. *The Elements of Herbalism.* New York: Barnes & Noble, 1997.

Jellin, Jeff M., Forrest Batz, and Kathy Hichens. *Pharmacist's Letter/Prescriber's Letter: Natural Medicines Comprehensive Database.* Stockton, Calif.: Therapeutic Research Facility, 1999. Also available by subscription at *www.naturaldatabase.com.*

Johnston, Barbara A. "*Prevention* Magazine Assesses Use of Dietary Supplements." *HerbalGram* 48 (2000): 65.

"The Mainstreaming of Alternative Medicine." *Consumer Reports* 65, no. 5 (May 2000): 17 – 25.

Morris, Charles A., and Jerry Avorn. "Internet Marketing of Herbal Remedies." *Journal of the American Medical Association* 290, no. 11 (September 2003): 1505 – 9.

"'Natural' or 'plant-derived' labeling can mislead." *National Consumers League* (January 17, 2002). *National Consumers League: www.nclnet.org/naturalpr0102.htm.* Accessed November 20, 2005.

Saper, Robert B., Stefanos N. Kales, Janet Paquin, Michael J. Burns, David M. Eisenberg, Roger B. Davis, and Russell S. Phillips. "Heavy Metal Content of Ayurvedic Herbal Medicine Products." *Journal of the American Medical Association* 292, no. 23 (December 2004): 2868 – 73.

Tindle, Hilary A., Roger B. Davis, Russell S. Phillips, and David E. Eisenberg. "Trends in Use of Complementary and Alternative Medicine by US Adults: 1997 – 2002." *Alternative Therapies in Health and Medicine* 11, no. 1 (January – February 2005): 42 – 49.

HOMEOPATHY

What It Is

German physician Samuel Hahnemann (1755 – 1843) was typical of many compassionate medical practitioners working during a time when medicine was harsh and unpleasant. Treatments could be quite severe, such as bloodletting, blistering, and purging. Worse, the efforts were usually ineffective and patients suffered needlessly.

Dr. Hahnemann wanted to find a milder, safer system. He and his assistants began experimenting on themselves in a series of tests called "provings."

For example, malaria had been a scourge in Europe for many years until cinchona bark was found to treat it effectively. Dr. Hahnemann noticed that if healthy people were given quinine, the active ingredient in cinchona, they developed malaria-like symptoms. Similar patterns with other treatments led him to develop his Law of Similars. According to this concept, if a substance produces a specific set of symptoms in a healthy person, it will cure people of the illness that has those same symptoms — provided it is diluted repeatedly. Since quinine given to healthy people produces symptoms similar to those experienced by malaria sufferers, extremely diluted solutions of quinine (called "homeopathic quinine") are believed to cure malaria. Likewise, belladonna given to healthy people produces fevers, flushing, and other flu-like symptoms, so homeopathic belladonna is used to treat colds and flu.

Over the course of his career, Hahnemann tested hundreds of substances and meticulously observed the symptoms elicited. He wrote the *Homeopathic Pharmacopoeia*, a text still highly respected by homeopaths and consulted regularly.

One of the reasons some patients like homeopaths is because the practitioner makes many of the remedies in the office, adding a sense of personal medicine. The remedies are made by dissolving plant, mineral, animal, or chemical products in water and alcohol. Unlike drugs and herbal remedies, though, extremely dilute solutions must be used. This is because Hahnemann's observations led him to propose another highly controversial law, the Law of Potentization.

The Law of Potentization claims that the more dilute a solution of a substance becomes, the higher its potency. Homeopathic remedies are diluted again and again in the belief that this increases their effect and effectiveness. This law contradicts the generally accepted finding in pharmacy and medicine that the more dilute a solution, the weaker its effect on the body.

Homeopathic remedies are labeled as so many "x" or "c." For example, a 15x potency means the substance was diluted fifteen times at a ratio of 1 in 10 (one drop of the original solution is mixed with nine drops of alcohol or water; then one drop of that solution is diluted by ten; and so on, fifteen times). A 12c potency means the substance was diluted twelve times at a ratio of 1 in 100. Some of these remedies are so diluted that homeopaths acknowledge there is practically no chance of even one molecule of the original substance remaining.

A variety of hypotheses are proposed to explain how such diluted solutions could have any effect on the body. A popular one, based on a 1988 article by

French scientist Jacques Benveniste and published in the prestigious journal *Nature*, claims that the substances leave some sort of electromagnetic imprint on the water molecules. Very few scientists accept this idea of "water memory," and no one has been able to repeat Benveniste's experiments. Such repetition of an experiment is an important test of any theory.

The more traditional explanation for homeopathic effectiveness is based on life energy theories and vitalism. Hahnemann used the term "vital energy" for the same life energy that is called *chi* in traditional Chinese medicine and *prana* in Ayurvedic medicine. Hahnemann explained this energy's role in his 1810 book, still regarded as the bible of homeopathy, *Organ of the Art of Healing* (also called *Organon*): "In the state of health the spirit-like vital force (*dynamis*) animating the material human organism reins in supreme sovereignty."

According to this view, the symptoms of an illness are signs that the body's life energy is fighting against an illness. Thus, a substance that produces those same symptoms works with the body's vital energy to promote self-healing. Eliminating those symptoms (a common goal in conventional medicine) is thus counterproductive, according to homeopathic theory. Thus, homeopathy does not seem to be compatible with conventional medicine because they are fundamentally at odds in their approaches to healing. (We should emphasize that we are willing to consider *any* therapy even if it has an approach fundamentally at odds with other therapies. However, we seek to base our recommendations on the best available evidence. Our questions are, "What is the evidence or proof that the therapy works?" "What is the strength of that evidence?" and even if it works, "Are there spiritual dangers of which you need to be aware?")

Hahnemann's explanation for his reports of the effectiveness of such diluted solutions focused more on the way the dilutions were done. At each dilution, the mixture must be shaken vigorously. Hahnemann believed this shaking released "the spiritual vital force" of the healing substance. Thus, more shaking allegedly releases more energy and gives stronger effects.

According to Dana Ullman, president of the Foundation of Homeopathic Education and Research, this energy is similar to the *prana* of Ayurvedic medicine, "the inherent, underlying, interconnective, self-healing process of the organism." Thus, although some claim homeopathy works through some unknown natural mechanism, its core principles are based on life energy beliefs. The scientifically questionable premises in homeopathy are understandable only by introducing life energy concepts.

Today, homeopathy is practiced in at least four different ways. Classical homeopathy requires consultation with a homeopath. Detailed descriptions of the patient's physical, emotional, and mental symptoms are collected. These are compared with the known effects of substances that have been collected in homeopathic proofings. These determine the specific homeopathic remedy for that individual's set of symptoms.

Clinical homeopathy differs in that the same remedy will be recommended for anyone with the same set of symptoms, much like herbal remedies or prescription drugs are recommended to treat a certain illness.

Complex homeopathy is similar to clinical homeopathy except that remedies are made using complex mixtures of homeopathic solutions.

Isopathy is a newer approach for allergies in which an extremely diluted solution of the agent that causes an allergic reaction is used to treat the allergy.

Claims

Homeopaths vary considerably in what they claim to be able to treat. Some limit their claims to chronic illnesses or those for which conventional medicine offers only limited symptom management. The most common are allergies, flu, cold, arthritis, and asthma. However, other homeopaths claim to be able to cure almost every known disease, including diabetes, cancer, heart disease, and other serious illnesses. Thousands of different homeopathic remedies are made from many different substances in accordance with the particular mixture of symptoms a patient reports.

Claims of effectiveness are often backed up by the consistent popularity of homeopathy in Europe (in particular, the long-standing endorsement by the British royal family). Ernst reported in 2005 that among family doctors in Europe, 20 percent in Germany are homeopaths, 42 percent in the United Kingdom refer patients to homeopaths, and 85 percent in Belgium are homeopaths.

The approach has been growing in popularity in the United States. Homeopathic sales increased rapidly during the 1980s and 1990s. Sales in mainstream retail outlets (as opposed to the Internet or multilevel marketing) grew by almost 50 percent in 2002. However, surveys by David Eisenberg and colleagues found that general use in the United States fell by half between 1997 and 2002 — from 3.4 to 1.7 percent of the population. At the same time, the proportion of those using homeopathic remedies under the care of a homeopath increased from 16.5 to 20.8 percent. In Britain, even while the National Health Service is paying for more alternative therapies, a number of local health authorities have stopped paying for homeopathic remedies because of a lack of evidence to support their effectiveness.

Study Findings

Some individual trials of homeopathy find beneficial effects (✓✓✓). However, a large systematic review of homeopathy trials published in August 2005 in the British journal *Lancet* did not. The researchers carried out a wide search and believed they had identified just about all published studies. They found 156 studies, although they carried out their analysis on 110 of these because of significant problems in the design of some trials. This was the largest and most comprehensive review to date. Some studies reported beneficial effects from homeopathy, but they found significant bias was involved in these reports. They showed that studies finding homeopathy better than placebo were smaller and of poorer quality. When poor-quality trials were excluded and only high-quality larger trials were considered, the reviewers concluded "there was no convincing evidence that homeopathy was superior to placebo" (✗✗✗).

These results appear to conflict with Klaus Linde and colleagues' 1997 conclusion to their review of eighty-nine studies (✓✓✓✓) that did not support the quotation frequently cited "that the clinical effects of homeopathy are completely due to placebo." However, two important qualifications must be made. Linde's review concluded that there was insufficient evidence that homeopathy is effective for any particular clinical condition. More important, no fewer than six re-analyses of this same data have come to the opposite conclusion (✗✗✗). Linde himself in 1999 published a reexamination of his 1997 study. He showed how higher-quality studies found homeopathy ineffective (✗✗✗), while low-quality studies tended to find it somewhat effective. The 2005 review has confirmed these findings on an even larger scale.

Yet some studies do report positive findings for homeopathy. One problem is that most homeopathy studies have different designs and examine different conditions. With any scientific study, it is important to repeat the study to make sure the findings can be replicated. In the small number of homeopathy uses where this has been done, Edzard Ernst reported in 2005 that either the results were negative or the studies were poorly designed (✗✗✗). Results like this make it difficult to accept that homeopathy works by anything other than a complex placebo effect.

In spite of the negative controlled research results, many people continue to believe that the remedies work. Some claim this comes from a powerful placebo effect stemming from the positive interactions patients have with homeopaths. The initial visit will involve an extensive interview to determine which preparation most closely matches the patient's combination of symptoms. Some homeopaths also believe it is important to classify a patient according to a set of constitutional types. The same problem might be treated with different remedies in people of different constitutional types, or the same remedy might be used to treat different problems in different people. The individualized attention needed to determine which remedy is used may itself be therapeutic.

Cautions

Since homeopathic remedies are extremely diluted (to the point of having no active ingredients at all), and only very small amounts are given, harmful side effects are not likely. However, there have been some reports of contamination of products. The lack of oversight of these products also raises concerns. Homeopathic preparations are not regulated like drugs in the United States under an exemption to the usual FDA drug regulations granted by law in 1938. They do not need to submit research evidence, nor must they adhere to all the good manufacturing practices required of drugs. They must list ingredients and their dilution. Conventional drugs are not permitted to contain more than 10 percent alcohol, but homeopathic remedies are exempt from this regulation and some contain much higher quantities of alcohol.

Although the relationship between patients and homeopathic practitioners is advantageous, most sales are directly to consumers by mail or from health food stores. A lot of people are self-diagnosing their problems and self-prescribing homeopathic (and herbal) remedies. The danger is in neglecting diagnosis and treatment of conditions that conventional medicine can cure or alleviate.

Recommendations

The scientific evidence that homeopathy works any better than a placebo is small and, in our opinion, very weak. For homeopathic remedies to work as proposed, core tenets of evidence-based science and reason would have to be completely overhauled — or thrown overboard. For this reason, most within the scientific community remain highly skeptical of homeopathy. Those who use homeopathy tend to believe very strongly that it works. Given that it is relatively safe and harmless, homeopathy might help those who believe in it because of the placebo effect. However, Christians who decide to use homeopathy must be discerning about the homeopaths they choose. Belief in homeopathy as a method of manipulating life energy is incompatible with Christian beliefs.

● Treatment Categories

Complementary

For any indication   ☹☹☹☹

Scientifically Questionable

For any indication   ☹☹☹☹

Spiritual

In the hands of some practitioners   👎

Quackery or Fraud

In the hands of some practitioners

● Further Reading

Ernst, Edzard. "Is Homeopathy a Clinically Valuable Approach?" *Trends in Pharmacological Sciences* 26, no. 11 (November 2005): 547 – 48.

Linde, Klaus, Michael Scholz, Gilbert Ramirez, Nicolas Clausius, Dieter Melchart, and Wayne B. Jonas.

"Impact of Study Quality on Outcome in Placebo-Controlled Trials of Homeopathy." *Journal of Clinical Epidemiology* 52, no. 7 (1999): 631 – 36.

Linde, Klaus, Nicolas Clausius, Gilbert Ramirez, Dieter Melchart, Florian Eitel, Larry V. Hedges, and Wayne B. Jonas. "Are the Clinical Effects of Homoeopathy Placebo Effects? A Meta-Analysis of Placebo-Controlled Trials." *Lancet* 350 (September 1997): 834 – 43.

"The Mainstreaming of Alternative Medicine." *Consumer Reports* 65, no. 5 (May 2000): 17 – 25.

Shang, Aijing, Karin Huwiler-Müntener, Linda Nartey, Peter Jüni, Stephan Dörig, Jonathan A. C. Sterne, Daniel Pewsner, and Matthias Egger. "Are the Clinical Effects of Homoeopathy Placebo Effects? Comparative Study of Placebo-Controlled Trials of Homoeopathy and Allopathy." *Lancet* 366 (August 2005): 726 – 32.

Ullman, Dana. *Discovering Homeopathy*: *Medicine for the 21st Century*, rev. ed. (Berkeley, Calif.: North Atlantic, 1991).

HYPNOSIS

● What It Is

Hypnosis (formerly called "hypnotism") has been seen by some as the illegitimate child of both medicine and psychology. Teenagers growing up in the 1950s would discover advertisements on the back of comic books where anything from 10 to 25 cents could buy a booklet that would teach them how to "control the minds of others" using "hypnotism." Earlier, in the 1930s, Dr. George Estabrooks, head of the Psychology Department at Colgate University, was adamant in his belief that hypnosis could be used to create a double agent or a secret assassin or be used for interrogation. Despite this seemingly sinister potential, many experts believe that only one in five individuals is a good subject for hypnosis no matter how it is used.

It is hard to get a firm grasp on exactly what hypnosis involves. Different methods are used to "induce" hypnosis, and there is some disagreement among experts about how to verify that someone is in a hypnotic trance as opposed to another similar state of altered consciousness.

Some question whether a unique state of hypnosis

even exists because many of its effects can be obtained without hypnosis. Disagreement also occurs over whether hypnosis is ever appropriate for Christians. There are Christian hypnotherapists, and there are Christians who vehemently oppose the practice. What almost everyone agrees on is that hypnosis is a method of inducing what is commonly called an "altered state of consciousness" — when the mind is not under the usual control of rational, logical faculties or consciousness. Daydreaming, tuning out, even sleeping can be types of altered states of consciousness. You're reading and find yourself drifting in and out of full awareness. You turn a page and realize you've no idea what you just read. Yet you were awake — reading — in an altered state of consciousness.

People under anesthesia, under the influence of drugs or alcohol, or engaged in various mystical experiences are in other forms of altered states of consciousness. Perhaps the most common experience of this type that most of us share is when we are deep in thought about some problem while driving or taking a long walk. Suddenly we find ourselves at our exit off the highway, several miles from our office, with no memory of getting there. Or we realize we have walked all the way around a park and cannot recall anything about what we've just done. In both instances, we were functioning effectively. We drove and walked safely, not endangering others or ourselves, yet our awareness was on our thoughts, the problem we were trying to solve. This, too, is a form of altered state of consciousness.

These altered states of consciousness can be objectively verified by measuring changes in breathing patterns, body temperature, and responses to stimuli and by using electroencephalography (EEG, which measures the electrical activity of the brain). Behavior can change, and a person responds differently to external stimuli. The student in class who has "drifted into another world" no longer hears the teacher's voice, though the voice is as loud and clear as before.

Hypnosis is a form of altered state of consciousness, though difficult to define. Some experts say people in hypnotic trances are alert and "in control," while others believe that people "in trance" are not fully alert, yet they are not asleep either. Rather than give a one-sentence definition of hypnosis, John Court, a Christian counselor and educator who uses hypnosis, describes the characteristic features of altered states of consciousness, and hypnosis in particular.

Court explains that having a person focus attention and filter out external distractions can induce hypnosis — or a hypnotic state or trance. Repetition helps — for example, the rhythmic drum beating used in religious ceremonies or therapists asking clients to count backwards. As the focus narrows, left-brain thinking (that which is logical and rational) becomes less dominant, and right-brain thinking is facilitated. This may leave a person open to imagery and visualization, which are commonly used during hypnosis. Therapists will often ask people to picture themselves in a relaxing scene, such as lying on a warm, pleasant beach.

While in the hypnotic trance, people are more passive than active. They wait and listen for things to happen rather than actively seeking to do something. They are very open to suggestion, to the ideas (and possibly the persuasion) of others.

And therein lies the basis for both the uses and the concerns of hypnosis. A therapist might tell someone during hypnosis that her arm is numb and insensitive, so she feels no pain while a physician is doing minor surgery on the arm. A psychologist may use hypnosis to help clients discuss painful memories they would not allow themselves to think about while fully conscious. Or a stage hypnotist may tell someone to act like a dog, so the person runs around barking.

Even those who practice hypnosis agree that it should be conducted only within a trusting relationship. Court acknowledges, "To be in a state of heightened suggestibility is to be at risk from any unscrupulous person who might seek to exploit the situation." During hypnosis, the person is under great pressure to respond to the expectations of the therapist. When hypnosis is being used to examine past memories, Court writes, "the hypnotist can find what is being looked for, whether grounded in reality or not."

Allegations of childhood abuse based on memories recovered during hypnosis have been very controversial. Even more controversy arises when the memories are said to come from past lives, and thus used as evidence for reincarnation.

A useful definition of hypnosis can be found in a Christian publication, the *Baker Encyclopedia of Psychology*:

> Hypnosis is clearly not a power or force that one possesses to control another. Rather, hypnosis appears to involve a shift in concentration, executed in a passive manner (such as occurs in daydreaming or sleeping), resulting in a state of consciousness distinguishably different from alertness or ordinary sleep. It is characterized by narrowing of attention, reduced rational criticalness, and increased responsiveness to suggestion. It appears to provide a clearer access to the functioning of the mind, allowing understanding of that which is subconscious or dissociated.

So, while hypnosis is induced in somewhat similar ways to how we fall asleep, the resulting state is distinguishable from sleep. During hypnosis people have greater "access" to their subconscious minds but are less under the control of their conscious minds. Because of how open to others' suggestions people become, hypnosis should never be entered into lightly.

History of Hypnosis

Hypnosis has been practiced for centuries in the Far East, but in the West, the first prominent promoter of hypnosis was Franz Anton Mesmer (1734 – 1815), an Austrian physician. He originally used magnets in his healings, believing that these assisted in the flow of "animal magnetism," a fluid he believed was present in all people. He later dropped the use of magnets, and his subjects were believed to be healed by being "mesmerized."

As mesmerism fell into disrepute, hypnosis gained some followers. Jean-Martin Charcot (1835 – 1893) used it to explore and alleviate hysteria in patients. He taught hypnosis to his students, including Sigmund Freud, who used it to explore hidden memories. Freud later stopped using hypnosis in favor of what would become known as psychoanalysis.

British physician James Braid (1795 – 1860) coined the term "hypnotism" (which has since been replaced by "hypnosis") and noted that people usually don't remember what happened during hypnosis. A British surgeon, James Esdaile, used hypnosis as an anesthetic during surgery. Hypnosis seemed poised to find a number of applications but faded rapidly after Freud's psychoanalytic methods replaced it as a psychological tool and drugs became available to induce anesthesia.

At the same time, Mesmer's form of hypnosis grew in popularity among a number of new spiritual groups, especially in the United States. Mesmerism was seen as a way to bring people into "harmony" with unseen spiritual forces. It was also seen as a useful technique to help people develop clairvoyant skills. Phineas Quimby (1802–1866) used mesmerism, and his results led him to believe that all sickness is illusory. His system developed into the New Thought movement and was taken up by Mary Baker Eddy, who had been treated by Mesmer at one time and became a part of Christian Science (although Eddy later rejected hypnosis).

All of these associations with unorthodox religious or spiritualist movements have left many Christians wary of hypnosis. More recently, the New Age movement adopted hypnosis as an important technique for spiritual enlightenment. When this use of hypnosis is coupled with stage hypnotists' entertaining (but somewhat alarming) scenes of people doing all sorts of strange and uncharacteristic things, there is no wonder some Christians see nothing but danger in hypnosis. Some even claim that the list of occult practices forbidden in Deuteronomy 18:10–11 includes hypnosis when it refers to one who "casts spells."

In light of these concerns, those considering hypnosis must look at both scientific and theological issues. Some might conclude that hypnosis can be embraced. Others might believe it should be rejected. Our answer is more complicated. After a careful examination of all sides of the argument, our conclusion is, "It depends!"

• Claims

The claims about hypnosis can be divided into four groups according to the primary goal of its use: entertainment, pain management, counseling, and spiritual growth.

Entertainment. Stage hypnosis involves entertainers getting people to do things they normally wouldn't do, all for the benefit of giving the audience some laughs. Stage hypnotists are highly skilled at recognizing who in the audience is most likely to enter a hypnotic trance. It is widely recognized that among any group of a hundred people, ten will be easily hypnotized, ten will be very difficult to hypnotize, and the rest fall somewhere in between. Some stage hypnotism is real, but some can be fraudulent or illusionary. John Court quotes from a training manual for stage hypnosis that admits, "Experience has shown down through the years that the hypnotic show must be faked, at least partially so, to hold audience interest and be successful as entertainment.... The successful hypnotic entertainer of today is actually not interested whether or not the subjects are really hypnotized — his basic function is to entertain. He is interested in his ability to con his subjects into a pseudo-performance that appears as hypnotism."

These shows and party "games" demonstrate how open to a hypnotist's suggestions people can be during a hypnotic trance. They show how a hypnotist can dramatically influence behavior. They show the power and the danger of naïvely becoming involved with hypnosis.

Pain management. Hypnotherapy in medicine is used primarily for the relief or prevention of pain, and for anesthesia, diverting attention from the pain. Some medical schools require all students to learn the practice and use it during minor surgery or labor and delivery, although in practice it is not widely used.

Counseling. Hypnotherapy is used psychologically to help people deal with phobias and unwanted habits, to uncover repressed memories, to treat dissociative conditions, and to enhance sports or arts performances. Hypnosis has been used abusively, according to John Court, as a "brainwashing" procedure.

Spiritual growth. The final area of interest in hypnosis is as a spiritual or religious practice. Those in favor of hypnosis, including Christian hypnotherapists, point to the similarities between the hypnotic trance and many religious practices and experiences. Worship services often include repetition, rhythmic singing or music, focused attention on an altar or pulpit, visual and verbal imagery, and distinctive odors. People report an openness to words in a sermon or song and often sense a spiritual presence. The Bible, for example, records people of faith having visions (Daniel, Peter, and many of the prophets), sometimes recorded as trances, as was the case with Peter (Acts 11:5; see also 10:11; 22:17).

The hypnotic trance is viewed by Christian hypnotherapists as a legitimate and natural way for anyone to achieve a greater sense of the transcendent and to become more open to spiritual encounters. The *Baker Encyclopedia of Psychology* puts it this way: "The value of hypnosis is that it provides a means of achieving a special state in which the person can go beyond the bounds of usual rational thinking to affect both mental and physical processes.... Such experience taps into the spiritual and unconscious resources of the individual and also into that part of the psyche that is open to the influence of God and the cosmos."

Study Findings

Studies of hypnosis for pain management have been conducted for more than thirty years. Much of the early research was not controlled effectively. More recent studies have found hypnosis beneficial, showing short-term improvements in pain intensity and headache frequency, along with reduced need for pain medication (✓✓✓). Hypnosis is increasingly available as a complementary therapy in pain management clinics. A 2005 review of hypnosis for pain found several studies in which effective pain relief was obtained (✓✓✓). The source of pain varied, with hypnosis being effective with burns, surgery, headaches, musculoskeletal pain, and fibromyalgia. Hypnosis was particularly effective in six studies involving pain from cancer and cancer-related treatment (✓✓✓). A systematic review of hypnosis used during labor found that women taught self-hypnosis required less medication for pain or to induce labor and more frequently had spontaneous vaginal deliveries (✓✓✓).

Many of these studies were carried out with relatively small numbers of patients. One of the largest studies to date of hypnosis for pain (✓✓✓) was reported in April 2000 in the British journal *Lancet*. More than two hundred patients were divided into three groups, one receiving normal treatment, another receiving hypnosis, and the third receiving extra attention from someone who ensured nothing negative was said during their surgery. All patients could give themselves as much pain medication as they needed. About half the patients in both the extra attention and hypnosis groups needed no pain medication, and those who took medication used half the amount used by those in the no-treatment group. Those receiving hypnosis reported that their pain did not get worse. They also had no blood pressure problems and their surgeries finished, on average, seventeen minutes earlier. The time savings was thought to have occurred because there were fewer complications.

While hypnosis was clearly beneficial, this study brings out another general problem with the evidence for hypnosis. This study did not compare hypnosis with a nonhypnotic relaxation group to determine if the benefits were specifically due to hypnosis or just to a general relaxation response. This leaves a question as to whether or not hypnotherapy is more effective than other psychological therapies such as meditation, guided imagery, stress-reduction techniques, and relaxation techniques.

Controlled studies on the use of hypnosis in psychological or behavior counseling are difficult to conduct. Most reports are case studies (✓✓) that usually find some benefit from hypnosis. Court's book describes cases involving patients with depression, phobias, and earlier traumatic incidences who improved with hypnosis, often in conjunction with counseling, medication, and prayer. As with any form of counseling or behavior modification, it is difficult to tease out the precise role of any one aspect of the treatment plan.

Hypnosis for smoking cessation demonstrates the difficulty of evaluating behavior modification programs. A Cochrane review, updated in 2005, found that among case reports and uncontrolled studies of hypnotherapy, the success rate for smoking cessation varied from 4 to 88 percent — an extremely wide margin. Nine randomized controlled studies were found, although with much variation in the hypnosis protocols. Overall, the percent of patients still not smoking six months after undergoing hypnosis was the same as after any other treatment or after no treatment. A couple of studies did find hypnotherapy more beneficial, but these were smaller and more poorly designed studies. The review authors concluded, "There is insufficient evidence to recommend hypnotherapy as a specific treatment for smoking cessation."

In another area, three meta-analyses of hypnosis for the treatment of obesity were published in the mid-1990s in the *Journal of Consulting and Clinical Psychology*. The first (✓✓✓✓) found that when hypnosis was added to cognitive-behavior therapy, obese patients lost significantly more weight than with therapy alone. The second (✗✗✗✗) reexamined the data from the first, added other studies that the first had not included, and concluded that there was no benefit from adding hypnosis. The third (✓✓✓) added new data obtained directly from the researchers (which had not been in the published research) and concluded that hypnosis was of benefit. These inconsistencies show how unclear research data can be. This is currently a difficulty in evaluating all psychological therapies.

Cautions

The use of hypnosis during medical procedures seems to be very safe, with few adverse effects reported. A very small percentage of research subjects report short-lasting drowsiness or headache. Probably the biggest concern about hypnosis arises from its use by inexperienced therapists and difficulties encountered during counseling. The latter are said to be related to counseling issues, not hypnosis.

Some believe that hypnosis gives control of one's mind to someone else. If this occurs, people may be deceived into doing things they don't want to do, they may be taken advantage of (sexually or spiritually), or they may even be exposed to evil spiritual beings. Court, the Christian hypnotherapist, warns, "The inherent dangers of a powerful technique that affects thinking, feeling, and behaviour cannot be discounted since anything powerful is open to abuse. The possibility of being open to demonic influence in this setting cannot be dismissed as fanciful if we believe in the presence of evil."

Kurt Koch, a widely respected Christian authority on the occult, has had much experience with hypnosis as practiced in East Asia. In his books, he recounts numerous cases of hypnosis bringing people into contact with occult spirits. While these sometimes occurred as part of religious practices, some occurred after people innocently engaged in hypnosis at parties and shows. During this type of hypnosis, people are unduly under the influence of others whom they may not know. They may not have the degree of control over their minds that is expected of Christians, who are called to be alert at all times. "So then, let us not be like others, who are asleep, but let us be alert and self-controlled" (1 Thessalonians 5:6). "Be self-controlled and alert. Your enemy the devil prowls around like a roaring lion looking for someone to devour" (1 Peter 5:8). For this reason, we believe that Christians should not engage in any form of hypnosis for entertainment purposes.

Christian hypnotherapists claim that fears about hypnosis arise largely from stage hypnosis and older authoritarian forms of hypnotherapy no longer commonly practiced. They claim that the primary purpose of hypnosis as a therapy is to give patients increased control over themselves and their behavior, not less control. Court says, "Most Christians will acknowledge that they have less control than they wish over some areas of their lives — habits, addiction, fears, sins — and are seeking to enhance control."

Hypnosis, for Court, is a way to help people develop self-control by empowering them: "This non-directive approach, involving conversation rather than formal induction, indirect allusion and metaphor rather than commands, together with agreed goals and purposes, provides quite a different environment from that which traditionally has been feared. It is based on the skillful use of communication at various levels, by words, gestures and metaphors." He points out that Galatians 5:23 calls us to practice self-control. We see hypnotherapy having a legitimate role, provided such an approach is taken with a trusted Christian therapist.

One other caution must be mentioned. The Federal Trade Commission (FTC) oversees the truthfulness of advertising claims in the United States. In September 2002, the FTC reported that 40 percent of the weight-loss ads they examined made false claims. The fraudulent claims were almost all in ads for dietary supplements or hypnosis. Keep in mind the precautions we described about fraud in chapter 5 and the entry on Diets and Dieting.

Recommendations

Christians are divided over the appropriateness of using hypnosis. It has been used successfully for pain control, allowing the avoidance or reduction of medication. It has been used to aid relaxation without resorting to sleep medication for individuals recovering from psychological and physical trauma. Its use is limited and always will be, even under the best of circumstances, because only one in five individuals is a good candidate for any type of hypnosis.

Case reports for the medical uses of hypnosis for anesthesia and analgesia are prolific, though there are questions about what is happening. Is it hypnosis that occurs or a deep state of relaxation? Does the difference even matter if the doctor using hypnosis is a Christian with no ulterior motives?

The fact that a form of self-hypnosis can occur naturally in an experience of religious ecstasy does not mean hypnosis should be artificially induced. It is never wise for a Christian to participate in stage hypnosis. Likewise, unless you know the practitioner and his or her methods and religious beliefs, it is unwise to experience any form of hypnosis. But if the practitioner is a Christian with no thought of anything other than using hypnosis to aid healing, there is evidence that the technique may bring positive changes in some, but not all, people.

Other areas associated with hypnosis are less certain. Age regression through hypnosis is a tool sometimes used to allow a patient to discuss early childhood traumas that might otherwise be forgotten or repressed. But how the hypnosis is induced, and how the individual is questioned, will determine whether the memory is real or created by suggestive questioning. This is an area that must be looked at with great caution and with the wisdom of mature Christian counsel.

Treatment Categories

Complementary

To induce anesthesia	☺☺☺
To manage pain	☺☺☺☺
To relieve headaches	☺☺☺
To manage pain during labor	☺☺☺
To manage chronic pain	☺☺

Scientifically Unproven

For psychological indications

Scientifically Questionable

To help with smoking cessation	☹☹☹
To help with weight control	☹☹
For any other indication	

Spiritual

When used by some practitioners to generate spiritual experiences	👎👎

Quackery or Fraud

In the hands of some practitioners

Further Reading

Abbot, N. C., L. F. Stead, A. R. White, and J. Barnes. "Hypnotherapy for Smoking Cessation." *The Cochrane Database of Systematic Reviews* 1998, no. 2. Amended February 17, 2005.

Benner, David G., ed. *Baker Encyclopedia of Psychology.* Grand Rapids: Baker, 1985.

Court, John. *Hypnosis: Healing and the Christian.* Carlisle, U.K.: Paternoster, 1997.

Cuellar, Norma G. "Hypnosis for Pain Management in the Older Adult." *Pain Management Nursing* 6, no. 3 (September 2005): 105 – 11.

Cyna, Allan M., Marion I. Andrew, and Georgina L. McAuliffe. "Antenatal Hypnosis for Labour Analgesia." *International Journal of Obstetric Anesthesia* 14, no. 4 (October 2005): 365 – 66.

Koch, Kurt E. *Occult ABC.* Grand Rapids: Kregel, 1986, 95 – 100.

Lang, Elvira V., Eric G. Benotsch, Lauri J. Fick, Susan Lutgendorf, Michael L. Berbaum, Henrietta Logan, and David Spiegel. "Adjunctive Non-Pharmacological Analgesia for Invasive Medical Procedures: A Randomised Trial." *Lancet* 355 (April 2000): 1486 – 90.

Pinnell, Cornelia M., and Nicholas A. Covino. "Empirical Findings on the Use of Hypnosis in Medicine: A Critical Review." *International Journal of Clinical and Experimental Hypnosis* 48, no. 2 (April 2000): 170 – 94.

IRIDOLOGY

What It Is

Iridology is a way of examining the iris of the eye to obtain health information. It is particularly popular in the United States and Germany. This method is at least one hundred years old and is based on the assumption that diseases manifest themselves in patterns visible in different parts of the iris. Its modern form was developed by Ignatz von Peczely, a Hungarian physician. He found an owl with a broken leg and noticed it had a dark stripe in the iris of one of its eyes. As the doctor nursed the owl back to health, the stripe faded. Von Peczely came to believe that similar associations exist between the iris and human illnesses. Veterinarians who specialize in bird care have never found the type of association alleged by von Peczely.

Iridologists believe the iris is divided into sections, each one connected in some manner to a particular body part. Very specific areas of the iris are assigned to each organ and tissue. For example, if the eye is looked at like the face of a clock, changes in the kidneys would manifest themselves in the right iris where the hour hand would be at about five thirty; thyroid changes would be seen where the hour hand would be at about two thirty.

Iridology seems to have a basis in scientific knowledge in that certain diseases, such as rheumatoid arthritis, do lead to changes visible in the iris. However, these are general changes throughout the iris, not the isolated changes described in iridology.

Claims

Iridologists claim to be able to diagnose the existence of a wide variety of diseases in the organs of the body. The diagnoses can be made by either examining the iris directly or by using photographs. Fulder's *Handbook of Complementary Medicine* claims that iridology is "the most valuable diagnostic tool of the naturopath." Iridologists claim they can determine if an organ has a tendency to develop an illness at some point in the future, believing that weaknesses or abnormalities will manifest as changes in the iris before any symptoms appear.

Other alternative practitioners use the same assumptions to claim they can make diagnoses by examining other parts of the body. For example, some practitioners make diagnoses based on the shape and pattern of the tongue, the soles of the feet, the palm of the hand, the pulse, or the ears.

Traveling iridologists visit health food stores and conventions, taking close-up instant photographs of customers' irises. Then they examine the photos and provide people with a list of concerns they have diagnosed. They often suggest herbal remedies they sell. The customer usually buys whatever is deemed appropriate to prevent development of a problem or to reduce an existing problem. Such traveling iridologists are often held in disdain by those who practice iridology in offices under what they believe to be more scientific and professional conditions.

IRIDOLOGY

Study Findings

A 2000 review identified seventeen studies of iridology. All of the uncontrolled studies, most of which were not blinded, concluded that iridology was a valid diagnostic tool (✓✓). However, the four controlled studies in this review came to the opposite conclusion. In a 1979 study (✗✗), three iridologists examined iris photographs of patients who were known to have either severe to moderate kidney disease or no kidney disease. One of the iridologists was a world-renowned expert who had written the authoritative book on iridology at the time. None of the iridologists correctly determined, with statistical reliability, which patients had kidney disease. Their results were no better than chance. The iridologist with the best results was correct only 2.5 percent of the time when he concluded that someone had kidney disease (as verified by other conventional tests). Three ophthalmologists with no experience in iridology examined the same photographs and had results similar to the iridologists. The best ophthalmologist correctly diagnosed kidney disease 3 percent of the time. In contrast, the standard conventional medical test at the time for kidney disease (plasma creatinine) had an accuracy level of 98 percent.

The three other studies cited in the review examined iridology objectively and found similar results (✗✗). One particular study (✗✗) tested three iridologists, and none of them noticed that one of the photographs was of a glass eye. Another study, published in 2005, arose from iridologists' claims to be able to diagnose cancer with the same accuracy as tissue biopsy — at very early stages. An experienced iridologist told the researchers which cancers he was best able to diagnose. Of the 110 participants, 68 had verified cancer of the five types listed by the iridologist. Forty-two other participants had no known cancer. The iridologist examined all the patients' irises and stated he had found 93 cases of cancer. His diagnosis of the type of cancer was correct in only three cases.

Cautions

Iridology itself is harmless, as the practitioner examines only the eyes. However, harm can occur if iridology is used in place of effective diagnostic tools. Of the 110 patients in the latest study, only three would have been correctly diagnosed. Subsequent treatments (or lack of treatment) based on iridology would have been inappropriate for almost everyone. Great harm would have resulted if these people were treated based on their iridology results.

In general, some people with serious illnesses will be told by iridologists they don't have an illness and may delay effective treatment. Others will be told they have illnesses when they don't and will go through the worry and expense of dealing with a misdiagnosis. Worse yet, the information may become a self-fulfilling prophecy given the power of suggestion. Misinformation has practical consequences — negative health effects and the inappropriate use of time and money. In addition, when iridology is used to sell herbal remedies, these may have adverse effects on the health of someone who did not need to take them.

Recommendations

Iridology is based on principles that go against well-established scientific knowledge and approaches. Objective tests have found clear evidence that it is unreliable. There is no reason to spend time and resources using iridology.

Treatment Categories

Scientifically Questionable

For any indication ☹☹☹☹

Quackery or Fraud

Always quackery, sometimes fraud

Further Reading

Ernst, E. "Iridology: Not Useful and Potentially Harmful. *Archives of Ophthalmology* 118, no. 1 (January 2000): 120–21.

Münstedt, Karsten, Samer El-Safadi, Friedel Brück, Marek Zygmunt, Andreas Hackethal, and Hans-Rudolf Tinneberg. "Can Iridology Detect Susceptibility to Cancer? A Prospective Case-Controlled Study." *Journal of Alternative and Complementary Medicine* 11, no. 3 (June 2005): 515–19.

LIGHT THERAPY

What It Is

Many factors affect the way we feel, but one of the more common involves the presence or absence of full-spectrum light. Psychologists and psychiatrists found a direct relationship between increased depression and periods of limited daylight. This connection was first observed with people living in northern climates where the winter hours of daylight are severely limited. Further studies indicated that people who work at night or stay indoors during daylight hours also suffer from depression more than those whose jobs and lifestyles regularly take them outdoors during daylight.

Light therapy evolved as an artificial way to help people who have inadequate exposure to daylight to achieve the same effect indoors. Full-spectrum lightbulbs, often placed in special multibulb holders, bring the equivalent of noonday light indoors. The bulbs are the same type of bulb sold by garden supply centers for growing warm-weather outdoor plants inside in the winter.

Light boxes are used as deemed appropriate in treating light deprivation symptoms. Someone who is severely depressed from being in an area where the winter days are extremely short may be suffering from seasonal affective disorder (SAD) and be told to use a multibulb light box for eight or more hours a day. Other people find that their mood improves when the office or factory lights are replaced with full-spectrum bulbs. These may be used in a desk lamp or overhead light.

More intense, shorter duration therapy is also carried out. In this type of light therapy, the person lies under intense full-spectrum lights for thirty to sixty minutes every morning immediately after wakening. Full-spectrum lightbulbs are quite safe, because, unlike a tanning booth that includes ultra-violet (UV) rays, full-spectrum lights emit very few UV rays. Research is examining whether only certain parts of the light spectrum are needed for light therapy. If this turns out to be the case, the light needed could be less intense and less uncomfortable to endure.

Other forms of therapy use light of different colors to treat specific illnesses believed to be associated with particular colors (also called "color therapy"). Sometimes UV radiation and even lasers are used in light therapy.

Claims

Probably the most common use of light therapy is to relieve depression that occurs during periods of little sunshine (called SAD). This approach has become standard therapy recommended by many psychiatrists, especially those practicing in areas with limited winter daylight hours. Light therapy is also considered standard therapy for a number of skin disorders, such as psoriasis (although in conventional therapy for psoriasis, the light includes UV rays).

There are many other claims concerning the therapeutic value of light. Light therapy has been recommended for depression other than SAD, in particular for depression associated with premenstrual syndrome (PMS). Another approach, color therapy, is based on the claim that each cell and tissue responds differently to different colors. Diseases are said to relate to energy imbalances in the tissues that can be rebalanced by light of different colors.

A radical form of cancer treatment involves injecting dyes into skin cancer cells based on the belief that the dyes absorb certain colors of light and kill the cancer cells.

Study Findings

Light is needed to produce vitamin D in skin and is used to treat jaundice in newborns (✓✓✓✓). Additionally, adequate light is important to avoid eyestrain and fatigue, especially when reading and working (✓✓✓✓).

Epidemiological studies (✓✓) have shown that people living in more northerly latitudes, where the winters are longer and darker, suffer more from depression. Elsewhere, people report more depression when their exposure to daylight is limited, both because of hours of available sunlight and because of when and how they work. Several studies (✓✓✓✓) have shown that introducing full-spectrum light boxes into people's homes can relieve this type of depression, called SAD. Basic research (✓✓) has shown that light affects the body's production of a hormone called "melatonin" (see the Melatonin entry). At night, in the dark, melatonin levels naturally increase, and this has been associated with winter depression. Light therapy therefore appears to reverse the overproduction of melatonin during long winter nights.

The use of light therapy to treat other forms of depression does not have the same degree of evidence. A 2005 review of light therapy to treat depression associated with PMS found four studies. All were small and were not double-blinded. When the results were combined in the review, a very small benefit was seen from light therapy (✓✓). However, each individual study reported favorable findings, and those conclusions have been widely disseminated in the media and on the Internet. The review noted that these conclusions were mistakenly based on comparing depression levels before and after light therapy (where there was benefit). The conclusions should have been based on comparing depression levels between the light therapy group and the control group. That comparison showed no significant improvement in three of the four trials (✗✗✗✗).

When light therapists claim to treat and cure other diseases, they have little or no evidence to support them. Color therapy is usually based on the principles of life energy and *chakras* and is thus part of energy medicine. Each *chakra* is said to be associated with certain tissues and emotions, but also with a particular color. Practitioners claim to be able to determine whether certain colors are missing. Light of specific colors is then believed to be useful in the treatment of those conditions. Crystals are sometimes used to direct light of different colors and energies to the person. In addition, some practitioners claim to be able to "send" healing colors to the person just by visualizing them. There is no scientific evidence to support the use of light to treat or cure illnesses in this way.

Cautions

Light therapy that increases someone's exposure to full-spectrum light is generally very safe. However, a small proportion of people experience agitation, headache, vision problems, dizziness, and similar adverse effects. These are probably brought on by the intensity of the light and are usually short-lasting. Standard light boxes filter out UV radiation, but if this is not done, overexposure can lead to sunburn, premature wrinkling, and skin cancer. While additional light can relieve some forms of depression, talking to others about the issues and seeking professional help remain important.

Color therapy should not be used instead of conventional treatment, especially for any serious illness. Christians should be particularly aware of color therapy practitioners who base their ideas on Eastern philosophy and life energy.

Recommendations

People thrive on an adequate balance of many natural substances. We realize the importance of rest, exercise, diet, and water for our health, but we also need adequate daylight. With our hectic lifestyles and increased time spent indoors and in cars, we need to plan to spend enough time outside in natural sunlight (whether cloudy or not). If this is not possible, making use of full-spectrum light boxes may bring some general relief to seasonal depression caused by lack of sunlight. However, the use of light or color therapy to treat or cure most diseases is not supported by the evidence.

Treatment Categories

Conventional

To treat seasonal affective disorder (SAD)	☺☺☺☺
To treat jaundice in newborns	☺☺☺☺
To treat some skin disorders	☺☺☺☺

Complementary

To treat depression	☺

Scientifically Questionable

Color therapy

Spiritual

As practiced by some, especially color therapists	👎

Quackery or Fraud

In the hands of some practitioners

Further Reading

Glickman, Gena, Brenda Byrne, Carissa Pineda, Walter W. Hauck, and George C. Brainard. "Light Therapy for Seasonal Affective Disorder with Blue Narrow-Band Light-Emitting Diodes (LEDs)." *Biology and Psychiatry* 59, no. 6 (March 2006): 502 – 7.

Krasnik, Catherine, Victor M. Montori, Gordon H. Guyatt, Diane Heels-Ansdell, and Jason W. Busse. "The Effect of Bright Light Therapy on Depression Associated with Premenstrual Dysphoric Disorder." *American Journal of Obstetrics and Gynecology* 193, no. 3 (September 2005): 658 – 61.

MAGNET THERAPY

What It Is

Magnet therapy is based on the belief that magnets have healing properties. Today there are two forms of magnet therapy. The one of most popular interest (and $5 billion in annual sales worldwide) involves permanent or static magnets. Magnets are strapped to the body, built into mattresses, or placed in shoes as insoles. They are mostly used to relieve all sorts of pain.

A second form of magnet therapy is pulsating electromagnetic field therapy based on the electromagnetic effect discovered by English physicist Michael Faraday. He noted that passing electricity through a wire coil produces a magnetic field. He also observed that by changing a magnetic field around an object, electric voltage could be generated. The pulsing of the magnetic field is essential for this effect.

Electrical signals are found throughout the body. For example, an EKG is a tracing of the electrical signals of the heart, and an EEG is a tracing of the electrical signals of the brain. Pulsating electromagnetic field therapy has been studied as a way to promote healing by generating electrical currents in the body. The most widely studied application of electromagnetic field therapy has been in the healing of broken bones. Results are promising, and the U.S. Food and Drug Administration has approved this therapy.

Pulsating electromagnetic field therapy is completely different from the popular use of permanent magnets that don't involve any pulsing electric current. The idea that a permanent magnet could have healing effects is ancient. The concept dates back to the 1500s, but its most famous proponent was Franz Mesmer, an eighteenth-century Austrian doctor. Mesmer later promoted hypnosis as a therapy and gave his name to the term "mesmerized." Mesmer claimed that all illness was caused by problems in the flow of "animal magnetism." He moved magnets around a patient's body to allegedly correct the flow of this magnetic energy.

Elisha Perkins was a prominent New England physician at the end of the 1700s who became a proponent of magnetic healing. He moved metallic rods, called "tractors," over an area where a patient was afflicted with a problem, such as rheumatism. He was convinced the rods worked because patients

M

spoke so highly of the relief they experienced. Perkins did not realize that the relief was due to what is now called "the placebo effect" (see p. 38 for more on Perkins and placebos). A person believes he or she feels better because of faith in the treatment, not because of anything the treatment itself does. Those who respond positively to an object that looks like medicine but has no possible biochemical effect on the body are said to be responding to the placebo.

The question is whether athletes wearing magnetic bands or people sleeping on magnetic mattresses to relieve pain are benefiting from the placebo effect or from the permanent magnets. A lot of money is passing through hands on the assumption that magnets do more than placebos.

Claims

The claims for permanent magnet therapy are very broad. It is most commonly promoted for the relief of aches, pains, headaches, and arthritis. For this purpose, magnets are placed within a variety of straps and wraps. Magnetic insoles are worn inside shoes to promote better overall health. Magnetic mattresses are recommended for people with generalized pain such as that associated with fibromyalgia.

Proponents of permanent magnet therapy say the magnets promote a better flow of charged electrolytes in the blood. This claim remains to be verified. The claim that permanent magnets influence blood flow by attracting iron in the blood is little more than a myth. Iron is enveloped in hemoglobin and would not be influenced by these types of magnets. Some manufacturers claim their magnets cure cancer, relieve enlarged prostates, and heal almost every ailment known to humanity.

Study Findings

Claims that permanent magnets increase blood flow are based on two studies, one done with saline (salt water) contained in glass tubes and the other with horses. However, these studies had a number of major flaws. Furthermore, many other studies have found no increase in blood flow. In addition, MRI scanners are widely used today, and these expose people to magnetic fields two to four times stronger than magnet pads. Yet no changes in blood circulation have been reported with the widespread use of this technology.

Magnets are most commonly promoted for the relief of aches and pain. A 2005 review found twenty-one randomized studies, all but two of which were double-blinded. Many of them were small, and some were poorly designed. A variety of types of pain were studied, including pain from arthritis, foot surgery, polio, fibromyalgia, and dysmenorrhea (painful periods), along with headaches, low back pain, and carpal tunnel syndrome. No one type of pain was examined in more than two studies. The magnets used varied a great deal, from mattresses, shoe inserts, and necklaces to pads strapped to the skin. In different studies, people wore the magnets for between forty-five minutes and six months, sometimes continuously and sometimes periodically. Such diverse study designs make general conclusions difficult.

Of the twenty-one controlled studies reviewed in 2005, eight found the magnet group had significantly greater pain relief than the placebo group, four found some positive and some negative results, and nine found the magnets no better than placebo. For example, one study (✓✓✓) with fifty postpolio patients with arthritis-like pain reported better relief after using a magnet pad for forty-five minutes compared to a placebo pad. Another study (✓✓✓) had forty-three patients with chronic knee pain wear knee pads with magnets or placebos. After two weeks, the group wearing the magnets had significantly less pain and increased walking speed compared to the placebo group. However, another study (✗✗✗) found no relief from shoulder and neck pain from wearing a magnetic necklace. Yet another study (✗✗✗) found no difference in relief of heel pain between patients wearing a magnetic insole or a nonmagnetic insole. In the latter study, 60 percent of patients in both groups reported improvement, which may have arisen from simply wearing an insole or from the placebo effect. It is important to note that treatments for pain are known to be highly susceptible to placebo effects, indicating that the mind is a major factor in coping with some forms of pain.

Another study (✓✓✓), published at the end of 2004, was one of the largest to date, with 194 participants. All participants had osteoarthritis of the knee or hip. They all wore a metal wrist bracelet for 12 weeks, being randomly assigned ones that were strongly magnetic (1,700–2,000 gauss), weakly magnetic (210–300 gauss), or placebo (0 gauss). Gauss is the unit used to measure magnet strength (or Tesla, where 1 Tesla = 10,000 gauss). Pain levels were the primary outcome of concern. This study showed that the strong magnet group had significantly more pain relief than the placebo group, but not compared to the weak magnet group. Leg stiffness and function measurements did not show significant differences among the groups. However, as a way to double-check their results, researchers measured the strengths of the magnets after the study ended. They discovered that more than half of the weak magnetic bracelets had been manufactured incorrectly and were much stronger. The strongest

"weak" magnet was of similar strength to the strongest "strong" magnet! In spite of this confusion, the trial did show some benefit from the strong magnets and provided evidence that magnet strength is important for pain relief.

The optimal strength of the magnets used in magnet therapy is uncertain. Most therapy magnets come in strengths of 200 to 10,000 gauss. By comparison, a refrigerator magnet has a strength of around 200 gauss. Most studies conducted with magnets less than 400 gauss have found little pain relief, whereas those with magnets stronger than 500 gauss have found significant pain relief. This could be taken as evidence that the magnets are having a real effect that is "dose" dependent. There is no agreement regarding minimal or optimal strength for magnet therapy.

Another issue is that the strength of a magnetic field falls off rapidly as you move away from the magnet (see the table below). Calculations have been done that raise significant questions as to whether any magnetism released from commercial products could penetrate the magnet's padding and the skin. You can verify this by checking how many pieces of paper an average kitchen magnet will hold up.

● Cautions

Magnets have not been found to cause any side effects. Those with heart pacemakers must avoid strong magnetic fields such as exist in MRI facilities, but the magnets used in magnet therapy are too weak to interfere with pacemakers. However, using them instead of effective therapies delays finding actual relief. With serious illnesses, this can have disastrous consequences.

There is another issue with the quality of magnets available commercially. Blechman and colleagues

Strength in Gauss	Magnet 1	Magnet 2	Magnet 3	Magnet 4	Magnet 5	Magnet 6	Magnet 7
Claimed	1000	2450	700	1000	2350	1500	2750
Measured at surface	38	137	80	385	1275	1270	1820
Measured 1 inch from surface	0.3	35	0.7	13.3	98.3	128.3	191.7

measured the actual strengths of the magnetic fields at the edge of seven magnets. The above table gives the average gauss values for the magnets. It contrasts the advertised strengths with the measured values as found on the surface of the magnet and one inch above it. Clearly, there are huge discrepancies between the claimed strengths of therapy magnets and the fields they emit. This raises even further questions as to whether any reported benefits are from the magnetism or the placebo effect.

● Recommendations

Many people are convinced that magnets help relieve a variety of conditions, which results in annual sales of over $5 billion. However, simply wearing a nonmagnetic belt, pad, or insert may be enough to produce a beneficial effect. In addition, the placebo effect is very powerful with the types of conditions for which magnets are commonly recommended. The results of randomized controlled trials are highly variable and inconclusive. The complete lack of adverse effects found with magnets makes their use on a trial basis reasonable. However, expending large sums of money on some of the available magnet products would be unwise. Even if magnet therapy under controlled conditions is shown to be beneficial, many products on the market are of questionable value given the discrepancies found between advertised and actual magnet strengths.

Magnet therapy has repeatedly come and gone in popularity over the last few centuries, suggesting that it becomes popular briefly because of the placebo effect, then loses support when patients do not get better. A number of physiological mechanisms have been proposed to explain how permanent magnets might be therapeutic, but not one has received general support.

Some proponents of magnet therapy use life energy ideas to explain how magnets might be therapeutic. David Eisenberg's frequently referenced surveys of alternative medicine use in the United States confusingly included magnets in his Energy Medicine category. In the eighteenth century, Mesmer stopped using magnets when he found he could influence people in similar ways by hypnotizing them. This led him to describe animal magnetism in terms very similar to life energy. Promoters of theosophy later used magnetism in this same way. (Theosophy is a philosophical-religious approach that blends ideas from the occult and Eastern religions and laid much of the foundation for the New Age movement.) Whenever people discuss magnets in terms of their influence on generalized energies of the body, Christians should be alert to the concerns we raise about energy medicine.

Treatment Categories

Scientifically Unproven

To relieve pain ☺

Scientifically Questionable

For other indications ☹

Spiritual

In the hands of some practitioners 👎

Quackery or Fraud

In the hands of some practitioners

Further Reading

Blechman, Abraham M., Mehmet C. Oz, Vijaya Nair, and Windsor Ting. "Discrepancy Between Claimed Field Flux Density of Some Commercially Available Magnets and Actual Gaussmeter Measurements." *Alternative Therapies in Health and Medicine* 7, no. 5 (September – October 2001): 92 – 95.

Eccles, Nyjon K. "A Critical Review of Randomized Controlled Trials of Static Magnets for Pain Relief." *Journal of Alternative and Complementary Medicine* 11, no. 3 (June 2005): 495 – 509.

Harlow, Tim, Colin Greaves, Adrian White, Liz Brown, Anna Hart, and Edzard Ernst. "Randomised Controlled Trial of Magnetic Bracelets for Relieving Pain in Osteoarthritis of the Hip and Knee." *British Medical Journal* 329 (December 2004): 1450 – 54.

MASSAGE THERAPY

M

What It Is

Mention massage to a group of people and you are likely to notice one of two reactions: Some think in terms of a soothing back rub by a loved one or in a setting such as a health club. Others think in terms of something sexual, knowing that advertisements for massage in some counterculture publications are really euphemisms for prostitution. When talking about massage therapies, neither is accurate, though the soothing back rub comes far closer to reality.

Massage therapy properly refers to a broad group of medically valid therapies that involve rubbing or moving the skin. Ancient writings and drawings document that massage has long been valued. The famous Greek physician Hippocrates wrote, "The physician must be experienced in many things, but assuredly in rubbing."

Massage played an important role at the foundation of the physical therapy profession. Nurses at the end of the nineteenth century incorporated massage into their practice, partly to offer something distinctive from physicians. Massage became very popular but was unregulated, with great variability in standards. Stories of massage leading to prostitution were rampant, resulting in a scathing 1894 editorial on English morality in the *British Medical Journal*. The journal called for the establishment of a professional society to oversee massage therapy. The Society of Trained Masseuses was founded six months later by four nurse/midwife masseuses. The society set up standards for training, practice, and surveillance. It adopted a biomechanical model to distance itself from the sensual side of massage. This organization gradually developed into the physical therapy profession.

Over the course of the twentieth century, massage faded from general health care. Some of this relates to the availability of other therapies, but the association of massage with sensual touching remained. Physical touch in general was seen as inappropriate in medical settings. However, by the end of the twentieth century, massage was receiving renewed interest and respectability because it was again understood as having a valid therapeutic role.

Today different types of massage are available, and massage is incorporated into a number of other therapies. The best-known form is probably Swedish massage, in which the hands move over the skin in long, gliding strokes (also called "effleurage"). The muscles may be kneaded, or light friction may be applied to the skin.

Massage is one of the most popular forms of alternative medicine practiced with children in the United States (see p. 78). In one survey, one-quarter of the parents who used alternative medicine with their children in the previous year reported massage as the therapy used. This was 3.5 times the frequency of the next most popular therapy (use of vitamins).

Rolfing is another form of massage that uses significant amounts of pressure to rebalance joints and restore elasticity to the fascia (the connective tissue surrounding all muscles). In addition, craniosacral therapy, reflexology, and acupressure involve putting pressure on specific parts of the body. Acupressure led to the development of Shiatsu massage, a much deeper and more aggressive form of massage. This developed in Japan but was strongly influenced by traditional Chinese medicine. Practitioners use what is called "*hara* diagnosis" to assess the flow of life energy, called *ki* in Japanese therapies. *Ki* is believed to be stored in the abdomen, so practitioners gently press on various parts of a person's abdomen. Treatment is carried out by massaging various acupoints using practitioners' fingers, thumbs, elbows, knees, or feet. A closely related practice, called *do-in* (or *daoyin*), is basically a self-applied form of Shiatsu. Given the life energy connections, there seems to be no reason for Christians to use Shiatsu massage when they can enjoy all the same benefits from a regular massage, without the spiritual overtones and dangers.

"Bodywork" is another name for various forms of massage that also tend to include life energy healing. Some of these are only slight modifications of Reiki, Healing Touch, and Therapeutic Touch (none of which necessarily involve physical contact).

Claims

Your skin is the body's largest sensory organ, and as such, touch in general is important to how you feel. The primary claim made for massage is that it relaxes people, directly leading to reduced muscle tension, lower heart rate, and lower blood pressure. Massage is also said to be helpful during infant development, for removing edema caused by swelling, and for relieving pain — and for all the comforts that come through physical contact.

Study Findings

Even though massage is one of the oldest therapies on record, research on its effectiveness is sparse. However, some studies are starting to verify what most people know through experience.

Studies (✓✓✓) with premature infants who were gently massaged showed that they gained weight more quickly and left the hospital earlier than those who were not deliberately touched in this manner. However, the quality of these studies is not the highest, leading the authors of a Cochrane review to question the reliability of their findings. Other studies (✓✓✓✓) have documented the relaxing effects of massage, including the lowering of anxiety levels and, to some degree, the reduction of some pain. Forms of chest massage have also been shown (✓✓✓✓) to help patients with respiratory problems. A Cochrane review (✓✓✓✓) of massage for low back pain found some evidence of benefit, especially if massage was combined with exercises and education. While all of these benefits are significant, no studies support any claims that massage can cure or treat more serious illnesses.

Cautions

Massage itself is very safe and effective for relaxation. The main danger arises when people think it actually cures an underlying disease. Some of the more aggressive forms of massage can cause bruising and pain afterward and should be used carefully on children and those who are frail. Given that some forms of massage can be intermixed with life energy therapies, Christians should inquire about all that will happen during a massage.

Recommendations

As a form of helping oneself to relax, massage is an old and valued therapy. Giving a massage or shoulder rub to a friend or family member can be a loving way to help him or her release some stress. Having a professional massage may bring extra relief so long as the underlying cause of the stress is also dealt with appropriately.

Treatment Categories

Conventional

To help development of premature infants	☺☺☺
To promote relaxation	☺☺☺☺
To reduce some types of pain	☺☺
To relieve respiratory problems, especially stress-related	☺☺

Complementary

For other indications involving stress reduction	☺☺☺☺

Scientifically Unproven

To cure any illness	☹☹☹☹

Spiritual

Shiatsu massage and massage as practiced by some practitioners	👎👎👎

Further Reading

Nicholls, David A., and Julianne Cheek. "Physiotherapy and the Shadow of Prostitution: The Society of Trained Masseuses and the Massage Scandals of 1894." *Social Science and Medicine* 62, no. 9 (May 2006): 2336 – 48.

Vickers, A., A. Ohlsson, J. B. Lacy, and A. Horsley. "Massage for Promoting Growth and Development of Preterm and/or Low-Birth-Weight Infants." *The Cochrane Database of Systematic Reviews* 2004, no. 2.

MEDITATION

What It Is

Meditation is a word that has been so broadly applied to an array of both healthy and harmful activities that it is difficult to get consistent agreement about its impact on health. For example, one person's idea of meditating may be to sit quietly while encouraging his body to relax. He will inhale deeply, exhale slowly, and create a moment of restful quiet in the midst of an otherwise hectic day. Another person's idea is to tune out everything while daydreaming or concentrating on something that is not the primary concern of the moment. One advertising agency employee talks of going on a long walk while she meditates on her client's problem, the focused attention helping her to develop creative solutions. And for others, meditation can be a deeply spiritual or religious practice, allowing some to relate intimately with the God of the Bible and others to contact spirit guides or even demons.

When discussing meditation, it is crucial to make sure that everyone knows what everyone means by the term. In general, it refers to a whole range of practices generally designed to take our minds off everyday business and stressful activities, helping us become more relaxed and reflective. Some use it to reduce or eliminate rational thoughts. The Bible's teaching on meditation will be examined below.

The type of meditation recommended as an alternative therapy sometimes has its origin in Eastern religions and mysticism. Transcendental Meditation (TM) is a recent adaptation of these older concepts. In general, the meditator wants to relax in a peaceful environment. Most sit comfortably, focusing their thoughts on something that minimizes troubling or distracting thoughts. Some focus on their own breathing, concentrating on the movement of air in and out of their lungs. Others repeat a mantra — a sacred word or formula given by a spiritual master — or just an ordinary phrase. With practice, people can consciously relax their muscles and learn to control other bodily functions not usually under their control.

Claims

The initial goal in meditation is to induce a state of relaxation. Herbert Benson has documented the many health benefits of what he calls the "relaxation response." This can bring about relief from much of the stress and anxiety experienced by people today. Since this stress can underlie numerous health problems, meditation has the potential to produce health benefits.

Eastern meditation and mystical meditation were not developed for their health benefits. They are primarily means toward spiritual enlightenment. The goal is to quiet or empty the rational mind so that people become more aware of their inner selves. This occurs as they enter a state of altered consciousness and come in contact with what adherents call the Universal Oneness (or other similar names). Here they claim to receive information about their health and the healing needed. Alternative therapies place great emphasis on intuition and the insight gained during meditation, encouraging people to trust their own intuition rather than the logic and reasons of others.

Study Findings

Clinical studies (✓✓✓✓) have confirmed that meditation can provide short-term benefits in reducing stress, relieving chronic pain, and reducing blood pressure. Studies (✓✓✓✓) also have shown that meditation can give some people a better sense of happiness and control of their bodies. However, what has not been shown is whether these changes have long-term health benefits. For example, a 2001 review found twenty-seven studies examining the impact of patients' anxiety levels before surgery on their recovery after surgery. These studies didn't examine the impact of any relaxation techniques, just whether anxiety was related to recovery. Clear connections were shown between pre-surgery anxiety and post-surgery mood and pain. However, no clear associations were found between anxiety and more objective measures of recovery such as length of stay in hospital or rate of wound healing. The field of research examining the impact of anxiety and relaxation on physical recovery and healing is relatively new, with evidence not yet available for many interesting issues.

Cautions

Meditation has been documented to cause problems. Transcendental Meditation, initially promoted by Maharishi Mahesh Yogi, was very popular in the 1960s and did much to familiarize Americans with meditation and Hinduism. But studies (✘✘) have found that its results are not always positive. Almost half of those active as TM trainers reported episodes of anxiety, depression, confusion, frustration, mental and physical tension, and inexplicable outbursts of antisocial behavior. Other studies (✘✘) have documented adverse effects as serious as psychiatric hospitalization and attempted suicide. Problems can arise when meditation is viewed as a simple exercise, when in fact it has considerable power to deeply impact a person psychologically and spiritually.

The spiritual enlightenment some maintain occurs in meditation can involve contact with spirit guides. The desire to rely more on one's own intuition contrasts with the biblical declaration that our intuition can lead to falsehood and deception. In many ways, humanity's problems stem from our reliance on ourselves to know what is best. God told Moses to have the Israelites sew tassels onto the corners of their garments to remind them of this important teaching. "You will have these tassels to look at and so you will remember all the commands of the LORD, that you may obey them and not prostitute yourselves by going after the lusts of your own hearts and eyes" (Numbers 15:39; see also Deuteronomy 12:8; Judges 17:6).

Insight received during meditation is especially problematic. Divination and visions are altered states of consciousness used to gain spiritual insight. Yet unless this insight comes from God, it only reveals the futility and deception of people's own minds. "Then the LORD said to me, 'The prophets are prophesying lies in my name. I have not sent them or appointed them or spoken to them. They are prophesying to you false visions, divinations, idolatries and the delusions of their own minds'" (Jeremiah 14:14; see also 23:16–17, 25–32). God spoke through the prophet Ezekiel to warn the Israelites about "those who prophesy out of their own imagination" (Ezekiel 13:2). What is learned during meditation must be evaluated, both medically and biblically.

● Recommendations

Christians should relax and reduce unnecessary stress in their lives. "Be still, and know that I am God; I will be exalted among the nations, I will be exalted in the earth" (Psalm 46:10). The Bible tells us to meditate: "Do not let this Book of the Law depart from your mouth; meditate on it day and night, so that you may be careful to do everything written in it. Then you will be prosperous and successful" (Joshua 1:8; see also Psalms 1:2 – 3; 19:14; 49:3; 104:34; 119:97, 99).

But Christian meditation is not emptying one's mind or focusing on one's inner self. Rather, it is filling one's mind with biblical truth while focusing on the Creator God of the universe. We will gain insight when we meditate on biblical truth. But this insight is based on the revealed Word of God and should lead to a life more in conformity with his ways.

Christians should make every effort to retain control over their thought life. "We demolish arguments and every pretension that sets itself up against the knowledge of God, and we take captive every thought to make it obedient to Christ" (2 Corinthians 10:5). Altered states of consciousness can open people to spiritual suggestion, making them vulnerable to demonic or other unwholesome influences. Meditation should therefore be seen as a method of promoting reasoned reflection on God and his Word.

● Treatment Categories

Complementary

To help in the short-term reduction of stress or anxiety	☺☺☺☺
To relieve some forms of chronic pain	☺☺☺
To reduce blood pressure	☺☺☺☺
To give a sense of happiness and control over life	☺☺

Scientifically Unproven

For any other indication

Spiritual

In the hands of many non-Christian practitioners	👎👎👎👎

● Further Reading

Haddon, David, and Vail Hamilton. *TM Wants You! A Christian Response to Transcendental Meditation.* Grand Rapids: Baker, 1976.

Heide, Frederick J. "Relaxation: The Storm Before the Calm." *Psychology Today* (April 1985): 18 – 19.

Munafò, Marcus R., and Jim Stevenson. "Anxiety and Surgical Recovery: Reinterpreting the Literature." *Journal of Psychosomatic Research* 51 (2001): 589 – 96.

NATUROPATHIC MEDICINE

● What It Is

Naturopathic medicine has developed from what was called "naturopathy" and is the system of health care practiced by naturopathic doctors (N.D.). Their focus is on "natural" means of preventing and curing illness as opposed to the use of "unnatural" pharmaceutical drugs and surgeries. The naturopathic approach is holistic, taking into consideration body, mind, and spirit. According to the National College of Naturopathic Medicine, illness demonstrates that the body is trying to heal itself via its "inherent vitality." This concept pervades the naturopathic approach to medicine but is defined in different ways. For some, it simply means a natural tendency toward health, but for others it reflects the same sort of life energy we have seen in Ayurvedic and traditional Chinese medicine. Regardless, naturopaths see their primary role as assisting nature to bring about healing or removing obstacles to healing.

In some ways, naturopathic medicine seems like a sensible approach to health and healing. The roles of diet, exercise, relationships, and other lifestyle issues in health are recognized. The emphasis on using only natural approaches to healing has a strong impact on many of the therapies recommended — herbal remedies, supplements, homeopathy, and Bach flower remedies. Instead of surgery, exercise and chiropractic therapy are used or recommended. Naturopaths often oppose immunization because it is not natural. In this way, while naturopathic medicine can address some important dimensions of health and healing, it often neglects other valid approaches.

Naturopathic training is varied. Some N.D.s have attended a four-year degree program available at four schools in the United States and one in Canada. Much training in the first two years is similar in content to that received by students in medical schools. The last two years focus on the "natural" treatments that N.D.s use most often — including homeopathy, herbal remedies, acupuncture, biofeedback, counseling, diet, and physical manipulations.

As of 2005, thirteen states in the United States license N.D.s, and the state of Washington requires health insurance to cover naturopathic medicine. A licensed N.D. is permitted to practice all therapies associated with naturopathy after passing certification examinations given after four years of training. Of great concern is that an N.D. degree can be obtained in much less rigorous ways. It is very important to determine how an N.D. degree was obtained.

● Claims

Naturopaths claim they can treat most general and chronic illnesses and say that they refer patients requiring complicated surgeries or high-technology treatments to conventional medical doctors. The emphasis in naturopathy is on preventive medicine and teaching people healthy lifestyles. However, some naturopaths have an antagonistic relationship with physicians and are reluctant to refer any patient to a physician. Likewise, some M.D.s and D.O.s are antagonistic toward N.D.s. Conventional physicians are concerned that since naturopaths receive much less training in medical diagnosis, they may not recognize some health problems — or may incorrectly diagnose them. In addition, prominent naturo-path educators recommend scientifically unproven treatments and sometimes scientifically question-able ones, such as hydrogen peroxide baths to treat asthma, St. John's wort and garlic to treat HIV-positive patients, ice packs to treat acute stroke, and pulse and tongue diagnosis (similar in many ways to iridology) to diagnose multiple sclerosis.

In spite of this, some health insurance plans cover naturopathic services, treating N.D.s as primary care providers in the same manner as a physician's assistant or nurse practitioner. The National College of Naturopathic Medicine describes its graduates as "primary care physicians." This same title is used by M.D. or D.O. primary care physicians who have com-pleted six to eight years of rigorous post-collegiate training.

Study Findings

Studies related to naturopathic medicine itself have not, to our knowledge, been published (✗✗✗). How-ever, studies related to specific therapies used by N.D.s are relevant and show much diversity. Recent research has affirmed the importance N.D.s place on diet, exercise, and relaxation (✓✓✓). Homeopathy has little scientific support (✗✗✗✗). Some herbal remedies and dietary supplements have a growing body of research support, but always for a limited number of specific uses (✓✓✓✓). The vast majority of the herbal remedies used by N.D.s are supported by only anecdotal evidence (✓✓), and for some the evidence shows that they don't work as recom-mended (✗✗✗).

Naturopathic literature places a much greater emphasis on anecdotal evidence than on controlled clinical trials. A long tradition of use within natu-ropathy counts as significant evidence of effective-ness for many N.D.s. For example, the Summer 2000 *Naturopathic Newsletter*, published by the Univer-sity of Bridgeport College of Naturopathic Medicine (owned by the Rev. Sun Myung Moon's Unification Church), lauded a number of alternative therapies on which little or no controlled research has been done. It stated that Bach flower remedies can treat "any emotional or mental condition," that Chinese herbs are effective for a huge variety of conditions ranging from infertility to allergies and asthma, that acupuncture should be considered along with herbs, and that chiropractic can assist with preg-nancy problems, heart conditions, and many other illnesses. The newsletter also promoted Ayurvedic medicine, hypnosis, and regression therapy. This type of uncritical promotion of everything "natural" concerns us and leaves us questioning the reliability of the recommendations made by many N.D.s. Not all N.D.s buy into every therapy, but patients must be very discerning in choosing an N.D.

Cautions

Naturopathic medicine as an approach has few dem-onstrated helpful effects or harmful side effects — if its limitations are accepted and adhered to. With se-rious illnesses such as cancer or emergencies such as heart attacks, a good N.D. will recognize the need to refer patients to others for specialized care. A good N.D. will focus on issues related to general healthy lifestyles and prevention of illness. However, if an N.D. fails to notice an illness (which may easily hap-pen given their limited training) or delays referral, serious harm could arise.

Some naturopaths claim illnesses arise from the accumulation of toxins in the body. These N.D.s rec-ommend cleansing, sometimes through diet or ex-ercise, but also with purgative methods or chelation therapies, some of which are very severe and can be both physically and psychologically harmful. In addition, since naturopathic medicine is tied in with beliefs about life energy, some naturopaths promote New Age approaches to health and spirituality. Discernment is needed when any practitioner moves into philosophical and religious discussions.

Recommendations

Naturopathic medicine emphasizes a holistic approach to health care that can be compatible with a scientific and biblical approach. However, it sometimes incorporates New Age spirituality and "life energy" concepts. In general, naturopathic medicine recommends some practices and lifestyle changes that can be beneficial. In our opinion, there is a risk with any N.D. who is antagonistic toward conventional medicine, because that antagonism could delay patients getting effective treatments for serious conditions.

Since some naturopathic treatments have not demonstrated clinical effectiveness, they should not replace therapies with established positive results. We would encourage naturopaths to apply the scientific method to their therapies. Furthermore, we believe that the publication of studies demonstrating both the safety and the effectiveness of any particular N.D. therapy will increase its acceptance both by the lay public and by conventional physicians.

Treatment Categories

Complementary

In some areas, such as diet,
exercise, and relaxation ☺☺

Scientifically Unproven

For many indications ☹☹

Scientifically Questionable

For some indications

Spiritual

In the hands of some naturopaths 👎👎👎

Further Reading

Atwood, Kimball C., IV. "Naturopathy: A Critical Appraisal." *Medscape General Medicine* 5, no. 4 (December 2003): 39. Posted December 30, 2003. *Medscape: www.medscape.com/viewarticle/465994.* Accessed November 4, 2005.

Pizzorno, Joseph E. "Naturopathic Medicine — A 10-Year Perspective (From a 35-Year View)." *Alternative Therapies in Health and Medicine* 11, no. 2 (March – April 2005): 24 – 26.

N

PRAYER FOR HEALING

● What It Is

Prayer for healing is by far the most popular "alternative therapy" used in the United States. We have serious reservations about calling prayer a therapy, but we'll discuss this below. In three large surveys carried out by David Eisenberg and colleagues at Harvard Medical School, prayer topped the list of most frequently used alternative therapies every time: 25.2, 35.1, and 45.2 percent in 1990, 1997, and 2002, respectively.

The latest of these, the 2002 CDC Survey, subdivided prayer to collect more detailed information. While prayer in general was the most popular "therapy," 43 percent prayed for their own health (making it the second most popular "therapy"), 24.2 percent had others praying for their health (the third most popular "therapy"), and 9.6 percent participated in a prayer group (the sixth most popular "therapy").

Amazingly, all three of Eisenberg's surveys left prayer out of their tallies on overall use of complementary and alternative medicine. We can think of only one reason for this. If prayer were included, the overall conclusion would have been that almost everyone in the United States is using alternative medicine. Such a conclusion reveals the problematic way alternative medicine is defined to include an overly broad range of health-related activities. At the same time, there appears to be a remarkable resurgence in prayer for health that is not receiving adequate attention.

People differ in what they mean by prayer. The Bible is very specific: prayer is communicating with God. It is talking to God and listening to his answers —

not a therapy as we normally understand that term. Requests made to God in prayer should, according to the Bible, always be saturated with humility, prayed in accordance with God's will and in the name of Jesus. "This is the confidence we have in approaching God: that if we ask anything *according to his will*, he hears us" (1 John 5:14, emphasis added).

The Bible certainly records numerous instances in which God, in answer to prayer, directly intervened to bring healing. King Hezekiah was near death when he prayed and received this reply from God: "I have heard your prayer and seen your tears; I will heal you" (2 Kings 20:5). A therapy implies that if you do something, you will get health benefits. While prayer can bring benefits, the Bible does not describe a simple cause-and-effect relationship to prayer. Ultimately, what we want will come about only if it is God's will.

Larry Dossey, the author of *Healing Words*, describes his view of prayer as "far different" from the "old biblically based views of prayer." He claims that biblical prayer arises from a worldview that "is now antiquated and incomplete" and constitutes a "uniquely 'pathological mythology.'" For Dossey, praying is a general attitude of leaving things in the hands of fate or some Universal Consciousness.

A researcher in the field of spirituality and healing, Elisabeth Targ, called prayer a form of "distant healing" that is "any purely mental effort undertaken by one person with the intention of improving physical or emotional well-being in another." Intercessory prayer is offered for a specific result to occur in someone else. But biblical prayer is more than "mental effort." We humbly ask God to intervene and cure Joe of cancer or speed Susan's recovery from surgery, if that is his will.

The emphasis in biblical prayer is not on what we must *do* to convince God to answer, but on God's *will*. An answer to prayer is dependent on God's power and God's will, not ours. Not so with many other forms of prayer in which the emphasis is on results. This has led to much interest in figuring out whether prayer works to bring about healing.

Study Findings

Interest in research involving intercessory prayer (which we will refer to as "prayer research") is not new. In 1872, John Tyndall proposed that all Christians pray for the patients of one London hospital for at least three years. Skeptical of Christianity, Tyndall believed his study would provide scientific evidence that prayer is ineffective.

The experiment was never conducted, but it generated a storm of controversy, with articles flying off the presses raising scientific, theological, and ethical concerns. Francis Galton, a cousin of Charles Darwin, noted that people frequently pray for clergy and royalty, in particular that they be granted long lives. He found they actually lived shorter lives than "less noble" professionals. To Galton, this was clear evidence that prayer doesn't work.

More recently, in 1988, Randolph Byrd, M.D., published a study (✓✓✓) on the effects of intercessory prayer on almost four hundred cardiac patients in an intensive care unit in San Francisco General Hospital. Half of the patients were prayed for by "born-again" Christians, and the other half made up a control group. The intercessors prayed for a rapid recovery, prevention of complications, and prevention of death. The prayed-for patients did significantly better in six ways than those in a control

group who received no prayer through the research. However, twenty-three other measurements made during this study showed no statistically significant differences. In fact, when all the results were grouped together, the prayed-for group did only a little better overall.

Measuring twenty-nine different outcomes, instead of only six, would seem to be a more thorough way of doing research, but it generates problems. The more outcomes measured, the greater the risk of finding a positive result just by chance. Also, if all twenty-nine outcomes are only slightly different (and not significant individually), adding them together could produce an overall result that is statistically significant. Byrd admitted that his individual results "could not be considered statistically significant because of the large number of variables examined." Only when the results were combined were they statistically significant.

Another team of researchers, led by William Harris, Ph.D., set out to repeat Byrd's study. This time 990 patients admitted to a coronary care unit in Kansas City, Missouri, were randomized into two groups. Half were prayed for by teams of five Christians (Protestant and Catholic) for twenty-eight days. Thirty-five different medical outcomes were measured.

Their study failed to reproduce Byrd's findings. Byrd had developed a research tool for ranking and evaluating his different measurements and producing an overall result. When Harris's team used Byrd's tool, the differences between the two groups were not significant (✗✗✗). They also found no statistically significant differences for any individual measurement. But then they developed a new tool that found that the prayer group scored 10 percent better than the control group. This difference is statistically significant (✓✓✓), but Harris concluded that "there is no known way to ascribe a clinical significance to it." In other words, they don't know how much difference being prayed for would make in people's actual lives.

In 2001, a third large randomized clinical trial was published. This time, as 799 patients were being discharged from a hospital coronary care unit, they were randomly assigned to receive prayer or not. Each patient was prayed for at least once a week by five individuals or groups for twenty-six weeks. The people praying were recruited from area religious and community groups, but the type of prayer was not specified. No significant differences (✗✗✗) were found between the two groups in various measures of cardiac health or illness. In 2006, the largest study of prayer for cardiac patients was published, this time involving 1,802 patients. In this study, no significant differences were found between those prayed for and those not receiving prayer.

Intrigued by these results, we searched for any controlled study of the health effects of intercessory prayer or related practices. We found twenty-five in all. Most of these were very different, using different types of prayer in patients with many different health conditions. We've grouped these studies as follows:

- small studies examining physical conditions (six studies).
- studies of psychological conditions (six studies).
- higher-quality studies of physical conditions (fourteen studies).

Small Studies of Physical Conditions

In this group of six small studies, all with less than ideal designs, two had positive results (✓✓✓) and four showed no benefits from prayer (✗✗✗). These studies were carried out between 1965 and 1994 and involved between sixteen and fifty-three subjects. They examined the effects of intercessory prayer on a range of conditions, such as diabetes, blood pressure, rheumatoid arthritis, pain and wound healing after hernia surgery, and leukemia. Three used Christian prayer; the other three used a variety of energy-directing forms of prayer. Of the two studies in which those prayed for did significantly better than the control group, one involved Christian prayer, the other a combination of Reiki and LeShan prayer.

Reiki calls on spirit guides to assist in a life-energy type of healing (see the Reiki entry). LeShan proponents believe the universe is interconnected and that when people achieve a certain state of consciousness, they can stimulate and enhance another person's natural capacity for self-healing. Although they claim their approach is not based on life energies, the concept is similar. LeShan is said to be completely natural, meaning it does not involve anything supernatural.

Studies of Psychological Conditions

In the studies of psychological conditions, four randomized double-blind studies showed no benefits (✗✗✗✗). One used LeShan prayer, the second used a general form of prayer to God, the third involved prayer by Jewish and Christian volunteers, and the fourth involved prayer by Christians. Two earlier studies showed some benefits, but both were poorly designed and were not controlled studies (✓✓). The improvements found in those who were prayed for could have been the result of a number of other factors.

Higher-Quality Studies of Physical Conditions

All fourteen studies in this group, which included the four cardiac studies addressed earlier, were designed according to current standards of high-quality clinical research. Most had large numbers of subjects. Two other studies involved a form of laying on of hands in addition to prayer. One of these, involving "paranormal" healers, showed no significant healing (✗✗✗). The second involved patients with rheumatoid arthritis and had two parts. Some patients reported much improvement after Christian prayer, laying on of hands, and Christian teaching. However, this part had no control group. The second part was randomized and double-blinded; the group prayed for showed no additional benefits compared to the control group (✗✗✗).

Another study randomly assigned kidney dialysis patients to receive prayer from Catholic women, visualized thoughts from psychology students, or no intervention. The three groups showed no significant differences in ten medical and ten psychological measurements (✗✗✗).

Two other studies examined "spiritual healing," a form of energy therapy, though even the researchers were unsure what the therapy involved. No significant benefits were found in either study (✗✗✗).

The next three studies in this group involved patients receiving a combination of Christian, Jewish, New Age, and Buddhist prayer. One was a pilot study of cardiac patients that had "encouraging" results but, because of the small number of participants, was not statistically reliable (✓✓). Named MANTRA I, it led to the much larger MANTRA II (748 patients at nine sites around the United States). Patients were first randomly assigned to receive prayer or no prayer. They were then randomly assigned a second time to receive either no additional complementary therapy or a combination of music, relaxed breathing, guided imagery, and Healing Touch therapy (a life energy – based therapy). No statistically significant differences were found among the four

groups of patients for the primary outcomes measured (✗✗✗). The complicated study design had advantages and disadvantages but showed no benefits for the prayed-for group.

The third study using a variety of prayer types included psychic, shamanistic, Jewish, Christian, and Buddhist approaches. They all directed positive healing energy to AIDS patients in the study. The results were mixed (✓✓). Of the eleven outcomes measured, those prayed for did significantly better in six. However, a writer with *Wired* magazine discovered some serious problems with the study after one of the researchers (Elisabeth Targ) died. The study was originally designed to measure the effect of prayer on death rates of AIDS patients. During the study, the AIDS "drug cocktail" became available, drastically reducing patient deaths. Only one patient died during the study, making it impossible to calculate any differences between the groups. The researchers then looked for other data they could use but still found no differences between the two groups. They ran another set of calculations, but the control group came out better. They decided to examine whether the frequency of various illnesses common to AIDS patients had been influenced by the prayer, but they hadn't collected data on these. So, after discovering which patients were in which group, they collected new data they had never intended to collect — and found differences that favored the prayed-for group. This was what was published, but with no mention of the tortuous path they had taken. Such a process is called "data mining" and is universally looked down on by researchers because it dramatically reduces the confidence one can have in the reliability of the evidence produced.

A particularly strange study on prayer was published in 2001 by Leonard Leibovici. He took 3,393 medical records for patients who had septicemia (an infection in their blood). He randomly assigned the names to two groups and said a short prayer for the well-being and full recovery of all those in one of the groups. However, all the infections had occurred four to ten years earlier. He called this "retroactive prayer." Leibovici then examined the patient records and discovered that the prayed-for group had statistically significant shorter stays in hospital and shorter duration of fever (✓✓✓). The death rates were not statistically different. Debate erupted in the journal *BMJ*. Did this show that prayer can impact the past? Or did it show that statistics sometimes give strange results? While we believe God can change the future, we don't believe he goes back and influences the past.

One last study must be examined as it demonstrates the serious problems that can arise when researchers do not adhere to accepted scientific and ethical standards. Although the results of this study have not been withdrawn, there are serious concerns about them. More than two hundred Korean women undergoing in vitro fertilization (IVF) were randomly assigned either to be prayed for by Christian groups in three countries or to a control group. The group being prayed for had double the pregnancy rate and double the implantation rate, both of which were highly significant differences. However, the study noted that the women had not been informed that they were being enrolled in the study. Columbia University, where the researchers were based, discovered that the study had never received ethical review. One of the three authors of the publication then admitted he didn't even know about the study until six months after it had been completed. A second author has since left Columbia University for Korea and refuses to comment on the study. The third author, Daniel P. Wirth, pled guilty to federal fraud charges in 2004. The investigation discovered that this is not his true name and that he

had been using it to collect Social Security payments for a man who died in 1994. He left a trail of fraud and embezzlement behind him. Wirth also published several papers on complementary therapies, including two of the studies in the group of small prayer studies. He published numerous studies on Therapeutic Touch. The institute where his publications stated all this research was occurring turned out to be just a post office box.

Jerry Solfvin, Wirth's mentor for his thesis research, and other researchers in this field wrote an open letter to Wirth asking him to respond to concerns about his research. He had failed to respond to their efforts to contact him privately. Meanwhile, they recommend that "Wirth's studies not be considered as scientifically valid until Wirth responds directly to these concerns."

Study Conclusion

From a purely scientific perspective, no clear conclusions can be drawn from these studies in spite of the improvements found in some. Two systematic reviews of prayer research have come to this same conclusion. The types of studies are very different, with some being highly complicated. But more important, we believe all these studies raise important theological questions, to which we now turn.

● Cautions

Prayer research is controversial. Some see it as a form of testing God and say it should not be done. We disagree. We do not believe this research is inappropriate, though we have reservations about its helpfulness. The story of Gideon's fleece in Judges 6:36–40 is an example of God answering a specific request for evidence of his reality and power.

When the disciples of John the Baptist asked Jesus if he was the Messiah, Jesus told them to believe him because of what they could verify by observation. "At that very time Jesus cured many who had diseases, sicknesses and evil spirits, and gave sight to many who were blind. So he replied to the messengers [from John the Baptist], 'Go back and report to John what you have seen and heard: The blind receive sight, the lame walk, those who have leprosy are cured, the deaf hear, the dead are raised, and the good news is preached to the poor'" (Luke 7:20–22).

Jesus' miracles were plain to see. The results of prayer research are far from conclusive. We disagree with those, either Christian or otherwise, who make these inconclusive results the primary pillars of their theological or philosophical claims. We also are concerned about those researchers who use these studies merely as an opportunity to find support for their particular beliefs about the nature of prayer — either to support or refute the power of prayer. Some of the investigations discussed above reveal the extent to which some have gone to find the results they wanted. Scientific research, to be valid, must be conducted in such a manner that results are not skewed by preconceived ideas.

Prayer research is not without risks. The inconclusive results might lead some people to turn away from prayer — and even from God himself — especially if they approach him strictly on the basis of scientific evidence or "results." The great variability in what people mean by prayer is problematic, not only scientifically but also spiritually. Nonbiblical types of "prayer" are often used.

In some research, such as the AIDS study, prayer meant sending impersonal healing energy to others. Elaine Harkness and colleagues claim healing from prayer comes "from the 'channeling' by the healer of an as yet undefined 'energy' from a 'source' to the patient." Those who view prayer this way often call it "distant healing" or "spiritual healing."

Various occult activities have also been defined as "prayer" to allow their inclusion in prayer research. Marilyn Schlitz and William Braud equate prayer with sorcery, shamanism, psychic healing, and telepathy. Harkness includes meditation, magic, and the use of mediums or "spirit doctors" as forms of distant healing. A popular author, Rosemary Guiley, believes prayer is a vibrating inner connection with the divine, which leads her to view prayer as control over esoteric powers.

People are being exposed to occult activities labeled as "prayer," possibly without their knowledge. Researchers tend to ignore or avoid these spiritual concerns, but they are crucial to how Christians should evaluate this research and make decisions about whether to get involved in various types of prayer offered in health care settings.

Theological Assessment

The fundamental theological flaw with all prayer research is the assumption that only humans impact the results. In this view, if prayer works, what people pray for will come about.

Dossey and others believe that prayer follows some natural law and that science will help us understand that law, just as it helped us understand the law of gravity. Under this view, negative results or inconclusive results count as evidence against the effectiveness of prayer.

Such an assumption holds true only if prayer is *impersonal*, based on some energy or thought power or unknown force. But that's not biblical prayer. Prayer, according to the Bible, is not an energy that, once emitted, takes on a life of its own with predictable outcomes. Scientific research could easily measure whether such an energy "works." But this is not what Christianity means by prayer. Biblical prayer is an inherently *personal* encounter with a personal and loving Father. And it is the Father who can choose to answer any prayer with "Yes," "No," or "Wait." In fact, inconsistent research results are *precisely* what the biblical teaching on prayer for healing would lead us to expect for two reasons — one theological and one scientific.

James 5:13 – 16 is an important passage on prayer for healing. It gives Christians instructions on how to respond to sickness, including praying and asking for prayer from others. James then presents Elijah as an example of a righteous man whose prayer was "powerful and effective." We can learn how to pray from Elijah's example and, in particular, from an incident involving him and the prophets of Baal (1 Kings 18:16 – 40).

This incident contrasts Elijah's effective prayer with the ineffective prayer of the prophets of Baal, a god worshiped by the nations around ancient Israel. At that time, the people of Israel were undecided about whether to follow God or Baal. Elijah proposed a test to show whose god was the true God. He told the prophets of Baal to sacrifice a bull, place it on a stack of wood, and then pray to Baal to send fire from heaven to burn up their offering. Elijah said he would do likewise, but pray to the God of Israel.

The prophets of Baal built their wooden altar, placed their sacrificed bull on it, and prayed to Baal. From morning until noon, they repeated, like a mantra, the words, "O Baal, answer us! O Baal, answer us!" They danced and leaped around the sacrificial altar, working themselves into a greater and greater frenzy. They eventually slashed themselves with swords and spears until blood gushed from their wounds. This continued until evening.

The narrator sums up the pathetic picture of their attempts to get an answer from the heavens: "But there was no response, no one answered, no one paid attention" (1 Kings 18:29).

Elijah took over. He repaired the altar of the Lord, which was in ruins. He arranged wood on the altar, sacrificed another bull, and placed it on the wood. He had the people soak everything with water, even filling a trench he had dug around the altar. Then Elijah prayed, "O Lord, God of Abraham, Isaac and Israel, let it be known today that you are God in Israel and that I am your servant and have done all these things at your command. Answer me, O Lord, answer me, so these people will know that you, O Lord, are God, and that you are turning their hearts back again" (1 Kings 18:36 – 37).

All of a sudden, everything on the altar burst into flames. Even the stones Elijah used to build the altar were consumed by fire. "When all the people saw this, they fell prostrate and cried, 'The Lord — he is God! The Lord — he is God!'" (1 Kings 18:39).

The theology in this story is particularly relevant to prayer research. It reminds us that the Bible forbids certain spiritual practices — and demonstrates their ineffectiveness in comparison to the power of God. Christians should refuse to participate in prayer research that involves non-Christian prayer.

The prophets of Baal believed that the more they prayed, and the louder they prayed, and the more they worked themselves into a frenzy, the more likely it was that their prayers would be answered. They focused on what they had to *do* to get an answer from Baal, their god.

A serious problem with prayer research is that it may foster such a mechanical approach to prayer. It uses and studies prayer as if it were just another impersonal "therapy" to try when needed. Prayer, spirituality, and even God himself can become viewed as things to be used to get what we want. Faith in God and his provision is thus trivialized and demeaned.

Prayer already becomes mechanical too easily. While we may not slash ourselves with swords to impress God, how often do we think God will be more inclined to answer our prayers if we do something extra or deny ourselves something? Do we think God will be more likely to hear us if we get up earlier, or stay up later, or pray longer? Do we hope some study will show us the best way to pray or the right words to say?

Elijah didn't relate to God through impersonal rituals or rote prayers. He prayed to God directly and personally. He asked God to let the people know that same day that he was the God of Israel. Elijah was concerned not so much that his prayer would produce certain results (e.g., flames from heaven) but that God would be glorified.

And God answered his prayer.

God is not interested in meaningless repetition. The Bible affirms persistence in prayer (Luke 18:1 – 5), but Jesus gave us the Lord's Prayer while rejecting rote prayer. "And when you pray, do not keep on babbling like pagans, for they think they will be heard because of their many words" (Matthew 6:7; see also Isaiah 29:13). Sadly, even the beautiful Lord's Prayer can be recited in meaningless ways. We should humbly make our requests to our Father in heaven and lay the burdens of our hearts at his feet.

From a scientific perspective, given that God can choose whether to answer a prayer or not and that this decision cannot be measured or controlled, no experiment is adequate to the task of answering our questions about prayer.

Think of it this way. If we wanted to study whether aspirin (or any other therapy) reduced the risk of heart attack, the best study design would be the double-blind, placebo-controlled study. However, if the aspirin could decide whether it would be absorbed or not, or even if absorbed whether it would work or not, then the experiment would no longer be controllable. There would be unmeasurable factors at work that would nullify any results obtained. Furthermore, if there were other unmeasurable factors at work, the study would be even less useful.

In the case of prayer, we cannot measure whether God chooses to say "Yes" or "No" or "Wait." Also, we cannot measure how many of the patient's friends and relatives are praying or if someone on the other side of the world is praying for everyone's health.

In other words, we contend that prayer can never be adequately subjected to the scientific method — simply because there are too many *un*controlled and *un*measured or *un*measurable factors. Further, if such experiments were carried out, *if* there were demonstrable benefits or harms, such effects would be inconsistent (which, by the way, is exactly what the results suggest to date).

Some Christians are discouraged by the inconclusive results of prayer research. Does this mean that God doesn't answer prayer? Or worse still, does he just arbitrarily pick and choose whose prayer to answer? Why would God not heal us physically in answer to our prayers for healing?

Adequate answers to these questions would take up a whole book. Often, though, the answer is that we don't know why God heals some and not others. God may choose not to heal people of great faith despite their prayers for healing. God may use an illness to assist us in our spiritual growth or to remind us of our need to depend on him. Paul's prayer to remove his "thorn in the flesh" was not answered the way he first wanted. This "thorn" is widely believed to have been a physical ailment: "Three times I pleaded with the Lord to take it [the thorn] away from me. But he said to me, 'My grace is sufficient for you, for my power is made perfect in weakness.' Therefore I will boast all the more gladly about my weaknesses, so that Christ's power may rest on me. That is why, for Christ's sake, I delight in weaknesses, in insults, in hardships, in persecutions, in difficulties. For when I am weak, then I am strong" (2 Corinthians 12:8 – 10). This doesn't give us an easy answer. But if we trust God, we must trust that he knows best.

As mentioned above, the inconclusive results from prayer research may also be due to the fact that researchers cannot ensure that those in a control group receive no prayer from others. Not only would there be ethical problems with any such attempt to block prayer, but we don't believe such attempts would be successful. A whole host of other people are likely praying for the research subjects in *both* groups. Because of such lack of controls, some scientists think this type of research will never reveal clear-cut answers. We tend to agree, for theological as well as scientific reasons.

Prayer research will never answer all of our questions about prayer. Clinical research on the effectiveness of prayer is designed to control the impact of human factors on the results. It cannot take into account God's decision — whether or not to answer a particular prayer — or even to delay an answer. Understanding the details of research design shows that the inconclusive results confirm our belief that God is personal and makes up his own mind about how to answer prayer. That should be encouraging, once we trust that God's decision is what is best for us.

Recommendations

The inconclusive results of these experiments should not be viewed as evidence against the power of prayer. God never promised to answer every prayer immediately or in the affirmative. Like any loving parent, God can answer "No!" and still be just, loving, and righteous. God can answer, "Just wait. Be patient." "Wait" and "No" are both answers to prayer that cannot be measured by the scientific method because they show up as if God didn't answer the prayer.

The inconclusive results of prayer research are consistent with the fact that God's will differs from one person to another. He may have a reason to heal someone in one situation but not heal someone else. As more studies are published, the results will continue to vary because God cannot be forced to act within the controls of scientific research.

We believe in the power of prayer because Scripture teaches us to pray. We recommend prayer for healing on the basis of our theological beliefs, not scientific research. This research makes it clear that Christians must be discerning about what is meant by "prayer" before welcoming it into modern health care or participating in its practice. But perhaps even more important, we believe in prayer for what it accomplishes in the one who is praying.

Prayer for personal comfort and endurance during illness and as death approaches is integral to Christian spirituality and health. The Bible promises comfort during sickness and pain. "Praise be to the God and Father of our Lord Jesus Christ, the Father of compassion and the God of all comfort, who comforts us in all our troubles, so that we can comfort those in any trouble with the comfort we ourselves have received from God" (2 Corinthians 1:3 – 4).

As we learn to cope with the illnesses, disorders, and disabilities that God chooses *not* to heal at the present time, and as we come to grips with the knowledge of our eventual death even when God does heal, prayer to God can make a huge difference in our lives. In fact, we would encourage those interested in researching prayer to pour their resources into studying the impact of prayer on those who pray.

But as we pray for healing, we must remember that God does not promise to heal us of every disease, though he does make a number of remarkable promises:

- salvation to anyone who is willing to believe in Jesus (Acts 16:30 – 31);
- a personal relationship with those who initiate one with him (Revelation 3:20);
- his unceasing presence in this life to comfort, protect, and provide for his people (John 10:7 – 15); and
- eternal life in his presence for those who put their faith in him (Luke 23:42 – 43).

We can and should pray for all of these promises when we are sick and suffering. We know that he will answer these prayers. He will give us the strength to endure what we must bear. We also can and should pray for healing. In spite of not having a guarantee of physical healing, we have something even greater: the knowledge that the Lord of the universe will be with us in our suffering. Knowing these promises and trusting in God, we will be able to say along with Paul: "I have learned to be content whatever the circumstances. I know what it is to be in need, and I know what it is to have plenty. I have learned the secret of being content in any and every situation, whether well fed or hungry, whether living in plenty or in want. I can do everything through him who gives me strength" (Philippians 4:11 – 13).

Treatment Categories

Complementary

In all situations, based on
biblical teaching ☺☺☺☺

Further Reading

Astin, John A., Elaine Harkness, and Edzard Ernst. "The Efficacy of 'Distant Healing': A Systematic Review of Randomized Trials." *Annals of Internal Medicine* 132, no. 11 (June 2000): 903 – 10.

Bronson, Po. "A Prayer Before Dying." *Wired* 10, no. 12 (December 2002). Posted December 2002. *Wired: www.wired.com/wired/archive/10.12/prayer_pr.html.* Accessed November 10, 2005.

Dossey, Larry. *Healing Words: The Power of Prayer and the Practice of Medicine.* New York: HarperSanFrancisco, 1993.

Galton, Francis. "Does Prayer Preserve?" *Archives of Internal Medicine* 125 (April 1970): 580 – 81, 587; excerpt from "Statistical Inquiries into the Efficacy of Prayer." *Fortnightly Review* 12 (1872): 125 – 35.

Guiley, Rosemary E. *Prayer Works: True Stories of Answered Prayer.* Unity Village, Mo.: Unity Books, 1998.

Myers, David G. "Is Prayer Clinically Effective?" *Reformed Review* 53, no. 2 (2000): 95 – 102. *David G. Myers: www.davidmyers.org/Brix?pageID=53.* Accessed September 6, 2006.

O'Mathúna, Dónal P. "Prayer Research: What Are We Measuring?" *Journal of Christian Nursing* 16, no. 3 (Summer 1999): 17 – 21.

Schlitz, Marilyn, and William Braud. "Distant Intentionality and Healing: Assessing the Evidence." *Alternative Therapies in Health and Medicine* 3, no. 6 (November 1997): 62 – 73.

Solfvin, Jerry, Jeff Leskowitz, and Daniel J. Benor, "Questions Concerning the Work of Daniel P. Wirth" [letter]. *Journal of Alternative and Complementary Medicine* 11, no. 6 (December 2005): 949 – 50.

Targ, Elisabeth, and Keith S. Thomson. "Can Prayer and Intentionality Be Researched? Should They Be? Point and Counterpoint." *Alternative Therapies in Health and Medicine* 3, no. 6 (November 1997): 92 – 96.

Wilkinson, John. *The Bible and Healing: A Medical and Theological Commentary.* Grand Rapids: Eerdmans, 1998.

PROGRESSIVE MUSCLE RELAXATION

What It Is

If you were asked to tense a particular muscle in your arm, you would probably be able to do it right away. What if you were asked to relax that same muscle? The assumption behind progressive muscle relaxation is that we often need to teach ourselves how to relax specific muscles. The goal is to be able to consciously relax any or all of the muscles of the body and thus induce a state of relaxation whenever it is needed. If we are tense before an examination or meeting or just from the day's activities, we can find relief by consciously relaxing our muscles.

Practically, the person lies down in a comfortable position. The procedure involves tensing specific muscles, holding the tension for a few seconds, and then releasing the muscles. As the muscles relax, the person focuses on the sensation in order to learn what it feels like. This tensing and releasing is repeated with different muscles of the body. The focus remains on sensing and recognizing the relaxation. With practice, the person should come to know the feeling of relaxation and be able to relax at will both individual muscles and the whole body.

Progressive muscle relaxation can be learned and practiced on one's own, though some prefer to work in groups or with an instructor. The technique is often combined with other relaxation techniques, such as visualization or deep breathing. Any approach can be added that helps bring the person into a deeper sense of relaxation.

Claims

The benefits claimed for progressive muscle relaxation relate to any condition in which stress or tension plays a role. Regular practice is said to be beneficial for improving one's overall well-being. Specific uses are to relieve chronic stress, tension headaches, anxiety, and other disorders. Back pain and sleep disorders are reported to benefit from the technique. People whose performances are negatively impacted by anxiety may benefit from progressive muscle relaxation. Thus, athletes and other performers may use the approach to relax.

Study Findings

Several small studies have been conducted on progressive muscle relaxation used with a variety of conditions, making generalizations difficult. A small number of studies (✓✓✓) found better pain relief compared to control groups. However, the results have mostly been short-term, with little evidence available on the long-term effectiveness of the approach. Two studies were found that supported the use of progressive muscle relaxation in asthma patients (✓✓✓). Use of progressive muscle relaxation with guided imagery for cancer patients receiving chemotherapy is one area in which a few studies have been completed (✓✓✓✓). These found that the incidence of nausea and vomiting is reduced in patients taught the technique.

Overall, although few studies are available, the evidence is positive that progressive muscle relaxation brings about relaxation. When the technique is compared with other relaxation techniques, results are variable as to which is more effective. Even when progressive muscle relaxation brings relief, it must be remembered that evidence is not available to support claims that this technique, in and of itself, will lead to cures of any illnesses.

Cautions

No adverse effects have occurred with progressive muscle relaxation. If visualization or guided imagery is to be added, the precise nature of the approach should be investigated for reasons discussed in the Visualization or Guided Imagery entry.

Recommendations

The technique of progressive muscle relaxation is relatively easy to learn. It can be taught quickly to patients who can use it in whatever circumstance they find themselves in. It may work directly by relaxing the body but also by shifting attention onto the muscles and away from the sources of tension. The technique can easily be combined with other relaxation strategies to enhance its impact.

Treatment Categories

Complementary

To promote relaxation	☺☺☺☺
To relieve stress-induced nausea and vomiting	☺☺☺
To relieve certain types of pain	☺☺☺
To relieve stress in asthma patients	☺☺

Further Reading

Huntley A., A. R. White, and E. Ernst. "Relaxation Therapies for Asthma: A Systematic Review." *Thorax* 57, no. 2 (February 2002): 127 – 31.

Yoo, Hee J., Se H. Ahn, Sung B. Kim, Woo K. Kim, and Oh S. Han. "Efficacy of Progressive Muscle Relaxation Training and Guided Imagery in Reducing Chemotherapy Side Effects in Patients with Breast Cancer and in Improving Their Quality of Life." *Supportive Care in Cancer* 13, no. 10 (October 2005): 826 – 33.

P

QIGONG

What It Is

Qigong (pronounced CHEE-guhng) literally means "energy work." Within traditional Chinese medicine (TCM), *qi*, or *chi* (both pronounced CHEE), is believed to be vital to keep a person healthy. There are Chinese hospitals where only Qigong is available, though most Chinese hospitals also have other health services, including an increasing amount of Western conventional medicine.

TCM focuses on preventive measures: physical moderation, exercise, diet, and breathing techniques. Each aspect has physical effects but also involves life energy, called *chi* in TCM. *Chi* is believed to be a mix of inherited energy, passed from parents to children at the time of conception, and energy derived from the food and air that sustain us throughout life. The transportation system for *chi* is believed by the Chinese to be a series of meridians that extend throughout our bodies and link our skin with our internal organs to assure our well-being. It is *chi* that is believed to provide protection from illness and to promote health.

Qigong consists of meditation, breathing exercises, and gentle repetitive movements that facilitate movement of *chi*. Tai Chi and other Chinese martial arts are based on these same principles except that the physical movements get progressively more active and assertive. Practitioners of Qigong focus on their breathing while doing the exercise movements and visualize *chi* flowing smoothly through their bodies or accumulating in areas that may be depleted.

Qigong exercises involve slow, rhythmic movements of parts of the body while sitting or standing. Legend has it that the movements were inspired by watching the instinctive movements of wild animals. The movements can also be done from a wheelchair or a bed, making this a type of exercise that almost anyone can do.

Qigong is practiced in two very different ways. Internal Qigong involves balancing and manipulating the flow of *chi* within oneself. External Qigong is a skill only master therapists can develop. Qigong masters are said to be able to direct *chi* externally to either heal other people or move objects without touching them. These Qigong masters allegedly perform great feats by what they claim involves manipulating and directing this nonphysical energy. Skeptics claim these are conjuring tricks, involving either sleight of hand or true magical powers.

Claims

Practicing internal Qigong is said to induce relaxation, promote general well-being, and reduce stress — effective as a complement to conventional therapies for patients with heart problems and cancer. The exercises can be a helpful and gentle regimen for those who are physically unfit or weakened by illness.

The claims made for external Qigong are much broader and more dramatic. Qigong masters are said to have cured every form of serious illness and even to have brought people back from the dead. This aspect of Qigong practice and belief raises significant concerns for Christians.

Study Findings

Many reports (✓) on Qigong have come from China, though Chinese studies on Qigong have not been systematically reviewed in the West. The studies that have been seen (✓✓) are often criticized for being nothing more than reports of one or two patients — anecdotes, case histories, or case reports too limited to be used as proof of effectiveness. They also lack the controls needed to assure that any observed changes were due to Qigong and not a host of other factors influencing people and their health.

A 2004 review of Qigong found ten scientific studies of relevance. However, most of them were small and many had design problems. They examined a variety of conditions and used both internal and external Qigong. The results were also variable, with some positive and some negative. At this point, the evidence regarding Qigong's relief of specific illnesses is weak and preliminary. There is also no clear evidence that Qigong increases resistance to illness or that it can cure any illness.

Evidence from other studies (✓✓✓✓) of gentle, regular exercise supports the beneficial effects of that component of the practice. However, randomized controlled studies of Qigong compared to other exercise regimens are needed to show whether Qigong has any benefits in the treatment of any illness or whether those benefits extend beyond those of exercise alone.

Cautions

In some ways, Qigong introduces people to the importance of taking time to relax and develop some sort of regular, gentle exercise routine. However, as with yoga, meditation, and other Eastern practices, we should never forget that the ultimate goal of such practices is religious. These practices are designed to help people become more unified with the universal energy field and develop their awareness of that energy. While the breathing and movement exercises may be innocuous at first, Qigong is an introduction to a worldview and religious system completely different from Christianity.

Qigong is not without problems. Numerous reports exist (✖✖) of people suffering side effects — from relatively mild symptoms of headache, dry mouth, and muscle twitching all the way to hallucinations and psychotic breakdowns. Most of these symptoms cease within months of stopping Qigong, although others have taken a couple of years to resolve. With the growing popularity of Qigong in China, specialized clinics have opened there to treat the increasing numbers of patients with what are now called "Qigong-induced mental disorders."

The Chinese book *Qigong: Chinese Medicine or Pseudoscience?* has been translated into English. The authors interviewed many of those involved in studies that allegedly demonstrated amazing feats using external Qigong. They concluded that most of these claims were based on hoaxes or conjuring tricks. If Qigong masters were able to do what they claim, in our opinion they would have to be tapping into some form of psychic or spiritual power. Since this clearly is not of God, it is most likely of the Evil One and antithetical to what Christians should be involved with. We can assume that the more benign manifestations of Qigong are simply less powerful examples of the same occult energy.

Recommendations

Christians should take a holistic approach to their health. This recognizes the importance of exercising, reducing stress, and taking time out of a busy schedule to allow our bodies and minds to recuperate. But since we can easily do all of these things without getting involved in practices and techniques that are infused with non-Christian beliefs and concepts, there should be no reason to practice Qigong. Given the alleged paranormal abilities of Qigong masters, Christians should be very reluctant to participate in their therapies at any level.

Treatment Categories

Complementary

As an exercise and breathing technique ☺☺

Scientifically Unproven

For any other indication ☹☹☹☹

Spiritual

In the hands of most practitioners 👎👎👎👎

Further Reading

Kemp, Carol A. "Qigong as a Therapeutic Intervention with Older Adults." *Journal of Holistic Nursing* 22, no. 4 (December 2004): 351–73.

Ng, Beng-Yeong. "Qigong-Induced Mental Disorders: A Review." *Australian and New Zealand Journal of Psychiatry* 33, no. 2 (April 1999): 197–206.

Zixin, Lin, Yu Li, Guo Zhengyi, Shen Zhenyu, Zhang Honglin, and Zhang Tongling. *Qigong: Chinese Medicine or Pseudoscience?* Amherst, N.Y.: Prometheus, 2000.

REFLEXOLOGY

What It Is

Reflexology is a very popular alternative therapy. Some European countries report that it is the most popular alternative therapy used there, while in the United Kingdom it is the most popular alternative therapy practiced by nurses. This recent popularity dates back to Dr. William H. Fitzgerald, an ear, nose, and throat physician who in 1915 created the American forerunner of reflexology. He had an idea that he described as "zone therapy." Various therapies similar to reflexology are said to have existed four thousand years ago in Egypt, India, and China. Originally, these were related to life energy concepts such as the Chinese *chi* or the Indian *prana*.

Reflexology, as it evolved from Dr. Fitzgerald's work, looks like a foot massage but is said to be much more. In its twentieth-century form, the body was divided into ten vertical zones running from the feet to the head and down each arm. The belief was that "energy" flows through each zone and must be balanced in order for the organs of that zone to be healthy. The zones on the left side of the body have reflex points on the left hand and foot; zones on the right correspond to reflex points on the right hand and foot. Imbalances in energy lead to the accumulation of waste material (uric acid and calcium crystals) at the reflex points.

Today the practice of reflexology involves the application of pressure at the reflex points to break up the granular accumulations. Practitioners claim this allows free and balanced flow of energy, which allegedly restores health.

In the 1930s, Eunice Ingham, a nurse and physical therapist, mapped out all the reflex points on the feet. She showed which part of each foot she believed corresponded to which organ. For example, she thought the brain can be assisted by putting pressure on the tips of the three largest toes on both feet. The left pelvis corresponded to the heel of the left foot, and so on. Today some reflexologists have come to believe that emotional problems can also be resolved by applying pressure to certain reflex points.

Claims

Practitioners claim reflexology aids almost every part of the body and relieves more than one hundred ailments. These include acne, asthma, cirrhosis of the liver, colds, fatigue, impotence, infections, and stress. It is said to work by improving the flow of blood to the corresponding parts of the body and eliminating toxic accumulations. Although this system sounds just like the energy therapies of traditional Chinese medicine (one of its historic roots), some proponents say it is based on a completely different type of energy. Others make no distinction, utilizing the same concept of life energy as used in Therapeutic Touch, acupuncture, and other energy therapies.

Study Findings

Reflexology may benefit people in the same way massage helps people relax and reduce their stress levels. However, little scientific evidence supports claims that the benefits exceed basic massage techniques. Most of the reports in the literature are case studies or anecdotal reports (✓). Two small studies (✓✓) found that reflexology helped reduce blood pressure and relieved migraine, but control groups were not used in these studies. Some small studies have examined reflexology for pain, but the results are inconclusive to date. A randomized controlled study with asthma patients found no benefit from reflexology compared to placebo massage (✗✗✗). Two other studies found reflexology better than placebo in relieving PMS symptoms and anxiety (✓✓✓). However, it was not possible to determine from these studies if reflexology offered any benefit over foot massage.

The zone maps of the feet are believed to be of central importance to reflexology. However, the maps vary considerably among authorities, which can lead to different therapists diagnosing different ailments. One study examined the reliability of two reflexologists' diagnostic skills. Eighteen patients with up to six known medical conditions were examined by two reflexologists. They neither diagnosed the correct conditions nor agreed with each other on each person's problems (✗✗✗). As a diagnostic tool, reflexology is not proven to be reliable.

Cautions

Reflexology is generally safe. A number of practitioners claim it can elicit a "healing crisis." This is a common claim in any therapy that involves "detoxification." Flu-like symptoms — light-headedness, disturbed sleep, and diarrhea — are said to result from the elimination of the toxic buildup that caused whatever problems led a patient to the practitioner. There appear to be no other serious side effects, though standard precautions should apply. Reflexology should not be used to diagnose illnesses, nor should it be pursued instead of proven effective treatment. It can be a welcome, relaxing adjunct to therapy, in much the same manner that massage can ease the stress of someone with heart problems, cancer, and the like.

Some reflexologists interpret their work in terms of life energy manipulation. Christians should be discerning about the beliefs being promoted by the person offering this type of foot massage.

Recommendations

Reflexology seems to be a form of therapy that may help with relaxation. But given its unproven efficacy and the potential for life energy involvement, caution is needed in choosing a therapist. An ordinary foot massage would be preferable.

Treatment Categories

Complementary

For relaxation, to relieve
anxiety or tension ☺☺☺

For relaxation, to relieve
headaches or pain ☺

Scientifically Questionable

For most indications,
especially to cure any illness ☹☹☹

Spiritual

In the hands of many practitioners 👎👎

Further Reading

Botting, Deborah. "Review of Literature on the Effectiveness of Reflexology." *Complementary Therapies in Nursing and Midwifery* 3 (1997): 123–30.

Stephenson, Nancy L. N., and Jo Ann Dalton. "Using Reflexology for Pain Management: A Review." *Journal of Holistic Nursing* 21, no 2 (June 2003): 179–91.

White, A. R., J. Williamson, A. Hart, and E. Ernst. "A Blinded Investigation into the Accuracy of Reflexology Charts." *Complementary Therapies in Medicine* 8, no. 3 (September 2000): 166–72.

REIKI

What It Is

Reiki comes from the Japanese *rei*, meaning "universal," and *ki*, meaning "vital force," and is pronounced "RAY-kee." *Ki* is the Japanese term for *prana*, or *chi*, the universal life energy. Proponents claim Reiki was practiced by Buddha and discussed in ancient Sanskrit writings that were lost. Some practitioners believe the therapy was in use in early first-century Rome and that it was the healing method practiced by Jesus, though there is no biblical or Sanskrit support for this claim.

Modern Reiki was developed out of an experience a Zen Buddhist monk had in the mid-1800s. The monk, Mikao Usui, had been meditating, fasting, and praying on Mount Koriyama in Japan for three weeks when he underwent a psychic experience. He reported that the secret to healing — Reiki — had been revealed to him. Subsequently, others have reported learning more details through channeling, which is the New Age term for a method of consulting spirit guides to obtain information from them. The website of the International Center for Reiki Training states, "It is the God-consciousness called Rei that guides the life force called Ki in the practice we call Reiki. Therefore, Reiki can be defined as spiritually guided life force energy." According to Pamela Miles, a Reiki master, Usui's teaching was "a system of spiritual practice." When Reiki was brought to the West, adherents "pragmatically reshaped the origins of Reiki, presenting Usui as a Christian minister."

All Reiki therapies have as their core concept that life energy pervades each person and that this energy is unconditional, divine, loving, and healing. Illnesses arise when the energy cannot flow properly through the person, usually due to blockages at the *chakras*, where life energy is converted from one form to another and ultimately into physical matter. The practitioner is a channel, allowing Reiki energy to flow through him or her, directing it toward the patient. Reiki has a number of variations, but the basic methods and beliefs are the same.

Training in Reiki consists of learning to open oneself to the energy so that it can flow freely through the practitioner. The energy itself is believed to know what each patient needs for healing. Reiki training requires involvement of a Reiki master. Until recently, Reiki training was carried out in secret ceremonies, the practitioners entrusted with knowledge they were not to reveal to others. Now Reiki is being openly promoted in popular alternative medicine books and nursing journals.

Practitioners of Reiki must go through various "attunements" during training. A Reiki master calls on the help of spirit guides to open students' *chakras* and fill them with life energy. Students report being able to feel the energy flow through them, which often leads to their hands getting hot. Students also intuitively receive special symbols that later become central to their healing practice. At the completion of this ceremony, a first-degree Reiki practitioner can detect and move life energy.

To become a second-degree Reiki, practitioners must learn both to use the symbols received in the first attunement and to send life energy over longer distances. They learn how to contact spirit guides and how to use them during healing.

The third level, the Reiki master, can only be attained through the invitation of a Reiki master. During this training, practitioners commit their lives to Reiki, come to embody life energy, and give complete control of healing sessions to their spirit guides.

The healing sessions themselves look very much like a Therapeutic Touch session. Practitioners place their hands, palms down, on or above the patient's body. The hands are kept in one place, and the practitioners attune themselves to the life energy. They are taught that they must not try to direct the energy but rather let it flow through them. They should initially focus their intention on bringing about harmony and healing, but once the energy starts to flow through them, they do not need to concentrate on what they are doing. The energy flow will cause sensations of hot, cold, tingling, color, or pain, and when these subside (after about five minutes) the practitioner moves to another area. A complete healing session can take an hour or more.

Practitioners also draw or visualize the special symbols to increase the power of the energy being directed. Second- and third-degree Reiki practitioners need not be present with their patients because they claim to be able to send life energy over long distances.

Claims

Most proponents of Reiki claim that it brings about relaxation, relieves pain, and brings enlightenment. Numerous hospitals and health care agencies in the United States have conducted Reiki in-services. One hospital in New England offers Reiki to all preoperative patients (except those of one dissenting physician) to promote relaxation and general well-being. However, some proponents claim it can cure and improve almost anything, from schizophrenia to cancer, marital problems to drug addictions. One Reiki master in India claims he can recharge drained batteries with Reiki.

Some claim Reiki is a way for Christians to live out their call to heal (for example, *www.christian reiki.org*). A few reasons are given for this perspective. One is the testimonies of Christians who say they have experienced benefits from receiving and practicing Reiki. A second is the claim that Reiki is a legitimate way to exercise the gift of healing. Yet no attempt is made to provide guidelines as to what may or may not be done in the name of healing. The third is the claim that life energy is the Holy Spirit. The website acknowledges that the term "Reiki" refers to life energy and the Universal Spirit. It then states that "Reiki means life energy that is guided by God. Some also feel this is just another way of saying Holy Spirit." In response to concerns about the spirit guides encountered in Reiki, the website says these may be such angels as Gabriel or Michael.

This approach, we believe, is spiritually naïve and potentially dangerous. The Bible has very clear teaching about spiritual evil. The Bible claims Satan is the father of lies (John 8:44) and a deceptive angel of light (2 Corinthians 11:14). Failure to acknowledge this leads to a lack of caution reflected in the website's claim that "those Christians who practice Reiki do so within the guidance and protection of God secure in the belief that they have been guided to follow Jesus' example to be a healer." This approach fails to recognize our responsibility to critically evaluate our actions. Such a principle could be used to justify any action a Christian felt called by God to carry out. God will not necessarily protect us if we drive 100 mph down city streets, and there is no guarantee he will protect us if we act as recklessly in the spiritual realm.

Study Findings

A small number of articles in professional journals report case studies (✓) in which an individual was said to have recovered or improved after receiving Reiki. In spite of the growing popularity of Reiki, few controlled studies have been published. Three small studies (✓✓) found that Reiki produced relaxation and relieved anxiety, but these had no control groups to compare Reiki with other relaxation techniques or placebo.

Five controlled studies were found in a comprehensive search. Two of these failed to demonstrate greater relaxation during Reiki compared to a mimic treatment acting as a placebo (✗✗✗). A randomized study (✗✗✗) with fifty stroke patients found no differences among the groups treated by a Reiki master, a Reiki novice, or placebo. Another study showed greater wound healing in a control group (✗✗✗) compared to a group receiving Reiki along with other complementary therapies. One study (✓✓✓) found greater pain relief in a group receiving Reiki compared to a control group. The latter two studies were carried out by Daniel Wirth and colleagues, whose whole research enterprise has been questioned since his conviction for fraud and embezzlement (see p. 240).

Cautions

Reiki is clearly antithetical to biblical Christianity. Communication with spirits is an integral part of the practice, during both training attunements and healing sessions. Contacting spirits is denounced in the Bible as sorcery, mediumship, and spiritism (Leviticus 19:26, 31; 20:6; Deuteronomy 18:9 – 14; Acts 19:19; Galatians 5:20; Revelation 21:8). Contacting spirit guides is dangerous spiritually, physically, and emotionally. "Be self-controlled and alert. Your enemy the devil prowls around like a roaring lion looking for someone to devour" (1 Peter 5:8). In their literature, Reiki practitioners sometimes claim

to seek what is called the "Kundalini experience," the pinnacle of psychic experiences, which can cause severe emotional and psychological disturbances (see the Yoga entry).

Recommendations

Christians should have nothing to do with Reiki. Those involved with Reiki, in our opinion, are engaging with evil spirits. In spite of the reasons given by those supportive of Reiki, we believe the clear biblical commands outlined above and the way Reiki is described by almost all practitioners show that practicing Reiki is inappropriate for Christians and not spiritually safe for anyone.

Treatment Categories

Complementary
To promote relaxation   ☹☹☹☹
To relieve pain   ☹☹☹☹

Spiritual
Certainly inappropriate,
  possibly occult   👎👎👎👎

Further Reading

Miles, Pamela, and Gala True. "Reiki — Review of a Biofield Therapy: History, Theory, Practice, and Research." *Alternative Therapies in Health and Medicine* 9, no. 2 (March/April 2003): 62 – 72.

O'Mathúna, Dónal P. "Reiki for Relaxation and Pain Relief." *Alternative Therapies in Women's Health* 5, no. 4 (April 2003): 29 – 31.

Stein, Diane. *Essential Reiki*. Freedom, Calif.: Crossing, 1995.

SHAMANISM

What It Is

Shamanism, or shamanic medicine, is possibly the oldest form of medicine still practiced today. Most tribal societies have or had their shamans, medicine men, witch doctors, sorcerers, or holy men. The shaman usually was both healer and priest for the tribe — highly respected. His or her work often involved lifelong learning. Even today practicing medicine men or women and shamans frequently combine the rituals specific to their culture with the use of plants that are known to have medicinal properties. Visualization techniques common to some alternative therapies are also included.

Modern-day shamans sometimes include conventional therapies, including various counseling techniques and pharmaceuticals. What is most distinctive about shamanic medicine is not the therapies involved but the means by which shamans determine what a particular patient needs. This emphasis goes back to the root meaning of the Siberian term "shaman," which is defined as "to know," with the emphasis on spiritual knowledge.

Shamans go through a long apprenticeship in which they learn how to contact and deal with the spirits of ancestors, animals, or demons. Within shamanism, healing involves becoming more under the influence of these spirits and allowing them to control more of one's life. To make contact with the spiritual realm, the shaman enters a trance, which can be induced by fasting, hallucinogenic herbs, or rituals that involve dancing, drumming, and chanting.

Once the spirits are contacted, the shaman acts as a mediator between the spirits and the patient to find out how the spirits have been offended and why they have sent this illness on the patient. Once this information is gathered, the shaman bargains with the spirits to find out what is needed to release the patient from the illness. Then the shaman returns to normal consciousness and carries out the magical practices needed to appease the offended spirits or demons.

Claims

Shamanism is actually a pagan religion in which it is believed that all illnesses are caused by spiritual events. This means that shamans believe they can cure all illnesses provided they can get the spiritual cooperation they believe is needed.

With recent interest in alternative medicine, even shamanism is becoming secularized. Some shamans now offer certain practices and therapies to nonbelievers. While some individual therapies practiced by shamans (visualization and herbal remedies) may be somewhat effective, each needs to be evaluated on its own merits.

Study Findings

Very little scientific research has been done on shamanism itself. However, study of the Bible reveals very clear advice. Shamanism incorporates occult and magical practices that are clearly forbidden in the Bible (Leviticus 19:26, 31; 20:6; Acts 19:19; Galatians 5:20; Revelation 21:8). In many ways, shamanism is equivalent to sorcery, which is frequently condemned. King Saul used a medium to contact the deceased spirit of Samuel (1 Samuel 28) and was explicitly condemned by God for doing so. "Saul died because he was unfaithful to the LORD; he did not keep the word of the LORD and even consulted a medium for guidance, and did not inquire of the LORD" (1 Chronicles 10:13 – 14). Occult practitioners (e.g., diviners, spiritualists, and mediums) and activities (e.g., sorcery, spells, and astrology) work to misdirect people in their greatest hours of need.

> Keep on, then, with your magic spells
>> and with your many sorceries,
>> which you have labored at since childhood. . . .
> All the counsel you have received has only
>> worn you out!
> Let your astrologers come forward,
> those stargazers who make predictions month
>> by month,
> let them save you from what is coming
>> upon you. . . .
> Each of them goes on in his error;
>> there is not one that can save you.
>
> *Isaiah 47:12 – 13, 15*

While God condemns occult practices (Deuteronomy 18:9 – 14), he recognizes that we need spiritual guidance. The message of the prophets and the apostles gives us the Bible, a divinely inspired book, unlike other books. "Above all, you must understand that no prophecy of Scripture came about by the prophet's own interpretation. For prophecy never had its origin in the will of man, but men spoke from God as they were carried along by the Holy Spirit" (2 Peter 1:20 – 21). However, God has revealed only part of what could be known of the spiritual world. "The secret things belong to the LORD our God, but the things revealed belong to us and to our children forever, that we may follow all the words of this law" (Deuteronomy 29:29). Shamans use occult practices in attempts to discover things that we have no need to know or should not know because the knowledge may harm us.

Cautions

During their training, shamans are possessed by either their spirit guides or the spirit of their "power animal" (a spirit with the form of an animal). These spirits are responsible for any healing that may occur through the shaman. Involvement with a possessed person may adversely affect others spiritually or even lead to their possession. Possession is not only spiritually dangerous but can lead to serious mental illness and physical suffering. A significant body of psychological research documents the increased prevalence of psychotic behavior among shamans, although some dispute this conclusion.

Increased global mobility and curiosity about other cultures have led some people to explore shamanistic practices. This has led to more than just spiritual concerns. More cases of toxicity from the beverage ayahuasca are being reported in the West as people experiment with shamanism. Ayahuasca, brewed by some shamans, contains powerful hallucinogenic drugs, including dimethyltryptamine (DMT), a Schedule I drug. Such drugs are not permitted for use in the United States because they lack any medical use and have serious adverse effects. Some groups are seeking permission to use ayahuasca as part of their religious ceremonies. The main adverse effects are intoxication and the psychological impact of "bad trips."

Some shamanic practices can be followed without committing oneself to shamanism, but these practices introduce people to this whole belief system and therefore may expose them to demonic oppression — or possession.

257

Recommendations

Christians should not dabble in the occult or adopt other religions, not even for the sake of health or healing. For this reason, Christians should not use the services of a shaman.

Treatment Categories

Complementary
For any indication ☹☹☹☹

Spiritual
Possibly occult 👎👎👎👎

Further Reading

Cassileth, Barrie R. *The Alternative Medicine Handbook*. New York: W. W. Norton, 1998, 314 – 17.

Halpern, John H. "Hallucinogens and Dissociative Agents Naturally Growing in the United States." *Pharmacology and Therapeutics* 102 (2004): 131 – 38.

TAI CHI

What It Is

Tai Chi, or Tai Chi Chuan, literally means "supreme ultimate power" and is part of traditional Chinese medicine. There are five major styles, with the *yang* form most commonly practiced in the West. As with Qigong, the purpose of the practice is to restore a balanced flow of *chi* and thereby promote health.

Most Westerners are familiar with Tai Chi as a martial art consisting of meditation, breathing exercises, and slow, graceful movements. It comes in short and long versions, lasting about ten or thirty minutes, respectively. Each session is composed of a series of specific postures combined into one long exercise. Many of these developed from watching animal and bird movements, as reflected in their names: "white crane spreads wings," "golden rooster stands on one leg," and "ride the tiger." Practicing outdoors is said to be better because it allows universal *chi* in the earth to rise up through one's feet to replenish the person's own *chi*.

The martial arts aspect of Tai Chi is little understood by practitioners of other forms of karate such as Tae Kwon Do, Kempo, and the like. The movements are so slow and smooth that they are comfortable for the elderly, which is not the case with other forms of martial arts that involve strikes and blocks. However, a skilled Tai Chi practitioner can speed up the movements to serve as a form of self-defense. Many Westerners are also unaware of, or unconcerned about, the spiritual aspects of Tai Chi.

Claims

Practicing Tai Chi is said to bring mental and spiritual clarity. It induces relaxation, benefits posture, and promotes a general sense of well-being (this much is true for more dramatic martial arts as well). It is used more to prevent illness than to help relieve symptoms once someone has become ill. Tai Chi is said to have many general health benefits, such as reducing blood pressure, cholesterol levels, tension, depression, fatigue, and anxiety. Others say it improves a person's circulation, digestion, and appetite.

Study Findings

Two reviews of Tai Chi were published in 2004. Both found a small number of randomized controlled studies (✓✓✓✓) that used Tai Chi to help people develop strength and balance so they fall less often. Falling is a significant and potentially fatal problem among the elderly. A small number of controlled studies (✓✓✓✓) found that Tai Chi increased flexibility and strength, although some did not. One study (✓✓✓) examined the number of falls people trained in Tai Chi experienced compared to those taught other balancing programs. The Tai Chi program cut the number of falls in half, a very significant improvement. However, whether these improvements stemmed from the life energy nature of Tai Chi or the exercise part of the program has not been addressed in the research published to date. Most practitioners would cite the life energy, while most Western students of Tai Chi credit the exercise and posture aspects because these lead to better balance.

Three other controlled studies have examined the psychological benefits of Tai Chi. Two studies (✓✓✓) found that those using Tai Chi scored better on tests of depression and well-being compared to a control group. In these cases, the control group involved no intervention. The third study (✗✗✗) compared Tai Chi to walking and a control group and found no psychological differences among the groups. Overall, the evidence is weak that Tai Chi is beneficial psychologically, with no evidence that it is more beneficial than other exercise programs.

Cautions

Tai Chi is a more demanding form of exercise than Qigong. People who are not used to exercising should be particularly cautious and have a general checkup by a physician before starting Tai Chi or any exercise program. The studies cited above were all done with healthy volunteers. People who are ill or weakened by age or disease should be cautious about starting any exercise program. The benefits from Tai Chi may not be as apparent with unhealthy patients.

The same cautions as expressed with all other life energy therapies apply to Tai Chi. The religious nature and goals of Eastern therapies should not be forgotten. In attempting to introduce people to the universal energy field — and help them become unified with the Universal Consciousness — these practices can be the door to the occult realm.

Recommendations

Tai Chi is frequently offered in the West as both an innocuous exercise regimen and a martial art, often with no religious aspects discussed with students. However, more serious practitioners are often committed followers of Eastern religions and may teach that these beliefs must be embraced to properly practice Tai Chi or experience its benefits. Thus, while there may be some general health benefits, Tai Chi may also bring spiritual harm.

Exercise programs have been designed for people at every point on the fitness scale and with a variety of preexisting ailments. We see no reason to adopt one immersed in religious connotations when nonspiritual alternatives are widely available.

Treatment Categories

Complementary

To help develop strength and
balance to prevent falls ☺☺☺☺

To increase flexibility and strength ☺☺☺☺

To improve mood or relieve
mild depression and anxiety ☺☺

Scientifically Unproven

For any other indication ☹☹

Spiritual

By its very nature 👎👎👎👎

Further Reading

Verhagen, Arianne P., Monique Immink, Annemieke van der Meulen, and Sita M. A. Bierma-Zeinstra. "The Efficacy of Tai Chi Chuan in Older Adults: A Systematic Review." *Family Practice* 21, no. 1 (February 2004): 107 – 13.

Wang, Chenchen, Jean Paul Collet, and Joseph Lau. "The Effect of Tai Chi on Health Outcomes in Patients With Chronic Conditions: A Systematic Review." *Archives of Internal Medicine* 164 (March 2004): 493 – 501.

THERAPEUTIC TOUCH

What It Is

Therapeutic Touch is an alternative therapy that has gained remarkable popularity and acceptability among nurses, though this disturbs some nurses. Close to one hundred nursing colleges teach the practice, and tens of thousands of health care professionals have been trained in it. A survey in 2000 – 2001 found that of hospitals in the United States offering complementary and alternative medicine, almost half provided Therapeutic Touch as an inpatient service.

Therapeutic Touch is said to be based on a number of ancient healing practices, with some practitioners including biblical laying on of hands in its heritage. Therapeutic Touch first became popular during a period when many members of the health care professions were looking for ways to show greater compassion for patients.

As first introduced, Therapeutic Touch seemed like an innocent, loving, compassionate, and perhaps healing therapy that allowed more contact with patients. What was not always understood was that the therapy is based on the manipulation of nonphysical human energies called *prana*, or *chi*. Therapeutic Touch practitioners work to sense the nonphysical energies through a form of meditation called "centering." The practitioners access their inner spirits, from which they receive guidance for the healing session.

Patients are asked to sit or lie comfortably, and practitioners pass their hands over the patients. The hands are usually kept two to four inches away from the skin, although practitioners sometimes do make physical contact. Some make the connection between touch and comfort or relaxation, especially for patients who are hospitalized and connected to various machines and monitors. The potentially deep personal interaction involved in touch can remind patients of their own humanity and the love of the caregiver. However, the theory behind Therapeutic Touch and the way it is taught by its main advocates stress that physical contact is not necessary — that Therapeutic Touch is an energy-based therapy.

The next phase of Therapeutic Touch involves practitioners assessing the patient's energy field for imbalances and disturbances, believed to be the precursors of illness. These are corrected in two ways. One is by "unruffling," a procedure in which the practitioner uses long sweeps, or passes, of the hands over the body. These are believed to smooth out the energy field. The other method is to direct energy to specific points of the body. If practitioners "sense" an energy field is "hot," they will send "cool energy" by visualizing coolness in their minds. If they sense a field is cold, they will visualize hotness. There is no way to objectively verify these evaluations or treatments. At the end of a session, the patient's energy field is reassessed. Then the patient is encouraged to relax for twenty to thirty minutes. During all these techniques, practitioners need to remain centered and intent on bringing healing.

Claims

The most common claims are that Therapeutic Touch elicits relaxation, relieves pain, promotes healing, and boosts the immune system. However, many other claims have also been made. For example, Therapeutic Touch is said to relieve premenstrual syndrome, depression, complications in premature babies, and secondary infections due to HIV; it is also said to lower blood pressure, decrease edema, ease abdominal cramps and nausea, resolve fevers, stimulate growth in premature infants, and accelerate the healing of fractures, wounds, and in-

fections. Dolores Krieger, one of the two developers of the practice, also claimed that in "several cases," premature babies who had been declared dead were resuscitated when given Therapeutic Touch. The babies, she claimed, went on to recover completely.

Study Findings

Therapeutic Touch has been the subject of much research. However, reviews of this research have generally found evidence supporting Therapeutic Touch to be very weak. For example, in the area of wound healing, it is frequently pointed out that two studies (✓✓✓✓) found that Therapeutic Touch hastened the healing of wounds. Less often cited were more recent studies (✗✗✗) that found opposite effects. There are now five studies in this area: two show faster healing with Therapeutic Touch, two show slower healing, and one shows no difference. To make matters more uncertain, all this research was published by Daniel Wirth, the controversial character discussed in the Prayer for Healing entry — the man convicted for fraud, his name that of a dead man, his research institution unlocatable. Thus, all his "studies" must be viewed with much skepticism. Regardless, the five published studies show a lack of clear support for Therapeutic Touch's effectiveness in wound healing.

Closer examination of all the other areas of research relative to Therapeutic Touch reveals inconsistency and weakness in research design. For example, systematic reviews of Therapeutic Touch research published in the late 1990s continue to be used to support the practice. Patricia Winstead-Fry and Jean Kijek found that a third of the twenty-nine studies they reviewed were negative (✗✗✗), and the others had either mixed or positive results (✓✓✓✓). They found other problems, such as lack of clarity in how the therapy was given and incomplete reporting of data. They also noted that using healthy participants in many studies "defies logic" when researching a healing therapy. They found that in many studies the researcher was also the therapist, raising concerns that this could potentially bias the research and influence the findings.

The review by Rosalind Peters included fewer studies (only nine) by limiting her interest to studies using the original Krieger/Kunz method of Therapeutic Touch. She again found many limitations with the research, concluding that it was not possible to draw more than tentative conclusions from the data. She found evidence of a "medium effect" (✓✓✓) on physiological outcomes (such as pain or wound healing) but insufficient evidence to support Therapeutic Touch as more effective than control interventions for psychological outcomes (✗✗✗). Therese Meehan, a Therapeutic Touch (TT) researcher, has concluded that "although it cannot be claimed with any confidence that TT is significantly more effective than a placebo, . . . some nurses in practice will remain convinced of its adjuvant effectiveness in facilitating comfort, peacefulness, and healing in a wide range of patients."

Some people will remain convinced of Therapeutic Touch's effectiveness because of misinformation about the practice. Dónal has published a study documenting numerous examples in professional journals of research conclusions being exaggerated or misrepresented. Sometimes people's belief in or enthusiasm for a therapy can overcome their professional obligation to report results accurately.

Cautions

Since Therapeutic Touch is a therapy based on spiritual life energy, Christians should avoid this practice.

Research shows that people feel better after Therapeutic Touch treatments. The question is whether this is due to the therapy itself or the care and attention given by the practitioner. Although frequently derided as "just" a placebo response, these effects are real and reflect the benefits of what used to be called "good bedside manner." However, Christians especially should know that all that feels good is not actually good for us.

The two founders of Therapeutic Touch were Dolores Krieger, a Buddhist, and Dora Kunz, then president of the Theosophical Society in America. The latter organization laid much of the foundation for the New Age movement and has been a major promoter of Eastern mystical and occult beliefs.

Buckland's Complete Book of Witchcraft describes a practice that is identical to Therapeutic Touch but is called "*pranic* healing." This has long been practiced within the Wiccan religion. Through involvement with Therapeutic Touch, people can get gradually drawn into these other religious systems. For example, Krieger recommends the use of divination and claims that her students learn to develop psychic means of communicating with trees, birds, and animals.

Therapeutic Touch easily leads into other practices such as Reiki and Barbara Brennan's Hands of Light, both of which involve contacting spirit guides. These have been combined under the broad heading of Healing Touch, an eclectic mix of energy healing therapies. These practices more clearly fall under the biblical prohibitions in Deuteronomy 18:9 – 14.

While the spiritual implications of Therapeutic Touch must be foremost in our minds, there are other concerns. Krieger has warned that patients can "overload" on Therapeutic Touch, leading to restlessness, irritability, anxiety, hostility, or pain. Others warn that it can make fevers worse or even stimulate the growth of cancer cells. Some of these effects may be due to the meditative state induced in patients, which has been known to cause problems.

Placebo effects are benefits arising from therapies that do not physically cause these effects. But adverse effects can be caused in similar nonphysical ways and are called the "nocebo effect" (see p. 40). Even if human life energy does not exist, telling people you are passing energy through them could cause negative effects.

Recommendations

Christians should spend time with those who are ill, praying for them, comforting, massaging, and laying hands on them. But they should connect their practices and motivations directly to Jesus Christ and their belief in his power, not to Therapeutic Touch — or any other therapy tied in with Eastern mystical beliefs or life energy practices. While there are superficial similarities between Therapeutic Touch and the Christian laying on of hands, these two ways of approaching spiritual healing are incompatible.

Treatment Categories

Scientifically Unproven
For any indication beyond
a placebo effect   ☹☹☹

Scientifically Questionable
For any physiological indication   ☹☹☹

Spiritual
In the hands of most practitioners   👎👎👎👎

Quackery or Fraud
In the hands of some practitioners

Further Reading

Meehan, Therese C. "Therapeutic Touch as a Nursing Intervention." *Journal of Advanced Nursing* 28, no. 1 (1998): 117–25.

O'Mathúna, Dónal P. "The Subtle Allure of Therapeutic Touch." *Journal of Christian Nursing* 15 (Winter 1998): 4–13.

_____. "Evidence-Based Practice and Reviews of Therapeutic Touch." *Journal of Nursing Scholarship* 32, no. 3 (Third Quarter 2000): 279–85.

O'Mathúna, Dónal P., and Robert L. Ashford. "Therapeutic Touch for Healing Acute Wounds." *The Cochrane Database of Systematic Reviews* 2003, no. 4.

Peters, Rosalind M. "The Effectiveness of Therapeutic Touch: A Meta-Analytic Review." *Nursing Science Quarterly* 12, no. 1 (January 1999): 52–61.

Winstead-Fry, Patricia, and Jean Kijek. "An Integrative Review and Meta-Analysis of Therapeutic Touch Research." *Alternative Therapies in Health and Medicine* 5, no. 6 (November 1999): 58–67.

T

TRADITIONAL CHINESE MEDICINE

● What It Is

When President Richard Nixon restored relations with China, taking journalists into an ancient culture they knew little about, the land and its traditions seemed both exotic and appealing. Reporters looked superficially at the unfamiliar lifestyles and created an appealing picture that lacked an explanation of the underlying philosophy. For example, there were images of young and old standing outside in parks, performing ritual movements (usually Tai Chi) that helped them remain supple and keep their balance and presumably helped them sustain mental and physical alertness. There was discussion of almost miraculous medical benefits from therapies such as acupuncture. And there was mention of a society in which moderation, balance, and harmony were the foundations of both medicine and lifestyle.

How uplifting and enlightening this all seemed to people in a culture where self-worth was sometimes determined by acquisitions. While China was in the news, the United States was starting to struggle with the beliefs that led to the bumper sticker, "He who dies with the most toys wins." Some churches were struggling with the idea of prosperity theology, which in its simplest form stated that God blesses good people with health and wealth. Of course, by this standard, Jesus Christ himself was a failure. Society was starting to find its modern lifestyle unsatisfying — not to mention unhealthy. And now here was a Chinese culture that didn't have all the mate-

rial benefits but appeared to have a better grasp on life in general. The attraction was immediate.

Medicine in the United States has since become embroiled in debates over the affordability of medical care, the value of health maintenance organizations, and the competition among hospitals to acquire the latest, ultraexpensive diagnostic technology. How seductively appealing, then, were the concepts of traditional Chinese medicine (TCM) that seemed to focus on wellness and harmony. Soon some of the practices were being introduced into wellness centers throughout the United States, and people were talking about the miracles of acupuncture, herbal treatments, and the like.

That first flush of excitement is more than a generation in the past, and we can talk objectively about a subject that has long been misunderstood. Written records about TCM date to between 200 BC and AD 100 in *The Yellow Emperor's Classic of Internal Medicine*. This book demonstrates that TCM is not just about physical health but is intertwined with Taoism, the ancient Chinese philosophy and religion. The moderation, balance, and harmony concepts of TCM are part of a deeply spiritual system quite removed from Christianity. To wholly embrace TCM is to accept a religion fundamentally at odds with what most Christians believe to be the Word of God.

Many who were drawn to TCM were not concerned about these inconsistent religious ideas. Many say Christianity is just another expression of Western greed and selfishness and pride. Yet what they rejected was often not an accurate representation of Christian faith. Materialism and selfishness are as erroneous for Christians as they are for those who adhere to Taoism, the underlying faith of TCM. Instead of embracing TCM, those Christians who were appalled by the inequity and materialism of their day should have worked to restore biblical values as given in God's Word. Unfortunately for many, that did not happen.

Just as Christianity was rejected in part because of its misrepresentation, TCM was embraced, to some degree, by accepting some misconceptions about it — some of which have remained to this day. It is important to clarify some of these by looking in detail at how TCM views life.

The ancient Chinese — and contemporary practitioners of TCM — believe that all of life is made up of opposites called *yin* and *yang*. Each needs the other, and they must always be in balance. Night and day, winter and summer — everything must come into balance with *yin* and *yang*. But just as day must adjust by shortening during the winter months, and night must shorten during the summer months, so *yin* and *yang* are constantly making adjustments to maintain harmony.

The body's internal organs are also said to have *yin* and *yang*. *Yin* organs are for storage; *yang* for elimination. A few parts of the body, such as the brain and blood vessels, have both *yin* and *yang* functions.

As there is stress or relaxation, subtle adaptations take place. So long as the *yin* and *yang* are in proper interrelationship, good health is assured. But when *yin* and *yang* cannot adapt and adjust, illness occurs.

TCM goes further. It teaches that the body has an invisible vital energy called *chi* or *qi* (both pronounced CHEE). *Chi* is a mix of inherited energy, passed from parents to children at the time of con-

ception, and energy derived from the food and air that sustain us throughout life. *Chi* is transported along an elaborate system of energy meridians, also invisible. As long as *chi* is flowing properly, you are said to be in good health. Disease occurs when the flow is interrupted.

There is a great deal more to TCM, too much to describe in any depth here. The major misconception regarding TCM in the West is that it involves the same general approach as conventional medicine except with the addition of such therapies as acupressure or acupuncture, breathing techniques, exercise regimens such as Tai Chi or Qigong, and some Chinese herbs. That is not the case. TCM is a completely different approach to health and life. Its beliefs are often in conflict with both the science of conventional medicine and the theology of the Bible. A complete shift in worldview is needed to fully embrace TCM.

Ironically, even the Chinese people had moved away from TCM until fairly recently. Over the centuries, its practice had waned in many parts of China. After the Cultural Revolution of Mao Tse-tung in 1949, TCM was revived, partly to reestablish Chinese culture and partly to cope with lack of availability of Western medicine during the years when China was closed to the outside world.

Practically, traditional Chinese doctors engage in extensive interviews with patients when they first visit them. In addition to asking questions, TCM practitioners make note of a patient's voice and breathing, as these are believed to be central to the movement of *chi* through the body. A physical exam may include smelling the patient's body, noting his or her "spirit" or overall complexion, and checking the tongue, which is believed to be the surface indicator of internal organ health.

Another distinctive diagnostic approach is pulse diagnosis. Conventional medicine uses the pulse to monitor the heart rate, but TCM uses it to monitor the flow of *chi*. Nine different pulses using different pressures are taken, the results believed to provide information about different organs. Iridology is another diagnostic approach, where the iris of the eye is examined for evidence of the health of organs throughout the body.

The primary goal of TCM is to restore or maintain a balanced flow of *chi* throughout the body. This is accomplished using a variety of therapies, all of which are chosen because of their expected impact on *chi*. Acupuncture is believed to work when needles are inserted into specific acupoints in the meridians, improving the flow of *chi*. The meridians do not correspond to nerves, blood vessels, or any other system known to science. Herbal remedies, moxibustion (the burning of the herb moxa), cupping (the placing of a cup over the injured area to create suction), acupressure, yoga, Tai Chi, and Qigong are all encouraged with a view to restoring balance between *yin* and *yang* and promoting the flow of *chi*.

Traditional Chinese medicine appears to have much in common with the contemporary concept of holism. More than two thousand years ago, traditional Chinese physicians began stressing moderation in all things and the importance of being in harmony, both with one's body and with nature. They stressed wellness, in part because they received money only if patients stayed healthy.

Claims

Traditional Chinese medicine is promoted as a complete health care system able to care for and treat all the health needs of patients. However, Westerners usually use it as a source of complementary therapies for promotion of health. While TCM uses all the diagnostic procedures and therapies, Western use often takes various TCM therapies in isolation. Thus, the claims made for acupuncture are usually made in isolation from the rest of TCM (a practice that would not happen in its original Chinese setting).

Study Findings

Research studies are usually based on one particular therapy, not the whole TCM system. Several of these therapies have been discussed separately in this book. Some aspects of TCM, such as acupuncture for certain types of pain, or Tai Chi as an exercise regimen, are producing beneficial results. Some Chinese herbal remedies, such as red yeast rice, are showing promise.

However, much of the system remains untested and unproven. A search of Chinese journals found reports of about three thousand randomized controlled trials of TCM. Over 90 percent of these were for proprietary TCM herbal mixtures that were compared with another remedy of unknown effectiveness. Most were short, incomplete reports leaving practitioners with little clear guidance.

One way to test TCM as a system is to compare the diagnoses and recommendations of different practitioners. A 2005 controlled study (✗✗✗) compared the recommendations of three TCM practitioners who each examined the same forty rheumatoid arthritis patients. On average, the TCM diagnoses were in agreement 31.7 percent of the time, which was no better than chance agreement. Similarly, the herbal remedies recommended to treat the conditions were in agreement 35 percent of the time. The practitioners were free to use any TCM diagnostic method and used pulse diagnosis 86.7 percent of the time. Similar variability has been found in several studies (✖✖✖) and demonstrates the highly subjective nature of TCM diagnosis and prescription.

Cautions

TCM is based on centuries of folk use, with little clinical evidence to support its claims as a medical system. The system promotes many therapies and diagnostic procedures of questionable value. Promotion of therapies on the basis of traditional widespread use has resulted in much harm throughout human history. When those therapies are all a culture has, their use is understandable but tragic. When other effective and safe therapies are available, TCM therapies need not be chosen and should not be promoted.

Questionable diagnostic approaches are likely to miss real illnesses and proclaim the presence of problems that may not exist. This causes pain and suffering that are avoidable. While some Western practitioners are lauding TCM as a better approach to health care, Chinese practitioners of TCM are adding Western procedures, such as surgery and pharmaceuticals. They retain the underlying religious beliefs of their culture, but when it comes to the delivery of health care, they are recognizing and adopting better approaches.

Physical harm can result from herbal remedies that contain toxic instead of beneficial herbs or from contamination of herbal products. TCM herbal products are unregulated in the United States, making them vulnerable to lax manufacturing and packaging standards. Quality is not consistent.

On top of the physical harm, psychological harm can result from involvement in consciousness-altering practices such as yoga, meditation, and Qigong. Finally, the spiritual harm that can result from introducing people to a religion other than Christianity cannot be minimized. While some of the underlying beliefs of TCM are compatible with biblical teachings, the central beliefs are different. Many of these therapies introduce practitioners to the occult realm, with all the dangers associated with demonic involvement.

Recommendations

Some of the general approaches to health within TCM are compatible with both Christianity and conventional medicine. The emphasis on balance through diet, exercise, and stress reduction is preferable to the fast-paced, high-stress Western lifestyle. Some particular therapies used for specific conditions have been shown to be of value. However, other TCM therapies recommended for specific ailments are often untested by Western standards, and some that have been tested are ineffective. Since these introduce people to Eastern religious ideas, without evidence of benefit, there seems to be little justification for their use, especially by Christians.

Treatment Categories

Complementary

Specific aspects of TCM (diet, exercise, etc.) can be useful.

Specific therapies for specific indications can be useful (see specific therapies).

Scientifically Unproven

As a medical system for preventive health care or therapy

Scientifically Questionable

To prevent or treat specific illnesses and diseases

Spiritual

In the hands of many practitioners 👎 👎 👎

● Further Reading

Cassileth, Barrie R. *The Alternative Medicine Handbook.* New York: W. W. Norton, 1998, 28 – 34.

Tang, Jin-Ling, Si-Yan Zhan, and Edzard Ernst. "Review of Randomised Controlled Trials of Traditional Chinese Medicine." *BMJ* 319 (July 1999): 160 – 61.

Zhang, Grant G., Wenlin Lee, Barker Bausell, Lixing Lao, Barry Handwerger, and Brian Berman. "Variability in the Traditional Chinese Medicine (TCM) Diagnoses and Herbal Prescriptions Provided by Three TCM Practitioners for 40 Patients with Rheumatoid Arthritis." *Journal of Alternative and Complementary Medicine* 11, no. 3 (June 2005): 415 – 21.

VISUALIZATION OR GUIDED IMAGERY

● What It Is

Mind-body medicine is based on the assumption that the mind can be used to influence physical conditions. Visualization describes a range of techniques by which the mind is used to influence the body. People usually sit or lie comfortably, close their eyes, and imagine some relaxing scene or image. As you picture yourself sinking into a relaxing environment, your body follows your mind and tension floats away.

Guided imagery can be done in groups or individually. Someone, either in person or recorded, describes an image to help others visualize a relaxing scene. Music is often added to enhance the setting. The assumption is that as the mind relaxes, the body will follow. Recent popularity in guided imagery stems from a method described by Roberto Assagioli in a popular book, *The Act of Will*, published in 1980.

Visualization can also be more active, as when athletes visualize themselves running the last lap of a race perfectly or hitting the ball with perfect form. Going through the behavior in one's mind is believed to improve the actions themselves. Some research has found a muscle reaction that matches what an athlete visualizes ahead of time. It is believed that the muscle memory from the visualization may help an athlete perform better if competition takes place shortly after the visualization technique.

Visualization in healing is somewhat similar. By imagining the cells and tissues of the body working optimally, some maintain that the cells will start to act this way and thus bring about enhanced healing. The Simonton visualization method, for example, is a popular technique whereby patients visualize their bodies' cells fighting and consuming cancer cells.

A number of alternative therapies incorporate more sinister forms of visualization. Some incorporate visualization as a way to find guidance from one's inner self or to contact spirit guides. A famous experiment described in a book called *Conjuring Up*

Philip started by having people "create" a person named Philip who had certain well-defined characteristics. In séances they visualized contacting this person and soon were receiving communications from him. This experiment is touted as evidence of the power of visualization, yet few mention the possibility that they may have contacted a spirit who was willing to play their game. Visualization can be an innocent way to relax or an occult activity.

● Claims

Visualization is said to be a way to improve performance, change behavior, cause relaxation, and relieve pain. While a medical resident at Duke University, Walt was taught visualization as a method for self-treating his severe migraine headaches — and found it quite effective. But others teach it as a way to directly cause healing, send life energy, or contact spirits. The more controversial aspects are tied in with the New Age and postmodern belief that people can create reality. Well-known proponents of Eastern healing techniques Shakya Zangpo and Georg Feuerstein say, "The thoughts and images that we hold in our minds are not just abstract, ineffectual ideas or neurons firing in our brains. They actively shape reality." As such, visualization is believed to demonstrate the power of the mind to change physical reality, including the body.

● Study Findings

Imagining things in our minds does cause physical responses. If we visualize food, we'll feel saliva beginning to flow; if we remember a scary situation, our hearts pump faster. Both of us were competitive athletes, and thinking of those days still causes our bodies to respond physically. Similarly, when we picture ourselves in our most relaxing hideaway, our bodies relax.

Research on guided imagery has focused mostly on whether such relaxation relieves pain. A 1999 review (✓✓) found "preliminary evidence" of effectiveness in this area. Better evidence published since then continues to support that conclusion. For example, one study (✓✓✓) enrolled 350 people who suffered from chronic tension headaches. Those who listened to a guided imagery audiotape daily for one month had significantly fewer and less severe headaches than a control group. Another study found that guided imagery did not reduce the frequency or severity of migraine headaches, but people using it reported an improved ability to cope with the headaches compared to a control group (✓✓✓). The number of studies in this area remains small, and a 2004 systematic review found that the benefit is relatively short-lasting. After five to seven weeks, the effectiveness of visualization on chronic pain decreased noticeably (✗✗✗).

Generalized relaxation responses and physiological reactions are very different from specific claims that visualizing cells fighting a disease will cause them to be more effective. Lots of anecdotal evidence (✓) backs up these types of claims. However, a number of well-designed but uncontrolled studies (✗✗) have found that while relaxation is produced, there is no evidence that visualization lessens any disease or complements other treatments.

● Cautions

Clearly, using visualization to call up spirits is prohibited in the Bible. Going deeper into one's own psyche can have adverse effects, just as occurs sometimes with meditation. Zangpo and Feuerstein, cited

V

above, who are not Christians but rather proponents of visualization and Eastern religions, claim, "By naively adopting certain visualization practices, we may well endanger our mental and physical health not only in this lifetime *but in future embodiments as well.* . . . Even if a person does not suffer any adverse side effects now, the connection with the lower realms has been made and will take effect in the future" (emphasis in original).

Recommendations

Visualization of neutral images — a peaceful brook, a flower garden, even a relaxing pattern — can be a helpful way to relax. Certain types of pain, especially those connected with stress and anxiety, can be relieved by guided imagery. Visualization may be a useful adjunct in professional counseling. However, there is no evidence to show that visualization itself helps cure any illness or bring about faster healing. Use of visualization to contact our "inner selves" or the spiritual realm is prohibited biblically — and dangerous. If visualization is recommended, ask for a complete description of what will be involved before participating. Avoid practitioners likely to involve other New Age therapies or practices.

Treatment Categories

Complementary
To promote relaxation ☺☺☺☺
To relieve tension-related pain ☺☺☺☺
To relieve acute pain ☺☺

Scientifically Unproven
For long-term relief of pain ☹☹

Scientifically Questionable
To treat or cure any illness ☹☹☹

Spiritual
In the hands of some practitioners 👎👎

Further Reading

Van Kuiken, Debra. "A Meta-analysis of the Effect of Guided Imagery Practice on Outcomes." *Journal of Holistic Nursing* 22, no. 2 (June 2004): 164 – 79.

Zangpo, Shakya, and Georg Feuerstein. "The Risks of Visualization: Growing Roots Can Be Dangerous." *The Quest* (Summer 1995): 26 – 31, 84.

YOGA

What It Is

Yoga in the United States has frequently been presented as a gentle exercise and relaxation therapy. It is frequently taught at health clubs, senior citizen centers, adult education programs, and similar locations. And it is increasingly available in Christian churches. It is also used for stress management and may be recommended to business executives.

However, yoga is more than an exercise program. The word *yoga* literally means "union." As an integral part of Hindu religion, it implies union with the "divine." It is fundamentally a spiritual exercise designed to bring spiritual enlightenment.

Yoga incorporates both *asanas* (physical postures) and *pranayamas* (breathing exercises). The *asanas* are assumed to relax the body and the mind and bring them into spiritual harmony. The *pranayamas*, while focused on physical breathing, are designed to regulate the flow of *prana*, the Hindu term for life energy. The exercises are to help bring a person into a meditative state from which union with the Great Unconscious occurs, leading to spiritual enlightenment.

Advancement in yoga is expected to bring moral and character changes, with the ultimate goal being the realization of one's divine nature. Given these Eastern roots, yoga is a deeply religious practice.

However, yoga is viewed by many as simply a set of breathing and posture exercises designed to improve strength and flexibility and promote relaxation. The different exercises address breathing, movement, and posture. Certain movements are done while exhaling, others while inhaling. The breathing is coordinated to help maintain various postures.

Different forms of yoga exist, each with its own set of positions of varying difficulty. The form most commonly practiced in the West is called "hatha yoga."

Claims

Most commonly, yoga is promoted as a way to reduce stress, increase flexibility, and promote better blood circulation. Other claims have been made that yoga can relieve back and neck pain and treat epilepsy and asthma.

Those committed to the spiritual roots of yoga claim it leads to spiritual enlightenment and union with the divine. The pinnacle of such enlightenment is called "Kundalini arousal." In Hindu mythology, Kundalini is the serpent goddess who rests at the base of the spine. When aroused, the serpent travels up the spine, activating a person's *prana* and clearing the person's *chakras* ("energy transformers"). The latter action releases psychic abilities, including healing powers. Ultimately, Kundalini reaches the head *chakra* that opens practitioners to enlightenment from occult sources and spirit guides.

Study Findings

Clinical research (✔✔✔) shows that yoga exercises can improve physical fitness. Studies (✔✔✔✔) have shown it can reduce stress and help relieve chronic pain. Numerous studies have been done with yoga

271

for specific conditions, but many of them have had methodological flaws. A few small studies examined the impact of yoga on asthmatic patients. The entry on Breathing Techniques gives more detail, but the results have been inconsistent (✓✓). Overall, these studies have not been able to determine whether any beneficial effects came from the stress reduction and breathing exercises or from the life energy and spiritual nature of yoga.

An important point to keep in mind when evaluating these studies is that the benefits came only with sustained, regular practice. The most encouraging study had asthmatic patients practice yoga daily for one hour for six weeks. If yoga is practiced less consistently or for shorter periods of time, there will most likely be less benefit, if any at all.

Cautions

Yoga, it must be remembered, does not cure illness. Using it in place of effective conventional therapies may exacerbate problems. If people believe yoga and meditation can prevent diseases, they may resist seeking help for serious illnesses until the disease has progressed too far. In addition, some of the postures and the physical exertion may cause physical problems. As with any exercise program, people should ensure they have no underlying health problems and start slowly.

The spiritual dimensions of yoga must also be kept in mind. People who start yoga as a form of exercise may find themselves exposed to its religious teachings. Gradually, people may find themselves seeking the spiritual enlightenment that yoga was originally designed to produce. Apart from the spiritual dangers, intense involvement with Eastern spiritual practices is known to cause psychological and emotional problems. People who have progressed to the point of Kundalini experiences have been known to have psychotic breakdowns.

Recommendations

Yoga is an alternative therapy that raises difficult questions for Christians. The physical and breathing exercises taught in yoga classes may improve general well-being. However, as a deeply religious practice with the goal of union with the divine, it is antithetical to biblical Christianity.

In spite of its reputation as a simple calisthenics program, reports of physical and spiritual harm continue to surface. A debate between Christian practitioners and opponents of yoga was triggered by Holly Robaina's 2005 article in *Today's Christian Woman*. The author interviewed a woman who was introduced to destructive beliefs through yoga. Robaina noted that terms commonly used in "secular" yoga have religious meanings. The "salute to the sun" posture used to begin many classes pays homage to the Hindu sun god, and *namaste*, used to end yoga classes, literally means "I bow to the God within you."

However, a faithful user of yoga responded that her faith in Christ is invigorated by yoga. As she goes through the positions, she reflects on Christ and his character. While some people's faith may be too weak to resist the temptation to explore the worldview behind yoga, this person's faith is strong and she claims she benefits from yoga. Robaina responded that the bottom line is not whether we are strong enough to practice yoga but whether we should refrain from yoga for the sake of those who may be too weak to withstand its spiritual lure (1 Corinthians 8:12 – 13).

We agree with Robaina's view. There may not be clear reasons for Christians to condemn all forms of yoga. Some people may be able to practice it beneficially and without spiritual problems. But the results are not all that matter. Paul gives some helpful advice in 1 Corinthians 6:12: "'Everything is permissible for me' — but not everything is beneficial." Given its origin and the potential for spiritual problems, the burden rests with the yoga advocate to demonstrate why this form of exercise should be chosen when so many other breathing, exercise, and stretching routines exist that have no spiritual underpinnings.

Treatment Categories

Complementary

To improve flexibility	☺☺☺☺
To improve physical fitness	☺☺☺
To reduce stress	☺☺☺
To relieve chronic pain	☺☺
To relieve asthma	☺☺

Scientifically Unproven

To treat or cure any illness

Spiritual

By nature and in the hands
of most practitioners ☞☞☞☞

Further Reading

Cassileth, Barrie R. *The Alternative Medicine Handbook.* New York: W. W. Norton, 1998.

Robaina, Holly Vicente. "The Truth about Yoga." *Today's Christian Woman* 27, no. 2 (March/April 2005): 40. *Christianity Today: www.christianitytoday.com/ tcw/2005/002/14.40.html.* Accessed September 16, 2005.

_____. "Take a Pass on Yoga." Posted June 7, 2005. *Christianity Today: www.christianitytoday.com/ct/ 2005/123/22.0.html.* Accessed September 16, 2005.

Tennant, Agnieszka. "Yes to Yoga." Posted May 19, 2005. *Christianity Today: www.christianitytoday.com/ct/ 2005/120/42.0.html.* Accessed September 16, 2005.

PART THREE

Herbal Remedies, Vitamins, and Dietary Supplements

CHAPTER 9

REVIEWS
OF REMEDIES

Herbal remedies, vitamins, and dietary supplements differ from the therapies covered in Part 2 in that most are consumed orally, though some are applied topically. Many occur naturally. They are used mainly in the same ways that people take pharmaceutical drugs (prescription or over-the-counter products) and should be viewed more like drugs and medicines instead of the way many people view them today.

Many people take herbal remedies, vitamins, and dietary supplements thinking they are mild ways to improve health. Eighty-six percent of those surveyed in 2002 believed that if a product was natural, this meant it was safe (*www.nclnet.org/naturalpr0102. htm*). Sometimes they are, but not always. The big problem in the United States is the lack of regulation and standards for these products. What's listed on the label is not necessarily in the bottle. Studies

have found missing ingredients, contaminants, prescription medications in what are sold as "natural" remedies, and differences in the content of a product from different manufacturers, sometimes even from the same manufacturer.

Although we separate these products into three categories in this section, in the United States they all come under the broad term "dietary supplement," used to identify how a product is regulated, not whether it has a certain beneficial effect or is free of adverse effects. Dietary supplements in the United States are defined by the 1994 Dietary Supplement Health and Education Act as any product (other than tobacco) that contains a vitamin, mineral, herb, botanical, or amino acid; a dietary substance used to supplement the diet by increasing total dietary intake; or a concentrate, metabolite, constituent, extract, or combination of any of the above ingredients.

So long as a product does not contain an ingredient regulated as a drug prior to passage of the 1994 act, it can be considered a dietary supplement.

This section includes some vitamins but not all. The importance of appropriate levels of vitamins in the diet has long been recognized by conventional medicine. Certain vitamins are included within complementary and alternative medicine (CAM) when they are popularly recommended to treat or prevent illnesses rather than to overcome a deficiency. Those vitamins used primarily to overcome deficiencies or treat specific diseases caused by those deficiencies are not included here.

Herbal Medicine

Herbal medicine is a lot more complicated than just picking some herbs and using them. Herbal remedies are products made from plants and used to promote health or to treat illness. Such products can include plant material itself or can be material extracted from the plant in various ways. Herbal remedies can be formulated as tablets, capsules, liquids, creams, and so on, so that they look like any other medication.

Virtually all herbs are potentially dangerous — some can be fatal. Many interact in negative ways with prescription and over-the-counter medicines, foods, other herbs, vitamins, supplements, and even some lab tests. There are many variables involved with herbal remedies — in the plants themselves, in their collection, in their preparation, and in the companies that make and sell them.

The same herb can affect people differently. Age, gender, physical condition, and other factors can influence a person's response to these remedies.

The elderly, the chronically ill, and women who are pregnant or breast-feeding should never take herbal remedies without careful coordination with their physician and pharmacist. What might be harmless for some can cause serious health problems or even death for others. And children are not little adults, to be given a smaller dose. Any parent considering an herbal remedy for a child should first seek competent medical advice.

The same herb can also be recommended for completely different purposes, depending on the medical system within which an herbalist is working. In Part 2, we examined in depth some of the traditional medical systems that developed in different parts of the world. Although practitioners in these systems use herbs, their beliefs influence the way they choose which herbs to use for which conditions. This leads to four very different approaches to herbal remedies.

The Four Primary Approaches to Herbal Remedies

- **Ayurvedic Medicine:** In Ayurveda, the traditional medicine of India, the biological reactions of herbs are not a major concern. Instead, the herbs fit into a complex system of energy medicine. There are the three *doshas*, or humors, consisting of *vata* (air), *pitta* (fire), and *kapha* (water). These evolve from the five elements of air, fire, water, earth, and ether. In this belief system, herbs are divided by their taste — astringent, bitter, pungent, salty, sour, and sweet. The taste relates to their healing properties. An herbal remedy is always meant to bring balance among the elements, a concept radically different from conventional medicine.

- **Traditional Chinese Medicine:** A medical system of balance between *yin* and *yang*, traditional Chinese medicine (TCM) categorizes elements in a similar way to Ayurveda, though based on different properties. The elements within TCM include wood and metal along with earth, fire, and water. TCM practitioners believe there is a direct relationship between an herb and one of the elements. Wood is sour, metal is acrid, fire is bitter, water is salty, and earth is sweet. The herbs are chosen for their taste, for their ability to restore balance, and according to an elaborate system in which the herbs are determined to relate to specific medical ills. It is a system that is quite foreign both to scientific understanding and to Christian belief systems.

- **Herbalism:** An herb is viewed in this system either as a means of transmitting life energy or as a way of allowing "nature spirits" to impact people's health. This approach is part of many nature religions, such as shamanism, Native American religions, and witchcraft (Wicca). While some herbs containing ingredients that impact the body or mind are used, herbalism teaches that the herbs are spiritually active. Some herbalists teach that healing occurs via spirits that reside in the plants. Herbs may be chosen because of the way the plants resemble the parts of the body that are ill or diseased. Herbalism represents a religious or magical approach to herbs rather than a scientific one.

- **Herbal Medicine:** Many modern pharmaceuticals originally were derived from plants but today are primarily available in synthetic preparations. Of the four approaches to herbal remedies, herbal medicine is considered the most scientific. This approach has led to clinical research which has revealed that some herbs should be considered when treating certain illnesses and conditions. Because herbal products are usually slower acting than pharmaceutical equivalents, patients who rely on conventional medicine are more likely to try herbs for conditions that last for years (chronic conditions such as asthma, low back pain, fibromyalgia, etc.) rather than for short-term illnesses.

The approach to herbal remedies used in this book will be in keeping with herbal medicine. When discussing an herbal remedy, we will not usually describe how it might be used within the other herbal systems. We have searched for the best evidence available regarding the effectiveness and safety of each herbal remedy. We have looked for controlled clinical trials that have tested the remedies as they are used to treat various conditions. We base our recommendations primarily on that evidence, when it is available.

Be Careful with Names

One big caution: look-alike drug names and doctors' bad handwriting have led to medication mix-ups in conventional medicine that have caused complications and even deaths.

The same problem of look-alike names exists with herbal remedies. Plants have both *common* names (e.g., feverfew) and one universally accepted two-part scientific Latin name (feverfew is *Tanacetum parthenium*). The first word gives the plant's genus, the second its species. Unfortunately, the same species of plant can have numerous common names, and sometimes the same common name refers to several totally different species. For example, the herbal remedy echinacea can be made from a number of different species: *Echinacea purpurea*, *Echinacea pallida*, or *Echinacea angustifolia*. The effect of each species is somewhat different, and no one knows if they have the same strength even when they act in the same way.

Occasionally a scientific name needs to be changed after scientists realize a plant was not classified correctly. As a result, the same plant can be referred to with more than one scientific name. Chamomile is a good example. It is most commonly identified as *Matricaria recutita*, but the same species has also been called *Matricaria chamomilla*, *Chamomilla recutita*, and a number of other Latin names.

Adding to the confusion on chamomile is the fact that some view chamomile as the same as yarrow. Yarrow (*Achillea millefolium*) is the European variety. And European yarrow was thought to be the same as the American variety, which now turns out to be a separate species (*Achillea lanulosa*). You get the idea.

Vitamins and supplements can have the same problem. For example, vitamin E comes in a variety of forms, known chemically as tocopherols. Some (specifically alpha-tocopherol) have been shown to be important for human health. There are natural (*d*-alpha-tocopherol) and synthetic (*dl*-alpha-tocopherol) forms. Gamma tocopherol may be the most potent but is not available in supplement form. Others have not even been studied. Yet they all are called vitamin E.

The supplement glucosamine also comes in different forms — glucosamine hydrochloride, N-acetyl glucosamine, and glucosamine sulfate — three completely different chemicals, although in all likelihood they have similar effects on the body. They all release glucosamine; however, they vary in how quickly and where the glucosamine is made available. That affects how well it is absorbed into the body and how quickly it will have its effects.

When referring to herbs, most people use the common English name. But even these common names can vary enormously from country to country — and sometimes even within different parts of the same country. And we have not even discussed brand names! Most herbs are now available in several brands made by different companies. Given how rapidly name brands come and go, however, we will not name specific products. It is important for you to check the labels for the specific species used in the preparation.

In our descriptions of herbal remedies, we'll try to make sense of the names by listing all of the most common names for an herb. We want to help you make wise decisions about what you should buy — and should *not* buy. We'll let you know which remedies are effective and which are not. We've also added a new symbol to highlight serious adverse effects, even if the remedy is effective. Whenever you're considering an alternative medicine remedy, remember these tips:

1. Know the specific scientific name for any herb or supplement as well as the common name.
2. Know which part of the plant has shown the best evidence for effectiveness (root, leaves, flowers, stem, or whole plant), and find a brand that specifies which part is used.
3. Don't trust the label on the bottle. The list of ingredients is no guarantee that the product actually contains those ingredients. Find products that state they have been independently tested, and verify those claims by visiting the websites of independent testing labs.

4. Choose brands on which (a) research has been conducted and (b) when possible independent quality testing has been performed. At times these will be European brands that are now becoming available in the United States.

Quality of Herbal Remedies and Dietary Supplements

A number of studies have found serious problems with the quality of dietary supplements, including herbal remedies that are available in the United States and around the world. Many studies have found that the concentrations on labels do not correlate at all with the quantities in the tablets or capsules. A study of Ayurvedic herbal remedies bought in the Boston area found that one in five products contained heavy metals such as lead, mercury, and arsenic. If used according to the labels, a person would ingest up to three times the EPA-recommended maximum dose. Several studies have found prescription drugs added to herbal remedies.

For these reasons, a small number of organizations are providing independent tests of the quality of herbal remedies and dietary supplements. One such company is ConsumerLab.com, which tests the most popular brands of dietary supplements, herbs, and vitamins. Their findings are sometimes very troubling. The lab found that a high percentage of products didn't contain the amount of key ingredients that the packages claimed. In some cases, the amount of active ingredient was *much* lower, which is a waste of your money. And some were much too high, which could be dangerous to your health.

To find out which products pass muster, consider subscribing to the ConsumerLab.com website (*www. consumerlab.com*). Their approach has some limita-

tions, since no one knows the active ingredients in some herbs. So even if the stated amount of an ingredient is in the product, that might not be the compound that makes the herb work. ConsumerLab. com reports on what's *in* a product, not whether that product is effective.

Another organization that evaluates supplements is the United States Pharmacopeia (USP) — an independent, not-for-profit organization. The USP-verified mark represents that USP has rigorously tested and verified the supplement to assure the following: (1) what's on the label is in fact in the bottle — all the listed ingredients are present and are in the declared amounts; (2) the supplement does not contain harmful levels of contaminants; (3) the supplement will break down and release the ingredients in the body; and (4) the supplement has been made under good manufacturing practices. This program has the advantage of ongoing testing of products to ensure continued compliance with the standards.

Products that pass the quality standards of ConsumerLab.com or USP or some other organization (e.g., *Good Housekeeping*) give manufacturers the opportunity to put the testing organization's Seal of Approval on their labels. For dietary supplements and herbal remedies, companies can voluntarily submit their products to be tested by these organizations. Those products that pass the rigorous testing process and stores that carry them are listed on the websites of the organizations (*www.usp.org/USPverified* or *www. consumerlab.com*). A small number of other organizations are developing similar quality assessment programs.

The entries in this part of the book will include recommended dosages. Often these are only educated guesses because of a lack of evidence. The safe and effective dose may also vary, depending on what other herbal remedies, dietary supplements, or pharmaceutical products are taken at the same time. For this reason, it is crucial to consult a health care professional before taking any remedies — natural or synthetic. Make sure you inform him or her about everything you are taking. When we can, we will give the doses in quantities of active ingredients. The units will be in grams. Note that 1 gram (g) weighs the same as 1000 milligrams (mg), which weighs the same as 1,000,000 micrograms (mcg). Doses given in mcg are therefore very small: 1 mcg = 0.001 mg = 0.000001 g.

Rating Scales

The following descriptions of the various herbal remedies, vitamins, and dietary supplements list what is known about each, the claims being made, the data available from high-quality research, the cautions, and our overall recommendations. We will use the abbreviated term "remedies" to describe this broad category. Each of the remedies listed is rated for effectiveness and safety. For a full explanation of the criteria used in rating the herbs, vitamins, and supplements, see pages 118 – 19.

Here, briefly, are the keys to the symbols we use.

Evidence for Using Remedies

If the evidence being discussed shows a remedy has benefit, we rated the *evidence* (the type of study itself) using a score of one to four ✓ symbols. The number of symbols was assigned according to the following criteria based on the amount of evidence and the type of evidence supporting the therapy.

Symbol	Type of Evidence
✓✓✓✓	Multiple high-quality randomized controlled trials demonstrate the efficacy and safety of this therapy.
✓✓✓	At least one randomized controlled trial or multiple nonrandomized trials support the efficacy and safety of this therapy.
✓✓	Nonrandomized series or numerous case reports in the peer-reviewed medical literature support the efficacy and safety of this therapy.
✓	Anecdotal evidence exists to support the efficacy and safety of this therapy.

Evidence Against Using Remedies

Studies can also provide evidence that a remedy should not be used for a particular condition. Those results could be evidence of either a lack of effectiveness or of harmful effects. To represent these sorts of studies, we developed a similar scale of one to four ✕ symbols. If the studies showed either no benefit, the potential for harm, or actual harm, we rated the *evidence* (not the potential for harm) using the following criteria:

Symbol	Type of Evidence
✕✕✕✕	Multiple high-quality randomized controlled trials demonstrate the lack of benefit or the significant potential for harm with this therapy.
✕✕✕	At least one randomized controlled trial or multiple nonrandomized trials support the lack of benefit or the significant potential for harm with this therapy.
✕✕	Nonrandomized series or numerous case reports in the peer-reviewed medical literature support the lack of benefit or the significant potential for harm with this therapy.
✕	Anecdotal evidence exists to support the lack of benefit or the significant potential for harm with this therapy.

Overall Recommendation Scale

As more research has been conducted, studies sometimes produced conflicting evidence. Therefore, we compiled the results of all the studies we located into a single guide. This rating scale is *our* "best estimate" of, or confidence in, a product's potential for physical benefit or harm for particular conditions. When a remedy is commonly used for a number of indications, we have developed separate recommendations. All of these are presented in the Treatment Categories section.

Overall Recommendation	Criteria
☺☺☺☺	75% – 100% confidence that the therapy is potentially beneficial (the potential benefits outweigh the risks)
☺☺☺	50% – 74% confidence that the therapy is potentially beneficial
☺☺	25% – 49% confidence that the therapy is potentially beneficial
☺	0% – 24% confidence that the therapy is potentially beneficial
☹	0% – 24% confidence that the therapy is of no benefit or potentially harmful (the risks outweigh the potential benefits)
☹☹	25% – 49% confidence that the therapy is of no benefit or potentially harmful
☹☹☹	50% – 74% confidence that the therapy is of no benefit or potentially harmful
☹☹☹☹	75% – 100% confidence that the therapy is of no benefit or potentially harmful

One of the new features in this expanded edition is a visual warning in the Treatment Categories sections, using one to four ⊘ symbols to highlight the risk of serious side effects. Even if evidence supports the effectiveness of a remedy, the risk of serious adverse effects may make its use unwarranted. If an entry has any of these symbols, read the Cautions section for that remedy carefully.

Categories of Remedies

Each remedy also is categorized to define how it can be viewed according to our present knowledge. Some fit into several categories. See pages 29 – 31 for definitions and explanations of the categories.

- Conventional
- Complementary
- Scientifically Unproven
- Scientifically Questionable
- Spiritual
- Quackery or Fraud

Further Reading

At the end of each remedy's entry, we list recommended further reading. We have used many resources to come to our overall conclusions. We would highly recommend three in particular for their thorough reviews of the clinical evidence regarding effectiveness and safety. We used all three with all remedies, so we won't list them again with each entry. The Cochrane Library systematic reviews are available in both detailed versions for health care professionals and as consumer summaries. The book by Fetrow and Avila is useful for health care professionals with direct patient contact and is designed to fit into a white-coat pocket. The third resource, the Natural Database, is not only thorough, but its Internet version is updated daily — ideal for those with clinical questions regarding remedies.

Cochrane Library. Available at *www.cochrane.org*.

Fetrow, Charles W., and Juan R. Avila. *Professional's Handbook of Complementary and Alternative Medicine.* 3rd ed. New York: Lippincott, Williams & Wilkins, 2003.

Jellin, Jeff M., Forrest Batz, and Kathy Hichens. *Pharmacist's Letter/Prescriber's Letter: Natural Medicines Comprehensive Database.* Stockton, Calif.: Therapeutic Research Facility. Also available by subscription at *www.naturaldatabase.com*.

ALOE

What It Is

Aloe vera is one of the most familiar of all the medicinal herbs. Of the more than three hundred species of aloe, only four are believed to have medicinal properties. The most potent medicinal effects are believed to come from *Aloe vera* (also called *Aloe barbadensis*), which is frequently produced in gel form.

Aloe is a drought-resistant succulent (a plant that retains juice in the leaves and stems) found in warm regions. The aloes mentioned in the Bible (Numbers 24:6; Psalm 45:8; Proverbs 7:17; Song of Songs 4:14; John 19:39) are actually fragrant woods burned as incense — unrelated to what is now called aloe.

Aloe has been known for its medicinal properties since at least 2100 BC. Many famous ancient healers wrote about aloe use by women for skin health or by soldiers to treat wounds. During the eighteenth and nineteenth centuries, aloe was one of the most popular prescribed and over-the-counter medicines.

Claims

Hand lotions frequently contain aloe. Some razor blades have a thin strip of aloe on them, and aloe is a common ingredient in many shaving creams. One reason: external use of aloe softens the skin. Aloe has been used for centuries in virtually every warm region of the world primarily as a topical preparation for cuts, burns, and skin diseases including acne, eczema, rosacea, psoriasis, and skin ulcers. Aloe is also used for dry skin, inflammation, itching, and hives.

Aloe has been taken internally for inner cleansing (gel or juice), irritable bowel syndrome and a variety of other gastrointestinal disorders (including ulcers, colic, and colitis), asthma, sinus congestion or cold, depression, diabetes, multiple sclerosis, seizures, menstrual complaints, and osteoarthritis — and also as a general tonic. It is used as a laxative (aloe latex), as an aid in elimination when a patient suffers from anal fissures or hemorrhoids, and for relief after rectal surgery.

Study Findings

Aloe gel contains a number of polysaccharides (complex sugars) that have moisturizing and soothing properties. Hence the inclusion of aloe vera in many cosmetics. In animal studies, topical preparations of aloe have been shown to promote wound healing and kill a variety of microorganisms. Aloe has been shown to produce anti-inflammatory and analgesic effects. Aloe contains a number of vitamins, including A, C, and E, and has been shown to contain magnesium lactate, which blocks histamine (which can cause pain and itching in the skin). Aloe also contains salicylic acid, the main constituent of aspirin. However, a small number of controlled studies (✖✖✖) of chronic wounds in humans found either no benefit from aloe gel or delayed wound healing.

Aloe gel contains compounds called "anthroquinones" that are known to be effective as laxatives (✔✔). Such compounds act by irritating the intestinal tract. Preliminary data suggests that aloe taken orally may reduce blood sugar levels. However, this is based on case reports and uncontrolled trials (✓✓).

Cautions

Aloe should never be taken orally by people with abdominal obstruction, Crohn's disease, ulcerative colitis, gastroenteritis, appendicitis, ulcers, or hemorrhoids. Long-term use of oral aloe has been reported (✗✗) to cause the loss of a number of electrolytes and in rare cases has led to heart arrhythmia, edema, neuropathy, or pigmentation of the bowels. In addition, you should never use aloe orally in combination with heart or blood pressure medications unless you do so under close medical supervision. The effects of those drugs can be changed by aloe because it affects the way the body handles potassium and thus can lead to serious health crises.

Aloe should not be taken internally during pregnancy. It has been implicated (✗) in causing miscarriage. Aloe should not be used by breast-feeding women, as a chemical that can harm babies (aloe-emodin) can pass into the breast milk.

Too large an oral dose of aloe can cause abdominal cramps (✗✗), especially in children. Though this problem is not too serious, the person must use a lower dosage in the future. Given the preliminary reports of oral aloe reducing blood sugar levels, people with diabetes should consult their doctors before taking aloe.

Taking aloe latex orally at a dose of 1 gram a day has caused kidney disease (nephritis), acute renal failure, and death (✗✗).

Note: Aloe gel is not the same as aloe juice. The juice is more likely to cause adverse effects if taken orally.

Recommendations

Aloe appears (✓✓) to be safe and effective as a topical gel for moisturizing the skin and treating a variety of acute skin conditions. A small amount of evidence (✗✗) suggests that aloe is not effective with chronic skin wounds and may even delay healing.

Little scientific data is available on oral use of aloe (juice or gel). Information remains largely anecdotal. Aloe is known to be potentially dangerous for people with high blood pressure or heart disease and should be used under a doctor's close supervision by anyone with such conditions. It should never be ingested by children under twelve years of age or by women who are pregnant or lactating or who could become pregnant.

Dosage

Used topically, aloe gel is applied liberally three to five times a day as needed. Oral use is not recommended.

Treatment Categories

Complementary

Topically to relieve acute skin wounds	☺☺☺
Topically to relieve psoriasis	☺☺☺
Orally as a stimulant laxative	☺☺☺☺

Scientifically Unproven

Topically to treat acne, eczema, or rosacea	☹☹☹☹
Orally to treat any other indication	☹☹☹☹

Risk of Serious Side Effects

Gel used orally	⊘⊘
Juice used orally	⊘⊘⊘

● Further Reading

Atherton, Peter. "Aloe Vera Revisited." *British Journal of Phytotherapy* 4, no. 4 (May 1998): 85 – 92.

Eshun, Kojo, and Qian He. "Aloe Vera: A Valuable Ingredient for the Food, Pharmaceutical and Cosmetic Industries — A Review." *Critical Reviews in Food Science and Nutrition* 44, no. 2 (2004): 91 – 96.

Gallagher, Joan, and Mikel Gray. "Is Aloe Vera Effective for Healing Chronic Wounds?" *Journal of Wound, Ostomy and Continence Nursing* 30, no. 2 (March 2003): 68 – 71.

ANDROSTENEDIONE

● What It Is

Androstenedione, also called "andro," became 1998's most famous and controversial dietary supplement in the United States. That's when baseball great Mark McGwire hit more home runs than anyone else ever had in professional baseball. McGwire beat the home run record of Roger Maris. A reporter noticed bottles of androstenedione and other dietary supplements in McGwire's locker. McGwire admitted he was taking the supplements and said he believed they contributed to his peak fitness.

The use of performance-enhancing drugs by athletes has become an ethical issue from the locker room to the halls of Congress. Andro has been banned by many sports organizations (but not by major league baseball). In part due to the criticism McGwire received regarding the example he was setting for younger athletes, McGwire announced the following year that he no longer took andro. McGwire retired in 2001, but the saga culminated in his appearance before a Congressional committee in March 2005. He and five other baseball stars were asked about drug use in baseball after a tell-all book by a former professional athlete alleged rampant misuse of performance-enhancing drugs. McGwire used his legal right to refuse to answer any questions, leaving only uncertainty about the origin of his phenomenal success as an athlete.

The use of steroids by athletes, especially the extent of use, remains controversial. Most sports organizations ban the use of steroids, usually because of their dangerous side effects and the inequity in performance they artificially generate. In 1990, the Anabolic Steroids Control Act made steroids more difficult to obtain without a prescription. Doctors who had been helping some athletes buy them began refusing such nonmedical requests. In response, some athletes turned to "natural" sources of steroids, commonly known in the gym as "prohormones."

Andro is found in Mexican yams and Scotch white pine, which means it can be sold almost unrestricted as a dietary supplement in the United States. After it was announced that Mark McGwire used andro, sales of the supplement increased fivefold. As a dietary supplement, adolescents have unrestricted access to andro. The belief circulated at gyms and workout fields: if you want to hit farther, run faster, or lift more, take andro.

● Claims

Andro is one of several products promoted as a "testosterone booster" to improve sports performance, increase energy, and speed recovery from exercise. Some take it to heighten sexual arousal and function. The human body naturally manufactures a variety of steroid hormones. Naturally made androstenedione is converted in the body into other, better-known hormones such as testosterone and estradiol. Some of these hormones are believed by many to enhance athletic performance.

Androstenedione is a steroid. Steroids are hormones that have numerous effects throughout the body, including what are called "anabolic and androgenic effects." Athletes look to steroids for the anabolic effects of increased muscle mass, decreased body fat, and physical aggressiveness. They hope to avoid any of the androgenic effects, which deal with the development of male organs and male characteristics. Some men do report undesirable androgenic side effects — such as acne, breast soreness and swelling, abnormal cholesterol levels, shrinking of the testicles, behavioral changes, decreased levels of the male hormone testosterone, and an increased risk of pancreatic and prostate cancer. In women, these steroids might cause masculinization with deepening of the voice, facial hair growth, acne, genital enlargement, abnormal bleeding, male-pattern baldness, and coarsening of the skin. Female athletes from behind the Iron Curtain of communism were regularly suspected of using steroids because of how masculine some of them appeared.

Pharmaceutical researchers have made hundreds of steroids, hoping to find anabolic products without androgenic effects, but have not been completely successful.

Study Findings

In spite of andro's popularity, there is little research to support its use. The earliest use of andro was with the former East German sports establishment. They developed a short-lasting nasal spray that could be used without detection when athletes were tested for drugs at competitions.

After the Berlin Wall fell, other countries gained access to the East German research and practices, leading one group of Germans to seek a patent for androstenedione. The patent application (✓) claimed andro led to higher blood testosterone levels but gave hardly any details. All of this early research was conducted with women, whereas recent research has been with men.

The first randomized controlled trial of oral androstenedione was reported in 1999. It contained two parts, reflecting the two changes sought by athletes. In the first part, ten men were given either 100 mg of andro or a placebo. Over the next six hours, the blood androstenedione levels of those given the steroid first increased and then returned to normal. However, testosterone levels did not increase (✗✗✗) compared to those taking the placebo. Since then, four other studies using 100 or 200 mg of andro (✗✗✗) found a similar lack of change in testosterone levels. Only one, in which 300 mg of andro was taken, showed a change.

The second part of the 1999 study and four other randomized double-blind studies (✗✗✗✗) examined the impact of 100 mg of andro supplements on muscle strength and lean body composition. None of them showed significant differences between those who took andro and those who took a placebo, nor did they differ in testosterone levels. However, those taking andro had much higher levels of estrogen (an important *female* steroid) and lower HDL cholesterol levels. HDL is the "good" form of cholesterol, with lower levels being associated with heart disease. These same findings were found in all studies conducted to date (✗✗✗✗).

Cautions

Although no visible adverse effects were reported in the above studies, elevated estrogen levels have been associated with some forms of heart disease and cancer. People who naturally produce larger amounts of androstenedione have been found in some (though not all) studies (✗✗) to have a higher risk of certain cancers. The long-term effects of taking andro have not been studied. Another study found several androstenedione products contaminated with another banned steroid, raising concerns about product quality.

Also of great concern is the extent to which people will go to achieve athletic success. As former competitive athletes, both of us understand the desire to win and the lure of accomplishment and approval athletically. But for Christians, the cost of pursuing fame and wealth must be evaluated in light of God's values. This is especially important when considering the lengths to which we will go as parents to help our children achieve sports success.

A gifted athlete may gain a competitive advantage from some drugs, although not from andro. However, the cost is high in terms of what andro use teaches about the importance of winning, no matter what. The moral, ethical, and physical toll can be extremely destructive. Spiritually, the hoped-for medal and other honors can easily become false gods.

Recommendations

Almost all major sports and sports medicine organizations see no reason for using androstenedione — and a number of significant reasons to avoid it. It is banned by the National Football League, National Collegiate Athletic Association, and International Olympic Committee. The American College of Sports Medicine has called for regulatory reform because drugs such as androstenedione are so readily available. The information available on androstenedione lends no support to its alleged value as a performance-enhancing agent but does raise concerns about its potential side effects, especially when taken long-term. Dangerous side effects are a risk with long-term use of most performance-enhancing drugs. Young athletes, who will not benefit from taking andro, are actually buying into false values. Andro should not be used by women who are pregnant or lactating.

Dosage

Athletes usually take 50 to 100 mg of androstenedione twice a day about an hour before exercise or first thing in the morning.

Treatment Categories

Scientifically Unproven

To improve sports performance, increase energy, speed recovery from exercise, or heighten sexual arousal or function   ☹☹☹☹

For any other indication   ☹☹☹☹

Risk of Serious Side Effects

With any use   ⊘⊘⊘

Further Reading

O'Mathúna, Dónal P. "Androstenedione for Performance Enhancement: New Research Reveals Only Harm." *Alternative Medicine Alert* 4, no. 9 (September 2001): 103–7.

Yesalis, Charles E., III. "Medical, Legal, and Societal Implications of Androstenedione Use." *Journal of the American Medical Association* 281, no. 21 (June 1999): 2043–44.

ANTIOXIDANTS

What They Are

Antioxidants are a diverse group of compounds that prevent or delay oxidation. Oxidation is a chemical reaction in which, most commonly, oxygen atoms are added onto other compounds. A familiar example of oxidation is the rusting of iron. Oxidation reactions, which are required for life, occur in every cell of the body.

The process by which food is broken down to release its energy involves numerous oxidation reactions, which is partly why we continually need to breathe in oxygen. Many biological compounds can undergo oxidation, but this is sometimes not desired in the body. Particularly sensitive to oxidation are proteins, lipids (fatty substances that make up all cell membranes), and DNA, the chemical of our genes. While we want to oxidize our food, we don't want to oxidize these other compounds. Inappropriate oxidation can destabilize healthy molecules, leading to what is known as oxidative stress, which can cause serious health problems and may contribute to various chronic diseases and the aging process.

When oxygen reacts with other compounds in our bodies, it sometimes produces what are known as "free radicals." Free radicals are unstable and often exist for but a fraction of a second before they react in one of two ways. They may be safely disposed of by the body's natural defense mechanisms, or they may react and form other free radicals. The latter chemical reaction can cause irreversible damage. For example, free radicals are able to oxidize LDL cholesterol, the "bad" variety that allows cholesterol to adhere to artery walls, possibly clogging the arteries and hindering blood flow. Oxidized LDL is more easily taken into blood vessel walls and can contribute to heart disease by damaging the blood vessels. Other damage caused by free radicals can lead to the development of other chronic diseases and plays a part in the aging process in general. Antioxidants can both slow production of free radicals and repair damage caused by oxidation.

A number of vitamins work as antioxidants in the body. These include vitamin C, vitamin E, and beta-carotene (which is related to vitamin A). These vitamins are found in many fruits and vegetables promoted for good health — carrots, tomatoes, citrus fruits, potatoes, green peppers, cabbage, spinach, sweet potatoes, kale, broccoli, and pumpkins, among others. Other compounds that act as antioxidants are some of the remedies we discuss in this book (for example, bilberry, grape seed extract, and selenium).

Claims

Free radicals are continually produced by the body and disposed of by the body's natural antioxidants. We also have enzymes that eliminate free radicals and other enzymes that can repair some of the damage they cause. However, parts of the body will still experience some free radical damage. This problem is increased for people who smoke or work in smoke-filled environments.

Some believe that aging is caused or accelerated, at least to some extent, by the gradual accumulation of damage from free radicals. This is why antioxidants are promoted to prevent the general deterioration of aging. Other more specific benefits are also being promoted.

Probably the area of greatest interest for antioxidant use is prevention of heart disease, especially atherosclerosis (clogging of the arteries), which can lead to heart attacks. Other age-related diseases involving oxidative damage for which antioxidants are being recommended include stroke, cancer, cataracts, and Alzheimer's disease.

● Study Findings

The role of antioxidants in the prevention of heart disease has been studied for decades. One of the underlying causes of heart disease is the buildup of plaque in the arteries. This begins when cholesterol is deposited on the inside of blood vessels. Cholesterol-transporting molecules (LDLs) are oxidized, causing them to release their cholesterol into the blood vessel walls. This hardens the vessels, restricts blood flow, and sometimes leads to blockage of the arteries. While a number of surgical treatments are now available to correct this, prevention is preferable. Antioxidants prevent oxidation of LDLs in lab experiments, and now they are being studied to see if they prevent heart disease in people.

Epidemiological studies are complex surveys in which people are asked about many factors related to their health. These (✓✓) have shown, for example, that increasing the amount of vitamin E or beta-carotene in the diet is associated with a lower risk of death from heart disease. Since both are antioxidants, some view this as evidence that antioxidants protect against heart disease. However, both compounds do several things in the body, and any one of these might protect the heart. Possibly those who consume vitamin E supplements do something else (or several other things) that protects the heart. For example, they might eat more fruits and vegetables, or they might exercise more regularly. It could be any combination of these factors that provides the protection.

As we will discuss in detail in the Vitamin E entry, randomized controlled trials have failed to show that vitamin E supplements reduce the risk of heart disease (✗✗✗). Other controlled trials did not produce the hoped-for benefits with heart disease from beta-carotene, selenium, vitamin C, or vitamin E supplements (✗✗✗). Because of these results, the American Heart Association stated in 2004 that the evidence does not justify using antioxidants to reduce the risk of cardiovascular disease.

Antioxidants are also recommended to prevent cancer. However, a 2004 Cochrane review, which identified fourteen large, high-quality studies of antioxidants (vitamins A, C, and E, beta-carotene, and selenium) used to prevent gastrointestinal cancers (✗✗✗), concluded that these supplements, alone or in combination, did not prevent cancer and in some cases increased the risk of cancer. A 2005 Cochrane review (✗✗✗) found no evidence of benefit from antioxidants in treating amyotrophic lateral sclerosis (ALS). Another 2005 Cochrane review (✓✓✓) found that antioxidant supplementation by pregnant women reduced the risk of preeclampsia and low birth weight. However, the studies conducted to date were of lower quality.

These apparently contradictory results can be explained by the differences between epidemiological studies and controlled clinical trials. People whose diets include foods high in antioxidants may prevent the development of certain diseases, whereas many of the clinical trials have tried to use antioxidants to treat these diseases. Antioxidants may be of little benefit to those who have already developed these diseases. Also, the health benefits of antioxidants may arise from a broad range of several antioxidants, whereas the clinical trials usually test one or a small number of antioxidants.

The Institute of Medicine (IOM) is the body charged with setting the recommended levels of various nutrients in the diet. It is part of the National Academy of Sciences, which is a private, nonprofit society of distinguished scientists with a congressional charter to advise the federal government on scientific issues. A new set of Dietary Reference Intakes (DRIs) for antioxidants was published in 2000 by the IOM, which expanded and changed what were previously called Recommended Dietary Allowances (RDAs). The RDA is now one of four types of DRIs, with nutrients being assigned a particular DRI depending on the quality of scientific evidence available for that nutrient. The RDA is the average daily dietary intake that will meet the nutritional needs of almost all healthy individuals.

For the IOM antioxidant report, experts from the United States and Canada reviewed all of the clinical research on vitamin C, vitamin E, selenium, and the carotenoids (such as beta-carotene). Their report concluded that "it has not been possible to establish that dietary antioxidants or other nutrients that can alter the levels of these [oxidative stress] biomarkers are themselves causally related to the development or prevention of chronic diseases." This position has not changed since the report was released.

• Cautions

Early studies seemed to indicate that beta-carotene reduced the incidence of some cancers, but later results raised important concerns. Studies (✘ ✘ ✘) have shown that smokers and people exposed to other cancer-causing agents such as asbestos who take beta-carotene supplements have even higher rates of cancer than people with the same risk who did not take the supplements. High doses of beta-carotene caused changes in enzyme levels in animals that made other cancer-causing agents more dangerous. Some studies (✘ ✘) suggest that too much vitamin C may have a pro-oxidative effect for some people — causing harm or disease.

For these and other reasons, some researchers urge caution in the number of antioxidant supplements people add to their diet. As with most good things, too much can have a detrimental effect. The IOM report on antioxidants contained a new feature establishing a Tolerable Upper Intake Level (UL) for supplements. The UL is the highest level likely to have *no* risk of adverse health effects for almost everyone. People taking more than the UL expose themselves to greater risk of adverse effects. The UL for vitamin C was set at 2000 mg per day based on the risk of serious diarrhea. The UL for vitamin E is 1000 mg per day based on the increased risk of bleeding because vitamin E can prevent blood from clotting. The UL for selenium is 400 micrograms per day based on the risk of selenosis, a condition associated with hair loss and nail sloughing. No UL was set for the carotenoids, but this was because of a lack of information, not because there is no risk of negative effects.

The Institute of Medicine has recommended that people not take over 2000 mg of vitamin C per day. Other studies have shown that several grams of vitamin C per day may be appropriate for reducing or eliminating the side effects of such high physical stress treatments as cancer chemotherapy. The problem is that what is appropriate varies with many factors, including the height, weight, age, and general health of the patient.

All these risks are associated with large amounts of antioxidant supplements. A diet rich in foods that contain antioxidants has not been associated with these risks. The only known risks of eating large quantities of these foods are those that come with overeating in general.

• Recommendations

A diet rich in fruits and vegetables will provide significant amounts of antioxidants. However, some recommendations made by people promoting the health significance of antioxidants require you to either take supplements or consume many pounds of certain fruits and vegetables, which is not a practical solution. The effects of consuming large quantities of antioxidant supplements over long periods of time are not known. In contrast to the complex mixture of antioxidants found in natural foods, antioxidant supplements are highly purified and concentrated. Some of them are manufactured just like drugs and other chemicals. Alternative therapists recommending supplements apparently do not realize they sometimes contradict their own recommendations for a return to a "natural" approach to health.

The best advice is to meet most of your antioxidant needs through a healthy diet supplemented by a single multivitamin. However, ConsumerLab.com published results on its subscription-based website in 2001 regarding twenty-seven multivitamin products. The results showed that half the products were of poor quality (see the entry on Megavitamin Therapy for more details). Particular individuals, such as those at high risk for cancer or heart disease, or pregnant women, may need supplementation. This should be monitored by a health care professional. Until more is known about these supplements, prudence demands caution.

• Dosage

The IOM report recommended new daily adult RDAs for vitamin C (75 mg for women and 90 mg for men — with an additional 35 mg per day recommended for smokers), vitamin E (15 mg alpha-tocopherol), and selenium (55 micrograms). Vitamin E recommendations are made more complicated because the vitamin has eight natural forms. The active form in humans is alpha-tocopherol. Only small proportions of other forms are converted into alpha-tocopherol. Many products do not clearly state which form they contain, making it difficult to know the amount of active material in the product. Regarding carotenoids, no recommendations were issued because there was insufficient data on which to base conclusions. These RDAs apply to both the United States and Canada.

• Treatment Categories

Conventional
To maintain recommended DRIs	☺☺☺☺
To prevent cardiovascular disease	☹☹☹☹
To treat cardiovascular disease	☹☹☹☹

Complementary
To prevent chronic diseases as part of a healthy diet	☺☺☺
To prevent preeclampsia	☺☺

Scientifically Unproven
To prevent gastrointestinal cancers	☹☹☹☹
To treat ALS	☹☹☹
To treat chronic diseases	☹☹☹☹

Quackery or Fraud
In the hands of some practitioners

Risk of Serious Side Effects

With large doses ⊘

• Further Reading

Frei, Balz. "Efficacy of Dietary Antioxidants to Prevent Oxidative Damage and Inhibit Chronic Disease." *Journal of Nutrition* 134, no. 11 (November 2004): S3196–S3198.

Institute of Medicine. *Dietary Reference Intakes for Vitamin C, Vitamin E, Selenium, and Carotenoids* (Washington, D.C.: National Academy Press, 2000).

Vivekananthan, D. P., M. S. Penn, S. K. Sapp, A. Hsu, and E. J. Topol. "Use of Antioxidant Vitamins for the Prevention of Cardiovascular Disease: Meta-analysis of Randomised Trials." *Lancet* 361 (2003): 2017–23.

BACH FLOWER REMEDIES

• What They Are

Edward Bach (1880–1936) was a thoroughly unconventional yet intensely compassionate man who began his career as a medical physician, then switched to homeopathy when he felt conventional medicine was not adequately helping his patients. He later concluded that homeopathy did not have the answer either and left his job in a London homeopathic hospital to find better treatments than either pharmaceuticals or homeopathic preparations. Increasingly, he came to believe that all illness is caused by emotional problems — "our fears, our anxieties, our greed, our likes and dislikes." He thought that if he could find a way to change a patient's emotions, good health would follow.

Bach moved to Wales and enjoyed walking through the woods. He appreciated the wildflowers and noticed his reaction to a new blossom. He concluded that different flowers elicit different emotional responses.

The doctor was convinced that he was highly intuitive. He is said to have used his psychic ability to determine which plants affect which emotions. For example, if he was feeling worried when he started his walk, he would hold his hand over the different plants he passed, sensing which one alleviated his concerns. If he was angry, he would use the same approach to find the plant that eased his tension. Over time he identified thirty-eight different plants that he said consistently affected his emotions. These formed the basis for his healing formulas.

Bach assumed that what affected him would work with others. He analyzed how best to obtain the healing power of the plant and settled on the collection of dew accumulating on flower petals just before dawn. He believed the early rays of sunlight transferred the flowers' healing power into the dew.

Dew collection was slow and limited. When Bach's practice began to grow, he needed a way to treat more patients. He settled on the idea of suspending flowers in clear springwater and exposing them to direct sunlight. This approach is used to this day. Remedies are supplied in concentrated solutions preserved with alcohol. These are diluted, and four drops of the appropriate flower remedy needed for emotional change are applied four times a day to the tongue.

Over time, other delivery methods were developed. Some flowers are boiled in a saucepan with two pints of springwater. The liquid is decanted, filtered through three layers of blotting paper, and mixed 1:1 with brandy. The final liquid can be dropped on the tongue or diluted within a glass of juice or water. It can also be rubbed on the knees or wrists, behind the ears, or on the temples, or even sprayed into the mouth with an atomizer. All methods are said to work equally well.

Bach's psychic abilities were also used in determining the emotional problems underlying a person's illness. He would intuitively decide that loneliness or anger or grief or some other emotion caused a patient's illness. He would choose the flower remedy accordingly, providing the drops and advising the patient to imagine that a healing light was penetrating his or her whole being, relieving the emotional problem. Bach felt that the flower remedies worked because the sun caused the transfer of healing energy from the flowers to the dew or water solution in which they were soaked. These energies, he believed, helped to restore the imbalances in people's "life energy" that he said were behind all emotional disorders.

Claims

Proponents have long lists of testimonials (✔) as to the benefits of the remedies. Case studies (✔✔) involving two patients were reported in 2003. Bach flower remedies are believed to cure all illnesses since these are all caused by emotional problems. Particular flower remedies are said to alleviate specific problems. For example, talkative people are said to be obsessed with their own troubles and experiences. They need heather blossoms to feel better. Someone who is going through a major life change — either biochemical, such as puberty or menopause, or psychological, such as divorce or a move to a new home — should be given walnut blossoms. Someone who is impatient with others will benefit from the impatiens plant. Someone with vague fears that constantly trouble them should use aspen, though those with extreme terrors will require rock rose. If you are overwhelmed by your work, perhaps becoming depressed by all you have to do, you will be helped by elm.

There is a five-flower combination remedy (Rescue Remedy) meant to be used as an emergency stress formula, such as following an accident or sudden loss of a loved one. The formula is available in the traditional form and as a cream, the latter to be used for stiff muscles, headaches, burns, insect bites, bruises, cuts, and sprains.

Some practitioners state that treatment must be individualized for each patient. This results in the same remedies being used for different symptoms in different patients.

Study Findings

Very few clinical tests have examined Bach flower remedies. Two uncontrolled trials (✔✔) for anxiety and depression found beneficial results. However, two other controlled trials (✗✗✗) found the benefit for anxiety and depression no better than that from placebo. The larger of these was a 2001 randomized double-blind trial (✘✘✘). One hundred healthy university students were given either Rescue Remedy or placebo, and their anxiety levels before examinations were measured using standard testing procedures. No significant differences were found between those taking the flower remedy and those taking a placebo. One other randomized double-blind study (✘✘✘) used Bach flower remedies for children with ADHD. The flower remedy was no more beneficial than placebo.

Chemical analysis of the remedies reveals only springwater and alcohol. Proponents accept this finding and claim that the remedies are effective because of life energy. Bach recognized the important role of mind-body influences in health. Taking the time to acknowledge and deal with one's emotional issues can benefit many people, regardless of whether they use these remedies.

Cautions

From a medical perspective, a real danger with these remedies is that people might use them in place of seeking effective medical or psychological help. From a theological perspective, the remedies seem to be steeped in psychic mysticism. Using them may expose the patient to teachings and practices that are contradictory to Christianity. Certainly if you have inadvertently used Bach flower remedies in the past, you need not fear that you have contaminated yourself with evil spirits. Paul's response to questions about whether Christians should eat meat sacrificed to idols applies here: "Eat anything sold in the meat market without raising questions of conscience, for, 'The earth is the Lord's, and everything in it' " (1 Corinthians 10:25 – 26). Nevertheless, we can envision no reason a Christian should knowingly use Bach flower remedies.

Recommendations

Unresolved emotional issues may play a role in people's illnesses. These issues should be addressed in appropriate ways. Some will be able to address them informally on their own or with family and friends, while others will need more formal help from trained professionals.

Christians should be building deep relationships with Christ and with other Christians to help one another with emotional and relational issues. Since these often involve areas of spiritual growth, we should acknowledge God's desire to help us mature in these areas. Often in helping others we will be helped ourselves. There should be no reason to turn to flower remedies to accomplish what the Spirit of God promises to do in us and through other Christians. Paul gave thanks for his Christian friends, "being confident of this, that he [God] who began a good work in you will carry it on to completion until the day of Christ Jesus" (Philippians 1:6).

Treatment Categories

Scientifically Questionable
For any indication ☹☹☹☹

Spiritual
According to how they
are alleged to work 👎👎👎

Quackery or Fraud
In the hands of some practitioners

Further Reading

Armstrong, N. C., and E. Ernst. "A Randomised, Double-Blind, Placebo-Controlled Trial of a Bach Flower Remedy." *Complementary Therapies in Nursing and Midwifery* 7, no. 4 (November 2001): 215 – 21.

Masi, Marl P. "Bach Flower Therapy in the Treatment of Chronic Major Depressive Disorder." *Alternative Therapies in Health and Medicine* 9, no. 6 (November – December 2003): 108 – 10, 112.

Pintov, Shai, Miriam Hochman, Amir Livne, Eli Heyman, and Eli Lahat. "Bach Flower Remedies Used for Attention Deficit Hyperactivity Disorder in Children — A Prospective Double-Blind Controlled Study." *European Journal of Paediatric Neurology* 9, no. 6 (November 2005): 395 – 98.

BEE PRODUCTS

What They Are

A number of products made by honey bees have become popular alternative remedies in recent years. The most popular of these are bee pollen, bee venom, honey, propolis, and royal jelly. Each of the products is used in different ways. They should not be confused with one another, nor should they be used interchangeably.

Bee Pollen

When honey bees collect nectar, pollen from the flowers collects on their legs and bodies. Bee pollen thus contains mostly flower pollen harvested from the bees when they return to their hives. Bee pollen is marketed as "the perfect food," containing essential vitamins, minerals, and enzymes. The precise composition of bee pollen varies, depending on which flowers the bees have visited.

While bee pollen may be nutritious, no clinical evidence is available to support its medicinal use. A small number of studies (✖✖) in the 1980s found that bee pollen did not improve the performances of athletes. There is no evidence that bee pollen alone has any therapeutic benefits. Bee pollen is relatively safe, although people allergic to pollens will most likely also be allergic to bee pollen. Since some allergies can be severe, caution should be taken when first using the product.

Bee Venom

Bee venom, or honeybee venom therapy (HBV), uses the stings of bees to treat various conditions. It is said to be particularly popular in Romania, China, and Russia. Proponents claim bee venom has an anti-inflammatory effect and is useful in the treatment of a wide variety of illnesses such as arthritis, multiple sclerosis, Bell's palsy, tendonitis, some muscle conditions, and irritable bowel syndrome.

Subcutaneous bee venom injections are FDA-approved for the treatment of severe allergies to bee stings. Early reports (✔✔) of bee venom suggested it had some benefit in the treatment of osteoarthritis. However, more recent controlled studies (✖✖✖) have not shown any benefit. Some people react to the injections with itchiness, swelling, and anxiety, which can lead to chest tightness, dizziness, asthma, and other allergic symptoms. Women, for some reason, have more frequent and more severe adverse reactions.

Honey

Bee honey has been used since ancient times as part of the care of wounds. Recently, such uses have been rediscovered and recommended. Honey used as a food is heat treated to remove bacteria. Honey used on wounds must be sterilized with gamma radiation, as heat destroys some of the therapeutic substances. The viscosity and pH of honey give it antimicrobial properties. Honey made by bees that feast on tea trees is approved in Australia as "therapeutic honey" because of the additional compounds from the tea trees.

Several controlled trials (✓✓✓) have demonstrated that honey improves the healing of wounds, especially those that have not responded to conventional therapy. However, most of these studies were small and of relatively poor quality. Adverse effects or allergic reactions have not been noted after topical application. However, using honey on large wounds in diabetic patients may result in elevated blood sugar levels. Much remains to be researched in terms of the optimal way to use honey on wounds, including the frequency.

Propolis

Propolis, or bee glue, is a sticky resin made by bees to repair holes in and to smooth the walls of bee hives. Bees make propolis from resinous materials collected from trees and leaves. Propolis has been used for a wide variety of indications throughout history. It is used orally to treat bacterial and viral infections and topically to cleanse wounds. One study (✓✓✓) found faster healing when a 3 percent propolis ointment was used to treat genital lesions caused by herpes simplex virus type 2. Antimicrobial properties have been seen in laboratory tests, but clinical trials have not been reported. The principal adverse effects are allergic reactions, which can range from mild to severe.

Royal Jelly

Royal jelly is a milky product secreted by those bees that care for developing larvae in the hive. It is the sole source of nutrition for the larvae that will develop into queen bees, which is how it got its name. It is sold as a general health tonic and recommended for a wide variety of ailments. Apart from some preliminary evidence that it may help reduce high cholesterol levels, there is no evidence of royal jelly alone having a therapeutic effect in humans.

A number of case reports (✗✗) have linked consumption of royal jelly to allergic reactions, with those allergic to other substances at particularly high risk. These reactions range from itchiness and swelling to asthmatic attacks and even death. A study in Hong Kong (✗✗✗) found that almost one-third of the people there had used royal jelly, and 7 percent tested positive to having an allergy to royal jelly.

● Treatment Categories

Conventional

Bee venom to treat severe bee allergies	☺☺☺☺

Complementary

Bee pollen to supplement a healthy diet	☺☺
Royal jelly to supplement a healthy diet	☺
Royal jelly to lower elevated cholesterol levels	☺
Propolis, topically, to prevent or treat infections	☺☺
Honey, topically, to treat burns and ulcers	☺☺☺

Scientifically Unproven

Bee venom for any indication ☹☹☹

Bee pollen for other indications ☹☹☹

Propolis for other indications ☹☹☹

Royal jelly for other indications ☹☹☹

Quackery or Fraud

In the hands of some practitioners

Further Reading

Burdock, G. A. "Review of the Biological Properties and Toxicity of Bee Propolis." *Food and Chemical Toxicology* 36, no. 4 (April 1998): 347–63.

Lusby, P. E., A. Coombes, and J. M. Wilkinson. "Honey: A Potent Agent for Wound Healing?" *Journal of Wound Ostomy and Continence Nursing* 29, no. 6 (November 2002): 295–300.

BILBERRY

What It Is

Bilberries, also called European blueberries (*Vaccinium myrtillus*), have long been a popular fruit for eating and cooking. The berries, which grow on a shrub closely related to the cranberry bush, are found most commonly in northern and central Europe as well as in the Rocky Mountains. They have great nutritional value, and it was as a result of their regular use in preserves that claims of medicinal qualities were made. Today bilberry fruit extract has become one of the most popular herbal remedies sold in the United States. The extract is also considered one of the standard medical tools by some European physicians when faced with treating a variety of eye disorders.

Claims

Bilberry has become popular primarily for its alleged ability to improve vision. During World War II, pilots in the British Royal Air Force enjoyed bilberry preserves with their meals. Those who ate the preserves felt they had better vision when flying night bombing runs. Since nothing else seemed to explain the changes in their night vision, the story spread and they concluded that the bilberries must have been enhancing their ability to see.

Today bilberry extract is used to treat a host of vision problems, including glaucoma, cataracts, diabetic retinopathy, poor night vision, and macular degeneration. Others recommend it for angina, heart disease, venous insufficiency, varicose veins, hemorrhoids, and atherosclerosis. Topically, it is used for mild inflammation of the mucous membranes of the mouth and throat. Bilberry leaf taken orally is used to treat diabetes, arthritis, dermatitis, and gout. Diarrhea and diabetes have long been treated in Europe with bilberries, but it is their impact on vision that has given the extract its American popularity.

Study Findings

The active ingredients in bilberry that seem to impact health are compounds called "anthocyanins."

These are part of the larger group of compounds called "flavonoids," which are known to have antioxidant properties. Bilberry leaves also contain high levels of chromium, which may lower blood sugar in some individuals.

Studies with animals have shown that anthocyanins stabilize collagen, make blood capillaries less porous after injury, and reduce swelling. They have also been found to improve circulation through the smallest blood vessels.

Bilberry fruit extracts have been tested in a number of studies (✓✓) on people with a variety of vision problems. However, almost all of these studies had few patients, no controls, and were of very short duration, making any firm conclusions difficult.

A 2004 review found twelve placebo-controlled trials of bilberry for night vision. Those of lower quality found some benefit from the herb (✓✓✓). Five higher quality randomized trials were found, of which four found bilberry no more beneficial than placebo (✗✗✗). All but one of these trials were conducted with healthy volunteers seeking to improve their night vision. No controlled trials have examined the effect of bilberry on those with eye diseases that impair night vision.

Commission E in Germany concluded that bilberry is possibly effective for acute diarrhea and circulatory problems and when used for mild inflammation of the mouth or throat.

Cautions

Although adverse effects from taking the extract have not been reported, some animals given bilberry fruit extract for prolonged periods developed anemia, acute excitatory states, and problems with muscle tone. Large doses were fatal to the animals.

Considering the extract's effect on blood flow, interactions with anticoagulant therapy could occur.

As with all dietary supplements sold in the United States, their quality varies enormously. A study was done of the anthocyanin concentration in fifteen bilberry extracts. The product with the most had over one hundred times as many anthocyanins as the product with the least, and the others had every level in between. Another study estimated that people need 50 mg of anthocyanins daily to see some benefit. Of the fifteen bilberry products tested, only five would give this amount of anthocyanins if taken as recommended. However, the latest recommendations regarding antioxidants include a Tolerable Upper Intake Level. This recognizes that taking too many antioxidants can cause adverse effects. This can be a real problem, given the great variation in antioxidant concentrations in bilberry extracts.

Recommendations

Very little clear evidence supports the use of bilberry fruit extract for the treatment of eye problems. Its popularity in Europe does not mean it should be a treatment of first choice. Given that many other effective treatments are available, standard therapy should not be avoided or delayed. Given the toxic effects found in animals, bilberry extract use should be limited to short periods.

Dosage

The dose varies considerably, with little known about how much is best or safe. Researchers have used 60 to 120 mg of bilberry extract twice a day for eye problems.

Treatment Categories

Complementary

To treat acute diarrhea	☺☺
To relieve circulatory problems	☺
To lower blood glucose	☺
To treat diabetic or hypertensive retinopathy	☺☺
To improve night vision	☹☹☹

Scientifically Unproven

For any other indication, including other eye problems	☹☹

Further Reading

Canter, Peter H., and Edzard Ernst. "Anthocyanosides of *Vaccinium myrtillus* (Bilberry) for Night Vision: A Systematic Review of Placebo-Controlled Trials." *Survey of Ophthalmology* 49, no. 1 (January – February 2004): 38 – 50.

Prior, Ronald L., and Guohua Cao. "Variability in Dietary Antioxidant Related Natural Product Supplements: The Need for Methods of Standardization." *Journal of the American Nutraceutical Association* 2, no. 2 (Summer 1999): 46 – 56.

BLACK COHOSH

What It Is

Native Americans referred to black cohosh as "squawroot" and used it both to treat menstrual cramps and to ease the pain of childbirth. The latter use has fallen into disfavor because of possible risks to the unborn child. The former use has remained popular and received a huge boost when studies reported potential problems with hormone replacement therapy (HRT) in 2001 and 2002. Up to that point, millions of women were given HRT to combat the symptoms of menopause. Women enter this stage of life as their natural production of estrogen and other hormones decreases. It made sense to replace those hormones to relieve menopausal symptoms. However, long-term studies in primarily older women found that the risks of HRT outweighed the benefits for many

women, who were advised to stop HRT. Many looked to natural approaches, of which black cohosh is one of the most popular. Even prior to the HRT problems, one survey of women in the United States aged forty-five to sixty-five years found that almost one-quarter had used alternative therapies to treat menopausal symptoms. Herbal remedies were the most popular approach used by these women, with black cohosh being the most popular.

Black cohosh, also known as black snakeroot, rattleroot, and bugwort, is an herbal remedy made from the underground parts (roots and rhizome) of a North American plant called *Cimicifuga racemosa*. Be aware that blue cohosh is a completely unrelated plant (*Caulophyllum thalictroides*), although both are called "squawroot" and used similarly. White cohosh is another unrelated plant.

Claims

One of the most common reasons given by women who use herbal remedies is to treat menopausal symptoms. Surveys have found that many women believed herbal remedies were better than HRT — even *before* the studies revealed the potential adverse effects of HRT. Native Americans used black cohosh for a variety of ailments, including rheumatism, sore throats, and menstrual problems. It continues to be popular as a way of decreasing hot flashes and as an alternative to hormone replacement therapy. Other uses are for premenstrual cramping, dysmenorrhea, and indigestion and as an insect repellent.

Study Findings

During the 1980s, at least eight clinical studies in Germany used a commercial product available there called Remifemin. This standardized extract is designed to deliver consistent amounts of triterpene glycosides (although whether these are the active ingredients is not clear). While positive results, and no adverse effects, were found, seven of the studies were not blinded — the participants knew what they were receiving. That means the results must be interpreted with some caution (✓✓). However, more recent studies have been randomized and double-blinded. Two compared two doses of Remifemin (39 mg and 127 mg per day) and found the women benefited equally (✓✓). Unfortunately, a placebo group was not included. A 2005 randomized trial (✓✓✓) found Remifemin significantly better than placebo in relieving menopausal symptoms, especially hot flashes.

One placebo-controlled study involved women who had been treated for breast cancer. The treatment often causes menopausal symptoms, and the women cannot take HRT because they are at higher risk of the hormones stimulating some cancers. In this study, women experienced similar benefits from black cohosh and placebo for seven of the eight symptoms measured (✗✗✗). Only with sweating (✓✓✓) was black cohosh more beneficial.

Cautions

Because black cohosh has some effect on menstruation and female sex hormones, it should not be used during pregnancy or breast-feeding. It increases the risk of miscarriage. (This advice is standard for virtually all herbs. The effect of most herbs on developing unborn children remains unknown. When herbs are deemed appropriate, their use should be monitored by a medical physician who is knowledgeable about herbal remedies.) There are midwives who use black cohosh to induce labor. Observational studies show no adverse effects on either the mother or the baby; however, it would take trials with large numbers of women and babies to see rare or uncommon side effects. Since there are no clinical trials to support the safety of this practice, we do not recommend it.

The most common side effects of black cohosh are intestinal problems, although little is known about its toxicity. Several cases of liver toxicity have been reported after women took black cohosh with or without other herbs. Although black cohosh has not been proven to have caused the liver damage, and the problem appears to be rare, careful monitoring of liver function when taking the herb may be warranted. Because of uncertainty about toxic effects, those who prescribe the remedy in Germany recommend that it be taken for no more than three to six months.

● Recommendations

Black cohosh appears to bring relief from some menstrual and menopausal symptoms, although very little is known about how it might do this. Almost all the clinical trials were conducted with one German product, Remifemin, which is now available in the United States. Another black cohosh extract (marketed as Menofem but currently not available in the United States or Canada) has some evidence to support its use in relieving hot flashes. There is no guarantee that other products will give the same results. ConsumerLab.com tested sixteen black cohosh products in 2005. All contained the amounts of black cohosh claimed on their labels and supplied at least 1 mg of triterpenes in the suggested daily dose. No contaminants were found.

Because of the general lack of information, especially on its toxicity, the use of black cohosh cannot be wholeheartedly recommended, although it certainly warrants further research. It should not be used by women who are pregnant or breast-feeding. For those women who cannot, or would prefer not to, use hormone replacement therapy during menopause, black cohosh may offer some benefit and be worth trying. Care should be taken not to confuse black cohosh with white cohosh or blue cohosh, the latter being much more toxic.

● Dosage

Most of the research has been conducted on Remifemin, available in tablet and liquid form. Dosage recommendations vary widely, but 40 mg per day is the most usual. Extracts standardized to contain at least 2.5 percent triterpene glycosides (or to deliver at least 1 mg of these triterpenes per daily dose) are recommended. However, evidence is not conclusive that triterpene glycosides are the active ingredients in black cohosh. Furthermore, Remifemin was recently reformulated and its current percentage of triterpene glycosides is not published. It is also important to distinguish between black cohosh products that are extracts and those that contain the whole herb or root. Extracts generally give a much more concentrated form of the active ingredients.

● Treatment Categories

Complementary

To manage menopausal symptoms
(short-term), especially hot flashes ☺☺☺
To manage menopausal symptoms in
women being treated for breast cancer ☺

Scientifically Unproven

For any other indication

● Further Reading

Huntley, Alyson, and Edzard Ernst. "A Systematic Review of the Safety of Black Cohosh." *Menopause* 10, no. 1 (January 2003): 58–64.

Osmers, Ruediger, Michael Friede, Eckehard Liske, Joerg Schnitker, Johannes Freudenstein, and Hans-Heinrich Henneicke-von Zepelin. "Efficacy and Safety of Isopropanolic Black Cohosh Extract for Climacteric Symptoms." *Obstetrics and Gynecology* 105, no. 5, part 1 (May 2005): 1074–83.

CAPSAICIN

What It Is

Capsaicin is the active ingredient in cayenne or chili peppers, also known as capsicum and hot pepper extract. Hot peppers have been cultivated for centuries, resulting in many varieties of the most common species, *Capsicum frutescens* and *Capsicum annum.*

Claims

Hot peppers are used primarily as a spice in cooking but also have a long tradition of medicinal use. Capsaicin is used both orally and topically. Orally it has been used for gastrointestinal problems (to stimulate digestion and for gas, colic, diarrhea, and cramps) and for circulation, high cholesterol, seasickness, fever, atherosclerosis, and heart disease. Topically it is used to relieve the pain of osteoarthritis, rheumatoid arthritis, and neuralgia (a sharp or burning pain that originates in nerves).

Capsaicin (like mustard plasters) was known as a "counterirritant," a substance placed on a painful area to cause further irritation, which somehow relieves the original pain. Others claim that capsaicin taken orally can reduce blood cholesterol and decrease the tendency of the blood to clot.

Study Findings

The counterirritant effects of capsaicin have been extensively researched (✓✓✓), leading to FDA approval of capsaicin as an external (topical) analgesic for pain from rheumatoid arthritis, osteoarthritis, psoriasis, and neuralgias, including shingles and diabetic neuropathy. However, studies showed it is not effective for all people. It cut in half musculoskeletal pain for about one in every eight patients treated with 0.025 percent capsaicin. For neuropathic pain, 0.075 percent capsaicin was effective after eight weeks in about one in every six patients.

Capsaicin is available in a number of over-the-counter creams and works well when used appropriately. It appears to work by causing depletion of Substance P, which is how peripheral nerves transmit painful stimuli back to the spinal cord. Capsaicin therefore prevents the brain from perceiving the pain. However, it takes a few days to use up the Substance P already in the painful area. Capsaicin is therefore most effective when used repeatedly for chronic pain such as with arthritis and neuropathy. It should be applied three to four times daily for at least four weeks.

Evidence to support the internal use of capsaicin is insubstantial, with the possible exception (✓✓) of its use as a digestive stimulant. Epidemiological evidence (✓✓) suggests that those who eat more chili peppers have fewer peptic ulcers. Preliminary evidence (✗✗) suggests that capsaicin does not relieve irritable bowel syndrome.

Cautions

Ironically, if all the Substance P in an area is not depleted, the intensity of the pain may increase. It is therefore very important that enough capsaicin cream be used. This can be a problem when people make their own creams, as the amount of capsaicin varies extensively among varieties of peppers. Capsaicin is extremely irritating to eyes, open wounds, and mucous membranes. After applying the cream to the skin, residual capsaicin is practically insoluble in cold water and only slightly soluble in hot water. It can be removed from the hands using vinegar. The cream may be helpful for shingles or psoriasis, but the skin should be monitored carefully for signs of excessive irritation.

Recommendations

Capsaicin is an effective analgesic for certain types of arthritis and chronic pain of the arms or legs. It has few side effects so long as it is kept away from the eyes and open wounds. Capsaicin may be unsafe when taken orally in amounts larger than in food, especially for children and women who are pregnant or breast-feeding. As those who have eaten hot peppers know, there is great variability in people's taste for peppers. These differences apply to skin tolerance as well as to taste buds.

Dosage

Capsaicin is very potent, so topical preparations often contain between 0.025 and 0.075 percent capsaicin, which should be applied no more than three or four times a day.

Treatment Categories

Conventional

Topically to relieve chronic musculoskeletal pain	☺☺☺☺
Topically to relieve chronic peripheral nerve pain (neuropathy) from shingles or diabetes	☺☺☺☺
Topically to relieve chronic peripheral nerve pain (neuropathy) from HIV/AIDS	☹
Topically to treat some forms of arthritis	☺☺☺

Complementary

Orally to stimulate the digestive system	☺☺
Orally to treat dyspepsia or peptic ulcers	☺
Orally to treat irritable bowel syndrome	☹

Scientifically Unproven

For any other indication

Further Reading

Foster, Steven, and Varro E. Tyler. *Tyler's Honest Herbal: A Sensible Guide to the Use of Herbs and Related Remedies.* 4th ed. New York: Haworth Herbal, 1999, 89–91.

Mason, Lorna, R. Andrew Moore, Sheena Derry, Jayne E. Edwards, and Henry J. McQuay. "Systematic Review of Topical Capsaicin for the Treatment of Chronic Pain." *British Medical Journal* 328 (April 2004): 991–95.

CASCARA

What It Is

Cascara is one of several herbal remedies used as a natural laxative to treat constipation. Native Americans in the Pacific Northwest used the bark and passed it on to Spanish explorers, who called it "cascara sagrada" (sacred bark). Extract of cascara is also used to flavor foods and beverages. The bark of the tree, *Frangula purshiana*, is used and is known to contain chemicals that stimulate the large intestine.

Claims

Cascara is used as a natural laxative for the treatment of acute and chronic constipation. Some also claim cascara can treat gallstones, liver problems, and cancer.

Study Findings

Cascara was listed as an FDA-approved over-the-counter laxative. That designation was removed in 2002 because no companies submitted evidence of its effectiveness. This doesn't necessarily mean it is not effective. Companies may have considered FDA approval unnecessary since cascara can still be marketed as a dietary supplement. A small number of studies (✓✓✓) have shown that cascara is an effective, safe, and relatively mild laxative for short-term use.

Cautions

Any laxative should not be used over extended periods of time because of the risk of dehydration and potassium loss. Use of cascara with other drugs or herbs with similar effects could exacerbate these problems. Cascara should not be used by people who have ulcers, intestinal obstructions, or abdominal pain of unknown origin. It is also not recommended for pregnant or lactating women or for children.

Recommendations

Cascara is a laxative of long-standing reputation. For short-term use in constipation, it may provide relief for some. Long-term use of any laxative is not recommended. An uncontrolled study was carried out in a retirement nursing home where almost half the residents were taking laxatives, including cascara. When the fiber content of the residents' diet was increased using powdered natural fiber, two-thirds of the residents were able to stop taking laxatives. The fiber was also less costly. The best approach to most cases of chronic constipation is to increase the fruit, vegetable, and fiber content of the diet.

Dosage

One teaspoonful of liquid extract can be used three times a day. Capsules of dried bark are also available, with one or two recommended at bedtime. These doses give about 20 to 30 mg of the active ingredients, but the smallest dose should be used.

Treatment Categories

Complementary

As a laxative to treat constipation ☺☺

Scientifically Questionable

As a laxative to help with weight loss ☹☹☹☹
For any other indication ☹☹☹☹

Further Reading

"Cascara Sagrada." *WholeHealthMD.com: http:// www.wholehealthmd.com/refshelf/substances_ view/1,1525,10013,00.html.* Accessed November 25, 2005.

Food and Drug Administration. "Status of Certain Additional Over-the-Counter Drug Category II and III Active Ingredients." *Federal Register* 67, no. 90 (May 2002): 31125 – 27.

Khaja, M., C. S. Thakur, T. Bharathan, E. Baccash, and G. Goldenberg. " 'Fiber 7' Supplement as an Alternative to Laxatives in a Nursing Home." *Gerodontology* 22, no. 2 (June 2005): 106 – 8.

CHAMOMILE

What It Is

Sometimes it seems that in the history of the Western world, there have been two consistent "Mom Medicines." The first is chicken soup, lovingly, though not always tastefully, prepared. Whatever the case, you always felt better after sipping it, because in many a home it represented all the love and concern you needed when you were afflicted with everything from colds and fevers to influenza and general malaise.

The second "Mom Medicine" is chamomile tea, a drink made from the daisy-like, apple-scented flower cultivated worldwide. Most Americans should be familiar with the form known as German, or genuine, chamomile; botanists have about a dozen different Latin names for it, with the most common ones being *Matricaria recutita* and *Matricaria chamomilla*. Roman, or English, chamomile (*Anthemis nobilis*) is a completely different plant. But no matter what the variety, one use has always been the same. It is the beverage served when you are tossing and turning in bed or anxiously pacing the floor, unable to sleep.

The pagan Anglo-Saxons were so delighted with the herb that they became convinced it was one of nine sacred herbs given to humans by the god Woden. What makes chamomile different from other Mom remedies is that after thousands of years of use, anecdotal evidence has been scientifically evaluated and somewhat validated — though not for every use. Roman chamomile, though widely used, contains ingredients that are similar, but not identical, to German chamomile. Most of the research has been conducted on German chamomile and is often assumed to apply to Roman chamomile. Whether or not this is appropriate is unclear.

German chamomile is an important example of how an herb's preparation affects its activity. The flower heads contain numerous compounds. Some are soluble in water; others are not. A tea made from the flower heads will contain mostly the water-soluble compounds. Making the tea in a closed container is said to capture more of the volatile oils, which are not very water soluble. Other remedies are made by soaking the flower heads in alcohol to obtain an extract that contains significantly more of the water-insoluble compounds. These alcohol extracts, or tinctures, have very different effects in the body and should only be used externally.

Claims

In contemporary German culture, chamomile is considered a cure-all and is used orally as a sedative and spasmolytic (for treating intestinal and menstrual cramps) and topically as an anti-inflammatory and wound-healing agent. The tea, made from the tiny flower heads, may suppress muscle spasms and reduce inflammation in the digestive tract. It is used for menstrual cramps, flatulence, and seasickness. Topically, chamomile oil or ointment may be applied as an anti-inflammatory for skin and mucous membrane problems, hemorrhoids, and leg ulcers. As an inhalant, it has been used to treat respiratory difficulties. A volatile oil is mainly responsible, so the tea must be made from fresh herb. When fresh, it is said to smell like apples; when old, it is said to smell like hay. It must be steeped long enough to release the oil, generally at least ten minutes in a closed container.

Study Findings

Animal studies support chamomile's traditional use as a wound healer and as an anti-inflammatory, antispasmodic, and antianxiety agent. One component, apigenin, binds the same receptors as antianxiety prescription drugs such as Valium and exerts anxiolytic and mild sedative effects in mice and relaxes intestinal spasms. However, very few human studies have evaluated these traditional uses. In one uncontrolled trial (✓✓), ten of twelve heart patients fell asleep after drinking chamomile tea.

Topical uses similarly have not been studied widely. The essential oil acts as an antioxidant and kills some skin bacteria (*Staphylococcus*) and yeast (*Candida* species). A number of studies (✓✓) have been done on a German product called Kamillosan, but these were mostly unblinded studies. Given this limitation, the preparation consistently brought improvements to a variety of skin disorders. However, other controlled trials have had less conclusive results. A recent controlled trial (✗✗✗) found no difference between chamomile and placebo in preventing inflammation of the mouth in patients receiving chemotherapy. In another randomized placebo-controlled trial (✗✗✗), radiation-induced skin reactions were less frequent and appeared later in chamomile-treated areas, but the differences were not statistically significant.

Cautions

The FDA considers chamomile safe, with no known adverse effects in pregnancy, lactation, or childhood. However, some experts believe German and Roman chamomile may damage the developing child before birth and stimulate the uterus. Since there is virtually no information on chamomile's use during lactation, it should not be used while breast-feeding. However, chamomile caused no adverse reactions in any of the human trials discussed earlier. Patients with severe allergies to ragweed should be warned about possible cross-reactivity to chamomile and other members of the aster family (e.g., echinacea, feverfew, and milk thistle). Roman chamomile causes more allergic problems than German chamomile.

Recommendations

While chamomile's therapeutic effects and safety remain to be definitively proven in human trials, its beneficial effects seen in animals and its good safety record in widespread traditional use by humans make it an acceptable short-term home remedy for soothing mild skin irritation, intestinal cramps, and agitated nerves. In the United States, it is commonly consumed as a tea or applied as a compress. The tea must be steeped for at least ten minutes in a closed container to have the maximum medicinal impact. It should not be taken in conjunction with other sedatives, such as benzodiazepines or alcohol. People allergic to ragweed or flowers in the daisy family could suffer allergic reactions. Alcohol extracts should only be used externally.

Dosage

When taken orally, about 3 grams of the dried flower heads are used to make a tea that can be taken up to three or four times a day. For topical use, ointments with 3 to 10 percent extracts can be used three times a day.

Treatment Categories

Conventional
To induce sleep	☺☺☺
To soothe mildly agitated nerves	☺☺
To soothe intestinal cramps	☺

Complementary
Orally to treat dyspepsia	☺☺
Topically to soothe skin irritation	☺☺
As a mouthwash to treat mild oral cavity mucosal infections	☺

Scientifically Unproven
For any other indication

Further Reading

Foster, Steven, and Varro E. Tyler. *Tyler's Honest Herbal: A Sensible Guide to the Use of Herbs and Related Remedies.* 4th ed. New York: Haworth Herbal, 1999, 105–8.

Patzelt-Wenczler, R., and E. Ponce-Pöschl. "Proof of Efficacy of Kamillosan Cream in Atopic Eczema." *European Journal of Medical Research* 5, no. 4 (April 2000): 171–75.

CHAPARRAL

What It Is

Chaparral is the favorite scenery of old cowboy movies. The term refers in general to an area dense in shrubs and small trees. However, chaparral as an herbal remedy refers to the creosote bush, the most common shrub found in the desert areas of the southwestern United States and Mexico. The botanical name of the bush is *Larrea tridentata*, although *Larrea divaricata* and *Larrea mexicana* also refer to either the same shrub or one that is very similar. The bush is a source of creosote, which has led to much interest in finding uses, especially medicinal uses, for the other plant material.

Claims

Native Americans have made a tea from the leaves and twigs and used it for a wide variety of conditions, including arthritis, cancer, venereal disease, tuberculosis, and colds and as a hair tonic. During the 1960s, interest focused on its anticancer properties, in particular the principal ingredient in the tea, nordihydroguaiaretic acid (NDGA). More recently, claims have focused on its antifungal, antibacterial, and antiviral properties. Because of these claims, chaparral has become a popular herbal remedy among those infected with HIV. Chaparral remedies are also marketed as liver tonics and blood purifiers and for weight loss.

Study Findings

Cancers in rats given NDGA did show slower growth, but when chaparral tea was studied in humans, the results were extremely variable. NDGA is a potent antioxidant, which may explain why it affects various living systems. However, no clinical studies support any of the alleged benefits of using chaparral. Although anecdotal reports (✓) of an "anticancer" effect may justify conducting controlled studies, chaparral has also been shown to stimulate the growth of certain tumors.

Cautions

When studies with rats were continued for longer periods of time, those given chaparral developed problems in their lymph nodes and kidneys. In humans, numerous cases of poisoning, acute hepatitis, and liver damage have been reported (✗✗) in people taking chaparral. Two of these people required liver transplantation. In 1992, the FDA issued a warning of the potential link between chaparral and liver toxicity. In addition, several cases of kidney failure were reported (✗✗) after ingestion of chaparral. This led to removal of many products from stores, although they have been reappearing in recent years. For example, one dietary supplement containing chaparral is being marketed for fever blisters with a claim that a patented manufacturing process renders the product nontoxic. To our knowledge, this claim has not been independently confirmed.

Recommendations

Since chaparral has not demonstrated effectiveness, and because it can have serious toxic effects, taking it in any form cannot be recommended. Chaparral should be avoided. Anyone already suffering from liver damage or jaundice should certainly avoid this remedy completely.

Dosage

No dose is safe.

Treatment Categories

Scientifically Questionable
For any indication   ☹☹☹☹

Quackery or Fraud
In the hands of some practitioners

Risk of Serious Side Effects
With any use   ⊘⊘⊘

Further Reading

Foster, Steven, and Varro E. Tyler. *Tyler's Honest Herbal: A Sensible Guide to the Use of Herbs and Related Remedies.* 4th ed. New York: Haworth Herbal, 1999, 109–11.

Sheikh, Nasreen M., Rosanne M. Philen, and Lori A. Love. "Chaparral-Associated Hepatotoxicity." *Archives of Internal Medicine* 157, no. 8 (April 1997): 913–19.

CHONDROITIN SULFATE

What It Is

Chondroitin sulfate naturally occurs in the cartilage of humans and other organisms, including sea cucumber and shark cartilage. It is a very large molecule made from modified carbohydrates. Chondroitin sulfate is one of a number of compounds called "proteoglycans" (formerly known as mucopolysaccharides) that act as lubricants within joints. Preparations are made by extracting chondroitin from animal cartilage, most commonly from bovine trachea.

Claims

Public interest in chondroitin sulfate skyrocketed after publication of the immensely popular book *The Arthritis Cure* (New York: St. Martin's Press, 1997). Studies of its effectiveness have been ongoing since the 1980s. Osteoarthritis is a degenerative disease in which cartilage and eventually bone are broken down, leading to pain, stiffness, joint swelling, and deformity. Treatment has primarily been limited to exercise and pain relievers. However, chondroitin sulfate, usually in combination with glucosamine sulfate, is now being promoted as an actual cure for "arthritis." Closer examination makes it clear that these claims usually refer to osteoarthritis. Chondroitin sulfate is said to reverse some of the cartilage damage that has already occurred. In some countries it is administered as an intramuscular injection.

Chondroitin sulfate is also used to treat ischemic heart disease, osteoporosis, and elevated cholesterol levels. Topically, it is used for dry eyes and as a medium for cornea transplantation.

Study Findings

Loss of proteoglycans and changes in the structure of chondroitin sulfate in joints have been shown to occur during the development of osteoarthritis. During the 1990s, controlled clinical trials (✓✓✓) were reported on the use of chondroitin sulfate for osteoarthritis. A 1998 study (✓✓✓) showed, with X-rays, what appeared to be the preservation of cartilage in the knees of patients with moderate to severe osteoarthritis who took chondroitin sulfate for more than one year. Another 1998 study (✓✓✓) using X-rays showed that chondroitin protected patients from severe finger joint damage.

A 2003 systematic review of research on chondroitin for osteoarthritis found eight high-quality controlled trials (✓✓✓✓). On all symptom measures, including mobility and pain, chondroitin was significantly better than placebo. This review also found evidence that glucosamine delayed narrowing of the joint space, which causes osteoarthritis. Studies on the impact of chondroitin on that measurement were not conclusive. The evidence therefore does not support claims that chondroitin prevents or reverses osteoarthritis. Nevertheless, these studies consistently showed that patients taking chondroitin sulfate had reduced pain, used less pain medication, and had improved mobility compared to those taking placebo. The subjects in all of these studies continued to use their usual analgesics as needed.

Controlled studies (✓✓✓✓) have shown that taking chondroitin sulfate and nonsteroidal anti-inflammatory drugs (NSAIDs) is significantly more effective than taking NSAIDs alone for reducing pain and improving function in patients with osteoarthritis of the hip and knee. Chondroitin may thereby allow patients to slowly lower the dosage of NSAIDs (or even discontinue them) after six to eight weeks.

Some trials have also been conducted using chondroitin sulfate in combination with glucosamine sulfate or glucosamine hydrochloride. When used in combination, lower doses of each can be given and the same benefits maintained. One particular product (Cosamine DS) contains chondroitin sulfate, glucosamine sulfate, and manganese ascorbate. In one controlled trial (✓✓✓), those taking the Cosamine DS reported significantly less osteoarthritic knee pain compared to those taking placebo. However, since the trial compared only the combination to placebo, we have no way of knowing which component in the Cosamine DS was the most helpful.

Chondroitin is a very large molecule, and studies show that only 8 to 18 percent of an orally ingested dose is absorbed into the bloodstream. However, it has been theorized, because of the studies showing its effectiveness, that it may be broken down in the digestive tract into smaller, more easily digested, medically active compounds.

Many chondroitin products sold in America may be inferior. In December 1999 and January 2000, ConsumerLab.com purchased brands of chondroitin and combined glucosamine and chondroitin products. These products were then tested to determine whether they possessed the claimed amounts of glucosamine and chondroitin. Nearly one-third of all the products did not pass testing. Among the glucosamine and chondroitin combination products, almost half (six out of thirteen) did not pass — all due to low chondroitin levels. The two chondroitin-only products also did not pass. In contrast, all ten of the glucosamine-only products passed the testing. One possible explanation for the low pass rate for chondroitin-containing products is economic — chondroitin costs manufacturers approximately four times as much as glucosamine.

In 2003, ConsumerLab.com retested two chondroitin products, eleven glucosamine/chondroitin products, and eight glucosamine/chondroitin/MSM products. Problems were found among only combination products, four of which were low in chondroitin sulfate. One product claimed to contain 500 mg per serving of "chondroitin sulfate complex." However, testing showed it contained less than 90 mg of chondroitin (less than 18 percent of the advertised chondroitin sulfate). Another product contained less than 85 percent of its claimed chondroitin sulfate. The brand names of products that passed testing can be viewed at the subscription-based ConsumerLab.com website (*www.consumerlab.com*).

Studies have shown that the benefits from chondroitin are usually delayed. They may take up to three months to appear after the product is started. However, there is also a lingering effect of up to three months of benefit after the product is stopped. Studies have shown that patients who take chondroitin sulfate (800 mg per day) for three months followed by three months of no treatment and then repeat treatment again for another three months retain a significant reduction in symptoms.

• Cautions

Side effects were infrequent in the studies (✗✗) that have been conducted. Some nausea and stomach and intestinal disturbances have been reported.

Chondroitin sulfate when given by injection can be painful. Some have raised concerns about bleeding because chondroitin sulfate is similar in structure to heparin, which prevents blood clotting. This has not been reported as a problem in clinical trials.

Recommendations

Research with chondroitin sulfate has produced promising results. Arthritis is a common and painful condition affecting millions of people around the world. The most common treatments for osteoarthritis usually involve pain relievers that are prone to serious adverse effects. A safe and effective remedy directed at the underlying cause of the disease would be a welcome addition.

Long-term studies are needed to ensure that the chondroitin sulfate benefits seen over a few months will last into years. This research also would help to determine whether there are any harmful effects from taking chondroitin for prolonged periods of time.

Glucosamine, along with chondroitin sulfate, is widely recommended, but the combination has not been as well studied in clinical trials. Since chondroitin sulfate is sold as a dietary supplement, products of different quality will remain available. Choose only reputable brands.

Dosage

The dose depends on the person's weight and is usually given along with glucosamine. An average daily dose would be 1200 mg of chondroitin and 1500 mg of glucosamine. This is usually divided into two to four doses, taken with food. Intermittent dosing has also been proposed where patients take chondroitin for three months, take three months off, and then take the supplement again. Few studies have examined this approach, but it appears to be effective.

Treatment Categories

Conventional
Topically after cataract extraction
or lens implantation ☺☺☺☺

Complementary
To relieve symptoms of osteoarthritis ☺☺☺☺
To relieve pain from osteoarthritis ☺☺☺☺
Topically to relieve dry eyes ☺☺

Scientifically Unproven
To treat heart disease, high cholesterol,
or osteoporosis
For any other indication

Further Reading

Leeb, Burkhard F., Harald Schweitzer, Karin Montag, and Josef S. Smolen. "A Meta-analysis of Chondroitin Sulfate in the Treatment of Osteoarthritis." *Journal of Rheumatology* 27, no. 1 (January 2000): 205–11.

Richy, Florent, Olivier Bruyere, Olivier Ethgen, Michel Cucherat, Yves Honrotin, and Jean-Yves Reginster. "Structural and Symptomatic Efficacy of Glucosamine and Chondroitin in Knee Osteoarthritis." *Archives of Internal Medicine* 163 (July 2003): 1514–22.

CHROMIUM

● What It Is

Chromium is known as a trace element, which means that very little is needed by our bodies. In fact, so little is needed that it was not recognized as being essential until 1959. Even now that it is better understood, much remains unclear. Many do not get the USDA estimated safe and adequate daily dietary allowance, but this appears to have no ill effects for most. So little chromium is needed that recommended daily intakes are given in micrograms, one of which equals one millionth of a gram.

Eating peanut butter on a regular basis will provide as much chromium as anyone needs. Chromium is present in peanuts as well as in wheat grain, dried yeast, and other whole grains. Foods such as liver, American cheese, cereals, and wheat germ also contain the mineral. These natural sources contain tiny amounts of chromium, and only 1 to 2 percent of that is absorbed into our bodies, but that appears to be enough for almost everyone. In spite of the tiny amounts needed, a growing number of proponents are recommending chromium, and many are buying more and more supplements containing the mineral.

● Claims

According to Barbara Stoecker, a researcher specializing in chromium, chromium is one of the two bestselling mineral supplements in the United States (the other is calcium). This is because the most popular uses for chromium relate to two areas of serious concern — to treat diabetes and to help people lose weight. In addition, chromium is said to increase people's energy, improve sports performance, reduce food cravings, cure acne, assist with sleep, relieve depression, reduce high blood pressure, and even increase how long people live. Is it any wonder that chromium is in such demand?

Chromium is usually sold as a complex called "chromium picolinate" because this form of chromium is said to be better absorbed from most people's intestinal tracts. It is often added to herbal combinations, especially those sold to help with weight loss. It is also available in chewing gum, sports drinks, and nutrition bars.

● Study Findings

Research on chromium as a treatment for diabetes must be considered separately from all other claims. Laboratory research has shown that chromium plays an important role in the way insulin works to regulate blood sugar. A number of clinical studies on the health effects of chromium were published in 1999 from an international conference sponsored in part by the U.S. Department of Agriculture. Foremost among these were several studies (✓✓✓) showing that chromium supplements did help some, but not all, people with type 2 diabetes mellitus. This form of diabetes, formerly called "adult-onset diabetes," is linked to overweight and can usually be controlled without insulin therapy (which is needed in type 1 diabetes).

In the clinical studies, some patients taking supplemental chromium were able to reduce the amount of prescription diabetic medications they took, but others showed no improvements. Most researchers believe that chromium benefits only those patients who lack chromium in their diet. They believe that if you already absorb enough chromium from your food, you will have no added benefit from a supplement. Unfortunately this knowledge is not as practical as it seems. Currently no test is available to easily and reliably determine if someone is chromium deficient.

While chromium may be helpful for some people with diabetes, there is very little evidence that it helps with weight loss. A 2003 review found ten randomized controlled studies. Eight of the ten studies (✗✗✗) found chromium to be of no more benefit than placebo. However, when all the results were combined, chromium supplements did produce significantly more weight loss than placebo (✓✓✓✓). The average weight loss with chromium was just over 1 kg more than with placebo over three months. The reviewers noted that while this was statistically significant, it was of questionable practical significance. People restricting calories or adding exercise would be expected to lose that much weight per week. Four studies (✗✗✗) involving athletes taking chromium showed no increase in muscle mass or decrease in body mass.

In 2005, ConsumerLab.com tested seven chromium-containing supplements and found that three failed their tests. One product had only 25 percent of the chromium claimed on the label — despite the fact that its label claimed it was "cGMP certified," "laboratory tested," and made with "pharmaceutical grade ingredients." Another product had 42 percent

more chromium than its label claimed. The third product had relatively high levels of hexavalent chromium, a potential carcinogen and toxin.

Cautions

One of the ongoing controversies in this area relates to the safety of taking chromium supplements. During the clinical research studies, no adverse reactions were reported. The United States EPA safe exposure dose is 350 times the recommended daily intake, and animal studies have found it very safe. The Institute of Medicine was unable to set a Tolerable Upper Intake Level because of insufficient data.

However, case reports (✗✗) of toxicity, especially involving kidney damage, have started to appear in the medical literature. At doses of 200 to 400 micrograms per day, chromium has been reported to cause mental and muscle disturbances. At doses of 1.2 to 2.4 grams per day, anemia and other blood system problems have been reported. Chromium when taken as a supplement does not increase the normal chromium level of normal breast milk. Therefore, the Natural Database has concluded that chromium is safe (in amounts not exceeding the adequate intake levels) for children and for women who are pregnant or lactating.

Two studies using tissues grown experimentally found that chromium picolinate can cause genetic damage, which could lead to cancer. Some experts believe this damage results from the chromium picolinate combination, not chromium itself, and are looking for other ways to administer chromium. Very little study has been conducted in this area, which should signal caution in using chromium for extended periods of time.

Recommendations

Chromium is an essential part of the diet, not a drug with a similar effect in everyone. A deficiency of chromium can cause problems.

The strongest evidence for the effective use of chromium supplements exists for treating diabetes in those patients who are chromium deficient. Since there is no reliable way to test for such a deficiency, people with type 2 diabetes might want to discuss a trial of chromium with their physician. Close monitoring of the blood glucose levels is essential. If the chromium helps, other medications may need to be reduced. If it doesn't, other medications would need to be maintained.

More important, exercise, diet, and weight-control play a very large role in managing diabetes and should not be neglected. If chromium supplements are beneficial, continued monitoring is important, especially of the kidneys, since the diabetes itself may lead to some renal problems that chromium might make worse.

Although chromium may be worth trying for patients with high cholesterol or triglyceride levels, much more effective options are available.

Dosage

The Institute of Medicine has set the adequate daily intake of chromium at 25 micrograms for women and 35 micrograms for men. Many products containing chromium picolinate recommend taking 200 micrograms of that formulation three times a day. However, studies have found no detrimental effects in people consuming diets with less than 20 micrograms of chromium daily.

Treatment Categories

Complementary

To prevent reactive hypoglycemia in diabetics	☺☺
To treat type 2 diabetes in those who are chromium deficient	☺☺☺
To treat type 2 diabetes in those who are not chromium deficient	☹☹☹☹
To lower cholesterol and triglyceride levels	☺

Scientifically Unproven

To treat patients with impaired glucose intolerance (prediabetes)	☹☹☹
To help with weight loss	☹☹☹
To improve athletic performance	☹☹☹☹
To increase energy levels	☹☹
For any other indication	

Further Reading

Althuis, Michelle D., Nicole E. Jordan, Elizabeth A. Ludington, and Janet T. Wittes. "Glucose and Insulin Responses to Dietary Chromium Supplements: A Meta-analysis." *American Journal of Clinical Nutrition* 76, no. 1 (2002): 148–55.

Pittler, M. H., C. Stevinson, and E. Ernst. "Chromium Picolinate for Reducing Body Weight: Meta-analysis of Randomized Trials." *International Journal of Obesity and Related Metabolic Disorders* 27 (2003): 522–29.

Stoecker, Barbara J. "Chromium." In *Modern Nutrition in Health and Disease.* 9th ed. Baltimore, Md.: Williams & Wilkins, 1999, 277–82.

COENZYME Q$_{10}$

What It Is

Coenzyme Q$_{10}$, also called "Co-Q$_{10}$" or "ubiquinone," is an antioxidant found in many foods, especially meat and seafood. Co-Q$_{10}$ is a fat-soluble compound chemically similar to the fat-soluble vitamins E and K. Co-Q$_{10}$ works like a vitamin in many ways but is not classified as one because it is produced in the human body (and vitamins are not). It is needed to allow the production of energy by the body's cells and to prevent oxidation within membranes. The Japanese government, in 1974, approved Co-Q$_{10}$ for treatment of heart failure. It is reported to be used extensively in Europe and Russia. Most Co-Q$_{10}$ is made by fermenting beets or sugarcane with a special strain of yeast.

Claims

A number of years ago, Co-Q$_{10}$ was an extremely popular dietary supplement said to prevent aging, cure cancer, and raise energy levels. The reasons for this were largely theoretical and anecdotal. For example, it was found that Co-Q$_{10}$ is present in greater levels among the young and vigorous than among the elderly and infirm. The theory was that perhaps a reduction in the antioxidant caused some of the ravages of aging. Taking this idea a step further, it was postulated that if people began taking the antioxidant, they could actually reverse aging by restoring the same chemical balance in their bodies that they had when young.

This type of postulating is the basis for much scientific research. However, it is nothing more than an idea. That was enough for some who touted the theory in the popular press as "fact." Next came advertisements with headlines along the lines of "Scientists Have Discovered the Fountain of Youth" and "The Miracle Pill That Can Add Years to Your Life." Even though the theory had *not yet been tested*, the implication was that the discovery was being confirmed.

Co-Q$_{10}$ is expensive, and its popularity has dropped off. Today Co-Q$_{10}$ is primarily promoted to prevent a variety of heart conditions, including congestive heart failure and angina. It is also used for diabetes, high blood pressure, Huntington's disease, muscular dystrophy, chronic fatigue, AIDS, and male infertility. Some use it topically for periodontal disease and to prevent wrinkles.

Study Findings

One of the original theories about Co-Q$_{10}$ was shattered in the early part of 2000 when test results (✗✗✗) failed to support claims regarding its antiaging properties. Yes, the antioxidant levels decrease with age. No, there seemed to be no direct cause and effect that could be countered by taking the supplements.

The issue of heart disease is less clear. A number of studies (✓✓) have shown that people with certain types of heart disease have lower levels of Co-Q$_{10}$. However, most studies (✓✓✓✓) show that long-term treatment (with up to 100 mg) of patients with congestive heart failure only slightly improves maximal exercise capacity and quality of life. In some clinical trials, the proportion of patients who showed improvements was similar to the proportion who benefited from conventional drugs such as ACE inhibitors and digoxin. A 2005 review (✔✔✔✔) of heart failure studies found five studies, four of which found Co-Q_{10} more beneficial than placebo. However, the review concluded that larger studies are still needed because all of the studies conducted to date have had problems in their designs. More clear-cut benefits have been found in a small number of studies (✔✔✔) in which Co-Q_{10} was combined with conventional heart failure drugs. Similarly, when Co-Q_{10} was combined with blood pressure–lowering drugs and anticholesterol drugs, additive effects were found (✔✔✔). The evidence that Co-Q_{10} is beneficial for those with angina is much weaker (✔✔).

There are reports (✔✔) of Co-Q_{10} reducing the cardiotoxicity of chemotherapy (with Adriamycin). Case reports (✔✔) exist of improved function in those with Huntington's disease or muscular dystrophy after use of Co-Q_{10}, but the first unblinded trial (✖✖) with Huntington's patients found no benefits. Early evidence (✔✔) suggests it may have some benefit in those with Parkinson's disease. It may (✔✔) improve immune system function in patients with AIDS. Small studies (✖✖) have shown no effect on blood sugar in diabetics. Studies (✖✖✖) have shown no improvement in athletic performance with Co-Q_{10} or, when applied topically, for periodontal disease. No studies have determined whether long-term improvements result with Co-Q_{10}, nor have any studies compared it directly to conventional medicines.

Co-Q_{10} may help patients with migraine headaches by decreasing the frequency by about 30 percent and reducing the number of days with migraine-related nausea by about 45 percent. These benefits can take up to three months to appear. However, taking Co-Q_{10} to prevent migraines does not reduce their duration or severity when they do occur.

Concerns about the quality and purity of Co-Q_{10} sold in the United States were addressed by ConsumerLab.com, an independent testing company that permits promoters to use its flask-shaped seal of approval on products that pass its criteria. In 2000, a significant number of products failed their testing. However, in 2004, retesting of thirty-two products showed that all but one contained the amount of Co-Q_{10} listed on the label (the one product that failed contained only 17 percent of what the label claimed). However, after release of the review, the manufacturer of the product that did not pass testing requested that ConsumerLab.com test a reformulated version of the product. The newer product passed testing. The results of these and other tests can be viewed by subscribing to their website.

• Cautions

In the clinical studies involving Co-Q_{10}, no significant adverse effects have been reported from taking 200 mg daily for six to twelve months or 100 mg daily for up to six years. Fewer than 1 percent of people report (✖) short-term nausea, vomiting, diarrhea, appetite suppression, heartburn, or epigastric discomfort. These side effects can be reduced if total daily doses that exceed 100 mg are divided and administered two or three times per day. Rarely, allergic rashes have been reported (✖). Furthermore, statins (drugs that reduce cholesterol levels) and some oral diabetes drugs (Micronase, Dymelor, and Tolinase) reduce levels of Co-Q_{10}. The clinical significance of this is not known.

Recommendations

Overall, early enthusiasm for Co-Q$_{10}$ as a cardiac supplement has diminished as more high-quality research has been reported. There is no proof that it reduces death rates from heart disease. The reported benefits may be due to Co-Q$_{10}$ being an antioxidant. However, it is a very expensive dietary supplement, especially given that it is readily available in fruits, vegetables, meat, and fish. In addition, much remains uncertain about how Co-Q$_{10}$ might work and how well it might work over the many years someone could be taking it. Furthermore, a number of well-established, conventional drugs are relatively inexpensive and reduce the risk of death in patients with heart failure. People at risk for cardiac problems may want to consider using Co-Q$_{10}$ but should consult their physicians first, especially if they are already taking another heart medication, a cholesterol-lowering drug, or an oral agent for diabetes — as Co-Q$_{10}$ could potentially react with each of these medications. Co-Q$_{10}$ may be useful when used along with conventional drugs, but its use should be carefully monitored by your doctor.

Dosage

Most studies have used 50 to 200 mg of Co-Q$_{10}$ divided into two or three doses during the day.

Treatment Categories

Complementary

To treat congestive heart failure	☺☺☺
To lower blood pressure	☺☺
To lower cholesterol levels	☺☺
To prevent migraine headaches ☺☺☺	
To relieve angina	☺
To reduce risk of harm to the heart from Adriamycin	☺☺

Scientifically Unproven

To counteract aging	☹☹☹
To improve sports performance	☹☹
To improve function in people with Huntington's disease	☺
To improve function in people with Parkinson's disease	☺
To treat type 2 diabetes	☺

Further Reading

Littarru, Gian P., and Luca Tiano. "Clinical Aspects of Coenzyme Q$_{10}$: An Update." *Current Opinion in Clinical Nutrition and Metabolic Care* 8, no. 6 (November 2005): 641 – 46.

Weant, Kyle A., and Kelly M. Smith. "The Role of Coenzyme Q$_{10}$ in Heart Failure." *Annals of Pharmacotherapy* 39, no. 9 (September 2005): 1522 – 26.

COMFREY

What It Is

Comfrey is a popular herb used both alone and in combination with many other herbs. The leaves, roots, and rhizome (a rootlike stem) of a number of *Symphytum* species are used in these preparations. The plants grow widely throughout North America, also going by the common names of blackwort, knitbone, and slippery root.

Claims

Comfrey has been lauded by some as a wonder herb and cure-all. Its most common use was in a cream believed to promote healing of cuts, bruises, burns, and wounds. It has been used as a gargle for periodontal disease and sore throats. For internal consumption, it was usually made into a tea (or a blended extract known as "green drink"). It was said to heal stomach ulcers, cleanse the blood, and relieve bronchial congestion. Some have recommended comfrey for excessive menstrual flow, diarrhea, persistent cough, rheumatism, bronchitis, cancer, and angina.

Study Findings

Analysis of the compounds contained in comfrey shows that about one-third of the root consists of a carbohydrate called "mucilage." This type of compound could form a thin film over the skin, providing some protection and soothing irritation. Another compound called "allantoin" is found in the roots and is known to stimulate cell proliferation, which would be useful in wound healing. Studies (✓✓✓) have shown comfrey to have some effectiveness when used topically on bruises and sprains. However, no other beneficial ingredients have been found in extracts of comfrey, while several compounds known to have serious toxic effects have been found.

Cautions

All comfrey species contain a variety of compounds called "pyrrolizidine alkaloids," with the roots containing about ten times as much of these materials as the leaves. All of these compounds are known to be toxic to the liver and may cause liver and lung cancer. In addition, some products labeled "common comfrey" (*Symphytum officinale*) have been shown to contain the more toxic prickly comfrey (*Symphytum asperum*) or Russian comfrey (*Symphytum x uplandicum*).

In animals given comfrey, liver and bladder tumors developed within six months, and other liver damage was clearly visible. Numerous cases (✗✗) of veno-occlusive liver disease (blood vessels in the liver become blocked, leading to death of liver tissue) have been reported after people ingested comfrey. One article in the British journal *Lancet* suggested that the most common cause of this particular disease is ingestion of plants containing pyrrolizidine alkaloids.

For these reasons, most medical authorities recommend that comfrey not be taken internally for any reason.

In addition, topically applied pyrrolizidine alkaloids have been shown to be absorbed through the skin. The American Herbal Products Association has recommended that *all* products with toxic pyrrolizidine alkaloids (e.g., comfrey) be labeled with the statement, "For external use only. Do not apply to broken or abraded skin. Do not use while nursing." In July 2001, the FDA asked manufacturers to remove comfrey from the market, but it is still available.

Recommendations

Comfrey may have some value when applied externally for the treatment of mild bruises or sprains. Since numerous other pharmaceutical and natural remedies are available for these conditions, we cannot think of any good reason to choose comfrey. If anyone insists on using comfrey, it should be used cautiously and for short periods since active ingredients in topical medications can be absorbed through the skin. Comfrey preparations should never be used on cuts or where the skin is broken. The risks of toxicity make any internal use of comfrey unwarranted and external use unwise.

Dosage

No oral dose of comfrey is safe, and few would recommend using it topically. Do not use comfrey ointment on broken skin or for longer than ten days.

Treatment Categories

Complementary

Topically on unbroken skin to treat bruises or sprains — yet because of its potential toxicity, we do not recommend its use. ☹

Scientifically Questionable

As a gargle to treat periodontal disease and sore throats ☹☹☹

Topically to promote healing of cuts or abrasions ☹☹

Orally for any indication ☹☹☹☹

Risk of Serious Side Effects

Orally ⊘⊘⊘⊘

Topically, especially if the skin is broken ⊘⊘⊘

Further Reading

Foster, Steven, and Varro E. Tyler. *Tyler's Honest Herbal: A Sensible Guide to the Use of Herbs and Related Remedies.* 4th ed. New York: Haworth Herbal, 1999, 121 – 25.

CRANBERRY

What It Is

Mention cranberries, and the first thought most Americans have is of the smooth or whole berry sauces served most frequently during holiday gatherings. Cranberry juice is also popular as a nonalcoholic beverage. Adding to its popularity is the claim that the juice may protect people from urinary tract infections (UTIs). As an herbal remedy, apart from the juice and the sauce, cranberry has been one of the ten bestselling herbal remedies for a number of years in the United States. The berries are widely available, growing throughout the United States on a small shrub (*Vaccinium macrocarpon*), also called the "trailing swamp cranberry."

Claims

In a study published in 1923, one healthy volunteer ate cooked cranberries and soon afterward had urine that was more acidic. Since bacteria causing UTIs do not grow as well in more acidic environments, cranberry products quickly gained a reputation for preventing and treating UTIs. This reputation continues to this day.

Additionally, cranberry juice is said to lessen the odor of stale urine. Odor is an especially problematic and embarrassing aspect of incontinence. Cranberry juice has also been used as a diuretic, as an antiseptic, and to treat cancer and fever.

Study Findings

After the earliest report (✔) found cranberry juice increased the acidity of urine, other studies (✘✘) found contradictory results. By the 1980s, it became clear that cranberry juice did not consistently change urine acidity. However, it was found to produce compounds that can prevent bacteria from adhering to the lining of the urinary tract. This action prevents bacteria from replicating and growing. A number of reports (✔✔) have noted a reduction in urine odor after incontinent people drank cranberry regularly.

The first controlled study (✔✔✔) of cranberry juice was published in the *Journal of the American Medical Association* in 1994. Elderly women drinking 10 ounces of cranberry juice per day had fewer UTIs than those drinking a similar-tasting red drink. However, a 1999 controlled study (✘✘✘) with children at high risk for developing UTIs found that drinking cranberry juice did not change the frequency of their infections. A 2004 Cochrane review identified seven controlled studies of cranberry. Five were very small, and many participants dropped out before completing the research. This suggests that long-term consumption of cranberry juice may not be appealing. The other two trials (✔✔✔) were larger, of high quality, enrolled only women, and found fewer UTIs in those drinking cranberry juice. Studies have not examined whether cranberry juice effectively treats UTIs.

Because long-term consumption of the juice may be problematic, many companies are marketing concentrated forms of cranberry extract in capsules or tablets. Unfortunately, there is virtually no reliable evidence that these have the same benefits as the juice. Therefore, experts recommend that women interested in trying cranberry for urine odor or UTI prevention use only the juice.

Cautions

No toxicity or adverse effects have been reported with cranberry juice until large quantities are consumed; drinking more than a gallon in one day causes diarrhea. However, many cranberry drinks contain lots of sugar, thereby adding many calories if consumed frequently.

Particular caution is needed with juice made from any other cranberries than the common North American variety (*Vaccinium macrocarpon*). Alpine cranberry (*Vaccinium vitis-ideae*), high-bush cranberry (*Viburnum opulus*, or cramp bark), and mountain cranberry (*Arctostaphylos uva-ursi*, or uva-ursi) are similar-looking bushes whose fruit is made into juices recommended for UTIs. These all contain compounds called "hydroquinolones," which can cause liver toxicity. These juices should not be used for extended periods by anyone and should never be given to children under twelve years of age. Women who are pregnant or breast-feeding should also avoid these forms of cranberries.

Recommendations

Cranberry juice and extracts may provide some protection against UTIs, although only a few studies with women support this conclusion. Since the juice is readily available and relatively inexpensive, it could easily be added to one's diet, especially for people who are prone to UTIs. The berries may also provide some benefit from their antioxidants, although they contain a small amount compared to other sources such as bilberry and grape seed. The high drop-out rate from studies suggests regular drinking of the juice may not be palatable for many. Once symptoms of a UTI develop, consult a physician about starting a course of antibiotics.

Dosage

Most studies use 10 to 16 ounces of juice a day, although little is known about how much is needed to prevent urinary tract infections.

Treatment Categories

Complementary

To prevent UTIs in women	☺☺☺
To prevent UTIs in children and men	☹
To deodorize urine in incontinent patients	☺☺☺
To treat diabetes	☹☹☹☹

Scientifically Unproven

For any other indication

Further Reading

Jepson, R. G., L. Mihaljevic, and J. Craig. "Cranberries for Preventing Urinary Tract Infections." *The Cochrane Database of Systematic Reviews* 2004, no. 2.

Lee, Yee-Lean, John Owens, Lauri Thrupp, and Thomas C. Cesario. "Does Cranberry Juice Have Antibacterial Activity?" *Journal of the American Medical Association* 283, no. 13 (April 2000): 1691.

CREATINE

What It Is

Creatine is a commonly used sports supplement that has become very popular with weight lifters and football players. A 2004 survey at one NCAA Division 1 university found that over one-third of its athletes were using creatine. Unlike steroids and stimulants, creatine is not banned by the International Olympic Committee or the National Collegiate Athletic Association (NCAA), in part because it is a normal constituent of people's diet. It is found in meat and fish and made by humans in the liver. However, NCAA institutions are not permitted to provide creatine supplements to their athletes, leaving them to find their own sources if they choose to use creatine.

The importance of creatine in exercise was noted as far back as 1847 when the meat obtained from wild foxes was compared with that of foxes raised in captivity. The wild fox meat had more than ten times the amount of creatine. It wasn't until the 1990s that creatine burst onto the athletic scene when British sprinters claimed it gave them a significant, and legal, boost in energy. Creatine has since been mass-marketed to such an extent that in 1999, 2.5 million kilograms were used as a supplement in the United States.

Claims

Many high school and college football programs openly or quietly support the use of creatine. When Mark McGwire broke Roger Maris's home run record in 1998, creatine was one of the supplements he ad-mitted he was taking (see entry on Androstenedione for more details). Some products claim creatine will make a well-trained athlete 5 percent stronger or faster. While that may not seem like a whole lot, it could turn a good athlete into a great athlete — if it is true. For the recreational runner or the person who lifts weights on occasion, creatine is said to provide more energy and delay the onset of fatigue. That would certainly be welcome — if it is true.

Study Findings

Creatine is one of the few alleged performance-enhancing substances that has been extensively studied. It plays an important role in providing energy for muscles during exercise. When we first start to exercise, energy stored in muscles is used up almost completely within a couple of seconds. To get us through the next few seconds, these stores are replenished using a substance made from creatine called "creatine phosphate" (CP). Creatine's role in fueling muscles is therefore during high-intensity exercise that lasts less than half a minute. Theoretically, by increasing the amount of creatine in the body, an athlete might be able to perform at high intensity for slightly longer periods of time. Also, since creatine is vital to replenishing energy stores, more creatine in the body might allow the muscles to recover more quickly for the next bout of exercise.

Studies (✓✓) have found that creatine supplementation increases the amount of creatine and CP stored in muscle cells. Athletes taking 20 grams of creatine daily for three days increased their levels by 17 percent, but more than half the creatine was excreted unchanged in their urine. There was also wide variation in how people responded. Those whose levels started the lowest (usually vegetarians) changed the most. This variability is thought to have influenced the results of studies examining whether supplementation improved people's athletic performance.

Since the 1990s, more than one hundred randomized, placebo-controlled, blinded studies have been conducted on creatine for performance enhancement or body composition. Many of these were relatively small and showed some variability in their results. Most used healthy male athletes and tested them running, swimming, bicycling, kayaking, and weight-lifting. A 2003 systematic review of these studies (✓✓✓✓) concluded that creatine effectively increases total and lean body mass and improves performance in high-intensity, short-duration, repetitive exercise regimens. For example, of the sixty-two studies examining exercise duration of less than 30 seconds, three-quarters found some benefit from creatine. Only eighteen studies examined exercise of 150 seconds or longer, with half finding creatine better than placebo and half not.

Other patterns emerged from this review of the studies. Benefits were greater when athletes began with a large "loading" dose for a short period and then continued at a lower dose. Few studies included women, and most of those found no benefits (✗✗✗). The benefits were greater with upper-body exercise than lower-body or overall body exercise. Most of the studies were conducted in controlled laboratory settings, such as on treadmills or with weightlifting equipment. When performance was examined in more usual sports situations, minimal improvements were found. The researchers noted that while creatine may promote strength gains, it often also leads to weight gain that may counteract any competitive advantage.

For recreational and endurance athletes (✗✗✗), creatine does not bring improvements in performance. This is to be expected since the creatine-CP system plays very little role in this sort of exercise. For one-time, high-intensity exercise (such as full-out exertion in sprinting or power lifting), no benefit occurs (✗✗✗). This type of exercise depends mostly on stored energy, not creatine. However, when athletes do repeated bouts of high-intensity, short-duration exercise, with rests under a few minutes long, studies (✓✓✓✓) show that creatine supplementation provides some limited benefits. Sports such as basketball and soccer involve this type of repetitive sprinting and resting. It is also important in what is called "interval training," where athletes do an all-out sprint, rest for a short period, and go again. Similarly, weight lifters may do an all-out lift, rest, and lift again. It appears that creatine may allow athletes to perform this sort of exercise at higher intensities and for more repetitions. This more intense training might better prepare the athlete for competition. However, there is also a risk that this more intense training could lead to injury or leave the athlete burned out.

Cautions

Many anecdotal reports (✗) of muscle cramps, gastrointestinal problems, and kidney problems exist. However, these adverse effects have not been recorded during controlled studies. Theoretically, long-term supplementation makes kidney problems likely, but we found only one study examining this issue. It monitored a small number of athletes (✓✓) taking 10 grams of creatine daily for up to five years and found no kidney problems. However, two case reports (✘) of kidney problems after creatine supplementation have been reported. These patients may have had kidney disease before taking the supplements, which would warrant people with kidney disease, or at high risk for it, being particularly cautious about taking creatine. Anyone taking other medication that might interfere with the kidneys should also be careful.

The only other established side effect of creatine (✘✘) is that it leads to weight gain of two to six pounds because of increased water retention in the muscles. This may be a problem for athletes competing in weight categories and might lead to unhealthy ways to reduce their weight for competition. Given the huge interest among high school athletes in creatine, it is disappointing that no information is available on its safety for younger athletes. For this reason, the American College of Sports Medicine recommends against creatine supplementation for those under eighteen years of age. Very little information is available on the effects of long-term supplementation for any age group. In addition, creatine should be avoided by women who are pregnant or lactating, as there is insufficient reliable information about its use in these situations.

There is some concern that creatine products sold in the United States may be of variable quality. ConsumerLab.com, an independent testing company that uses German testing standards to test herbs, vitamins, and supplements sold in the United States, tested thirteen creatine products purchased in 2000. Most of the products met the standards. One failed because it contained less than the claimed amount of ingredients, and a significant amount of impurities was found (see *www.consumerlab.com*). However, when ConsumerLab.com retested creatine products in 2003, they found that only half of them passed the testing. Both liquid products failed, with one containing less than 1 percent of the claimed amount of creatine. An effervescent product and a chewable wafer product failed for containing less than 90 percent of their claimed creatine. All of the standard powdered products passed testing. The NCAA has warned athletes that creatine supplements may be contaminated with banned performance-enhancing agents that could lead to positive drug tests.

Note: Creatine is broken down in the body to creatinine and excreted in the urine. Creatinine levels are regularly checked by physicians as a way to detect problems such as kidney diseases. Creatine supplementation leads to elevated creatinine levels, mimicking kidney disease, even though the kidney function may be normal. Anyone taking creatine should alert health care professionals if giving them a urine sample for testing.

Recommendations

For athletes whose training involves high-intensity repetitions, creatine supplementation may provide some benefits. But people vary a lot in how much they respond, and the improvements are not large. For example, in one study with power lifters (✔✔✔), those who took creatine lifted 7.8 kg more after supplementation, but those who took a placebo were able to lift 7.0 kg more. The difference was statistically significant but may not make a practical difference, especially with the unknown potential for adverse effects.

As Christians, we must also be concerned about how far we go in promoting athletic achievement. Both of us were competitive athletes and have been blessed in many ways from our experiences in sports. But the desire to win must be balanced against other important values. Taking supplements of uncertain benefit and safety is not warranted. It too easily communicates to others, especially youngsters, that winning is all-important, no matter what the cost.

For recreational athletes and those who exercise aerobically, creatine supplementation will be of no benefit. Given the lack of data on long-term safety, it would be advisable not to take the supplements for extended periods of time. Creatine is readily available in meat and fish, so these foods will provide adequate amounts for almost everyone.

Dosage

Athletes usually start with a "loading" dose of 20 grams per day for four to six days (usually taken in 5-gram portions four times a day, often mixed in sugary drinks). Following this, a 2-gram daily dose is taken to maintain the elevated levels. However, researchers have found that the same amount of creatine can be stored in the muscles after taking 3 grams per day for 30 days. This second regimen is considered to be easier on the kidneys.

Treatment Categories

Complementary

To enhance performance during
brief, high-intensity, anaerobic
exercise ☺☺☺☺

To enhance muscle function in those
with muscular dystrophies ☺

To improve exercise tolerance in those
with congestive heart failure ☺

Scientifically Unproven

To enhance performance during
recreational or aerobic exercise ☹☹☹☹

To enhance endurance
or performance in most
highly trained athletes ☹☹☹

To treat those with ALS ☹☹

To treat those with rheumatoid
arthritis ☹☹☹

Further Reading

Branch, J. David. "Effect of Creatine Supplementation on Body Composition and Performance: A Meta-analysis." *International Journal of Sport Nutrition and Exercise Metabolism* 13 (2003): 198 – 226.

Volek, Jeff S., and Eric S. Rawson. "Scientific Basis and Practical Aspects of Creatine Supplementation for Athletes." *Nutrition* 20, no. 7/8 (2004): 609 – 14.

DHEA

What It Is

Dehydroepiandrosterone (DHEA) is a steroid hormone, meaning it is a chemical messenger carrying information around the body. It is found in high concentrations in the brain. Our bodies produce it in particularly high quantities during two periods of our lives. The first is during fetal development, with the production almost stopping at birth. The second period begins around the age of seven and rises to a maximum in the mid-twenties before gradually dropping off. By the time you are in your sixties, you will typically have only 10 to 20 percent of your youthful peak values of the hormone.

This drop-off rate has led people to speculate that DHEA may be the elusive fountain of youth. Yet the actual function of DHEA is unknown. All that is certain is that our bodies normally use it to make many of the other hormones we need.

Claims

Daily DHEA supplements are supposed to slow aging, burn fat and build muscle mass, strengthen the immune system, treat lupus, and help prevent heart disease, cancer, diabetes, Alzheimer's disease, and Parkinson's disease. DHEA allegedly boosts libido, alleviates depression, and increases general feelings of strength, stamina, and well-being. It is said to be able to slow down the mental deterioration that can accompany aging and improve memory. The latest claim is that it will be a natural alternative to hormone replacement therapy in postmenopausal women and will treat vaginal dryness and increase bone strength.

Other alternative medicine providers promote DHEA supplements for conditions such as chronic fatigue and immune dysfunction syndrome and fibromyalgia syndrome. Most of these providers will first check either serum or salivary levels of DHEA and then supplement with small amounts of DHEA (10 to 50 mg per day) and monitor DHEA levels.

Study Findings

The last couple of decades have produced studies suggesting that DHEA may actually play a role in many of the conditions listed in the above claims. However, most of these studies were done on animals. In general, animal studies are an important step to developing safe and effective treatments for humans. However, there is a very significant caution needed with animal studies — and those with DHEA in particular. Humans and a few primates are the only species known to produce DHEA naturally and to have such high blood levels. This means that the results of these animal studies are not directly applicable to humans. They help move research along but should not be used to make confident claims about the effect of DHEA in humans.

Unfortunately, because marketers have seized on the results of early studies that may or may not turn out to be applicable to humans, abundant unfounded claims circulate about the benefits of DHEA. Since 1994, it has been widely advertised and freely available as a dietary supplement, which has helped to promote widespread use before its effectiveness and safety have been fully investigated.

These early, positive studies stimulated research into DHEA in humans, the results of which are starting to appear. Some studies (✓✓) in older people have shown preliminary evidence that DHEA can enhance people's mood and can have antidepressant effects. A 2001 Cochrane review examined studies using DHEA to improve mental function and boost memory. The review found four studies (✗✗✗) with inconclusive results and concluded there was no evidence to support the use of DHEA in normal older people to improve mental performance.

Research results released in 2000 (✓✓) showed that low DHEA levels are associated with an increased risk of heart disease in middle-aged men — those with the lowest DHEA levels had a 59 percent higher risk. However, these data do not answer the question of whether taking DHEA will bring up these levels or reduce cardiovascular risk in men.

DHEA has been recommended for systemic lupus erythematosus (SLE), a chronic inflammatory autoimmune disease that affects many tissues, especially the skin, joints, kidneys, nervous system, and mucous membranes. The symptoms come and go in intensity. Research showed that those with SLE had reduced DHEA levels. DHEA was then used to treat SLE in a small number of clinical trials. Although preliminary, the results have been generally positive (✓✓✓), with flare-ups being less severe and less frequent. Patients were also able to reduce the doses of other medications they were taking. None of these studies lasted more than one year, which is an important limitation given the cyclic nature of SLE. This means that the improvement may have been due not to DHEA but merely to the normal course of the disease.

Some athletes who use DHEA claim it increases testosterone levels to allow muscle building and more vigorous training. Very few studies have examined these claims, but one study (✗✗✗) with young, healthy men given DHEA found that it neither increased testosterone levels nor gave the men any more muscle or strength gains than when they took a placebo.

Overall, DHEA has some useful therapeutic actions. However, it has been proposed to treat a huge range of conditions. A search for research studies carried out on DHEA shows that it has been tested for many conditions but often with only one or two studies on each illness. Until a clearer picture emerges of what DHEA helps and what it doesn't help, only tentative recommendations can be made for most indications.

Cautions

One of the biggest concerns about DHEA arises from it being a natural steroid. These compounds are powerful, with a wide range of actions. When taken orally, at doses of 50 mg per day or less, adverse effects with DHEA are infrequent and generally mild. At doses of 200 mg per day, DHEA frequently causes adverse effects.

High blood levels of DHEA have been linked (✗✗) to a number of cancers, especially breast cancer in women and prostate cancer in men. DHEA can be converted in the body into testosterone, estrogen, and other sex hormones. This leads to fears that high doses will have negative effects on the many functions influenced by these other hormones. High levels of these hormones have also been implicated in a number of cancers and heart disease. This is of special concern if DHEA is used for extended periods of time.

In addition, DHEA use is associated (✖✖) with acne, increased facial hair, loss of scalp hair, deepening of the voice, weight gain, decreased HDL cholesterol ("good" cholesterol), abnormal liver tests, insulin resistance, and mild insomnia. Mania is rarely reported in people taking daily doses ranging from 50 to 300 mg. However, the mania may not begin until two to six months after starting DHEA. DHEA is not considered safe for use in children or in women who are pregnant or lactating.

Another problem with DHEA arises from its availability since 1994 under the Dietary Supplement Health and Education Act. These products are no longer regulated by the FDA or any other federal agency. So, for example, a 1998 study of DHEA products found that fewer than half of them contained the amount of DHEA stated on the label; some contained none at all. Other products claim to contain plant steroids that can be converted into DHEA. However, this chemical conversion process does not occur within the human body!

ConsumerLab.com tested seventeen DHEA-containing supplements. Fourteen products were DHEA only, and three included other herbal, vitamin, or mineral ingredients. The tests found that three of the seventeen products (18 percent) contained significantly less DHEA than claimed. One product claimed it was "Pharmaceutical Quality" yet was found to have only 19 percent of what its label claimed. Another product had only 79 percent of the claimed DHEA yet indicated that it met "USP standards."

Recommendations

At this point, research does not conclusively support the use of DHEA supplements for most of the purposes for which they are marketed. Although it may not be unreasonable for a health care provider to use this supplement while monitoring blood or salivary levels, there is still virtually no compelling evidence that this type of intervention is effective — and there are significant theoretical risks from DHEA since it is a steroid hormone that can impact numerous biochemical processes in humans and may stimulate cancer. Therefore, some researchers have commented that use of DHEA outside of a carefully monitored clinical trial is unwarranted. Those interested in eternal youth should look elsewhere (Revelation 21:4).

Dosage

Most studies use 50 mg a day for DHEA treatment. Higher doses have been used for specific conditions.

Treatment Categories

Conventional

To treat documented DHEA deficiency	☺☺☺
To treat adrenal insufficiency	☺☺☺

Complementary

To treat systemic lupus erythematosus	☺☺
To treat some menopausal symptoms	☺☺
To treat aging skin	☺☺
To increase bone density (osteoporosis or osteopenia)	☺
To treat some forms of erectile dysfunction	☺
To improve mood and general well-being	☺
To treat chronic fatigue syndrome	☹
To treat sexual dysfunction	☹

Scientifically Unproven

To improve mental performance	☹☹☹

To improve sports performance ☹☹☹☹

To treat Alzheimer's disease ☺

Quackery or Fraud

In the hands of some practitioners

Further Reading

Chang, Deh-Ming, Joung-Liang Lan, Hsiao-Yi Lin, and Shue-Fen Luo. "Dehydroepiandrosterone Treatment of Women with Mild to Moderate Systemic Lupus Erythematosus: A Multicenter Randomized, Double-Blind, Placebo-Controlled Trial." *Arthritis and Rheumatism* 46, no. 11 (November 2002): 2924–27.

Parasrampuria, J., K. Schwartz, and R. Petesch. "Quality Control of Dehydroepiandrosterone Dietary Supplement Products." *Journal of the American Medical Association* 280, no. 18 (November 1998): 1565.

Pepping, J. "DHEA: Dehydroepiandrosterone." *American Journal of Health System Pharmacy* 57 (2000): 2048–56.

DONG QUAI

What It Is

Dong quai (*Angelica sinensis*) has been used for centuries in traditional Chinese medicine (TCM) for a variety of gynecological problems, including relief of menopausal symptoms. The remedy is a dried extract made from the roots of the plant. Traditionally, it is combined with other herbs, but it has become popular in the West as a single-herb product for relief of menstrual symptoms. Dong quai was one of the herbal remedies many women turned to after problems were revealed with hormone replacement therapy in 2001.

Claims

In TCM dong quai is said to strengthen the life energy associated with blood. The symptoms associated with this are very similar to those of menopause. Dong quai is said to relieve problems with menstrual flow, hot flashes, nervousness, dizziness, insomnia, and forgetfulness. It is also recommended more generally as a tonic for women.

Study Findings

Animal studies have shown that dong quai does not act as a replacement for the hormone estrogen. The only published clinical trial (✗✗✗) involved seventy-one postmenopausal women with bothersome night sweats or hot flashes. The randomized double-blind study lasted twenty-four weeks. No significant changes occurred in the women's endometrial thickness or with vaginal smears, indicating the herb did not have an estrogen-like action. The number and intensity of hot flashes and night sweats decreased equally in both the dong quai and placebo groups. The most likely explanation is that dong quai worked via the placebo effect.

In one controlled clinical trial (✓✓✓), a topical cream (called SS Cream) containing nine herbs, one of which was dong quai, was tested in men with lifelong premature ejaculation. The treated group had significant improvements compared to those using the placebo cream. However, there is no way to know which of the ingredients in this cream were effective.

Cautions

A 2005 laboratory study showed that a dong quai water extract mildly stimulated the growth of breast cancer cells, raising concerns that it should not be used in women susceptible to breast cancer. Dong quai also contains chemical compounds called "psoralens," which may cause the skin to become sensitive to sunlight and result in dermatitis. Dong quai contains about 40 percent sugar, which should be noted by those who are diabetic. In TCM, dong quai is classified as a "heating" herb that may increase sweating and hot flashes in some women. Analyses of dong quai extracts have found that it contains several compounds known to interfere with blood clotting. Women taking anticoagulants, such as warfarin or aspirin, could be at increased risk of bleeding if they take dong quai. It is considered unsafe in pregnancy. Since no studies show that it is safe to use in children or in lactating women, its use is not recommended.

Recommendations

In spite of a long tradition of use in TCM, the only clinical evidence available does not support the use of dong quai for menopausal symptoms. The one clinical trial has demonstrated no effectiveness beyond a placebo effect. Other evidence suggests that dong quai may cause adverse effects for women who are diabetic, take blood-thinning medication, or are at higher risk of breast cancer.

Dosage

The usual dose is 3.5 to 4 grams of dried root per day, or 200 mg three times daily of an extract standardized to contain 1 percent ligustilide. In TCM, an individualized preparation will be made using other herbs.

Treatment Categories

Scientifically Unproven
To treat pre- or postmenopausal symptoms ☹☹☹☹
To treat premature ejaculation ☹

Scientifically Questionable
For any indication ☹☹☹☹

Spiritual
In the hands of some TCM practitioners 👎

Further Reading

Hirata, Janie D., Lillian M. Swiersz, Bonnie Zell, Rebecca Small, and Bruce Ettinger. "Does Dong Quai Have Estrogenic Effects in Postmenopausal Women?" *Fertility and Sterility* 68, no. 6 (December 1997): 981–86.

Huntley, Alyson L., and Edzard Ernst. "A Systematic Review of Herbal Medicinal Products for the Treatment of Menopausal Symptoms." *Menopause* 10, no. 5 (September–October 2005): 465–76.

ECHINACEA

What It Is

Echinacea was widely used by various Native-American tribes living in the central plains, where the plant grows wild. The type known as purple coneflower (*Echinacea purpurea*) was the treatment of choice for insect bites, snakebites, colds, sores, toothaches, and a variety of infections.

Today there are three varieties of the herb in common usage, and it has become one of the bestselling herbs in the United States. Among those who took part in the 2002 CDC Survey, echinacea was by far the most commonly used herbal remedy. Of those using herbal remedies, 40 percent said they used echinacea (the next most popular being ginseng, used by 24 percent).

Echinacea purpurea is the species most commonly used in echinacea herbal remedies. However, *Echinacea angustifolia* and *Echinacea pallida* are also used, sometimes interchangeably. Each species has somewhat different effects in the body, and no one really knows if they are equally effective. All species grow naturally in the central and eastern United States.

Claims

The knowledge and use of *Echinacea purpurea* was passed from Native Americans to Europeans gradually settling farther and farther west. However, its use dropped off after the development of antibiotics in the middle of the twentieth century.

Interest in echinacea was revived after reports emerged from Germany that a number of clinical trials found it helped prevent and treat cold and flu. Today echinacea is marketed as a natural cure for the common cold. Historically it has been used for many problems, including, but not limited to, pyorrhea, tonsillitis, boils, rheumatism, migraines, dyspepsia, wounds, eczema, bee stings, hemorrhoids, psoriasis, and varicose ulcers.

Study Findings

From a standpoint of evidence, the expressed juice from the tops of *E. purpurea* and the roots of *E. pallida* and *E. angustifolia* are the best-tested preparations and those most likely to be efficacious (*E.* is short for *Echinacea*). The other parts of the various species of *Echinacea* may be helpful, but we are not aware of any research to support their use.

Early interest in echinacea was generated by a small number of clinical trials in Germany (✓✓✓) that found that people taking echinacea got about one-third fewer colds than those taking a placebo. Those taking echinacea in these studies also reported less severe symptoms when they did get a cold and stated that the symptoms went away sooner. Laboratory tests have found that echinacea stimulates the immune system, which could help people fight off infections. However, all these results were from a relatively small number of studies that, while being randomized and controlled, were not designed as rigorously as possible.

A 1999 Cochrane review (✓✓✓✓) found sixteen controlled studies. Overall, a consistent, though small, benefit was found from taking echinacea. Since that time, several randomized double-blind trials have been published. Approximately one-third of these studies (✗✗✗) found echinacea no more beneficial than placebo. However, about two-thirds of the studies (✓✓✓✓) found that those taking echinacea immediately after cold symptoms began had somewhat reduced severity and length of symptoms. The more recent higher-quality trials show improvements of about 10 to 30 percent. For example, the 2004 trial by Vinti Goel found that for the echinacea group, average scores on a cold symptom scale were 23 percent lower and the symptoms were gone 27 percent sooner (about a day and a half).

However, the 2005 review (✗✗✗) by Thomas Caruso and Jack Gwaltney examined the results of trials in light of their quality. They found that the only two trials that met all their predetermined quality criteria found echinacea to be no better than placebo for the common cold, and all the trials that found it to be of benefit had at least one significant methodological flaw. They also noted that the common cold is one of the conditions for which placebos are highly effective.

The results from a smaller number of trials for the prevention of the common cold or flu (viral upper respiratory infection, or URI) were not positive (✗✗✗). Overall, the evidence does not support the use of echinacea to prevent colds.

Much uncertainty remains about echinacea, in particular because of the many different plants and preparations that are on the market. In the United States, there are an estimated eight hundred different products made from echinacea. Concerns have also been expressed about poor product quality, which may explain poor consumer satisfaction with echinacea. A *Consumer Reports* survey in May 2000 found that only 21 percent of echinacea users said

it helped with upper respiratory infections. When eleven products were tested by ConsumerLab.com in 2004, five failed. One had excessive lead contamination. Four products were low in phenols, the plant chemicals used to judge the quality of echinacea. One product contained less than 5 percent, another 50 percent, and the third 75 percent of the *claimed* amounts of phenols. Despite the availability of laboratory methods to identify echinacea, products claiming to contain it are frequently mislabeled, and some contain no echinacea at all. The term "standardized" on the label should bring some reassurance of quality but is not a guarantee with echinacea products.

• Cautions

When echinacea is taken in reasonable doses, side effects have been relatively mild and reversible. In clinical trials, some people have reported nausea or constipation as well as skin reactions. *Echinacea* species are members of the daisy family, so people with ragweed allergies should be cautious when taking these preparations. The most common negative reaction is to echinacea's unpleasant taste.

Some people take echinacea throughout the winter months to prevent cold and flu. No studies have been done on the safety of long-term echinacea use. There is some evidence (✗✗) that taking it for more than eight to ten weeks may weaken the immune system, leaving the person more susceptible to infections. Those who already have diseases of the immune system (such as multiple sclerosis, AIDS, or tuberculosis) could have further deterioration if echinacea is taken for more than a month or two.

There is some preliminary evidence that an *Echinacea purpurea* juice extract is safe in children ages two to eleven years when used for up to ten days.

However, echinacea has been reported to cause rashes in children. Echinacea should be avoided during pregnancy and lactation, as there is a lack of evidence regarding its safety during these times.

Recommendations

Echinacea may provide some help in relieving the symptoms of cold and flu. Many of the controlled studies have been conducted with European products that are known to be of high quality. Some of these are now available in the United States, but many other products are also available whose quality is not known or regulated. Three cases of adverse effects from echinacea products have been reported to the FDA, which determined that the remedies were contaminated with lead, arsenic, and selenium. Given its apparent safety, echinacea may be a helpful option when a cold or flu begins but should not be used for extended periods of time. Long-term use cannot be recommended, given the lack of benefit for preventing infections and the lack of long-term safety studies. It should not be used by pregnant or breast-feeding women.

Dosage

The juice is sometimes used (6 to 9 ml a day), but in tablet form up to about 1 gram of dried material is taken three times a day. There is great variability in the types of preparations available.

Treatment Categories

Complementary

To minimally reduce the severity and duration of the common cold	☺☺☺

Scientifically Unproven

To treat flu	☹☹
To prevent or treat colds in children	☹☹
To prevent colds and flu in adults	☹☹
For any other indication	

Further Reading

Caruso, Thomas J., and Jack M. Gwaltney Jr. "Treatment of the Common Cold with Echinacea: A Structured Review." *Clinical Infectious Diseases* 40 (2005): 807–10.

Goel, V., R. Lovlin, R. Barton, M. R. Lyon, R. Bauer, T. D. G. Lee, and T. K. Basu. "Efficacy of a Standardized Echinacea Preparation (Echinilin™) for the Treatment of the Common Cold: A Randomized, Double-Blind, Placebo-Controlled Trial." *Journal of Clinical Pharmacy and Therapeutics* 29, no. 1 (February 2004): 75–83.

Huntley, Alyson L., Joanna Thompson Coon, and Edzard Ernst. "The Safety of Herbal Medicinal Products Derived from Echinacea Species: A Systematic Review." *Drug Safety* 28, no. 5 (2005): 387–400.

ELDERBERRY

What It Is

Elderberries have long been the subject of both myth and medicine. Archaeologists have traced the cultivation of the shrub back at least to the Stone Age, and there have been stories throughout Europe concerning the connection of the bush with spirits and witches.

The berries grow on a variety of elder shrubs from the *Sambucus* genus and have been enjoyed in pies, preserves, and, of course, wine. The edible berries have to be cooked to prevent nausea, vomiting, and diarrhea. The most popular species used in herbal medicine include the flowers and cooked fruit of the American elder (*Sambucus canadensis*) and the cooked fruit of the European elder (*Sambucus nigra*).

Claims

Ripe elderberries have been used for centuries as flavorings and to makes juices and elderberry wine. The medicinal remedies have primarily been made from extracts of the flowers.

Traditionally, elderberries have been used most commonly for their diuretic and laxative effects. Many other uses have been reported, ranging from treating measles, cancer, and toothaches to repelling insects. Another use has been to treat diabetes. Others recommend American elderberries for epilepsy, gout, headaches, neuralgia, psoriasis, rheumatism, sore throats, and constipation. European elder flowers have been used for cough, cold, laryngitis, flu, and sinusitis. European elderberries have been used for the flu, constipation, sciatica, neuralgia, and cancer.

Elder flowers, usually mixed with yarrow and peppermint leaves, are often brewed into a tea to act as a mild stimulant.

Study Findings

Very little clinical support exists for the vast majority of the uses of elderberry extract. However, very recent research on animals did find that the extract lowered blood glucose levels through insulin-like activity. In addition, three small human studies (✓✓✓) showed that a product containing the European elderberry juice (Sambucol) shortened the duration of influenza and relieved some of the symptoms of the flu in adults and children. In a 2004 study, flu symptoms were relieved on average four days earlier in the group taking elderberry extract compared to placebo. The specific compounds causing this, or any of the other alleged effects, have not been identified. This anecdotal evidence and promising early studies need to be explored in greater depth.

Cautions

All parts of the American elderberry contain cyanogenic glycosides that can release cyanide. These compounds are more prevalent in the leaves, stems, and unripe fruit and therefore should not be used in preparing elderberry juice. The flowers and ripe fruit usually are free of these compounds. Children using the stems as peashooters (✖) have suffered cyanide poisoning. Other adverse reactions, which may also be related to the cyanide, include diarrhea and vomiting. The European elder is not reported to contain cyanogenic compounds. One elderberry product, Sambucol, has been used safely in children, but little is known about its use during pregnancy or lactation.

Recommendations

Elderberries have been used to make juice and wine for centuries. These beverages may provide some health benefits, but these are very mild. Medicinal use of many of these products seems unwarranted, at least with the American elder, given the risk of cyanide poisoning and the availability of other pharmaceutical and natural remedies to effectively treat the conditions for which elderberries are recommended. The European product, Sambucol, appears to be useful in treating the flu. Other than nausea, vomiting, and diarrhea if the fruit is not cooked sufficiently, elderberry products appear to have few adverse effects when used for up to five days. No adverse effects have been reported for adults or children.

Dosage

No consensus exists. The studies of Sambucol used 15 ml of syrup four times daily.

Treatment Categories

Complementary
To relieve flu symptoms by about half (with Sambucol) ☺☺

Scientifically Unproven
For any other indication

Further Reading

"*Sambucus nigra* (Elderberry)." *Alternative Medicine Review* 10, no. 11 (March 2005): 51 – 54.

Zakay-Rones, Z., E. Thom, T. Wollan, and J. Wadstein. "Randomized Study of the Efficacy and Safety of Oral Elderberry Extract in the Treatment of Influenza A and B Virus Infections." *Journal of International Medical Research* 32, no. 2 (March – April 2004): 132 – 40.

E

EPHEDRA

What It Is

Ephedra is unique in many ways. After seven years of trying, the FDA succeeded in 2004 to ban sales of ephedra as a dietary supplement. Prior to this, almost two-thirds of all herb-related adverse events reported at U.S. poison control centers involved ephedra, even though its sales made up less than 1 percent of all dietary supplement sales. One study reported on 16,000 adverse events associated with ephedra. Ironically, while ephedra was by far the most adverse event – prone herb, it was also one of the most popular. In 1999, it was estimated that 12 million people in the United States used 3 billion doses of ephedra. Given this popularity, and in spite of the recent ban, ephedra products are likely to remain available to those who really want them. The FDA has seized millions of dollars' worth of illegal ephedra products. Manufacturers are now finding replacement herbs (e.g., bitter orange) that contain the same, or similar, chemicals.

Ephedra gained notoriety as the herb of choice for people trying to get the most out of life. It was recommended for everyone from young adults seeking to maximize their work, school, and intimate lives with minimal sleep, to sleep-deprived parents of new babies, to older individuals hoping to regain their youthful vigor. If all the anecdotal stories were to be believed, the herb could serve as a stimulant, increase sexual pleasure, and help people lose weight. Of greater interest to those with breathing problems is the fact that ephedra has long been used as a treatment for asthma, bronchitis, and the common cold.

Some users claim that it also eases suffering from arthritis.

Ephedra is also known as "herbal ecstasy" because of its stimulant ability, as "herbal fen-phen" for its alleged ability to help people shed unwanted weight, and by the Chinese names Ma Huang and Ma Huanggen. Ma Huanggen, made from the rhizome and root of Chinese ephedra (*Ephedra sinica*), is rarely used except by those who are troubled by night sweats. Ma Huang, made from the stem and branches of this same plant, has been the source of most of ephedra's alleged benefits.

The genus *Ephedra* contains more than forty different plant species. Other than Chinese ephedra, the most common medicinal species of ephedra include intermediate ephedra (*Ephedra intermedia*) and Mongolian ephedra (*Ephedra equisetta*). Each species has its own characteristic mixture of compounds called "alkaloids." The most common alkaloid is ephedrine, first isolated in 1885. In its purified form it has been used within conventional medicine as a bronchodilator (for the relief of asthma), decongestant, and vasopressor (a drug that increases blood pressure and heart rate).

Claims

Ephedra has been used traditionally in China for more than five thousand years, primarily for the treatment of asthma. Just the stems and branches were used, not the entire plant. Later in China, Ma Huang was used to treat bronchitis, hay fever, the common cold, and other ailments. The *Ephedra* species native to North America (*Ephedra nevaden-*

sis), often called American ephedra or Mormon tea, contains none of these alkaloids; therefore, it lacks both the therapeutic benefits and the risks of other *Ephedra* species.

The alkaloid ephedrine is widely used in conventional medicine as a decongestant and asthma remedy. Other ephedra alkaloids commonly prescribed by physicians include pseudoephedrine and norephedrine. Phenylpropanolamine is a manufactured mixture containing two ephedra alkaloids that was sold as an over-the-counter weight-loss product until it was taken off the market because of its side effects.

All the ephedra herbal remedies are said to provide natural ways to control asthma, lose weight, boost energy levels, and increase sexual pleasure. Some claim ephedra can be used for a natural, legal high. Many ephedra manufacturers add caffeine to their products to enhance the effects. Some herbalists recommend it as an appetite suppressant, cardiovascular stimulant, and central nervous system stimulant.

Study Findings

Decades of research with the purified alkaloids ephedrine and pseudoephedrine have shown that these are effective nasal decongestants and relieve bronchial asthma. They also increase blood pressure, heart rate, constriction of blood vessels, bronchial dilation, and central nervous system stimulation. They can suppress coughing and are anti-inflammatory in animal studies. They have been available in a number of over-the-counter pharmaceutical preparations since the 1930s. These drugs act by stimulating the central nervous system, which explains why they simultaneously affect numerous body systems.

This also means they must be carefully monitored to ensure the correct dose is taken.

Positive results with *ephedrine* do not necessarily mean that *ephedra* products are as effective. Since alkaloid content in the various *Ephedra* species varies, the amount of ephedrine in any herbal remedy will vary, making careful dosing impossible with herbal remedies. Very few clinical studies with ephedra alone could be found. A small number of studies (✓✓✓) of ephedra combined with caffeine (and sometimes also aspirin) found a minimal amount of weight loss. Although statistically significant, those receiving ephedra and caffeine lost less than 1 kilogram more than those taking placebo and had two to four times as many side effects (✗✗✗).

Studies of athletic performance were even less supportive of a beneficial effect. A couple of studies of ephedra alone showed no exercise improvements (✗✗✗). Some studies (✗✗✗) used combinations of ephedra and caffeine and had inconsistent results. However, all these studies reported significant increases in heart rate and blood pressure compared to placebo. Thus, athletes may experience increased exertion, but that has not translated into improved performances in these studies.

Cautions

Ephedra products contain drugs demonstrated (✗✗✗✗) to affect the body in a wide range of ways. Their side effects include high blood pressure, increased heart rate, heart palpitations, anxiety, restlessness, headache, psychoses, stroke, heart attack, cardiac arrhythmias, and death. For this reason, ephedra products are likely to interact with other drugs taken to influence these systems. As of 1998, forty-four deaths (✗✗) had been reported to the FDA that were associated with ephedra. The sudden death in 2003 of a professional baseball player was linked to ephedra and drew much public attention to the adverse effects of the supplement. Thousands of other instances of adverse effects (✘✘) associated with ephedra products had also been reported to the FDA. Many of these occurred in teenagers using the products to get high, lose weight, or enhance athletic performance. Ephedrine is notorious for causing kidney stones, an effect that has also been reported (✘✘) after taking herbal ephedra.

Of concern also is the great variability in ephedra products. A 1997 study examined nine products labeled "Ephedra extract." Two contained no ephedrine. If people followed the directions on the labels of the other products, they would have consumed anywhere from 5 mg to 89 mg of ephedrine alkaloids daily. Anyone who had been taking one brand and switched to another could easily take too much.

Another problem was discovered when four of the products showed a pattern of alkaloids that does not occur in any known *Ephedra* species. The most likely explanation is that these products were spiked with synthetic drugs. Similar studies published in 1998 (with nine Ma Huang products) and in 2000 (with twenty ephedra products) found the same problems. In half the products tested in the 2000 study, researchers found at least a 20 percent discrepancy between the alkaloid quantity in the product and the amount listed on the label. One product contained no ephedrine alkaloids at all.

Recommendations

Ephedra is now a banned dietary supplement and should not be used. The active ingredients in ephedra are powerful drugs with a broad range of effects throughout the body. However, these same substances are readily available in standardized phar-maceutical preparations. Using herbal remedies to obtain these compounds "naturally" only adds uncertainty and danger. There is no reason to use these remedies.

Beware, however, of some stimulant supplements being marketed as "Ephedra-free." Some of these contain bitter orange (*Citrus uranium*), which contains an alkaloid called "synephrine." This substance is closely related to ephedrine and has many of the same effects on the body. That means it may also carry all the same risks as the banned products.

Dosage

Since ephedra is banned, no dose should be used.

Treatment Categories

Conventional

Only pharmaceutical ephedrine for short-term therapy under medical direction

Complementary

Ephedra products for any indication   ☹☹☹☹

Risk of Serious Side Effects

Ephedra herbal products
for any indication   ⊘⊘⊘⊘

Further Reading

Andraws, Richard, Preety Chawla, and David L. Brown. "Cardiovascular Effects of Ephedra Alkaloids: A Comprehensive Review." *Progress in Cardiovascular Diseases* 47, no. 4 (January – February 2005): 217 – 25.

Betz, Joseph M., Martha L. Gay, Magdi M. Mossoba, Sarah Adams, and Barbara S. Portz. "Chiral Gas Chromatographic Determination of Ephedrine-Type

Alkaloids in Dietary Supplements Containing Ma Huang." *Journal of AOAC International* 80, no. 2 (March – April 1997): 303 – 15.

Gurley, B. J., S. F. Gardner, and M. A. Hubbard. "Content Versus Label Claims in Ephedra-Containing Dietary Supplements." *American Journal of Health System Pharmacy* 57, no. 10 (May 2000): 963 – 69.

Shekelle, Paul G., Mary L. Hardy, Sally C. Morton, Walter A. Mojica, Marika J. Suttroop, Shannon L. Rhodes, Lara Jungvig, and James Gagné. "Efficacy and Safety of Ephedra and Ephedrine for Weight Loss and Athletic Performance." *Journal of the American Medical Association* 289, no. 12 (March 2003): 1537 – 45.

EVENING PRIMROSE

What It Is

The evening primrose is a North American wild-flower (*Oenothera biennis*) whose fragrant yellow blooms, lasting just one night, have long delighted hikers and lovers out for an evening stroll. The fruit pods contain many small seeds from which an oil is extracted.

Evening primrose oil (EPO) contains a relatively high proportion of essential fatty acids (EFA). EPO from commercial strains of the flower contains about 72 percent of one particular EFA called "cis-linolenic acid" (LA) and 9 percent of gamma-linolenic acid (GLA). LA belongs to the group of omega-3 fatty acids. EPO is one of the richest plant sources of GLA. Only borage oil (24 percent GLA) and black currant seed oil (16 percent GLA) contain more. These two compounds (GLA and LA) play an essential role in the inflammatory and immune responses of the body.

Claims

EPO has been called the King's Cure-All in England, where it is enormously popular. One survey in 2005 found it was the most commonly used herbal medicine in one region of England. In the United Kingdom, it was approved, prescription only, for allergy-related eczema, although the regulatory body there withdrew the product's marketing license in 2002 after reviewing new studies.

EPO has gained interest as a treatment for pre-menstrual syndrome (PMS) and menopause in the wake of the adverse effects reported for hormone replacement therapy. More generally it is recommended by herbal medicine practitioners for everything from calming hyperactive children to speeding wound healing and curing cancer. In Canada it is approved as a dietary supplement to increase essential fatty acid intake.

What has made EPO one of the most popular herbal remedies in the United States has been the connection established between GLA and inflammatory diseases. Thus, EPO is recommended for the treatment of rheumatoid arthritis, dermatitis, eczema, psoriasis, and asthma. It is also commonly promoted for cardiovascular disease, fibrocystic breast disease, and multiple sclerosis. Others recommend it for breast pain, high cholesterol, Raynaud's phenomena, Sjogren's syndrome, post-viral fatigue syndrome, diabetic neuropathy, neurodermatitis, and some pregnancy-related problems.

Study Findings

Research into the role of EFAs in inflammation is proceeding at a rapid rate and producing interesting results. These compounds will be discussed more thoroughly in the entry on Omega Fatty Acids. Studies have shown that supplementing the diet with sources high in these fatty acids can result in increased levels of anti-inflammatory EFAs and improvements in people's health. However, many of these studies (✓✓) have been relatively small and of poorer quality, and their results must be interpreted cautiously.

The important role of GLA in the diet has been clearly demonstrated, though primarily in epidemiological studies (✓✓). Certain diseases are connected to low dietary EFA or impairments in the body's ability to make GLA (e.g., depression, arthritis, cardiovascular disease, inflammatory bowel disease, and insulin resistance). In studies of these sorts of conditions, EPO theoretically could be expected to bring some relief, or more likely play a role in their prevention.

However, very few high-quality studies have been conducted using EPO for specific conditions in humans. In treating eczema, a 2000 review (✗✗✗✗) found that the larger and better studies demonstrated no benefit. A 2003 randomized study (✗✗✗) used 1 gram of GLA (from borage oil, believed to be identical to that from EPO) and found no benefit for eczema. A few studies (✓✓✓) involving people with rheumatoid arthritis and osteoarthritis have found that patients used less pain medication when taking EPO compared to those taking placebo. However, the EPO did not change the severity of the disease itself. EPO also appears to have no effect on allergic asthma or psoriasis.

Several randomized controlled trials (✗✗✗) have shown EPO to be no better than placebo for the treatment of premenstrual syndrome. One study (✗✗✗) on its use in treating hot flashes during menopause found no benefit. A large trial (✗✗✗) with breast pain (mastalgia) found that GLA was no better than placebo, including when it was given along with antioxidant vitamins. While earlier trials (✓✓) found some benefit, these were small and of lower quality. EPO has also been found to be no more effective than placebo (✗✗✗) in preventing preeclampsia or in shortening the length of labor.

European trials have looked at EPO for a number of medical indications. Effectiveness has been reported (✓✓) for a variety of chronic, painful conditions, including Sjogren's syndrome, diabetic neuropathy, rheumatoid arthritis, and irritable bowel syndrome. However, none of these conditions have been examined in controlled trials.

Cautions

Overall, evening primrose oil (and other sources of the "good" essential fatty acids such as nuts, cold-water fish oil, and black currant oil) appears to be safe and well tolerated. EPO can sometimes cause indigestion, nausea, soft stools, abdominal pain, and headache. However, the effects of long-term use, as would be required for many of the conditions for which it is recommended, have not been examined. Studies of this aspect of use are especially important since 4 to 8 grams daily are often suggested. This amount of oil is also relatively expensive and has led to efforts to find other sources of gamma-linolenic acid. Some concerns have been expressed about product quality. However, ConsumerLab.com tested four EPO products in 2005, and all passed the tests by containing what their labels claimed and by meeting the standards set by ConsumerLab.com for omega-3 fatty acid products.

The medical license in the United Kingdom was withdrawn purely for lack of evidence of effectiveness, not concerns about safety. EPO may be associated with pregnancy complications and therefore should not be used by pregnant women. However, EPO is considered safe in children and lactating women.

Recommendations

While certain people can clearly benefit from supplementing their diet with gamma-linolenic acid, this does not mean that everyone needs to take evening primrose oil. By analogy, your car won't run any better on a full tank of gas than it will on a half tank. But if you're out of gas or if the gas cap is locked, you need some other way to get the gas into the gas tank. In the same way, if your body doesn't make enough gamma-linolenic acid or if you're getting very little in your diet, evening primrose supplements would be a good option to try for overall general health. However, its usefulness in treating any particular condition is very limited.

Dosage

Daily doses in the range of 2 to 4 grams of evening primrose oil are commonly used, though much higher doses are sometimes recommended.

Treatment Categories

Conventional

In Canada, to increase essential
fatty acid intake ☺☺☺

Complementary

To treat osteoporosis, along
with fish oils and calcium ☺

To treat eczema ☹☹☹☹

To relieve mild breast pain
(mastalgia) ☺☺

To relieve severe breast pain
(mastalgia) ☹☹☹

To relieve premenstrual
or menstrual symptoms ☹☹☹

To prevent preeclampsia ☹☹☹☹

To shorten the duration of labor ☹☹☹☹

To relieve various painful
inflammatory conditions ☹

Scientifically Unproven

For any other indication

Further Reading

Haimov-Kochman, Ronit, and Drorith Hochner-Celnikier. "Hot Flashes Revisited: Pharmacological and Herbal Options for Hot Flashes Management. What Does the Evidence Tell Us?" *Acta Obstetricia et Gynecologica Scandinavica* 84, no. 10 (October 2005): 972–79.

Williams, Hywel C. "Evening Primrose Oil for Atopic Dermatitis." *British Medical Journal* 327 (December 2003): 1358–59.

FEVERFEW

• What It Is

If you lived in Greece during the time of Jesus, you would have encountered feverfew as a medicine for hot inflammations and hot swellings. Historians believe that these terms refer to what we today would call arthritis joint discomfort.

Over the years, feverfew has had numerous botanical names, including *Tanacetum parthenium* and *Chrysanthemum parthenium*. It is a member of the daisy family, a perennial seen in fields and along roadsides. The flowers have yellow disks and ten to twenty white-toothed rays. The leaf, either fresh or freeze-dried, is generally used in herbal preparations.

• Claims

Feverfew has been grown in gardens in Europe for centuries. Currently feverfew is a popular herbal remedy for the prevention and treatment of migraines. In traditional and folk use, feverfew is reported to help in the treatment of fever, arthritis, menstrual difficulties, cough, chest colds, "melancholy," "sadness of spirit," vertigo, headache, colic, flatulence, indigestion, worms, hysteria, and difficulty urinating. It has also been promoted as a topical treatment for insect bites and as an insect repellent when planted around a house or garden. By far the most common use is for migraine headache prevention and treatment.

• Study Findings

A 2004 Cochrane review located five randomized placebo-controlled trials of feverfew for preventing migraine headaches. The reviewers were less positive about their conclusions than when they published an earlier review in 2000. They found the studies variable in their conclusions. The two studies of highest quality (✘✘✘) showed no benefit from feverfew, while the three others (✔✔✔) found it more beneficial than placebo. A problem with these studies is that very different feverfew products were used. Some studies used feverfew leaves, and others used extracts made in various ways. It is also known that the assumed active ingredient in feverfew, parthenolide, is relatively unstable. This means that the way the products are made will affect their quality significantly.

To overcome such problems, a German product (MIG-99) uses carbon dioxide to make an extract of the herb. A 2005 randomized double-blind trial (✔✔✔) carried out in several medical centers found the extract effective. The number and severity of migraines were reduced significantly compared to placebo. The researchers noted that the proportion of people who responded well to feverfew was lower than with conventional drugs, but so too was the number of adverse effects. They concluded that feverfew has a place in preventing migraines if first-choice medications are not suitable.

All these studies were conducted with migraine sufferers who took feverfew to see if it reduced the number of attacks. Although the studies are sometimes cited to support using feverfew to treat migraines, none of them directly examined this effect. Although those using feverfew experienced migraines during the studies, the severity of the migraines was usually no different than that of the migraines experienced by those taking placebo.

Apart from clinical studies with migraine prevention, one randomized controlled trial (✘✘✘) has been conducted that showed feverfew was not helpful for rheumatoid arthritis.

Cautions

Occasional mouth ulcerations and gastric irritation (in 5 to 15 percent of users) have been reported (✘✘) with the use of fresh feverfew leaves (especially when using the traditional method of feverfew administration — chewing fresh feverfew leaves). These effects have not been reported with the use of dried leaves in capsules. Other reported adverse effects include skin rashes, rapid heart rate, indigestion, colic, and weight gain. Feverfew is a member of the daisy family and should not be used by people with known allergies or sensitivity to other members such as ragweed, chamomile, or yarrow. Other adverse effects reported include dizziness, light-headedness, slightly heavier periods, heartburn, skin rash, and diarrhea.

Those who had used feverfew for several years and then abruptly stopped taking the herb experienced the recurrence of incapacitating migraines (what are called "rebound headaches").

Feverfew has been said (✘) to cause miscarriage, to increase menstrual flow, and to cause uterine contractions in pregnant women at term. Although there is little evidence on this issue, it would be wise not to use feverfew during pregnancy. However, there is no information on feverfew excretion in breast milk. There is no data concerning the use of feverfew in children, but some experts say it should not be used in children twelve or younger.

Feverfew has been reported (✘✘) to decrease the blood's ability to clot, so it is prudent for patients on aspirin to avoid feverfew until safety studies are available.

As with all herbal remedies, products vary widely in their quality. One study examined three feverfew products (*Tanacetum parthenium*) and found that only one contained the active ingredient of feverfew — parthenolide. This chemical may be the major antimigraine constituent, but even if it is not, its absence indicates problems with the quality of these two products.

Recommendations

Evidence from clinical trials is not conclusive but suggests that feverfew, taken daily for at least a month or two, can be effective and safe in reducing the incidence of migraine headaches in a certain proportion of people. However, it is not as effective as standard prescription medications used to prevent migraine headaches, though it may have fewer side effects. Feverfew has not been tested for the treatment of migraine headaches.

Dosage

Studies have used daily doses of 50 to 100 mg of feverfew extract. The new German extract, MIG-99, is taken as a 6.25 mg dose three times daily.

Treatment Categories

Conventional

As a second-line agent to prevent
migraine headaches   ☺☺

Complementary

To treat migraine headaches   ☹☹☹

To treat rheumatoid arthritis   ☹☹☹

Scientifically Unproven

For any other indication

Further Reading

Diener, H. C., V. Pfaffenrath, J. Schnitker, M. Friede, and H.-H. Henneicke-von Zepelin. "Efficacy and Safety of 6.25 mg t.i.d. Feverfew CO2-Extract (MIG-99) in Migraine Prevention — A Randomized, Double-Blind, Multicentre, Placebo-Controlled Study." *Cephalalgia* 25, no. 11 (November 2005): 1031 – 41.

Pittler, M. H., and E. Ernst. "Feverfew for Preventing Migraine." *The Cochrane Database of Systematic Reviews* 2004, no. 1.

GARLIC

What It Is

According to some reports, garlic is the herb most commonly taken by Americans. It has been credited with many things, both real and imagined, yet its uses are occasionally at cross-purposes with one another. For example, everyone who has gone on a dinner date and wanted to maintain kissing-fresh breath has heard the warning not to eat anything with garlic. The lingering odor puts an instant damper on romance. Yet garlic is also said to increase sexual prowess.

The ancient Egyptians, Greeks, Romans, Babylonians, and Chinese all wrote about the healing properties of garlic. In 1722, French citizens reported protection from the plague if they drank garlic vinegar. In 1858, Louis Pasteur reported the antibacterial activity of garlic. Garlic was administered as an antiseptic poultice during World War I. Lovers of horror stories and low-budget drive-in movies know the importance of hanging garlic around the neck if you venture out during a full moon. This may be folklore's only protection against vampires, though whether it has magical properties when confronting the undead or simply offends their sense of smell is unclear.

Apart from myth, garlic, whether slivered, minced, used as whole cloves, or crushed, is one of the most common aromatics used in cooking. *Allium sativum*, also known as poor man's treacle or clove garlic, is said to have originated in Central Asia. Eventually it was introduced into the Mediterranean area. It is now cultivated worldwide.

The medicinal parts of garlic are the whole fresh clove, the dried clove, and the oil prepared from the clove. It is a member of the allium plant family, which includes onions, shallots, and leeks. These plants contain sulfur-rich derivatives of the amino acid cysteine that are thought to have medicinal benefits.

When raw garlic is cut or crushed, the enzyme alliinase interacts with the cysteine compound alliin, inside the clove, to produce allicin. Allicin gives garlic its typical aroma and taste but is volatile and usually breaks down either in a few hours at room temperature or after twenty minutes of cooking. More stable compounds such as ajoene and dithiins are formed when garlic is macerated in oil. These compounds may be stable for more than a year.

Allicin is also thought to be one of the most important medicinal substances in garlic, although little or no allicin is present in the intact garlic clove. The garlic plant produces allicin as a natural defense against bacteria and other organisms. Allicin is highly irritating and has been shown to kill bacteria in laboratory studies.

The instability of allicin makes it difficult to study its clinical effects and those of its derivatives. Numerous investigators are studying allicin's blood-thinning activity, antibacterial or antifungal properties, and antioxidant potential. Most clinical studies have used dried garlic powder tablets.

Claims

Recent interest has focused on garlic's alleged ability to lower serum lipid levels and to prevent age-dependent vascular changes. Garlic has long been thought to be effective in the prevention of heart disease by lowering cholesterol and acting as a mild blood thinner. Herbalists use garlic for high blood pressure, diarrhea, ringworm, hypersensitive teeth, cold, flu, cough, headache, athlete's foot, gout, rheumatism, cancer and snakebites and also as an aphrodisiac.

Study Findings

Animal and laboratory studies have indicated that the sulfur-containing compounds in garlic may in-terfere with the liver's cholesterol-making enzyme, HMG-CoA reductase. This is the same enzyme affected by prescription medications called "statins." These products are known to occur naturally (as in red yeast rice), although pharmaceutical statins result in much larger reductions in cholesterol levels.

Clinical studies as early as 1926 examined the beneficial effects of garlic on cardiovascular diseases and noted reductions in cholesterol levels. However, these early studies were carried out with people eating between seven and twenty-eight cloves of garlic per day. During the 1980s and 1990s, many clinical trials (✓✓✓✓) reported that garlic lowered cholesterol levels, but most of these have had only a small number of patients. A 1993 meta-analysis — a way of combining the results of several similar studies — (✓✓✓✓) found an overall average 9 percent reduction in cholesterol levels in those given garlic. A similar 1996 meta-analysis (✓✓✓✓) reported a 12 percent reduction in total cholesterol levels.

Soon after that, two larger controlled trials (✓✓✓✓) reported reduced cholesterol levels of about 6 percent, although with no changes in triglyceride levels. Another meta-analysis (✗✗✗✗) published at the end of 2000 led the authors to conclude that the cholesterol-lowering benefits of garlic were so small it was questionable whether they would make any difference to patients' health. After that, six new randomized controlled trials found no significant reductions in cholesterol or triglyceride levels compared to placebo. A 2002 review (✗✗✗✗) noted that in spite of earlier beneficial results, in the last five years, no randomized, double-blind, placebo-controlled study could be found in which the results indicated a clear beneficial effect of a garlic preparation alone on blood lipids. Recent reviews have also noted that while some studies found benefits after one and three months, no studies lasting six months or longer showed significant reductions in cholesterol levels.

Animal studies have shown that garlic's sulfur compounds can inhibit the development of atherosclerosis (hardening of the arteries). Studies in humans, though, have had conflicting results. Even those with positive effects have been small. The benefits here may be due to an antioxidant effect, but again the results are not conclusive. A 2002 review (✗✗✗) located almost thirty studies of garlic's use in lowering blood pressure. Most were small, of short duration, and not conducted to the highest methodological standards. Of these, almost three-quarters found the garlic preparations of no greater benefit than placebo. In general, much remains uncertain about garlic's contribution to the prevention and control of cardiovascular disorders.

A meta-analysis of eighteen epidemiological studies (✓✓) revealed that eating raw garlic cloves may have a beneficial effect in preventing stomach and colorectal cancer. However, epidemiological studies are not controlled studies, and there was much variability among the studies, with some of very low quality. Most of the studies were conducted in China, where garlic cloves release significantly more allicin than garlic from anywhere else in the world (three times as much as garlic grown in the United States). The authors were cautious in their conclusions. The anticancer properties of garlic are currently under investigation.

Fresh garlic may be the only preparation that allows a person to get a significant amount of allicin. The odor and stomach upset that may be caused by chewing raw garlic, however, make it a poor choice for a cholesterol-lowering agent. Cooked garlic may be better tolerated, but prolonged cooking will also inactivate the sulfur-containing compounds thought to be beneficial. No well-designed long-term studies using raw or cooked garlic are available.

Because of the variability among products, manufacturers currently usually show the allicin content or allicin potential as a way to estimate strength. There are significant technical difficulties in the commercial preparation of garlic supplements, however, because of the rapid breakdown of the volatile sulfur compounds.

Manufacturers have devised methods to attempt to preserve allicin. Most of the clinical studies showing benefit from garlic have tested the brand-name product Kwai, which contains freeze-dried fresh garlic in coated tablets. Once ingested, the surface coating of the tablet dissolves in the stomach, allowing the enzyme alliinase to convert inactive alliin to the active allicin. The tablet is odorless because it is coated, with the active ingredients released sufficiently far along in the digestive tract to avoid a garlic odor.

Another method uses rapid drying of cut garlic, presumably before allicin is produced. The rapid degradation of these compounds following drying minimizes the allicin content in standard garlic powder. Yet another method involves inactivating alliinase and adding the enzyme back to the final dried product. Unfortunately, alliinase is easily denatured by stomach acid. Products using distilled garlic oil or garlic powder have shown conflicting results in humans and cannot be recommended at this time.

One study in Germany reported that only about 25 percent of the garlic products available had an amount of allicin equivalent to one clove of fresh garlic. Some odorless products did not contain any active compound. ConsumerLab.com purchased fourteen garlic products to test and could not rate them on its usual pass/fail basis. While some products contained what their labels claimed, the recommended serving sizes would not have delivered what research shows is needed for beneficial effects. Conversely, one product that did *not* meet its claim for allicin yield still provided an adequate daily amount of allicin. A number of products significantly exceeded their label claims.

Cautions

Garlic is generally considered safe. The most common problems are an undesirable garlic taste and smell, something that unfortunately can also occur with the so-called "odorless" preparations on the market. Some people can be hypersensitive to garlic and should avoid these products. Those who have stomach ulcers or other gastric problems should avoid them also.

Raw garlic can cause stomach upset, reflux, and gas symptoms and may also be highly irritating to some people's skin. Garlic may interfere with blood clotting, so it is not recommended for patients taking drugs such as aspirin or warfarin. It may enhance the effects of other antiplatelet drugs, oral diabetic drugs, or insulin. There have been reports of garlic causing uterine contractions, so it should be avoided during pregnancy. For use in children and in women who are pregnant or lactating, garlic is considered safe in the amounts normally found in food; however, it is considered possibly unsafe in medicinal amounts.

Recommendations

Evidence from a number of studies suggests that garlic may have a mild cholesterol-lowering and blood-pressure-lowering effect. This effect seems to be more evident in individuals with elevated cholesterol or blood pressure levels. The beneficial results were found with a German product, Kwai, or a Japanese product, Kyolic. Both products are now available in the United States. A number of well-designed trials, especially more recent ones, have failed to show any significant benefit from garlic supplements. High-dose garlic may prevent or stimulate the regression of the cholesterol plaques that cause atherosclerosis, but the evidence here is not strong. The varying quality of garlic preparations may account for some of the different results among studies.

Fresh garlic can certainly be recommended as a component of a plant-centered diet and as part of an overall strategy of lifestyle modification to lower cholesterol levels. Powdered garlic products may be used as well; however, there are concerns about limited shelf life for these products as well as a lack of knowledge about consistency in the manufacturing process.

Garlic may be lightly cooked to avoid the side effects of raw cloves, but too much cooking will deactivate the sulfur-containing compounds that may be the active agents.

For those with high cholesterol levels, the lowering effect of garlic is not great. Conventional statin drugs have significantly greater effects, and garlic should not be substituted for medical therapy without first discussing your plans with the health care professionals overseeing your care.

A diet containing garlic may have some benefit in preventing cancer, but benefits from using garlic to treat cancer have not been demonstrated.

Dosage

For effects related to heart disease, most studies use 600 to 900 mg per day, usually divided into three doses. This corresponds to about 4 grams of fresh garlic or 8 mg of garlic oil per day. The cancer prevention effects were seen with a diet containing one clove of garlic a day. There is great variability in garlic product strengths.

Treatment Categories

Complementary

To lower elevated cholesterol levels	☺☺
To reduce high blood pressure	☺
To prevent atherosclerosis	☹
To slow development of atherosclerosis	☺
As dietary garlic to prevent stomach and colorectal cancer	☺
As supplements to prevent stomach and colorectal cancer	☹
To reduce the risk of prostate cancer	☺
To reduce the risk of breast or lung cancer	☹☹
To treat or reduce the risk of diabetes	☹☹

Scientifically Unproven

For any other indication

Further Reading

Banerjee, Sanjay K., and Subir K. Maulik. "Effect of Garlic on Cardiovascular Disorders: A Review." *Nutrition Journal* 1 (2002): 4. *Biomed Central: www.nutritionj.com/content/1/1/4.* Accessed November 10, 2005.

Brace, Larry D. "Cardiovascular Benefits of Garlic (*Allium sativum* L)." *Journal of Cardiovascular Nursing* 16, no. 4 (July 2002): 33–49.

Fleischauer, Aaron T., Charles Poole, and Lenore Arab. "Garlic Consumption and Cancer Prevention: Meta-analyses of Colorectal and Stomach Cancers." *American Journal of Clinical Nutrition* 72, no. 4 (October 2000): 1047–52.

Jakubowski, Hieronim. "On the Health Benefits of *Allium* sp." *Nutrition* 19, no. 2 (2003): 167–68.

Stevinson, Clare, Max H. Pittler, and Edzard Ernst. "Garlic for Treating Hypercholesterolemia: A Meta-analysis of Randomized Clinical Trials." *Annals of Internal Medicine* 133, no. 6 (September 2000): 420–29.

GINGER

What It Is

Ginger (*Zingiber officinale*) is a perennial plant with thick, underground stems called "rhizomes" that are used for medical and culinary purposes. The above-ground stem can grow to a height of twenty-four feet. Ginger is native to southern Asia but is now cultivated extensively throughout the tropics. The very best quality ginger is said to grow in Jamaica, but more than 80 percent of the ginger imported into the United States is reported to come from China and India.

Claims

The perceived medicinal qualities of ginger have been broadly documented in cultures as diverse as Indian, Chinese, Arabic, Greek, and Roman. It is cited in ancient Ayurvedic, Sanskrit, and Chinese texts as early as the fourth century BC for conditions such as stomachache, diarrhea, cholera, toothache, and nausea. First-century Roman herbalist Dioscorides included ginger in his herbal text, which became the basis for much of the practice of medicine throughout the Middle Ages.

In addition to its medicinal applications, ginger is also widely used as a spice in foods, beverages, candies, and liqueurs and is commonly used in many cosmetic products. The Chinese use fresh ginger in many dishes, not only for its spicy flavor and perfume but also as a *yang* ingredient to balance cooling (or *yin*) dishes. Five-spice powder and many curries contain dried ginger.

Ginger has many reported beneficial pharmacological effects, including antioxidant properties, prevention of abnormal blood clotting, and reduction of high prostaglandin levels, which cause inflammation. It is also used for loss of appetite and indigestion. Herbalists will also recommend ginger for colic, dyspepsia, gas, rheumatoid arthritis, baldness, snakebites, and rheumatism.

Study Findings

A small number of studies with very different designs (✓✓✓) found that ginger provided relief from pain and swelling caused by osteoarthritis and rheumatoid arthritis. Most studies (✓✓✓✓) have examined ginger's ability to prevent and treat nausea in a variety of clinical settings, including postanesthetic nausea. Studies (✓✓✓) were done on vomiting in pregnancy, motion sickness, and seasickness as well as on chemotherapy-induced nausea (✗✗).

The way ginger works for the prevention and treatment of nausea is not clear. The effect appears to be directly on the gastric system, unlike some conventional drugs that impact the central nervous system (CNS).

Sigrun Chrubasik and colleagues' 2005 review of studies using ginger to treat postoperative nausea and vomiting found five studies with conflicting results. Most people took 1 gram of ginger. Two studies found ginger to be similar in effectiveness to 10 mg of metoclopramide (Reglan), with both being more effective than placebo. However, metoclopramide is not regarded as an effective antiemetic in postoperative situations. Combining the results of similar studies (✗✗✗✗) led the reviewers to conclude that overall, ginger is no more beneficial than placebo in the treatment of postoperative nausea and vomiting.

Multiple studies have been performed using ginger to prevent motion sickness. About the same number of studies found ginger more effective than placebo (✓✓✓✓) as found ginger no better than placebo (✗✗✗). In one study, a group given ginger tolerated being spun around on a revolving chair significantly better than a group given Benadryl or another group given placebo. However, other studies found ginger of no significant benefit, and the results must therefore be seen as inconclusive.

Only one study (✗✗) evaluating ginger for nausea associated with chemotherapy has been reported. This study involved a nonrandomized unblinded protocol called a "case series." Eleven patients with a history of chemotherapy-induced nausea were undergoing chemotherapy for lymphoma. They were given 1,590 mg of ginger thirty minutes prior to chemotherapy, and their symptoms were carefully monitored and recorded. Those given ginger had slightly less nausea, but this difference was not significantly different from the control.

A 2005 review (✓✓✓✓) of randomized double-blind studies involving women in the first trimester of pregnancy found six relevant studies. Two of these found ginger about as beneficial as vitamin B_6, and four found it more beneficial than placebo for nausea. Patients received a variety of preparations of differing doses. Ginger did not appear to negatively affect the women in terms of miscarriages, early births, or other adverse effects.

We should point out that the inconsistency of the results discussed above is also found in studies of conventional medications for nausea and vomiting. This inconsistency is due, in part, to the difficulty of measuring symptoms such as nausea. In addition, the effect of antinausea medications and herbs is often subtle and difficult to discern unless tested in a homogenous population with a high prevalence of nausea. Also, a relatively small improvement requires a large number of participants to detect, and many of these studies involved small numbers.

Ginger is less effective when given to a patient who is already nauseated. All food forms of ginger can be used, but dried capsules are preferable. Candied ginger is usually not dried well enough to be therapeutic, and the pickled and candied forms have not been tested in controlled studies. The liquid sources of ginger (ginger ale or ginger tea) generally have such low concentrations of ginger that large quantities would have to be consumed for the ginger to have an effect.

When buying ginger tablets or capsules, look for the amount of ginger in each capsule, and look for a lot number and expiration date. Although some products are standardized, the smell and taste of ginger are better guides to freshness and, therefore, efficacy.

● Cautions

Ginger is generally well tolerated when taken orally in typical doses. However, doses greater than 5 grams per day are associated with increased side effects such as heartburn, diarrhea, abdominal discomfort and an irritant effect in the mouth and throat. Also, ginger used topically can cause a form of dermatitis.

The use of ginger during pregnancy for hyperemesis gravidarum (a severe form of morning sickness) is controversial among botanical experts. Ginger's effect on a woman's hormones and blood clotting warrant caution in recommending ginger for pregnant women. The risk of bleeding is slight but real. On the other hand, studies involving pregnant women have not reported adverse effects. Given the small numbers of women involved in these studies, and assuming serious adverse effects would be relatively infrequent, the safety of taking ginger during pregnancy remains unclear. Caution should prevail when using ginger during pregnancy. Large doses should not be used during pregnancy until better safety data has been collected. There is insufficient evidence for the use of ginger in amounts greater than those found in foods by lactating women and by children.

Ginger also is not recommended for patients with gallstones, as ginger increases the flow of bile and may lead to gallbladder obstruction or colic. Finally, large doses of ginger have been known to cause heartburn and may cause central nervous system depression and cardiac arrhythmias. Concerns have also been raised about ginger interacting with blood-thinning medications, but reports of these problems have not been made.

patient has a history of bleeding disorders, gallbladder disease, or miscarriage.

The data on ginger for prevention and treatment of chemotherapy-induced nausea and motion sickness are too poor to draw definitive conclusions, with the exception that there is evidence that oral ginger may help prevent chemotherapy-induced nausea when given following administration of intravenous (IV) prochlorperazine (Compazine). The data on prevention of postoperative nausea are mixed. Some evidence suggests that oral ginger is as effective as metoclopramide (Reglan) for reducing postoperative nausea and vomiting in patients not receiving anesthesia or narcotic analgesia at the same time. However, once a patient has received a narcotic, ginger does not prevent postsurgical nausea and vomiting.

Anyone considering taking ginger prior to chemotherapy or surgery should discuss this with his or her physician well in advance. In some cases, patients should not take any form of medication before surgery or other medical procedures.

Recommendations

Ginger is an ancient spice that has a reputation for preventing nausea and vomiting in several situations. The data are not conclusive in any of these settings, but it seems reasonable to use a trial of ginger for the prevention of motion sickness and seasickness for two reasons (1) there is data to support its efficacy and safety, and (2) it is relatively inexpensive and readily available.

Despite common food and folk use, experts debate whether ginger should be recommended for nausea during pregnancy. However, this caution becomes a generally agreed-on warning if the pregnant

Dosage

Different doses are recommended for the different uses of ginger. Usually between 0.5 and 1 gram (tablets or capsules) of dried, powdered ginger root is recommended. For motion sickness, a dose of 1 gram of dried, powdered ginger root thirty minutes to four hours before the journey has been used. For morning sickness, a dose of 250 mg of ginger four times daily has been used. For chemotherapy-induced nausea, a dose of 2 to 4 grams of powdered ginger daily is commonly recommended.

For any condition, it is generally recommended that doses not exceed 4 grams per day.

● Treatment Categories

Complementary

To prevent nausea from seasickness	☺☺
To prevent nausea from anesthesia	☺
To prevent or treat morning sickness during pregnancy	☺
To prevent nausea from motion sickness	☺
To treat vertigo	☺
To relieve pain from rheumatoid arthritis	☺
To relieve pain from osteoarthritis	☺
To prevent nausea from chemotherapy	☹

Scientifically Unproven

For any other indication

● Further Reading

Boone, Sarah A., and Kelly M. Shields. "Treating Pregnancy-Related Nausea and Vomiting with Ginger." *Annals of Pharmacotherapy* 39, no. 10 (October 2005): 1710 – 13.

Chrubasik, S., M. H. Pittler, and B. D. Roufogalis. "Zingiberis Rhizoma: A Comprehensive Review on the Ginger Effect and Efficacy Profiles." *Phytomedicine* 12, no. 9 (September 2005): 684 – 701.

GINKGO BILOBA

● What It Is

Look into the shopping basket of older health food store shoppers, and chances are you will see one or more of three herbal remedies — saw palmetto for prostate and sexual function, St. John's wort for minor depression, and ginkgo biloba for memory. Usually these are not taken because of the suggestion of a physician, though increasingly St. John's wort is being suggested for some patients. Instead, the popular press has helped make these "the big three" for helping an increasingly aging population cope with age-related health issues.

Products such as ginkgo biloba are symbols of people's awareness that mental decline is an unnatural state of aging, not the norm of a person's last two or three decades of life. This may help to explain why, according to the 2002 CDC Survey, ginkgo is the third most commonly used herbal remedy in the United States. Almost one-quarter of those who use herbal remedies stated that they use ginkgo. It is also very popular in Europe and is approved in Germany for the treatment of dementia.

Ginkgo biloba is a tree native to Southeast Asia, where such trees can be more than a thousand years old. The species is believed to have survived from the time of the dinosaurs and has been described as a "living fossil." It is also an extremely hardy tree, being one of the first forms of life to reemerge near the sites where the atomic bombs were dropped in Japan. The leaves, the part used to make the herbal remedy, have a distinctive fan shape. An extract is made from these using alcohol, then dried and made into capsules.

Claims

The claims for ginkgo center on improvements in mental capacity. It is recommended for general memory loss related to aging, advancing Alzheimer's disease, and cognitive problems occurring after a stroke or with depression. It has also been used for several types of dementia, including vascular dementia. Ginkgo contains a variety of antioxidants that prevent oxidation reactions known to play a role in diseases of brain tissue. Herbalists have been known to recommend ginkgo for depression, headache, tinnitus, dizziness, difficulty concentrating, mood disorders, peripheral vascular disease (especially claudication), hearing loss related to vascular disease, PMS, heart disease, high cholesterol, and dysentery. Ginkgo has also been used to reverse sexual dysfunction caused by antidepressants (especially the SSRIs such as Prozac). More generally, it has become the main ingredient in a number of "memory boosters."

Study Findings

A number of animal studies have found that ginkgo does help with learning and memory. The first controlled clinical trial (✓✓✓) in the United States (by Le Bars) found the extract helpful for patients with mild to moderate symptoms related to Alzheimer's disease or multi-infarct (vascular) dementia. After six months to a year of ginkgo, patients' symptoms had remained stable or slightly improved, while the symptoms of those taking a placebo had worsened. The same research team published a second trial in 2000 (✓✓✓) finding similar benefits. A 1998 review of nine randomized controlled trials (✓✓✓✓) found that ginkgo was more effective than placebo in delaying the onset of dementia. Other small studies (✓✓✓✓) continue to report beneficial effects on memory in healthy young to middle-aged people as well as those with age-related memory loss and various forms of dementia.

However, at the end of 2000, a study (✗✗✗) was published which found that older people with mild to moderate dementia (due to Alzheimer's or other causes) did not benefit from taking ginkgo. Another study in 2003 (✗✗✗) similarly found ginkgo no more beneficial than placebo in treating elderly people with dementia or age-related memory impairment. Such contradictory findings demonstrate why more studies of ginkgo are needed before firm recommendations can be made. They also point to the importance of accurately diagnosing patients' conditions prior to involvement in research. In general, studies in which participants began with impaired memory tended to report significant improvements compared to studies that enrolled healthy people. A 2002 study (✗✗✗) with more than two hundred healthy older adults found no differences in memory between those taking ginkgo (40 mg three times daily) and those taking a placebo.

A 2005 review (✓✓✓✓) found six small studies of the effects of ginkgo on healthy adults lasting less than two days and nine lasting longer. Overall, about two-thirds of the studies found beneficial effects in the area of attention, memory, and speed in memory tasks. However, there was quite a bit of variability in the results. The results also appeared to be less beneficial as studies continued beyond a few weeks, suggesting that people may become used to ginkgo's effects. It should also be noted that the tests were very specific and structured. Performance on examinations or everyday mental activities were not examined.

Ginkgo is believed to work by increasing the flow of blood through arteries and veins in various tissues, including the brain and the arms and legs. In keeping with this, small clinical trials (✔✔) have shown that ginkgo can improve overall functioning in patients with peripheral arterial disease, improve certain aspects of memory in people in their fifties, and even improve some asthmatic symptoms. More than fifteen European trials (✔✔✔) have shown improvement in claudication (pain in calf muscles that people with narrowed or blocked arteries get when walking).

Ginkgo has also been tested with a wide variety of other conditions. A systematic review (✘✘✘✘) of ginkgo for tinnitus (ringing in the ears) found six studies that revealed no overall benefit. Ginkgo has been recommended to relieve depression. Eight small studies of ginkgo's impact on mood, including depression, were found, of which six found the herb to be no more beneficial than placebo (✘✘✘✘). Ginkgo has been reported to reduce the sexual dysfunction that can occur as a side effect of some antidepressants. However, a 2004 trial (✘✘✘) found ginkgo no more beneficial than placebo. Interestingly, some people reported spectacular improvements with their problems, but this occurred with both ginkgo and placebo.

Ginkgo's antidementia effects are similar to those of currently available prescription drugs. However, while these effects are statistically significant in clinical studies, it remains unclear whether this is enough to make a noticeable difference in people's lives. So far, while ginkgo has been shown to delay the onset of dementia, it has not been shown to prevent or treat dementia.

• Cautions

Ginkgo seeds can cause fatal neurological and allergic reactions and should never be taken. The extract, made from ginkgo leaves, has led to relatively few side effects. In the Le Bars research, twice as many patients taking ginkgo reported intestinal problems compared to those taking a placebo. Bleeding problems (✘✘) have occurred in patients also taking blood-thinning drugs (such as aspirin or warfarin). However, a controlled study of the interaction between ginkgo and warfarin found no negative effect on blood clotting. Some studies have raised concerns that ginkgo might inhibit an enzyme called "monoamine oxidase" (MAO). This would mean that it could cause problems with a number of other antidepressant drugs that act the same way. People taking the above medications may also be concerned about memory loss and should consult their physician before taking ginkgo or any other herbal remedy.

Most clinical studies have been conducted with an extract made according to specific German specifications (called EGb 761). Because there are no precise standards for the preparation of herbal products sold in the United States, what you buy may not have been made in the same way. ConsumerLab.com's review of ginkgo products in 1999 found that nearly one-quarter of the thirty brands tested did not have the expected levels of chemical marker compounds, despite claims to have been "standardized." Further testing in 2003 found that seven of nine ginkgo products lacked adequate levels of certain key ingredients. A 2006 review of memory-enhancing supplements included thirteen ginkgo products, only six of which passed. One product made from dried ginkgo leaf (not the more usual extract) had the highest level of lead encountered in any dietary supplements tested by ConsumerLab.com. One of the other products that failed testing was immediately recalled by its manufacturers. These reports can be viewed by subscribing to *www.consumerlab.com*.

There is no reliable data on which to determine if ginkgo is safe to use in children or in women who are pregnant or lactating.

Recommendations

Ginkgo has been the subject of many clinical trials, although most of them have been relatively small. Apart from studies related to memory, a wide variety of other conditions have been examined in a few studies each. Many studies used the standardized extract, EGb 761, now available in a few brands. Many other brands are available whose quality is uncertain.

While ginkgo looks promising as a means of delaying the memory loss related to a variety of diseases, some studies have found no benefit. Studies have found memory benefits only for about six months. Ginkgo may prove helpful for retarding age-related memory loss, dementia, and peripheral arterial disease. However, studies have not examined the benefits or safety of taking ginkgo long-term.

Many healthy people also take the herb in the hope of boosting their memory or increasing performance on examinations. While some studies have reported ginkgo beneficial in these areas, the research has been highly structured and not carried out in real-life circumstances. Continuous usage of ginkgo for these benefits does not appear to be warranted. Most studies involved short-term memory tests, not recall of material typically examined in school or college tests. The work and study needed for those exams cannot be replaced by any pill.

Dosage

The usual dose is 120 to 240 mg daily, divided into two or three doses.

Treatment Categories

Complementary

To stabilize or slightly improve cognitive function, at least for the short term, in those with Alzheimer's disease ☺☺☺

To slightly improve cognitive function in those with multi-infarct (vascular) dementia ☺☺☺

To increase walking distance for people with peripheral arterial disease or claudication ☺☺☺

To relieve cognitive symptoms of other types of dementia ☺☺

To retard age-related memory loss ☺☺

To improve memory and concentration in healthy people ☺☺

To prevent symptoms of dizziness ☺☺

To relieve headaches ☺☺

To treat age-related macular degeneration ☺

Scientifically Unproven

To relieve tinnitus ☹☹☹

To relieve mild depression or SAD and to improve mood ☹☹☹

To reverse sexual dysfunction associated with SSRI antidepressants ☹☹

Further Reading

Crews, W. David, Jr., David W. Harrison, Melanie L. Griffin, Katherine D. Falwell, Tara Crist, Lesley Longest, Laura Hehemann, and Stephenie T. Rey. "Ginkgo Preparations in Healthy and Cognitively Intact Adults: A Comprehensive Review." *HerbalGram* 67 (2005): 43 – 62.

Gertz, H.-J., and M. Kiefer. "Review about Ginkgo Biloba Special Extract EGb 761 (Ginkgo)." *Current Pharmaceutical Design* 10, no. 3 (2004): 261 – 64.

Le Bars, Pierre L., Martin M. Katz, Nancy Berman, Turan M. Itil, Alfred M. Freedman, and Alan F. Schatzberg. "A Placebo-Controlled, Double-Blind, Randomized Trial of an Extract of Ginkgo Biloba for Dementia." *Journal of the American Medical Association* 278, no. 16 (October 1997): 1327 – 32.

Sierpina, Victor S., Bernd Wollschlaeger, and Mark Blumenthal. "Ginkgo Biloba." *American Family Physician* 68, no. 5 (September 2003): 923 – 26.

GINSENG

What It Is

If it can be said that there is a "fountain of youth" in any one herbal remedy, ginseng would be first in line to claim the title. In China, during the time of Jesus, medical texts identified ginseng as leading to longevity, wisdom, and enlightenment. While few today would claim you can gain wisdom from a bottle, the connection between ginseng and longevity continues to be made both in the United States and in many parts of the world where the herb is used. Some Chinese still refer to ginseng as "the root of immortality."

Ginseng preparations are made from five different plants, the most popular being Asian ginseng (*Panax ginseng*) and American ginseng (*Panax quinquefolius*). Siberian ginseng is made from the botanically unrelated *Eleutherococcus senticosus* and contains a completely different set of chemicals.

Red ginseng is steam-cured prior to drying, which leaves a reddish color in the product. White ginseng is produced when the roots are bleached and dried quickly.

Claims

The 2002 CDC Survey reported that almost one-quarter of those using herbs were using ginseng, making it the second most popular herbal remedy in the United States. It is consistently one of the most popular herbal remedies used.

Ginseng is most widely used as an "adaptogen," an herbal remedy that allegedly restores a wide variety of bodily functions to normal. This is not a term that fits easily into the biomedical model in which a remedy is presumed to have a more specific effect. Ginseng has been used to treat nervous disorders, anemia, wakefulness, dyspnea (difficulty breathing), forgetfulness and confusion, prolonged thirst, decreased libido, chronic fatigue, angina, diabetes, and nausea.

In traditional Chinese medicine, it is believed to restore deficiencies in a person's *chi*, or life energy.

Asian ginseng is said to have more *yin* and to be better suited for women, while American ginseng is said to be better for men because it has more *yang*.

• Study Findings

A vast number of studies on ginseng have been conducted over several decades, but the results are not consistent. Many individual components, called "ginsenosides," have been isolated from ginseng and found to have multiple and opposing actions in the body. For example, ginsenoside Rb-1 depresses the central nervous system (CNS), while ginsenoside Rg-1 is a CNS stimulant. Ginsenoside Rg-1 stimulates the heart, while ginsenoside Rb-1 depresses the heart. Given the natural variability of all plants, different ingredients will be present in different proportions from one crop to another, making it difficult to get consistent findings.

European references, including German Commission E reports, cite human studies (✓✓✓) indicating that ginseng may improve mental alertness, memory, physical endurance, sleep pattern, and appetite. These reports also say ginseng may be helpful in treating hyperlipidemia, treating type 2 diabetes, improving resistance to stress, improving immune response, protecting against some toxins, and in treating congestive heart failure. However, while individual studies may support these actions, many of the studies have had very few participants and were poorly designed. Some studies (✓✓✓) report some helpful results, but many others (✗✗✗✗) found no benefits from ginseng.

Using ginseng as a general tonic to improve well-being and mental abilities has the best supportive evidence. The ginsenosides have demonstrated antioxidant properties that may lead to general health benefits, especially if part of a healthy diet and lifestyle. Even here, though, few studies have been published. One three-month randomized controlled trial (✓✓✓) showed a significant increase in subjective "quality of life" scores among 625 ginseng users. Another similar study with college-aged volunteers (✓✓✓) who took 100 mg of ginseng twice a day for twelve weeks found that they experienced a statistically significant improvement in the speed at which they were able to perform math calculations. A combination ginseng and ginkgo product (Gincosan) was tested in five small studies (✗✗✗✗), but only one found it more effective than placebo in improving people's mood.

Studies in animals and a few clinical trials (✓✓✓) have suggested that Asian ginseng may be effective in treating type 2 diabetes. One small Canadian trial (✓✓✓) evaluated the effect of American ginseng on blood sugar levels after people consumed glucose. The researchers found that when nondiabetic subjects took ginseng forty minutes before the glucose challenge, significant reductions were observed in their blood sugar levels. In subjects with type 2 diabetes mellitus, the same was true, whether capsules were taken before or together with the glucose challenge. The researchers concluded that for nondiabetic subjects, to prevent unintended hypoglycemia, it may be important that American ginseng be taken with the meal. However, a 2002 Cochrane review of Chinese herbs used to treat type 2 diabetes concluded that overall, the evidence does not support the use of ginseng to treat diabetes.

One area where studies have been conclusive is with athletes using ginseng. In the 1980s, reports emerged from Germany that athletes had improved performances after taking ginseng. This led to nine well-controlled, though small, studies (✗✗✗✗) in which performance was not improved by ginseng.

With increased interest in herbal treatments for menopausal symptoms, one recent study (✘✘✘) examined the impact of ginseng on these symptoms. No benefits beyond placebo were seen. The same result occurred with the ginseng-ginkgo combination product.

Overall, most human studies show no benefit from ginseng. The inconsistency between ginseng's huge popularity and its poor results in research may have to do, at least partially, with the poor design of some studies, the lack of adequate controls, and the failure to standardize the ginseng administered. In addition, the literature reveals considerable confusion about the different species of ginseng, with little concern for the fact that Siberian ginseng is from a completely different genus. Among the few human trials that are of good quality, the results can be considered only suggestive, not conclusive. On the other hand, ginseng's reputation may be the source of a strong placebo effect that benefits many users.

● Cautions

A number of side effects have been found (✘✘) when people take large doses of ginseng for extended periods of time (in the past this was called the "ginseng abuse syndrome," although experts now discount the existence of such a syndrome). The supposed symptoms include diarrhea, weakness, tremors, palpitations, nervousness, decreased libido, and high blood pressure. Side effects with ginseng are not rare and include insomnia, breast pain, vaginal bleeding, fast heart rate, decreased appetite, diarrhea, headache, vertigo, and skin reactions. Some medical studies in Russia (✘✘) have led practitioners there to recommend that patients not use large doses of ginseng for more than two weeks at a time without a break.

However, no specific formula for use and abstinence has been developed.

Ginsenosides are steroidlike, which can cause menstrual problems as well as increase the serum levels of hormones such as testosterone. People with diabetes should be very cautious when taking ginseng, as it has led to hypoglycemia (very low blood sugar levels). Ginseng also may hinder blood clotting, which is especially problematic in patients taking blood thinners (such as aspirin or warfarin).

In addition, ginseng products are notorious for being mislabeled and adulterated, which can cause a whole host of other problems. One study found that one in four ginseng products contained no ginseng. In another study of fifty-four ginseng products, 85 percent were evaluated as being "worthless," containing little or no ginseng. Also, *Eleutherococcus senticosus*, usually labeled "Siberian ginseng," actually contains no true ginseng. Drinks and chewing gum made from ginseng are now available, but the quantity and quality of the herb they contain are unknown.

In 2000, ConsumerLab.com purchased twenty-two brands of Asian and American ginseng sold in the United States. Only nine products met all of the testing criteria for quality and purity. Even more problematic, eight products contained unacceptable levels of pesticides, with two products having pesticide levels more than twenty times the allowed amount. One of the pesticides found (hexachlorobenzene) is banned from use with food crops throughout the world because of cancer-causing concerns. Two ginseng products also contained lead above the acceptable level.

ConsumerLab.com retested ginseng products in 2003. A high amount of hexachlorobenzene was found in one of the five products labeled "Korean ginseng." This type of ginseng consistently fails quality tests more than others. Another product that failed in 2003 was a liquid labeled "extra strength," which contained less than 10 percent of the expected ginsenosides.

The 2003 ConsumerLab.com tests overall showed considerable improvement in only three years. No products were contaminated with heavy metals and none contained undeclared caffeine. In summary, sixteen of the eighteen products met the ConsumerLab.com criteria for ginseng quality, label claims, lack of contaminants and adulterants, and disintegration.

Insufficient reliable data exists to conclude that ginseng is safe in childhood, pregnancy, or lactation; therefore, ginseng should be avoided during these periods.

Recommendations

When taken orally in moderate amounts for less than three months, quality ginseng products appear to be relatively harmless for most people except during those stages of life mentioned above. It may have some benefits in helping type 2 diabetics and may help some people feel better and more energetic, although none of the "well-being" benefits have been conclusively verified in research. Therefore, people who take ginseng risk paying a high price without proven benefit, as preparations cost up to $20 per ounce and vary tremendously in quality. If you are going to purchase ginseng, make sure you use a reputable brand that can demonstrate that it contains the correct amount of the appropriate plant and is free of cancer-causing compounds.

Dosage

For most indications, 0.25 to 0.5 grams of the root are taken twice a day. Large quantities, up to about 3 grams two or three times daily, have been recommended by some.

Treatment Categories

Complementary
(all apply to *Panax* ginseng species)

To give a general feeling of well-being or improved energy	☺
To lower blood glucose levels slightly	☺
To improve mental alertness, memory, and cognitive functioning	☺
To treat insomnia, fatigue, and depressed mood in menopause	☺
To reduce high cholesterol levels	☹
To improve the immune response	☹
To protect against congestive heart failure	☹

Scientifically Unproven

To improve athletic performance in healthy young adults	☹☹☹☹
To relieve hot flashes in menopause	☹☹☹
For any other indication	

Further Reading

Bahrke, M. S., and W. R. Morgan. "Evaluation of the Ergogenic Properties of Ginseng: An Update." *Sports Medicine* 29, no. 2 (February 2000): 113–33.

Vogler, B. K., M. H. Pittler, and E. Ernst. "The Efficacy of Ginseng: A Systematic Review of Randomised Clinical Trials." *European Journal of Clinical Pharmacology* 55, no. 8 (1999): 567–75.

Yeh, Gloria Y., David M. Eisenberg, Ted J. Kaptchuk, and Russell S. Phillips. "Systematic Review of Herbs and Dietary Supplements for Glycemic Control in Diabetes." *Diabetes Care* 26, no. 4 (2003): 1277–94.

GLUCOSAMINE

What It Is

Glucosamine is an important component of proteoglycans and other compounds used to make connective tissue. Proteoglycans act as lubricants within joints and are integral to the makeup of healthy cartilage. Glucosamine is available on its own or in a number of salt forms, including glucosamine sulfate and glucosamine hydrochloride. All are converted into glucosamine in the stomach and are therefore believed to be equivalent.

Claims

Glucosamine sulfate came to widespread public attention as part of the "medical miracle" promoted in the book *The Arthritis Cure* (New York: St. Martin's Press, 1997). The subtitle of the book claimed that a combination of glucosamine and chondroitin sulfate "can halt, reverse, and may even cure osteoarthritis." Since then, glucosamine has become available in many formulations as a way to treat and cure arthritis. According to a *Consumer Reports* survey done in 2000, nearly 36 percent of the people surveyed who had arthritis were using glucosamine regularly. Over-the-counter dietary supplements and prescription products are available.

Study Findings

A 2005 Cochrane review (✓✓✓) found twenty randomized controlled trials using glucosamine on its own for osteoarthritis. Osteoarthritis is the most common form of arthritis, leading to joint pain and stiffness, especially in the knee and hip. All the research on glucosamine that we found was conducted with patients who had osteoarthritis and does not necessarily indicate whether glucosamine will help people with other types of arthritis.

Of the twenty studies, eighteen followed people for an average of nine weeks. The two other studies were conducted for three years. Since osteoarthritis lasts for many years, people will take medications for it for prolonged periods, and long-term assessment of remedies is essential.

Overall, glucosamine was significantly more beneficial than placebo. The average benefit compared to placebo was 28 percent more pain relief and 21 percent greater improvement in overall functioning. The two three-year studies found X-ray evidence that physical joint deterioration was slowed by glucosamine.

Five of the studies compared glucosamine to conventional drugs used to treat osteoarthritis. Glucosamine sulfate appears to work as well as the nonsteroidal anti-inflammatory drugs (NSAIDs) ibuprofen (Advil, Motrin) and piroxicam (Feldene) for symptom relief. However, NSAIDs work within a week or two, while glucosamine can take four to eight weeks to relieve symptoms. Other researchers have found that glucosamine sulfate (1500 mg a day) may be more effective than acetaminophen (Tylenol). The results were similar for effectiveness, but glucosamine had a lot fewer adverse effects. Glucosamine sulfate was not found to be very effective for more severe, long-standing osteoarthritis or in patients who were older or overweight.

A more detailed analysis of the research revealed other important findings. In spite of the overall benefits of glucosamine, five studies found it no better than placebo. None of these studies used a patented Italian product made by Rotta Pharmaceutical Company. This product is approved as a prescription drug in the European Union and regulated like other prescription drugs.

Products available in the United States are available as dietary supplements and vary widely in quality. One study of glucosamine dietary supplements found that products had anywhere between 41 and 108 percent of what the labels stated. Another study found glucosamine products with no glucosamine in them. ConsumerLab.com tested glucosamine products in 2003 and found no quality problems with the ten products that contained glucosamine only. Among thirty-three combination products (adding chondroitin and/or MSM), problems were found only among four products that were low in chondroitin sulfate — a particularly expensive ingredient.

Glucosamine is sold in many forms, including glucosamine sulfate, glucosamine hydrochloride, and N-acetylglucosamine. Evidence regarding which products are best is not readily available. A small number of studies used glucosamine hydrochloride and did not have as beneficial an effect as studies using glucosamine sulfate. No research evidence supports the use of N-acetylglucosamine for osteoarthritis. Glucosamine hydrochloride is less expensive than glucosamine sulfate, which is the naturally occurring form. Some products are labeled "glucosamine sulfate" but actually contain glucosamine hydrochloride with added sulfate.

Cautions

Adverse reactions to glucosamine have been mild and infrequent, with gastrointestinal problems being most frequently reported. All of these went away once people stopped taking the medication. However, glucosamine is involved in a number of metabolic processes, warranting close monitoring of patients taking it for long periods. For example, animal studies and at least one human study (✗ ✗) have found that glucosamine can play a role in worsening insulin resistance, which underlies some cases of diabetes. People with osteoarthritis tend to gain weight, which also makes them susceptible to type 2 diabetes mellitus.

Therefore, people with diabetes, or at risk for developing it, should be cautious when using glucosamine and at the very least inform their physicians if they are taking glucosamine. Blood sugar problems have not been reported in the other clinical trials of glucosamine, although this problem would only be expected after prolonged use.

Furthermore, there is a theoretical concern that glucosamine derived from marine exoskeletons may cause allergic reactions in people allergic to shellfish. However, no such reactions have been reported. Unfortunately, most producers of glucosamine do not list the source of the product on the label.

There is insufficient reliable information about the use of glucosamine in childhood, pregnancy, and lactation, and therefore it should not be used during these periods.

Recommendations

Overall, there is some evidence to suggest that glucosamine sulfate may provide relief from the symptoms of osteoarthritis. Timothy McAlindon's 2000 review concluded that although the positive effects of glucosamine are "exaggerated," "some degree of efficacy appears possible." There is no evidence to suggest that it cures arthritis, as has been suggested in popular literature.

Many recommend using glucosamine in combination with chondroitin sulfate, but this has not been studied well to date. Glucosamine alone appears to produce a smaller benefit than chondroitin alone. However, chondroitin products in the United States are often substandard. Only reputable brands, certified by independent labs, should be used (you can find a list of approved products at *www.consumerlab.com*). There is no information on the safety or effectiveness of taking glucosamine for longer than three years.

● Dosage

The most frequently recommended dosage of glucosamine alone is 500 mg three times daily. The dose depends on the person's weight and is often in combination with chondroitin. An average daily dose would be 1200 mg of chondroitin and 1500 mg of glucosamine. This is usually divided into two to four doses taken with food.

● Treatment Categories

Complementary

As glucosamine *sulfate* to relieve pain and increase mobility in those with osteoarthritis ☺☺☺☺

As glucosamine *hydrochloride* to relieve pain and increase mobility in those with osteoarthritis ☺☺

As glucosamine *sulfate*, in combination with chondroitin, to relieve pain and increase mobility in those with osteoarthritis ☺☺☺

As glucosamine *hydrochloride*, in combination with chondroitin, to relieve pain and increase mobility in those with osteoarthritis ☺

As glucosamine *sulfate* to relieve pain and improve function in those with tempomandibular joint (TMJ) arthritis ☺

Scientifically Unproven

To cure any form of arthritis ☹☹

● Further Reading

McAlindon, Timothy E., Michael P. LaValley, Juan P. Gulin, and David T. Felson. "Glucosamine and Chondroitin for Treatment of Osteoarthritis: A Systematic Quality Assessment and Meta-analysis." *Journal of the American Medical Association* 283, no. 11 (March 2000): 1469–75.

Richy, Florent, Olivier Bruyere, Olivier Ethgen, Michel Cucherat, Yves Honrotin, and Jean-Yves Reginster. "Structural and Symptomatic Efficacy of Glucosamine and Chondroitin in Knee Osteoarthritis." *Archives of Internal Medicine* 163 (July 2003): 1514–22.

GOLDENSEAL

What It Is

Goldenseal is one of the more popular herbal remedies in the United States, being native to the woodland areas of the eastern and midwestern states. It was standard antiseptic medicine for both Native Americans and the pioneer families who settled the West, learning the indigenous ways as they traveled. The Cherokees used goldenseal for stomach ailments, an idea that the settlers adopted much later in a patent medicine for intestinal upsets. Other traditional uses were as an eyewash, a mouthwash, a treatment for stomach ulcers, and a dye. It was included among official lists of medicinal herbs in the United States until 1955.

Goldenseal (*Hydrastis canadensis*), part of the buttercup family, is a small herb with a bright yellow underground stem, from which it gets its name. Other names for it include golden root, eye root, and ground raspberry (because it has a small red fruit).

Claims

The most popular current claims are that goldenseal is a natural antibiotic, antiseptic, and antidiarrheal. Its most popular use is for colds, especially combined with echinacea. It is recommended for any upper respiratory tract infection and all cold symptoms. Some Internet promoters market it as a panacea, claiming it can cure almost everything. Herbalists use goldenseal as an eyewash for conjunctivitis and as a diuretic and laxative. It is also recommended for soreness and infections in the mouth and gastrointestinal tract. Topically it has been used for eczema, itching, acne, dandruff, ringworm, fever blisters, and wounds. Goldenseal has also received a boost in popularity from the faulty but prevalent belief that it can mask illicit drugs in urine drug screens.

Study Findings

We found no clinical studies on goldenseal (other than those examining whether goldenseal could mask illicit drugs in the urine). However, the herb contains a drug called "berberine" that has been shown to have broad antimicrobial activity. Berberine is found in many herbs with antimicrobial reputations, including barberry, Oregon grape root, goldenthread, and a number of Chinese herbs. In one randomized controlled trial, a single dose of berberine (400 mg) significantly reduced stool volume and duration of diarrhea among patients with bacterial dysentery. In another trial, berberine was more effective than placebo and as effective as a standard prescription antibiotic in treating children with the parasite *Giardia*.

However, the studies of berberine used quantities far greater than the amount found in goldenseal and its products. It has been estimated it would take twenty-five or more commercially available goldenseal capsules to obtain the same amount of berberine used in these studies. These studies did not examine berberine's effects within the body, and there is evidence showing it is very poorly absorbed from the digestive tract. No reports show that berberine is active against viruses, which cause the colds and flu that goldenseal is said to prevent and cure.

Cautions

A 2005 study (✖✖✖) examined the impact of several herbs on enzymes the body uses to break down drugs and other compounds. Goldenseal had the most powerful inhibitory effect of the herbs studied. Drugs that are normally broken down by these enzymes would therefore remain at higher concentrations, which could lead to adverse effects.

Large amounts of goldenseal cause nausea, vomiting, numbness, high blood pressure, and breathing problems. A few fatalities have been reported, and goldenseal has also caused abortions. It should therefore be completely avoided during pregnancy or when a woman might become pregnant. Nor should goldenseal be given to babies or nursing mothers.

Berberine increases bilirubin levels in the blood, and bilirubin causes jaundice. While there is little or no indication that goldenseal can cause jaundice, the fact that one of the active ingredients increases bilirubin means that goldenseal is likely to cause someone who has jaundice to worsen.

The popularity of goldenseal has led to its overcollection. It is difficult to cultivate and is becoming increasingly rare in its natural habitats. This has driven prices up and has led some producers to use other, less expensive berberine-containing herbs in their goldenseal products. Some of these herbs are more toxic than goldenseal.

Recommendations

Goldenseal may have some use as an antibiotic when applied externally to the body or used orally to treat diarrhea. There is no evidence that it works against viral infections. The long list of adverse effects and its potential for drug interactions as well as the plant's endangered species status make its popular use for diarrhea, colds, and flu unwarranted.

The use of goldenseal for colds should be discouraged for other reasons. We turn to drugs and remedies for all sorts of minor, short-lasting ailments. Overuse of antibiotics has led to antibiotic-resistant organisms. Resorting to natural products just extends the concerns. If you have a cold, take plenty of liquids and rest, letting the minor ailment run its course. Then when you truly need medication, you will have a better chance it will work at the lowest dose possible.

Dosage

A wide variety of oral doses are recommended, with 0.5 to 1 gram three times a day being most common.

Treatment Categories

Scientifically Unproven
To treat cold and flu   ☹☹
For any other indication

Scientifically Questionable
To mask illicit drugs in urine
drug screens   ☹☹☹☹

Risk of Serious Side Effects
Interacting with other drugs   ⊘⊘

● Further Reading

Gurley, Bill J., Stephanie F. Gardner, Martha A. Hubbard, D. Keith Williams, W. Brooks Gentry, Ikhlas A. Khan, and Amit Shah. "In Vivo Effects of Goldenseal, Kava Kava, Black Cohosh, and Valerian on Human Cytochrome P450 1A2, 2D6, 2E1, and 3A4/5 Phenotypes." *Clinical Pharmacology and Therapeutics* 77, no. 5 (May 2005): 415–26.

O'Mathúna, Dónal P. "Goldenseal for Upper Respiratory Infections." *Alternative Medicine Alert* 3, no. 5 (May 2000): 56–58.

GRAPE SEED EXTRACT

● What It Is

Grape seed extract was one of the ten bestselling herbal remedies at the turn of the millennium but has since dropped off in popularity. Interest arose from what has been called the French Paradox. Studies in the 1970s showed that when a country's citizens enjoyed a diet that contained relatively high proportions of fat, they also suffered a higher than average incidence of and deaths from heart disease. The one extreme exception to all this was France and, to a lesser degree, Mediterranean countries. They had relatively high amounts of fat in their diet but a relatively low incidence of heart disease. When researchers looked to see how the French high-fat meals differed from similar high-fat meals in countries plagued with heart disease, the one consistent difference was not on the plate but in the glass. French men, women, and children tended to drink one or more glasses of wine with their meals, something citizens of other countries did not.

However, recommending a daily glass of wine raised concerns about negative effects and the potential for abuse. Certainly the myth of the safety of wine consumption was shattered when it was found that the French have a relatively high incidence of alcoholism. In fact, the higher alcohol-related death rate in France completely eliminates any benefit due to the lower death rate from heart disease. Others are now questioning whether the "French Paradox" is actually just a statistical anomaly due to the way the original surveys were conducted. In spite of this, interest in grape products remains high, with grape seed extract identified as the most likely candidate to have potentially beneficial effects.

Pycnogenol is another name used for some grape seed extract products, although the name is also used for pine bark extracts that contain compounds similar to those in grape seed extract. Interestingly, the French are again credited with discovering this possible remedy. In 1534, Jacques Cartier, a famous French explorer, was trapped by ice on the Saint Lawrence River. He and his men had plenty of stores of biscuits and salted meat to survive the harsh winter. Although they were able to eat their fill, they developed scurvy, a disease we now know is caused by vitamin C deficiency. Some of Cartier's men died. Those who survived recovered when they met Native Americans who advised them to drink a tea made from the bark and needles of pine trees.

No one knew why this helped, but four centuries later, Professor Jacques Masquelier of the University of Bordeaux in France determined that the pine bark and needles contained vitamin C. He then found bioflavonoids and other components he termed "pycnogenols." Grape seed extract contains these same types of components.

• Claims

Proponents claim that grape seed extract improves circulation, in particular bringing relief for varicose veins (technically called "chronic venous insufficiency"). Grape seed extract is reported to protect against heart disease, treat arthritis and allergic reactions, and fight cancer. Most of these effects are said to result from the extract's antioxidant activity. These effects have been traced to a group of compounds called "flavonoids." The particular ones found in grape seed extract are also called "procyanidins" or "OPCs." These are present in much greater amounts in red wine compared to white wine or grape juice. They are believed to work via the same general antioxidant effect discussed in the Antioxidants entry.

• Study Findings

The epidemiological studies continue to be the primary evidence connecting cardiac benefits with grape seeds — and these studies examined wine, not grape seed extract. Grape seed extract contains antioxidants, and studies have shown that these can have beneficial effects on the hearts of animals fed high-fat diets. However, very few studies examined grape seed extracts given to humans. Double-blind studies from the 1980s (✓✓✓) did show improvements in blood flow. One more recent study (✓✓✓) showed that the concentration of antioxidants in the blood was increased after five days of taking the supplements. However, the longest of these studies lasted just one month. No studies have examined whether taking grape seed extract leads to lower incidence of heart disease.

A few small clinical trials (✓✓✓) have examined grape seed extract and pycnogenol (from sources other than grape seed) with varicose veins. These studies found consistent reductions in swelling, pain, and feelings of heaviness in people's legs. One randomized controlled study (✗✗✗) examined the effect of grape seed extract on hay fever symptoms due to ragweed allergy. No differences were found between the extract and placebo.

• Cautions

No adverse effects or drug interactions have been reported from grape seed extract. Rats and mice fed very large quantities suffered no ill effects. One theoretical concern is that grape seed extract may increase the blood-thinning effect of warfarin because of the presence of vitamin E in the extract. These issues have not been investigated. Caution should be exercised since beta-carotene is another antioxidant of natural origin that was promoted widely until large-scale studies showed it could have harmful effects when taken by long-term smokers.

As with all dietary supplements, quality is a concern. One study examined the quality of six grape seed and pine bark products. The total flavonoid content of these products ranged from 2 to 804 mg per gram of extract. When the researchers tested the ability of these products to prevent oxidation, the flavonoid content ranged from 16 to 8,392. The units are not particularly relevant (technically, micromole trolox equivalents per gram). What is remarkable is the 525-fold difference in strength!

Grape seed extract should be avoided in amounts greater than found in food sources during childhood, pregnancy, and lactation, as insufficient reliable information is available.

Recommendations

Antioxidants appear to play an important role in preventing heart disease and other illnesses. The Bible recognizes the value of a little wine for stomach problems (1 Timothy 5:23). Grape seed extract is a potentially useful product of this type and appears to be very safe. However, there is little evidence that taking antioxidants from one particular source has the same benefit as eating a diet rich in a variety of antioxidants. Until properly designed clinical trials show that grape seed extract prevents the incidence of heart disease or affects its severity, it should only be taken as part of a balanced diet rich in fruits and vegetables.

Dosage

Doses vary considerably, with 25 to 300 mg daily being suggested for up to three weeks. After this, 40 to 80 mg daily is recommended. One clinical trial used 720 mg daily.

Treatment Categories

Complementary

As a dietary source of antioxidants	☺☺☺
To relieve the symptoms of varicose veins	☺☺
To prevent cardiovascular disease	☺
To improve night vision	☺

Scientifically Unproven

To treat cardiovascular disease	☹☹
To treat high blood pressure	☹☹
To prevent hay fever	☹☹☹☹
For any other indication	

Further Reading

Bernstein, David I., Cheryl K. Bernstein, Chunqin Deng, Karen J. Murphy, I. Leonard Bernstein, Jonathan A. Bernstein, and Rakesh Shukla. "Evaluation of the Clinical Efficacy and Safety of Grapeseed Extract in the Treatment of Fall Seasonal Allergic Rhinitis: A Pilot Study." *Annals of Allergy, Asthma and Immunology* 88, no. 3 (March 2002): 272–78.

Law, Malcolm, and Nicholas Wald. "Why Heart Disease Mortality Is Low in France: The Time Lag Explanation." *British Medical Journal* 318 (May 1999): 1471–80.

Prior, Ronald L., and Guohua Cao. "Variability in Dietary Antioxidant Related Natural Product Supplements: The Need for Methods of Standardization." *Journal of the American Nutraceutical Association* 2, no. 2 (Summer 1999): 46–56.

GREEN TEA

What It Is

Apart from water, tea is the most widely consumed beverage on the planet. Black, oolong, and green tea all originate from leaves of *Camellia sinensis*, but they are prepared in very different ways. Green tea is produced from leaves that are withered, steamed, and dried. This gives a tea with lesser amounts of polyphenols, which are the compounds giving black tea its stronger, tannic flavor. Green tea may contain 1 to 4 percent caffeine (about 20 to 50 mg per cup), which is similar to black tea. Green tea is the main traditional tea in China, Japan, India, and parts of the Middle East. It has been growing in popularity in the West. The health benefits of drinking tea have been mentioned in traditional Chinese medicine sources for hundreds of years.

Claims

Green tea has been consumed mostly as a social beverage and stimulant because of its caffeine. Recent interest has arisen because of epidemiological studies that noticed reduced occurrences of cancers in cultures where green tea consumption was high. Chemical investigations have found a number of ingredients that are active in laboratory tests of cancer cells.

More traditional uses of the tea are to treat stomach disorders, vomiting, and diarrhea. Regular consumption is said to lower cholesterol levels and protect against cardiac diseases. This is said to be due to the presence of many antioxidants. Green tea (either the extract or used tea leaves and bags) is also used externally to prevent and treat a variety of skin problems ranging from sunburn to skin cancer.

Study Findings

The processing of tea produces compounds called "polyphenols." One group of polyphenols is called the "catechins." Green tea contains about ten times more catechins than black tea. In purified form in laboratory tests, catechins have been shown to inhibit cancer cell growth. Evidence that green tea might protect people against cancer comes from epidemiological studies (✓✓). For example, a 2005 review of epidemiological studies found four studies that together showed that people who regularly consumed several cups of green tea every day had a lower risk of breast cancer. The risk was reduced by about 10 percent, which is statistically significant. In comparison, the risk of breast cancer in regular drinkers of black tea was found unchanged or even slightly increased in thirteen epidemiological studies.

Similar findings (✓✓) have been reported for bladder, esophageal, pancreatic, gastric, colorectal, and ovarian cancers. For example, a Chinese study found that women who consumed ten or more cups of green tea per day lowered their risk of cancer of the colon, rectum, and pancreas by 18, 28, and 37 percent, respectively. For men, the risks were lowered by 33, 43, and 47 percent, respectively. These results must be viewed cautiously. Lowering of risk is not the same as prevention of cancer. Reduced risk in these studies relates to the statistical chances of getting cancer. Also, it must be remembered that epidemiological studies do not prove that something prevents or cures an illness, only that there seems to be some connection between the two. Evidence is not available to demonstrate that green tea prevents or cures any cancer.

In 2005, Japanese researchers reviewed studies of green tea and stomach cancer. In some studies in which patients were asked about past practices, green tea consumption was associated with reduced risk of stomach cancer. The researchers also reviewed "prospective" studies in which patients were questioned about their activities on an ongoing basis. These studies are held to be more reliable since people easily forget what they did in the past. Six prospective studies (✗ ✗ ✗) were located, and none of them found any benefit from green tea consumption. This points to the importance of controlled studies in this area.

The catechins in green tea are antioxidants, which may explain how they contribute to protection against cancer. Some cancers arise because of oxidative damage. Increasing the proportion of antioxidants in the diet is part of why people are advised to increase the number of fruits and vegetables they consume.

Antioxidants are also known to have cardiac benefits. Again, epidemiological studies (✓✓) have found that green tea drinkers have better lipid and cholesterol levels. However, in a small number of controlled studies (✗ ✗ ✗) in which green tea or its extracts were added to people's diets, no changes were found in lipid or cholesterol levels. Similar patterns of evidence have emerged for incidence of heart attacks and atherosclerosis (hardening of the arteries).

Topically, animal studies suggest that green tea or some of its components may protect against damage from UV radiation in sunlight. Some laboratory studies with human skin cells have supported this; controlled studies with humans have not been conducted.

ConsumerLab.com has performed a preliminary review of two green tea products. Both passed as they contained the expected amount of catechins. Green tea supplements used to treat cancer were the subject of a full product review by ConsumerLab.com in 2006. Of the seven products tested, three failed the independent company's tests. Two were contaminated with lead, and one had only 71 percent of the amount of active ingredient listed on the label.

Cautions

Some people are allergic to green tea and susceptible to what is called "green tea asthma." Those considering adding green tea to their diet should do so gradually and cautiously, especially if they are allergic to other plants. Green tea contains vitamin K, which will counteract the blood-thinning effects of warfarin. Green tea contains caffeine, and therefore large doses will lead to all the adverse effects of caffeine: headaches, nervousness, agitation. Women who are pregnant or breast-feeding should be particularly careful about their caffeine intake. Green tea is used widely in other cultures, and its potential to cause problems in pregnancy is unknown.

Recommendations

Green tea is a source of antioxidants that carry general health benefits. For those who enjoy tea, green tea may have some additional health benefits compared to black tea. Green tea contains about the same amount of caffeine as black tea. Therefore, it will act as a stimulant to overcome sleepiness. The connection between green tea and cancer or cardiovascular diseases is intriguing. Read our entry on Vitamin E to see why supplement recommendations should not be based on epidemiological studies alone. Given the lack of controlled studies, green tea should not be used in place of medical checkups or advice.

● Dosage

Most epidemiological studies find benefits in people who report drinking at least six to ten cups per day. Extracts are also available, and three capsules per day are recommended.

● Treatment Categories

Complementary

To provide antioxidants as part of a healthy diet	☺☺☺
To improve mental alertness (because of the caffeine content)	☺☺☺
To protect against a wide variety of cancers (such as bladder, esophageal, stomach, ovarian, and lung [but not breast, pancreatic, colon, or rectal] cancers)	☺

To reduce the risk of breast cancer recurrence	☺
To lower levels of cholesterol and other blood lipids	☺
To reduce the risk of high blood pressure	☺☺

Scientifically Unproven

To treat cancer	☹☹☹
To treat heart disease	☹☹☹

● Further Reading

Cooper, Raymond, D. James Morré, and Dorothy Morré. "Medicinal Benefits of Green Tea: Part I. Review of Noncancer Health Benefits." *Journal of Alternative and Complementary Medicine* 11, no. 3 (June 2005): 521–28.

———. "Medicinal Benefits of Green Tea: Part II. Review of Anticancer Properties." *Journal of Alternative and Complementary Medicine* 11, no. 4 (August 2005): 639–52.

Sun, Can-Lan, Jian-Min Yuan, Woon-Puay Koh, and Mimi C. Yu. "Green Tea, Black Tea and Breast Cancer Risk: A Meta-analysis of Epidemiological Studies." *Carcinogenesis*. October 10, 2005. *http://carcin. oxfordjournals.org/cgi/reprint/bgi276v1*. Accessed November 25, 2005.

GUARANA

What It Is

Guarana is of Brazilian origin and is a dried paste made from the crushed seeds of *Paullinia cupana*. The shrub is widely cultivated in Brazil and the Amazon basin as a valuable cash crop. It is highly sought after as an ingredient in stimulant drinks and herbal remedies. Pieces of the seed husks that remain in guarana give the preparation a bitter chocolate taste. Guarana contains significant amounts of caffeine. Typically, guarana seeds contain up to 7 percent caffeine, compared to coffee beans, which contain 1 to 2 percent. Some guarana can have as much as 10 percent caffeine.

Claims

Traditionally, guarana was used throughout South America as a stimulant, an aphrodisiac, and a treatment for a variety of disorders. Guarana is used today as a "natural" source of caffeine in stimulants and weight loss products. Since the 2004 ban of ephedra, many producers have replaced ephedra with guarana (or increased the concentration of guarana in products that had previously included it). In spite of this, possibly because of consumer alerts and concerns about guarana, sales in 2004 plummeted by about 77 percent.

Study Findings

No studies were located that studied the effect of guarana itself. One study examined an herbal remedy containing a mixture of guarana, yerba maté, and damiana. The herbal remedy is recommended for losing weight. In the controlled study, those taking the herbal mixture had significantly delayed stomach emptying. After forty-five days, they had lost 5.1 kg (about 11 pounds), compared to 0.3 kg (less than a pound) for the placebo group. Participants who chose to continue taking the mixture for one year showed no further weight loss or any regain.

The caffeine in guarana is a stimulant, and guarana contains other closely related compounds that may enhance this effect. It is reported that the stimulant effects of guarana last longer than those of coffee or caffeine alone. However, there is no evidence to support claims that guarana helps people lose weight or perform better athletically.

Cautions

Guarana appears poised to take over from ephedra in both its widespread use in stimulant drinks and supplements and its reputation as a cause of adverse effects. A young Australian woman died after drinking some of a 55 ml bottle of "Race 2005 Energy Blast with Guarana and Ginseng." She had been diagnosed with mitral valve prolapse, a fairly common cardiac complaint that rarely leads to sudden death. She had agreed to limit caffeine intake to one cup of coffee per day since caffeine stimulates the heart. A postmortem revealed that her system contained the caffeine equivalent of fifteen to twenty cups of coffee. The deaths of an eighteen-year-old Irish basketball player and three young Swedish people have similarly been linked to stimulant drinks with high caffeine contents (of various origins).

HERBAL REMEDIES, VITAMINS, AND DIETARY SUPPLEMENTS

The FDA wrote to producers of health drinks in 2001 reminding them that herbs could not be added to foods and drinks to have a stimulant effect. Such products remain widely available, especially on the Internet. Guarana increases blood pressure and therefore must be used cautiously, if at all, by people with high blood pressure or other cardiac problems. Caffeine interacts with a large variety of pharmaceutical drugs.

Guarana should not be used long-term on a consistent basis. Caffeine toxicity occurs with consistent consumption of more than 1 gram per day. Its symptoms include insomnia, nervousness, irritability, and heart palpitations and can lead to more serious problems such as delirium, convulsions, and seizures. Acute doses of 5 to 10 grams can be fatal, usually from ventricular fibrillation (which occurs when the heart's electrical signals are disrupted, leading to little pumping of blood out of the heart).

Recommendations

A small amount of guarana is likely to be similar in its stimulant effects to coffee or tea. The problem is that it is very difficult to know when you are getting a small or large amount. Guarana is a relatively expensive source of caffeine, and there are concerns about product quality. Many people who should or want to limit their caffeine intake will not associate guarana with caffeine. For some, this can be dangerous. If products were adequately labeled and regulated, guarana would pose few difficulties beyond those of tea or coffee. Given the current situation, some companies are using large concentrations of guarana to make products that are highly stimulating. Without adequate knowledge of how much caffeine is in these products, some people will be put at risk. We therefore recommend that, for now, guarana products be avoided, especially by the elderly, people

with chronic disease, children, and women who are pregnant or nursing. Even for healthy adults, its use should be approached very cautiously.

Dosage

A suitable dose is not known. Many recommend 200 to 800 mg of guarana, up to a daily maximum of 3 grams. The latter contains about 250 mg of caffeine, which is acceptable for adults.

Treatment Categories

Complementary
As a stimulant drink, but only
if the caffeine content is known ☺

Scientifically Unproven
To help with weight loss ☹☹☹☹

Scientifically Questionable
To improve athletic performance ☹☹☹☹

Quackery or Fraud
In the hands of some practitioners

Risk of Serious Side Effects
In large quantities and for those
who should limit caffeine intake ⊘⊘⊘

Further Reading

Cannon, Marianne E., Clive T. Cooke, and James S. McCarthy. "Caffeine-Induced Cardiac Arrhythmia: An Unrecognised Danger of Healthfood Products." *Medical Journal of Australia* 174, no. 10 (May 2001): 520–21.

Hess, Aleda M., and Donald L. Sullivan. "Potential for Toxicity with Use of Bitter Orange Extract and Guarana for Weight Loss." *Annals of Pharmacotherapy* 39, no. 3 (March 2005): 574–75.

HAWTHORN

What It Is

Hawthorn might be called a "living fence." The name is a corruption of the translation from the German, in which it was called the "Hedgethorn." This spiny shrub grows to a height of thirty feet if not regularly trimmed and was used in Germany to mark off plots of land. The bush provided beauty and, because of its spiny nature, security from trespassers.

Hawthorn is the name given to a number of *Crataegus* species. The most popular one used for medicinal purposes is *Crataegus laevigata*; however, many of the *Crataegus* species are interchanged in remedies. The leaves, flowers, and fruit of most species contain a number of biological substances that may dilate blood vessels and lower blood pressure. Antioxidant flavonoids are found in the highest concentrations in the young buds and leaves. Hawthorn is best known in many parts of the world as a heart or cardiac tonic. It is available in Germany as a prescription medicine.

Claims

Hawthorn berries have been used for centuries in Europe and the Orient for their beneficial effects on the cardiovascular system. Hawthorn extracts have been used to treat various heart diseases, particularly angina and congestive heart failure (CHF). The active ingredients are said to relax smooth muscle in coronary vessels and thus may help prevent angina. In Europe, hawthorn has been used for many varied conditions, including anxiety, digestive problems, and infections. Topical applications were used for boils, sores, and ulcers. Hawthorn berries have also been used in some foods, including jams, jellies, and preserves.

Study Findings

Laboratory studies in animals have shown that *Crataegus* extracts contain antioxidants and are able to prevent abnormal blood clotting. The extracts have also been shown in animals to improve abnormal cholesterol levels and atherosclerosis via a variety of mechanisms. In several animal studies, highly concentrated extracts have been shown to have a protective effect on the heart without increasing cardiac blood flow. Animal studies have also shown that hawthorn dilates blood vessels and inhibits angiotensin-converting enzyme (thereby making it an ACE inhibitor, similar to prescription ACE inhibitors). It has also been shown to have a mild diuretic effect.

In humans, case studies (✓✓) have shown that hawthorn increases the strength of the contraction of the heart and increases coronary blood flow while decreasing the heart rate and the consumption of oxygen. A 2003 review (✓✓✓) found thirteen randomized placebo-controlled studies with patients with chronic heart failure. Most of the studies showed a clear improvement in cardiac function in patients taking an extract of *Crataegus*. A number of symptoms were improved in different trials. Four studies used an objective measurement of maximal exercise. When the results were combined, a clear improvement was visible. Most studies allowed patients to continue their conventional heart medications, making it difficult to know if hawthorn is effective on its own or only in combination with other medications.

Cautions

Hawthorn has been shown to be relatively free of adverse effects and, when compared with other drugs that increase heart function, may have benefits for the heart. Concerns have been raised that hawthorn may increase the effect of another heart failure medication called "digitalis." However, a 2003 controlled study found no differences in heart tests given to people when they were taking digitalis with hawthorn or digitalis alone. Nevertheless, people taking any heart medication should consult their physician before trying hawthorn so that any changes can be monitored carefully. Hawthorn might be safe for long-term use; however, no studies have been performed for longer than sixteen weeks. Hawthorn has not been shown to be safe for use by children or women who are pregnant or nursing.

Recommendations

Further studies of hawthorn in humans with heart disease are now ongoing at a number of medical centers. Hawthorn appears to be most effective for milder cases of heart failure and may be inappropriate for more advanced stages. Physicians use a system called the New York Heart Association (NYHA) stages to describe the severity of heart disease. In Stage I, heart disease patients have symptoms only with strenuous activity, and in Stage II the symptoms occur with less strenuous activity. More advanced heart disease leads to symptoms with moderate ac-

tivity (Stage III) or any activity (Stage IV). Symptoms experienced include palpitations, trouble breathing, fatigue, or chest pain. Because of its favorable side-effect profile, hawthorn is probably safe to be used with NYHA Stage I or II heart failure; a physician should be involved in treatment decisions with NYHA Stage III or IV heart failure, but hawthorn is probably not an appropriate treatment.

Dosage

A powder containing 300 to 1800 mg of dried extract is usually taken orally, divided into two or three doses during the day or used to make a tea.

Treatment Categories

Complementary

To improve symptoms associated with
NYHA Stages I and II heart failure ☺☺☺☺
To treat coronary artery disease ☺☺

Scientifically Unproven

To improve symptoms associated
with NYHA Stages III or IV heart failure ☹

Further Reading

Degenring, F. H., A. Suter, M. Weber, and R. Saller. "A Randomised Double-Blind Placebo-Controlled Clinical Trial of a Standardised Extract of Fresh Crataegus Berries (Crataegisan) in the Treatment of Patients with Congestive Heart Failure NYHA II." *Phytomedicine* 10, no. 5 (2003): 363–69.

Pittler, Max H., Katja Schmidt, and Edzard Ernst. "Hawthorn Extract for Treating Chronic Heart Failure: Meta-analysis of Randomized Trials." *American Journal of Medicine* 114, no. 8 (June 2003): 665–74.

HORNY GOAT WEED

What It Is

Anyone using the Internet these days will be flooded with unsolicited advertisements for various products. Foremost are remedies said to promote sexual performance. For men, a popular herb added to many products is horny goat weed. The name refers to several species of the genus *Epimedium*, but especially *Epimedium sagittatum*. The extract itself is sometimes called "epimedium."

The story behind the name is that a long time ago a goat herder in China noticed that his herd was incessantly sexually active. He carefully watched the goats and discovered that their promiscuity increased after eating a particular weed. The Chinese call it Yin Yang Huo, and soon it had a reputation as a human aphrodisiac. In 2004, horny goat weed reached the top twenty in herbal remedy sales in the United States.

Claims

Horny goat weed is alleged to be an aphrodisiac and to treat impotence, premature ejaculation, mental and physical fatigue, heart disease, and various infections. The main claim is that the extract works like testosterone, which has generated further interest in the bodybuilding community, where it is said to be a stimulant.

Study Findings

Laboratory studies have shown that horny goat weed and some of its active ingredients act to cause vaso-dilatation and increased blood flow. They appear to work by a number of different mechanisms, including the blocking of calcium channels. Some pharmaceutical antihypertensive drugs also work this way. Animal studies have supported these effects and found that animals become more sexually active after being fed the extract.

Although animal studies show some interesting results, controlled trials in humans are completely lacking. A 2001 review found four studies (✔✔) in Chinese language journals that the reviewers had translated. Two of the studies used horny goat weed alone, and the other two used it in combination with other Chinese herbs. Only one of the studies had a control group. In the three uncontrolled studies, patients were given the herb and their symptoms were examined as time went on. One uncontrolled study enrolled patients with erectile dysfunction, and 92 percent reported that the herb improved their condition. The three other studies enrolled patients with kidney disease, and the majority of patients had improvements in their sexual performance. Few details were given regarding how the improvements were measured.

Cautions

In animal studies, the herb has been shown to have few adverse effects. Extended use has been reported to lead to dizziness, nausea, vomiting, dry mouth, and nosebleed. In humans, large doses of Japanese epimedium have caused respiratory arrest and muscle spasms. Given the vasodilating ability, those taking medications to prevent blood clotting or lower blood pressure should be concerned that horny goat weed may add to their effect and cause adverse effects.

ConsumerLab.com purchased five epimedium (horny goat weed) products for testing. Four of the five were not compliant with FDA label requirements because of incomplete information about the plant material. In the laboratory, the one product that passed labeling requirements was found to contain only 45 percent of the claimed marker compound. None of the products passed testing.

Recommendations

In spite of horny goat weed's widespread promotion, especially on the Internet, little is known about its effectiveness or safety. A small number of poorly described Chinese studies lend some support to its ability to overcome erectile dysfunction. However, it is marketed primarily to healthy men to increase their sexual performance and overall energy levels. No evidence was found to support that use.

Horny goat weed is promoted as part of a culture focused on sexual performance as just another physical activity. As such, it is viewed mechanistically with drugs and other devices touted to improve performance. Overlooked are the relational and spiritual dimensions of sexuality. Although Christians are sometimes said to be prudish about sexuality, this should not be the case. God made humans as sexual beings and gave intercourse as a wonderful blessing to be experienced within marriage. Following God's design for sexuality will provide married couples a path toward improved sexual relations, just as God offers to improve all areas of our lives.

For some people, sexual difficulties require medical interventions. When effective, these can bring much relief and are to be welcomed. But medicine, conventional or alternative, should not be used to promote a licentious or exploitative sexuality. Many pills and potions claim to offer unbounded, unlimited sex with anyone and everyone. Such marketing strategies feed the flesh nature that opposes our spiritual lives. "Those who belong to Christ Jesus have crucified the sinful nature with its passions and desires. Since we live by the Spirit, let us keep in step with the Spirit" (Galatians 5:24–25).

Dosage

No standard dosage is apparent because of lack of information.

Treatment Categories

Scientifically Unproven

To treat any form of
sexual dysfunction ☹☹☹
To improve sexual performance ☹☹☹☹

Spiritual

In terms of sexual corruption
through the ethos promoted
by marketers 👎👎👎

Quackery or Fraud

In the hands of some practitioners

Further Reading

Cirigliano, Michael D., and Philippe O. Szapary. "Horny Goat Weed for Erectile Dysfunction." *Alternative Medicine Alert* 4, no. 2 (February 2001): 19–22.

HORSE CHESTNUT

What It Is

Chestnut roasting brings warmth on cold fall nights. Many a child looked forward to collecting horse chestnuts and to finding the shiny brown nut inside the fleshy green seed. These come from the tree *Aesculus hippocastanum*. Although closely related, this tree is not the same as that revered by Ohio residents and brought to life in Brutus Buckeye, the Ohio State University mascot. The Ohio buckeye is *Aesculus glabra*, and the California variety is *Aesculus californica*. Each tree is reported to have different medicinal properties.

Claims

Different parts of *Aesculus hippocastanum* have been used for very different effects. The bark of young branches has been used to treat malaria and dysentery. However, older bark contains toxic materials and should not be used orally. A topical preparation of the bark has been recommended for lupus and skin ulcers. An extract of the leaves is recommended for arthritis, eczema, and a variety of skin conditions.

Most interest has been expressed in an extract of the seeds. This extract must be prepared carefully, as the seeds contain a toxic compound called "aesculin." This compound is a member of the coumarin family, as is warfarin. Extracts containing aesculin will increase bleeding times. The seeds also contain a glycoside called "aescin," which is recommended to treat varicose veins (also called "chronic venous insufficiency").

Varicose veins are a common and painful condition afflicting 10 to 15 percent of men and 20 to 25 percent of women. The veins do not function properly and leak fluid into the tissues, especially in the legs. This leads to swelling, pain, and hardening of the skin. Conventional care is often limited to compression stockings, which can be uncomfortable and unattractive. A major concern is that the condition can lead to the production of blood clots, which has more serious consequences.

Study Findings

Laboratory and animal studies have been carried out on horse chestnut seed extract and purified preparations of aescin. These revealed that the extracts have anti-inflammatory activity and can cause veins to contract better, making it more difficult for water and other materials to pass through the walls of blood vessels. This could be beneficial in the treatment of varicose veins.

A 2004 Cochrane review (✓✓✓✓) found sixteen randomized double-blind studies of horse chestnut seed extract used in people with varicose veins. Some studies measured different symptoms, but overall the results were generally beneficial. Six out of seven studies found significant relief of pain compared to placebo. Four out of six studies found significant reductions in leg swelling. In eight studies that examined pruritus (itching), only four found the extract significantly more beneficial than placebo. Most studies also showed significant reductions in the volume and size of people's legs.

In a different type of study, doctors surgically removed small pieces of veins from people with varicose veins. In the laboratory, researchers examined the effect of aescin on the veins and found that aescin led to contraction of veins from regions of the leg with early stages of disease. However, no effect was seen in veins from areas with later stages of the disease. The researchers suggested that horse chestnut seed extract may only be beneficial in the early stage of varicose veins. However, controlled studies have not confirmed this finding.

Such laboratory findings suggest that the extract may be beneficial in a variety of conditions in which blood vessels are leaking or damaged, such as with hemorrhoids and leg ulcers. One controlled study (✓✓✓) was found in which aescin was given orally to patients with hemorrhoids. Significant improvements were found after two months when patients evaluated their symptoms. Physical examination revealed significantly more improvements in bleeding and swelling compared to placebo. These improvements were visible after two weeks, and the subjective improvements were noted after six days.

Cautions

Many of the controlled studies found no adverse effects. In those that did, gastrointestinal effects were most common, but dizziness, headache, and pruritus were also reported. Postmarketing studies in Germany found that less than 1 percent of users had adverse effects. Standardized horse chestnut seed extract seems to be safe when used for two to twelve weeks. However, long-term usage has not been examined, nor has the extract been evaluated in pregnant or breast-feeding women or in children. The raw seed, bark, flower, and leaf are unsafe when used orally because of the toxin aesculin. The dose can be lethal. Poisoning has been reported of children drinking tea made with chestnut twigs and leaves.

Great care must be taken in selecting a high-quality product. A 2004 study found high levels of the toxic metals cadmium and lead in a small proportion of horse chestnut products purchased in Brazil. Unfortunately, independent labs have not tested horse chestnut products.

Recommendations

Horse chestnut seed extract can be recommended for the short-term treatment of varicose veins. However, since treatment for this condition will continue for many years, long-term studies are needed. The extract has been very safe in short-term studies. Given the lack of other satisfactory treatments, horse chestnut seed extract should be considered for varicose veins. Other uses, apart from those listed below, do not have supportive evidence.

Dosage

The usual dose is 300 to 600 mg of horse chestnut seed extract, which is usually equivalent to 50 to 100 mg of aescin. It is usually taken once or twice a day.

Treatment Categories

Complementary
To treat varicose veins	☺☺☺☺
To treat hemorrhoids	☺☺
To treat ulcers	☺

Further Reading

Brunner, Friedrich, Christine Hoffmann, and Sanja Schuller-Petrovic. "Responsiveness of Human Varicose Saphenous Veins to Vasoactive Agents." *British Journal of Clinical Pharmacology* 51, no. 3 (March 2001): 219–24.

Sirtori, Cesare R. "Aescin: Pharmacology, Pharmacokinetics and Therapeutic Profile." *Pharmacological Research* 44, no. 3 (September 2001): 183–93.

KAVA

• What It Is

The history of kava is a blend of myth, magic, marketing, and reality. It has been the ceremonial drink of choice in the Pacific islands since before their history was recorded. Kava is said to have been first reported by Captain James Cook, who called it "intoxicating pepper." Kava drinking was the equivalent of happy hour, the liquid used in the manner of friends taking their first, slow sips of their favorite alcoholic beverages at the end of a hard day's work.

The actual preparation of the ceremonial drink, at least by the eighteenth century, was not a pleasant one. The root of a species of pepper tree was cut into small pieces and passed among the islanders preparing the drink. They chewed the pieces to gain the juice and a rather pulpy mass, all of which was spit into a bowl. None of the juice was consumed by the "cooks." Coconut milk was then poured over everything, and the mixture was strained through coconut fibers. The pulpy pieces were squeezed to get as much of the juice mixed in with the milk as possible, then set aside. Finally, the coconut milk and kava juice mix was poured into a second bowl and quickly consumed. Fortunately, contemporary kava preparation is far more sanitary.

Nowadays, kava, or kava-kava, or "intoxicating pepper," is an herbal remedy made from the shrub *Piper methysticum* that grows primarily in the South Pacific islands. The underground parts (roots and rhizome) are used to make the extract.

• Claims

Herbal manufacturers claim kava is "nature's stress buster" and a natural way to relieve anxiety (as an alternative to such drugs as Valium). It is also used to promote sleep. One promoter claims it is the herbal equivalent of having a soak in a hot tub and a massage. Others recommend kava for promoting wound healing; for treating headaches (including migraines), colds, rheumatism, tuberculosis, chronic cystitis, and menstrual problems; and as an aphrodisiac.

• Study Findings

More than a dozen compounds isolated from the plant have been shown to cause muscle relaxation and pain relief in animal and laboratory studies. A 2003 Cochrane review (✓✓✓✓) found twelve randomized double-blind, placebo-controlled studies of kava used to treat anxiety. All of them found kava at least somewhat better than placebo. Seven of the studies used the same test to measure anxiety levels, which allowed their data to be combined into a meta-analysis. This showed a significant improvement for kava over placebo. However, the effect size was small and the studies were limited by being small and short-lasting (between one and twenty-four weeks).

The evidence indicates that kava is somewhat effective at relieving generalized anxiety. One study (✓✓✓) found that kava was as effective as oxazepam, a Valium-like drug. Another study (✓✓✓) found no significant differences in either effectiveness at reducing anxiety or side effects between kava and two conventional drugs used to treat anxiety (opipramol and buspirone). All the clinical studies that have shown kava to be effective have used formulations containing 30 to 55 percent of kava lactones, the compounds thought to be the active ingredients. Extracts containing 70 percent kava lactones exist, and some claim they may be more effective.

● Cautions

The safety of kava preparations is a topic of much controversy, especially in relation to liver toxicity. On the one hand, controlled trials have found no evidence of liver damage, nor has post-marketing surveillance in Europe. Traditional users of the kava beverage in the South Pacific islands do not report liver problems. On the other hand, Canada and many European countries have banned the sale of kava since 2002 because of concerns about the potential risk of severe liver-damaging effects from kava preparations. Germany was the leading importer of kava, and its ban influenced many other countries to follow suit. The FDA issued a warning letter in March 2002 highlighting concerns about the potential risk of serious liver damage from kava. As a result, kava sales in the United States have plummeted. Almost one hundred cases (✖✖) of liver problems have been reported worldwide. Six people have required liver transplants, and three people have died.

Controversy rages as to how clearly a connection can be established between kava and these serious liver injuries. The University of the South Pacific in Fiji reported on recent developments in this area in May 2005. Close examination of the case reports has revealed that the people requiring liver transplants were taking other herbs and drugs. Some of them

were predisposed to damage because of a deficiency in an enzyme that eliminates drugs from the body. Experts have also pointed out that the traditional beverage is prepared as a water extract, while products sold as dietary supplements use organic liquids to extract material from the plant. This results in the beverage containing 4 to 6 percent kava lactones, while dietary supplements contain 30 to 50 percent. Some sociologists are claiming that Western interests are hijacking the traditional usage, which is negatively impacting the South Pacific cultures.

The World Health Organization has set up a panel to investigate all these issues and report on how best to resolve them. As of June 2006, the Fijian government was encouraging Western countries to lift their bans on kava because of their economic impact on the region.

Apart from the rare but serious liver problems, reported side effects of kava are relatively mild, with the most common being intestinal disturbances, muscle weakness, and allergic reactions. Other less common side effects include headache, dizziness, enlarged pupils, disequilibrium, and (rarely) allergic skin reactions. Drowsiness can be a problem, especially when kava is taken along with alcohol or other depressants, although one randomized controlled trial showed no side effects from combining kava and alcohol. Nevertheless, those driving or operating machinery while taking kava should be cautious and alert to any possible changes it may induce. As with any medication affecting the brain, an abuse syndrome can develop. As with all herbal remedies, there can be great variability in the strengths of different kava preparations.

Chronic abuse of kava leads to a syndrome called "kawaism," which is characterized by reddened eyes, dry and scaly skin, and a yellowish discoloration of the skin, eyes, and nails. If kava use is stopped, the signs of the syndrome are slowly resolved.

The Natural Database rates kava as "possibly unsafe" when used orally for more than three months and as "possibly unsafe" during pregnancy or lactation. We do not believe kava should be used by children or teenagers.

Recommendations

Kava holds out some promise as a mild way to treat anxiety. However, very little clinical research has been conducted on it, and no studies have examined its long-term effects. Generalized anxiety is a common disorder but can have many causes. Using herbs or drugs exclusively may result in relief of symptoms without addressing the underlying emotional and spiritual causes. Use of kava usually results from self-diagnosis, which may not be reliable or accurate. Anxiety is also one of the conditions for which placebos are most effective, which may contribute to kava's overall effectiveness.

Dosage

Most studies have used a dose of about 100 mg of kava extract three times a day. However, products vary widely in the concentration of kava lactones they contain.

Treatment Categories

Complementary

Note: The current widespread ban on kava products in many countries should be taken into consideration when deciding whether to use kava products.

To relieve anxiety	☺☺☺
To relieve stress	☺☺
To relieve restlessness	☺☺
To relieve menopausal anxiety	☺
To relieve social anxiety	☺
To treat anyone with any liver problems or at risk of liver damage from infections, alcohol abuse, or certain drugs	☹☹☹☹

Scientifically Unproven

For any other indication

Risk of Serious Side Effects

Serious liver problems from kava are rare but potentially fatal ⊘⊘

Further Reading

Clouatre, Dallas L. "Kava Kava: Examining New Reports of Toxicity." *Toxicology Letters* 150 (2004): 85–96.

Stevinson, Clare, Alyson Huntley, and Edzard Ernst. "A Systematic Review of the Safety of Kava Extract in the Treatment of Anxiety." *Drug Safety* 25, no. 4 (February 2002): 251–61.

University of the South Pacific. "Academic Questions Ban on Kava Products." Posted May 10, 2005. *USP News: http://www.usp.ac.fj/news/story.php?id=57.* Accessed December 3, 2005.

LICORICE

● What It Is

Most of us think of ropelike red and black candy when we think of licorice. However, the candy is not licorice but anise-flavored "sticks." European licorice is more likely to be the "real thing." In America, the most common use for licorice is as an ingredient in tobacco products to counteract the bitter flavor and add some sweetness.

Commercial licorice is extracted primarily from the roots and rhizomes of what is called Italian or Spanish licorice (*Glycyrrhiza glabra typica*), along with a number of other closely related species — including Persian or Turkish licorice (*Glycyrrhiza glabra violacea*), Russian licorice (*Glycyrrhiza glabra glandulifera*), and Chinese licorice (*Glycyrrhiza uralensis*). The plant grows in subtropical areas, with most commercial licorice coming from eastern Mediterranean countries.

● Claims

Licorice has been used for centuries in China, Egypt, Greece, and Rome as an expectorant and carminative (antiflatulence agent). It has also been used to mask bitter flavors (it is still added to pharmaceutical cough and cold preparations). The primary medicinal use was as a natural treatment for peptic ulcers. Others recommend licorice for bronchitis, gastritis, colic, arthritis, lupus, tuberculosis, and hepatitis and in formulations to increase fertility in women with polycystic ovarian syndrome. It has been used intravenously to treat hepatitis B and C and topically as a shampoo for a number of scalp disorders.

● Study Findings

Licorice root contains between 5 and 9 percent glycyrrhizin, a compound fifty times sweeter than glucose (a form of sugar). Glycyrrhizin can be broken down (chemically or during digestion) to glycyrrhetic acid, which is not sweet. It is thought that glycyrrhetic acid is the compound that is active in the body, having mild anti-inflammatory effects and stimulating the secretion of mucous in the stomach. A number of randomized controlled trials (✗✗✗) looked at the effect of deglycyrrhizinized licorice in treating gastric and peptic ulcers. In general it was no more effective than placebo — although it had significantly fewer side effects than glycyrrhizin. Glycyrrhizin's potential for treating ulcers led to much research and even the development, in the 1960s, of a semisynthetic derivative called "carbenoxolone." While clinical studies (✓✓✓) showed that the licorice derivatives were effective, they were less effective than standard drugs such as cimetidine. Glycyrrhizin also had much more serious side effects (✗✗✗), including edema, high blood pressure, and excessive secretion of potassium.

There are at least two randomized controlled trials (✓✓✓) of intravenous glycyrrhizin in hepatitis C patients. In both studies, glycyrrhizin lowered serum liver enzyme levels that had been elevated by the infection. This means it might relieve some of the liver damage that hepatitis C can cause. Clinical trials (✓✓✓) have also shown benefit in patients with hepatitis B. However, during treatment there were no changes in the hepatitis virus levels in the blood. In these studies, which were very small, the treatment appeared to be safe and well tolerated. Qualified professionals administered the sterile intravenous preparations, a formulation that is not available over-the-counter and should not be administered without medical supervision.

Licorice is added to many multiherb preparations. One of these was found to be more effective than placebo in relieving dyspepsia (a more severe form of heartburn). Another relieved menopausal symptoms. Yet another was found to be no more beneficial than placebo in treating eczema. However, the role licorice played in these effects could not be determined from these studies.

Cautions

Licorice contains compounds that interfere with the normal breakdown of corticosteroids. These occur naturally in the body and play important roles in inflammation, healing, and electrolyte balance. This may explain the wide range of adverse effects reported for licorice, especially with prolonged use. Headache, lethargy, water retention, electrolyte imbalances, high blood pressure, and heart failure have been noted (✗✗) in people consuming about 1 gram of glycyrrhizin daily. These symptoms have occurred in people eating a quarter pound of some European licorice candy daily or swallowing their saliva while continuously chewing tobacco. The symptoms may accumulate gradually and may not be recognized as being connected with licorice consumption.

While corticosteroids are not sex steroids, one study (✗✗) found that seven young men given 0.5 gram of glycyrrhizin daily had reduced testosterone levels and other changes in their steroid levels. These could have far-reaching health effects.

Licorice, taken chronically, can theoretically interact with a number of prescription and over-the-counter drugs (such as aspirin, NSAIDS, steroids, female hormones, diuretics, heart drugs, insulin, and MAO inhibitors). Individuals taking prescription drugs should not take licorice without first consulting their physician.

Licorice can have abortifacient, estrogenic, and steroid effects in humans and has been shown to stimulate the uterus in animal studies. Licorice, in amounts greater than in foods, should not be taken by women who are pregnant or breast-feeding. Licorice has not been shown to be safe in children.

Recommendations

Licorice candy in the United States will provide a lot of sugar and little or no licorice. If you enjoy licorice, it is probably the anise flavoring you like. Products that contain real licorice extract (more common in European candy) should not be used for extended periods of time. The extract may have some expectorant and antiulcer effects, but conventional medicine provides more effective treatments that do not carry the same risks. The use of glycyrrhizin for hepatitis B or C should be coordinated with a hepatologist (expert in liver disease).

Dosage

A typical dose of licorice is whatever gives a person 200 to 600 mg of glycyrrhizin. A tea made from 1 to 4 grams of powdered root gives roughly this amount of glycyrrhizin.

Treatment Categories

Complementary

To treat some forms of cough	☺☺
To treat peptic ulcers	☺
Intravenously under medical supervision to treat hepatitis B or C	☺☺
To treat gastric ulcers	☹
To treat indigestion (dyspepsia and acid reflux)	☹☹

Scientifically Unproven
For any other indication

Risk of Serious Side Effects
With high doses for prolonged periods ⊘

Further Reading

Foster, Steven, and Varro E. Tyler. *Tyler's Honest Herbal: A Sensible Guide to the Use of Herbs and Related Remedies.* 4th ed. New York: Haworth Herbal, 1999, 241–43.

LUTEIN

What It Is

According to Kelly and colleagues' survey of more than eight thousand adults published in 2005, lutein has become the most popular dietary supplement or herbal remedy used by Americans. Among men over sixty-five, it is three times more popular than the second most widely used supplement (glucosamine).

Lutein is a member of the chemical family of carotenoids, of which beta-carotene is better known. Many carotenoids are effective antioxidants. Lutein and a closely related compound, zeaxanthin, are unique in the way they accumulate in specific parts of the human eye. They are the only carotenoids found in the macula, a small area of the retina that is very important for vision, especially its sharpness. The macula is also called the "yellow spot." Purified lutein is yellow in color. Lutein and zeaxanthin are also the only carotenoids found in the lens of the eye. Lutein concentrations are naturally higher in people with darker-colored eyes, while blue eyes have the lowest concentrations. Lutein occurs throughout the human body, not just in the eye. It is the second most common carotenoid found in human serum.

Large amounts of lutein occur in dark leafy green vegetables, such as broccoli, spinach, kale, and Brussels sprouts. High concentrations are found in yellow foods such as corn and egg yolks. Commercial lutein is usually isolated from the leaves of marigold plants (*Tagetes* species). The average intake of lutein has been dropping in the United States and Europe, probably because of reduced consumption of dark leafy greens. The recommended daily intake is 6 mg, while the average intake is 1.7 mg in the United States and 2.2 mg in Europe. This has led to much interest in the addition of lutein to foods and beverages and the use of lutein dietary supplements.

Claims

Antioxidants in general play an important role in preventing tissue damage after injury or even due to normal metabolism. The most widespread claim for lutein supplementation is that it can prevent age-related macular degeneration and cataract formation. The former can lead eventually to blindness. Lutein is known to protect the eye from high-energy blue light, which is the most damaging part of visible light. This protection has also been claimed for the skin, with lutein being added to products that protect the skin from UV damage. Lutein, like most antioxidants, is also claimed to protect people from a range of chronic diseases, especially cardiovascular disease.

Study Findings

In epidemiological studies (✓✓), those with the lowest blood serum levels of lutein had higher risks of developing age-related macular degeneration (AMD). This finding has been reported in at least five studies since 1994, although one study found no connection between intake levels of dietary lutein and AMD. Most epidemiological studies found that higher lutein intakes were associated with reduced occurrence of cataracts, but some studies found no association.

A small number of controlled studies (✓✓✓) have been conducted in which lutein intake was increased either through dietary supplements (usually 15 mg of lutein per day) or leafy green vegetables. A 2004 review identified five such studies in which all reported increased serum lutein levels. One study found that people taking lutein supplements developed darker pigmentation in their eyes compared to those not taking the supplement. However, these studies do not show that higher lutein levels prevent AMD or other eye diseases.

A series of case studies (✓✓) showed that individual patients put on lutein-rich diets had improvement of up to 92 percent in AMD symptoms. The first double-blind study (✓✓✓) of AMD and lutein was published in 2002. Ninety AMD patients were randomly assigned to take either 10 mg of lutein, 10 mg of lutein plus other antioxidants, or placebo. After one year, those taking lutein had significant improvements in several objective vision measurements and a 50 percent increase in macular pigment. Those taking lutein plus other antioxidants had slightly better improvements than those taking lutein alone. A very small pilot study (✓✓) with five patients has found similar vision benefits for those with cataracts taking lutein. Another small study (✓✓✓) found beneficial effects for those suffering from another eye disease called "retinitis pigmentosa." Lutein supplements may therefore be beneficial for general eye health.

Animal and epidemiological studies (✓✓) have shown a connection between lutein levels and cardiac diseases. One study found that those with the highest levels of lutein had their risk of stroke reduced by about one-third. In that same study, vitamin E, vitamin C, and other carotenoid intakes did not change the risk of stroke. However, no controlled studies of the effect of lutein on heart disease were found.

Research on the role of lutein in skin health is more limited. There are theoretical reasons to link lutein levels with protection of the skin from damaging UV rays. Some animal models have confirmed that dietary lutein can have a protective role. Evidence from human studies is not yet available.

Associations have also been made between lutein intake and the occurrence of several cancers. Again, the evidence is preliminary at this point.

Cautions

No adverse effects have been reported. Lutein is likely to be safe in pregnancy and lactation given that it has been granted "generally recognized as safe" (GRAS) status. When ConsumerLab.com purchased nineteen products for testing in 2004, huge variations were seen in the suggested daily dose of lutein. These ranged from 0.25 mg to 22.5 mg of lutein, nearly a ninety-fold difference. Of the products tested, all but one contained the amounts listed on the labels.

Recommendations

Lutein's "generally recognized as safe" status means it can be added to foods and beverages, which has already occurred in some cereals, margarine, baked goods, candy, and milk products. Lutein supplementation can be recommended for eye health in general, especially as people age and become more susceptible to eye disease. Lutein may also be beneficial for preventing other illnesses such as heart disease and some cancers. Studies with lutein demonstrate again the importance of increasing the amount of fruits and vegetables in the diet.

Dosage

Huge variation exists in the doses recommended. In the products tested by ConsumerLab.com, the most common recommendations were 6 mg and 20 mg daily. An official RDA has not been established. Controlled studies have used supplements with 2 to 15 mg of lutein. Capsules are usually taken two or three times daily. A dose of 6 mg is understandable as it approximates the amount found in the diets of populations with lower risks of macular degeneration and cataracts. It is not clear whether a higher dose provides any more benefit. A cup of cooked kale contains 44 mg of lutein, while there are 26 mg in a cup of cooked spinach. Multivitamins with a daily dose of 25 micrograms (mcg) of lutein likely have too little lutein to offer any benefit; 25 mcg is the same as 0.025 mg.

Treatment Categories

Complementary

As a source of dietary antioxidants	☺☺☺☺
To prevent and treat age-related macular degeneration	☺☺☺☺
To promote general health of the eye	☺☺☺
To prevent and treat cataracts	☺☺
To prevent cardiovascular disease	☺☺
To improve skin health	☺☺
To prevent diet-related cancers	☺
To treat retinitis pigmentosa	☺

Further Reading

Alves-Rodrigues, Alexandra, and Andrew Shao. "The Science Behind Lutein." *Toxicology Letters* 150, no. 1 (April 2004): 57–83.

Bartlett, Hannah, and Frank Eperjesi. "An Ideal Ocular Nutritional Supplement?" *Ophthalmic and Physiological Optics* 24, no. 4 (July 2004): 339–49.

Kelly, Judith P., David W. Kaufman, Katherine Kelley, Lynn Rosenberg, Theresa E. Anderson, and Allen A. Mitchell. "Recent Trends in Use of Herbal and Other Natural Products." *Archives of Internal Medicine* 165 (February 2005): 281–86.

MANGOSTEEN

What It Is

Mangosteen juice is made from a tropical fruit that many view as particularly exquisite, including Queen Victoria of Britain. Its nicknames include "Queen of Fruit" and "Food of the Gods," and it is the national fruit of Thailand. Its botanical name is *Garcinia mangostana*, which is where the term "mangosteen" comes from. This fruit should not be confused with either the mango or other *Garcinia* supplements. Regulations did not permit the importation of mangosteen into the United States until 2002. Within a couple of years, it broke into the top ten among *Nutrition Business Journal*'s list of bestselling natural products.

Mangosteen contains a group of compounds called "xanthones." These are found in a very restricted group of plants. Their chemical structure is similar to that of the antioxidant compounds called "flavonoids" (such as are found in grape seed extract and hawthorn). Mangosteen also contains lycopene, a member of the carotenoid group of antioxidants. Lycopene intake has been associated with reduced cancer risk, but that is only supported by epidemiological studies. Tomatoes, especially processed tomato products, have much larger quantities of lycopene.

Claims

Mangosteen has been used for centuries in traditional Chinese and Ayurvedic medicine for a wide range of conditions. Uses have included treatment of diarrhea, inflammation, wounds, infections, burns, and pain. Recent popularity has broadened these claims to include use against diabetes, allergies, atherosclerosis, depression, aging, and cancer.

Study Findings

No clinical trials have been conducted on mangosteen. Most published reports identify particular xanthines that have been isolated from mangosteen. A small number of laboratory studies have been conducted on these compounds, but no controlled studies of their impact on humans are available.

Cautions

No adverse effects have been reported. Since virtually no reliable information is available about the safety of mangosteen (especially in the elderly, people with chronic diseases, children, or women who are pregnant or lactating), we recommend that these people not use it.

Recommendations

Mangosteen fruit and juice are popular and tasty. As a way to increase consumption of fruits and vegetables, they can be highly recommended. For whatever reasons, mangosteen is also being touted as having specific healing properties. There is no reliable evidence to support these claims. Promoters use questionable tactics to increase sales of supplements containing mangosteen. After listing many alleged

M

uses of mangosteen, the Phytoceutical Research organization states on its website, "We have only just begun to understand [the] variety and number of ways this fruit can be used to treat serious medicinal conditions." Yet further on, the same website states, "The mangosteen is a food and not a drug with the intrinsic danger inherent in all drugs. Therefore, complex human studies (randomized trials) have not been necessary to establish either safety or efficacy." Yet all the studies they cite in support are chemical studies of the chemical nature of the chemicals contained in mangosteen.

Enjoy the fruit. Avoid the hype.

Dosage

None known.

Treatment Categories

Complementary

As a tasty fruit and source
of antioxidants ☺☺☺☺

Scientifically Unproven

To prevent or treat any condition

Quackery or Fraud

In the hands of some practitioners, especially
when sold as supplement capsules

Further Reading

Phytoceutical Research. Various webpages. *Phytoceutical Research, LLC: www.mangosteenMD.com*. Accessed December 3, 2005.

Setiawan, Budi, Ahmad Sulaeman, David W. Giraud, and Judy A. Driskell. "Carotenoid Content of Selected Indonesian Fruits." *Journal of Food Composition and Analysis* 14, no. 2 (April 2001): 169 – 76.

MARIJUANA

What It Is

Marijuana hardly needs any introduction. Whether it's called cannabis, pot, grass, weed, Indian hemp, or any number of other names, the plant in question is *Cannabis sativa* (sometimes called *Cannabis indica*). In some ways it could be viewed as the most popular herbal remedy of them all, even though in most jurisdictions it is illegal to grow marijuana, illegal to have it in your possession, illegal to use it, and illegal to sell it. We have great concern about the illegal use of marijuana and the attempts to legalize the use of unsafe forms of marijuana. The experiment with legalized medical marijuana in ten states received a very negative review in June 2005 when the U.S. Supreme Court found that California's law was likely to increase the supply of marijuana for recreational use. The ruling basically stated that federal laws banning marijuana trump state laws that allow its use. Apart from those covered by such laws, only a small number of people are legally allowed to use marijuana during research. However, given the popularity of this herb, we have included it here to explore the medical claims being made and to provide a scientific evaluation of its active ingredients.

Marijuana's illegal use in the United States peaked in the 1960s, but it remains very popular. About half of all people living in the United States are believed to have tried marijuana (most illegally) at some time in their lives. The 1992 National Household Survey on Drug Abuse found that approximately 5 million Americans illegally use marijuana on a weekly basis. Nearly 70 percent of high school students reported using it illegally in the previous month. A 2005 survey in the United Kingdom found that 24 percent of teenagers had used marijuana, and 15 percent had used it in the previous month. Use drops off dramatically as people enter their thirties.

Marijuana differs from all of the other herbal remedies we discuss because of its illegal status. Marijuana has been very difficult to obtain medically since passage of the Marijuana Tax Act of 1937. It is currently regulated in the United States as a Schedule I drug, which means it is viewed as having a high potential for abuse, as lacking any accepted medical use, and as being unsafe for use under medical supervision. This means marijuana is unavailable even for physicians to prescribe.

Starting as far back as the 1970s, efforts were made to reclassify marijuana as a Schedule II drug, which would allow doctors to prescribe it for certain conditions. These efforts were quashed by the Drug Enforcement Agency in 1992, which led to proponents going directly to voters to change the laws. In 1996, voters in California and Arizona passed ballot initiatives permitting the use of marijuana as a medicine. Arizona's referendum was invalidated, but by the time of the 2005 U.S. Supreme Court ruling, ten states had legalized the medicinal use of marijuana. Concerns have been expressed, even by some supporters of these initiatives, that in practice marijuana clinics simply make marijuana more easily available for anyone who wants it.

Marijuana has a very long history of medicinal use, being mentioned in ancient records from China and India. It was first introduced into Western medicine by an Irish doctor, William O'Shaugnessy, who returned from India in 1842. Both its illegal and medicinal uses involve smoking or eating the unpurified leaves and flower tops. As with all herbs, there is great variability in the strength and quality of samples. However, it is generally acknowledged that the potency of marijuana available today is much higher than that of what was available on the street a couple of decades ago.

The active ingredients in marijuana are a group of about thirty compounds called "cannabinoids." The most abundant and active of these is THC (delta-9-tetrahydrocannabinol, or delta-9-THC). A manufactured form of THC has been available since 1985 as a Schedule II drug called Marinol, or "dronabinol." Marinol is FDA-approved for the treatment of chemotherapy-induced nausea and vomiting and for AIDS-induced weight loss. In 1999, this product was reassigned to Schedule III, meaning it is viewed as having less potential for abuse and dependence. (Schedule II drugs include narcotics, amphetamines, and barbiturates, which are viewed as highly susceptible to abuse with severe dependence.) Some of the marijuana research has been conducted on pure THC and other cannabinoids and must be distinguished from that done on whole marijuana itself. Unless otherwise stated, "marijuana" in this entry refers to smoking or eating marijuana plant material.

Claims

During the nineteenth century, medical journals and pharmacopeias recommended marijuana as an appetite stimulant, muscle relaxant, pain reliever, hypnotic agent, and anticonvulsant. Most of marijuana's current use centers around its ability to induce euphoria, relaxation, sexual arousal, and a general "high." Although some would like to see

marijuana legalized as a recreational drug, we will address only the controversy about its medical use.

On the one side are those who claim marijuana should be available under medical supervision to relieve nausea and vomiting associated with chemotherapy, to lower intraocular pressure in glaucoma, to stimulate appetite in AIDS patients who have difficulty maintaining their weight, to treat multiple sclerosis, to act as an anticonvulsant and muscle relaxant with certain spastic disorders, and to relieve chronic pain.

On the other side of this issue are those who might agree that marijuana has some of these effects but would argue that it should still not be legalized for three reasons:

1. More effective treatments are available for all these conditions.
2. Marijuana, especially smoking marijuana, can have negative effects, not the least of which is dependence. For this reason, they would prefer that purified substances such as Marinol be used, not marijuana joints.
3. Marijuana is believed to be a "gateway" drug. Those who use other illicit drugs have usually tried marijuana earlier. The claim is that marijuana acts as a "gateway" to these other drugs and that making it available medically would lead to patients and others trying other illicit drugs.

The debate about whether marijuana has a legitimate medical use has similarities to the debate about other herbal remedies. Some give compelling anecdotal reports of people with cancer or AIDS or multiple sclerosis being helped by smoking marijuana, who then have to face the anxiety and embarrassment of obtaining marijuana from drug dealers. Even if its medical use were legalized, the familiar questions arise concerning quality and consistency. But this herbal debate is complicated by claims that marijuana is addictive and harmful.

Equally compelling stories exist of people's lives being ruined by marijuana. Some of these people started using marijuana out of curiosity or because of peer pressure. Some are concerned that legitimizing the herb in any way will lead to more people getting hooked on it. However the legal and political situation gets resolved, the first step is to resolve the medical debate, and that centers around the results of research on marijuana and its cannabinoids.

Study Findings

After California voters legalized medical marijuana in 1996, the White House Office of National Drug Control Policy asked the Institute of Medicine (IOM) to review the scientific evidence concerning marijuana. The IOM is the same organization that issues the Recommended Dietary Allowances for vitamins and nutrients. It is a private, nonprofit organization that advises the federal government on medical issues, especially those involving controversy over scientific evidence.

In March 1999, the IOM released a report, *Marijuana and Medicine: Assessing the Science Base*, that has become the focus of much of this controversy. The report concluded, "Until a non-smoked, rapid-onset cannabinoid drug delivery system becomes available, we acknowledge that there is no clear alternative for people suffering from chronic conditions that might be relieved by smoking marijuana, such as pain or AIDS wasting. One possible approach is to treat patients as 'n-of-1' clinical trials." The n-of-1 design means that each individual patient acts as his or her own control and is carefully monitored while given different test substances. The patients and re-

searchers can be "blinded" to which substance the patient is taking at any particular time. This design allows greater individualization of care but makes it very difficult to generalize the results across groups of patients. It also makes it impossible to know how much the individualized care contributed to any changes observed.

The first of such n-of-1 trials with a sublingual spray was published in 2004. These sprays contain a liquid extract of marijuana and deliver a precisely measured amount of cannabinoid under the tongue. The thirty-four patients had chronic pain that had not been helped by many other conventional treatments. Some patients found the sprays ineffective or the study too burdensome. Others found the sprays helpful. Eight patients had pain due to failed spinal surgery, and all reported benefits. Common side effects were dry mouth, dizziness, and euphoria or dysphoria (a term for generalized "bad" feelings). The benefit of the pain relief was viewed as much greater than any negative effects. Being able to use the spray in public, compared to smoking marijuana, was viewed as a major advantage.

Much progress has been made in recent years in understanding how the compounds in marijuana might help patients. Researchers discovered that THC interacts with very specific proteins in the brain called "receptors." Many different types of receptors are found throughout the body carrying out a wide range of activities. Researchers have discovered that THC works in the brain on what is now called a "cannabinoid receptor." We naturally make at least one compound that interacts with this receptor, called "anandamide" (the name comes from *ananda*, which means "bliss" in Sanskrit).

This research is showing that the human brain has a cannabinoid system that is naturally involved in controlling pain, movement, and memory. This system is overactive in obesity, which may open up a way to treat obesity if a receptor blocker is discovered. However, cannabinoids stimulate this system. There is great excitement about research in this new area. Traditional use of marijuana is based on real interactions between cannabinoids and this system in people's brains. This research may lead to new treatments in various areas, but much remains unknown. The fact that our brains have a cannabinoid system means that marijuana may influence us in many ways that we currently are unaware of or don't understand.

The second area of research has been with pure cannabinoid drugs, such as THC or Marinol. Marinol is FDA-approved for two indications. Anorexic AIDS patients who took Marinol in randomized controlled trials recovered their appetite significantly better compared to those taking placebo. They also experienced less nausea and improved mood and regained some of their lost weight. Marinol was not as effective as another pharmaceutical drug used to stimulate the appetite (megestrol acetate, or Megase). One small study found Marinol of no benefit in anorexia nervosa.

Other studies with chemotherapy patients have shown significant benefit in reducing nausea and vomiting. However, when researchers compared THC to another antiemetic drug (metoclopramide, or Reglan), three times as many patients receiving metoclopramide reported effective relief. So, while Marinol works, it is not as effective as other available drugs. In addition, the researchers noticed that different people responded very differently to the same dose of Marinol. A lot of people also reported unpleasant feelings while taking Marinol. Recreational users of marijuana report these same unpleasant effects. This drug therefore has to be closely monitored until individualized doses are determined.

The use of THC for pain relief has very little controlled research. The IOM reviewers could find only one study conducted since 1981 using THC, and none with marijuana. The studies conducted prior to then were poorly designed. The results of studies with acute pain were contradictory, and in some cases those taking THC reported feeling increased pain. Studies of THC for chronic pain were more encouraging, though still limited. Three small double-blind studies reported significantly more pain relief for cancer patients. A 2001 review still found no studies of smoking marijuana for pain relief, but examined nine randomized controlled trials of THC and other pure cannabinoids. The review concluded that these drugs were about as effective as codeine in relieving cancer pain or postoperative pain, but with significantly more adverse effects. The cannabinoids were much less effective than conventional analgesics.

A report released in December 2005 by the Royal College of Physicians in Britain could add only two studies using oral sprays of pure cannabinoids: the n-of-1 trial described earlier and one randomized controlled study. The latter study tested two cannabinoid sprays against a placebo spray. A standard for measuring effectiveness of pain treatments is a 2-point improvement over placebo on an 11-point scale. Although both sprays were significantly better than placebo, the improvement was only 0.6 point.

This same report found some evidence that THC may be helpful for patients with multiple sclerosis. Mounting laboratory and animal studies show that cannabinoid receptors are involved in multiple sclerosis, though much remains unclear. A few small randomized controlled studies have shown some benefit from purified products such as Marinol. The largest study to date was funded by the Medical Research Council (MRC), Britain's governmental funding agency. Published in 2003, it found significant improvements in muscle spasticity with Marinol compared to placebo, but not with an oral cannabis extract. Patients took the capsules for fifteen weeks, and the findings led the MRC to fund a three-year study of THC for multiple sclerosis that started in 2005.

Note that the studies cited so far have used purified cannabinoid drugs. Controlled studies of smoking marijuana have not been conducted widely, yet this is the use that receives most attention. One study with cancer patients found smoking marijuana similar in effectiveness to THC capsules for controlling nausea and vomiting. Other studies comparing marijuana to antiemetic drugs have found marijuana effective in about one-quarter of the patients and much less effective than pharmaceutical drugs. During the 1970s, when interest in medical marijuana increased, acute nausea and vomiting occurred in almost 100 percent of chemotherapy patients. Since then, and especially in the 1990s, much more effective drugs have been developed that control these side effects in 70 to 80 percent of chemotherapy patients. However, some patients remain unresponsive to these newer drugs.

Medical marijuana use is probably more popularly reported to counteract the wasting syndrome experienced by AIDS patients. However, this area has received very little controlled research, with most of the claims being based on anecdotal reports. The only controlled evidence is that for Marinol.

Overall, there is little evidence to support the claim that smoking marijuana is medically useful. However, a small proportion of patients do not respond well to pharmaceutical agents. The euphoric effect of marijuana also might help some people feel better. These factors will be taken into consideration in our conclusion.

Cautions

Advocates of medical marijuana point out that no one has ever reported a lethal overdose from marijuana. Estimates based on animals have put the amount needed to kill someone at about 20,000 times the amount normally used medically. This compares with some drugs whose lethal dose is only a few times the amount commonly prescribed. While this may be the case, it would be analogous to claiming that since few people die from an alcohol overdose, no serious problems arise with the use of alcohol below its toxic levels.

Marijuana use can lead to problems after both acute and chronic use. The high for which marijuana is used recreationally has many similarities to intoxication. A 2005 study of car accidents in France found that the chances of drivers being responsible for a fatality were more than three times higher if they had been using marijuana compared to those who had not. At least 2.5 percent of fatal crashes were due to marijuana, compared to 28.6 percent due to alcohol use. Marijuana leaves people sedated and less coordinated, making it unwise to drive or operate equipment while under its influence. Coordination problems may last up to twenty-four hours, long after the person no longer feels high. Many people report euphoria and positive feelings from the high, but 40 to 60 percent report unpleasant experiences. This has been the case with marijuana smoked for medical reasons, with sublingual sprays of marijuana extracts, and with Marinol.

About 10 percent of regular recreational users of marijuana develop dependence, according to the Royal College of Physicians' report. When people stop using marijuana after chronic use, they can have withdrawal symptoms such as restlessness, insomnia, nausea, and cramping. Compared to the withdrawal symptoms of other abused drugs, these can be mild and short-lived. The IOM report found no conclusive evidence that marijuana is a "gateway" drug. The frequent finding that users of illicit hard drugs report having earlier used marijuana can be explained by the fact that marijuana is so commonly used. Underage tobacco smoking and alcohol drinking act as "gateway" drugs just as much as marijuana. The 2005 survey in the United Kingdom also identified reduced time spent with parents and increased time spent with drug-using peers as the most significant factors leading to teenagers' use of illegal drugs. At the same time, no evidence counteracts the fear that allowing medical use of marijuana might lead to greater illicit use.

Other physical effects of smoking marijuana are of significant concern. All-out efforts are under way to reduce tobacco smoking because of its widely acknowledged dangers. Marijuana smoke does not contain nicotine but has a significantly higher tar content that is usually not filtered, except when water bongs are used.

The first study to conclude that marijuana smoking puts people at higher risk for cancer was published in December 1999. This epidemiological study compared the rate of marijuana use among adults with head and neck cancer to similar people without cancer. The researchers found that after they made allowances for other risk factors such as smoking cigarettes and drinking alcohol, those who had used marijuana at any time had 2.6 times the risk of these cancers compared to those who had never used marijuana. However, later studies have not found any increased risk of these cancers from smoking marijuana. Similarly conflicting results have been published from other epidemiological studies of marijuana and lung cancer risk — although clear evidence of lung damage is visible. Marijuana smoke

contains carcinogens, but it also contains compounds that have been found to prevent the spread of cancer cells in laboratory tests. At this point, it is unclear how marijuana affects someone's risk of cancer, although there are good reasons to be concerned about the connections.

Other negative effects have been reported. Students regularly using marijuana have lower grades, more traffic accidents, higher use of alcohol and sex as coping mechanisms, and more psychiatric problems than nonusers. These conclusions come from epidemiological studies that do not establish cause and effect, but they have been cited as evidence of what is called "amotivation syndrome."

More serious is growing evidence of a connection between marijuana use and psychosis. Cannabis can precipitate psychosis, and continued cannabis use in psychotic patients makes their illness worse. The relationship between the two is complicated, with considerable debate over whether marijuana causes psychosis or whether people with psychosis tend to experiment with marijuana. The evidence is moving toward a consensus that daily use of marijuana causes psychosis and precipitates schizophrenia, especially if use begins before age fifteen. A study in New Zealand monitored marijuana use in people for twenty-five years and published its results in 2005. It found that daily marijuana users had a 1.6 to 1.8 times greater chance of developing psychosis even after all other known causes were taken into account. Evidence from animal and brain studies has shown a connection between the natural cannabinoid system in the brain and the neurotransmitters believed to be involved in psychosis, though much remains to be learned here .

Other concerns have been expressed that marijuana may negatively impact the immune system, increasing the risk of infection. This would be particularly problematic since the people for whom medical marijuana is most frequently recommended (AIDS and chemotherapy patients) are already at very high risk for infections. Research is not as yet clear about this connection.

The Natural Database rates marijuana as "possibly unsafe" for adults and children, "unsafe" for pregnant women, and "likely unsafe" (orally or inhaled) for breast-feeding women. The Royal College of Physicians' report states there is no evidence that cannabis use damages the unborn.

Recommendations

Obey the law. That is first and foremost. Marijuana in most states and countries is illegal — to grow, possess, use, or sell. Our recommendations in no way ignore this most important aspect of any discussion on marijuana.

Recommendations about marijuana use must be carefully subdivided. First, there is clear evidence that marijuana contains powerful drugs with much potential for relieving nausea, vomiting, loss of appetite, pain, and muscle spasticity in those with multiple sclerosis, and also for elevating mood. Very few preparations currently deliver these components safely. Marinol (dronabinol) is available in the United States for these conditions, and another, nabilone, is available in the United Kingdom. Extracts of marijuana are now available as sublingual sprays. However, other much more effective pharmaceuticals with fewer side effects are usually available for all these conditions and should be tried first. If they fail, you may benefit from your doctor prescribing one of the cannabinoids. One reviewer of our book has much experience prescribing Marinol. This doctor found that a few people gained striking benefits with nausea or anorexia that was poorly controlled in other ways.

However, there was no way to predict ahead of time who would gain such benefits. Research is needed to develop more effective and safer products.

Our second recommendation concerns patients for whom purified cannabinoids and other pharmaceuticals do not work well. For example, patients who already have nausea might not be able to tolerate any oral medicine. Should doctors be able to prescribe marijuana smoking for patients in these situations? The evidence does not indicate that large numbers of people would benefit from smoking marijuana, although a few might. The serious adverse effects of smoking marijuana must also be taken into account. The most reasonable compromise seems to us to be to allow seriously ill patients who do not respond to conventional drugs to try marijuana as part of a short-term clinical trial (probably of the n-of-1 design).

However, as Christians we should obey the laws of our governments unless they conflict seriously with our faith. Paul stated it succinctly: "Everyone must submit himself to the governing authorities, for there is no authority except that which God has established. The authorities that exist have been established by God. Consequently, he who rebels against the authority is rebelling against what God has instituted, and those who do so will bring judgment on themselves" (Romans 13:1 – 2; see also Matthew 22:21). Considering the availability of other medical approaches in most cases, we see no need for anyone to break the law to provide marijuana for medical reasons, and we strongly urge that the law be upheld.

This general approach to highly restricted availability of marijuana for medical use was allowed in thirty-six states between 1978 and 1992 under an FDA program called the Compassionate Investigational New Drug (IND) application. The

IOM review recommended that this program be restarted. Patients would need to be fully informed that they were enrolling in an experimental study and being given a potentially harmful drug delivery system. Meanwhile, research is urgently needed to develop new products that deliver the active ingredients in marijuana in effective, standardized, fast-acting systems that are legal.

Our third recommendation is that marijuana not be licensed as a medical drug. We reiterate the conclusion of the IOM review: "If there is any future for marijuana as a medicine, it lies in its isolated components, the cannabinoids and their synthetic derivatives. Isolated cannabinoids will provide more reliable effects than crude plant mixtures. Therefore, the purpose of clinical trials of smoked marijuana would not be to develop marijuana as a licensed drug but rather to serve as a first step toward the development of non-smoked rapid-onset cannabinoid delivery systems." In this way, the issue of medical marijuana would quickly become a thing of the past.

Our fourth recommendation is that a consistent effort should be maintained to discourage all use of marijuana even if at some future time its illegal status is changed. The risks of using marijuana are great. Every year, about 100,000 people seek help in kicking the marijuana habit. The church could play a significant role here as only Jesus Christ can fill the void that marijuana abusers experience.

Dosage

Marinol is usually prescribed by physicians in doses of 5 to 15 mg every two to four hours for nausea and vomiting due to chemotherapy, or 2.5 to 10 mg twice a day for appetite stimulation in people with AIDS.

Treatment Categories

Conventional

Orally as pure cannabinoid (not the marijuana plant) to bring about moderately effective relief of nausea and vomiting with chemotherapy and AIDS-related weight loss

Complementary

If the following four requirements are met, a short supervised trial with medical marijuana may be justified:

1. no currently legal therapy is effective;
2. marijuana is legal in that jurisdiction;
3. the physical and mental risks are understood by the patient; and
4. the possible benefits exceed the risks.

To relieve chronic disease-related nausea and vomiting or to treat appetite loss associated with weight loss

To produce a euphoric effect in some people with a terminal or severe chronic disease

To treat anorexia and appetite loss associated with AIDS wasting

To relieve muscle spasticity in those with multiple sclerosis

Scientifically Unproven

For any other indication

Risk of Serious Side Effects

From smoking marijuana   ⊘⊘⊘

● Further Reading

Best, D., S. Gross, V. Manning, M. Gossop, J. Witton, and J. Strang. "Cannabis Use in Adolescents: The Impact of Risk and Protective Factors and Social Functioning." *Drug and Alcohol Review* 24, no. 6 (November 2005): 483–88.

Campbell, Fiona A., Martin R. Tramèr, Dawn Carroll, D. John M. Reynolds, R. Andrew Moore, and Henry J. McQuay. "Are Cannabinoids an Effective and Safe Treatment Option in the Management of Pain? A Qualitative Systematic Review." *British Medical Journal* 323 (July 2001): 1–6.

Fergusson, David M., L. John Horwood, and Elizabeth M. Ridder. "Tests of Causal Linkages Between Cannabis Use and Psychotic Symptoms." *Addiction* 100, no. 3 (March 2005): 354–66.

Joy, Janet E., Stanley J. Watson, and John A. Benson. *Marijuana and Medicine: Assessing the Science Base.* Washington, D.C.: National Academy Press, 1999.

Laumon, Bernard, Blandine Gadegbeku, Jean-Louis Martin, and Marie-Berthe Biecheler. "Cannabis Intoxication and Fatal Road Crashes in France: Population-Based Case-Control Study." *British Medical Journal* 331 (December 2005): 1371–76.

Melamede, Robert. "Cannabis and Tobacco Smoke Are Not Equally Carcinogenic." *Harm Reduction Journal* 2 (October 2005): 21. *BioMed Central: www.harmreductionjournal.com/content/2/1/21.* Accessed December 22, 2005.

Notcutt, William, Mario Price, Roy Miller, Samantha Newport, Cheryl Phillips, Susan Simmons, and Cathy Sansom. "Initial Experiences with Medicinal Extracts of Cannabis for Chronic Pain: Results from 34 'N of 1' Studies." *Anaesthesia* 59 (2004): 440–52.

Royal College of Physicians. *Cannabis and Cannabis-Based Medicines: Potential Benefits and Risks to Health.* London: Royal College of Physicians, 2005.

MEGAVITAMIN THERAPY

What It Is

Megavitamin therapy, also called "orthomolecular therapy," involves taking large doses of vitamins, minerals, and amino acids to treat a variety of physical and psychological illnesses. The therapy is based on the belief that some individuals within any group will absorb fewer nutrients than others, even if all are given an identical diet, rich in nutrients and everything needed to sustain good health. The inability of these people to absorb adequate nutrients from a proper diet is believed to lead to the development of different illnesses.

Some proponents of megavitamin therapy maintain that vitamins and minerals can cure illnesses in the same manner as drugs. Instead of thinking of them as nutrients required in small amounts for normal metabolism, the practitioners prescribe vitamins and minerals tailored to what they believe are an individual's medical needs. The doses recommended are vastly higher than any Recommended Dietary Allowance (RDA). Advocates respond that RDAs are arbitrary values that are always changing, and they are simply recommending another change.

There is some truth in the claim that RDAs for vitamins were originally determined in large part by arbitrary measurements. Our knowledge about vitamin supplements, our bodies' nutritional needs, and the long-term impact of various quantities of nutrients has increased over the years. Current recommendations differ, in some cases, from the original RDAs. Solid evidence may support claims that what was once considered safe is actually causing problems for some. Other substances, such as chromium, are being added to the list of required nutrients.

But these changes and developments are not what megavitamin therapy recommends. For example, in the 1960s, Nobel Prize winner Dr. Linus Pauling, a biochemist, promoted his belief that the use of megadoses of vitamin C could do everything from cure the common cold to treat some forms of cancer. At that time he was taking at least 10 grams (10,000 mg) of vitamin C per day. Studies later indicated many benefits from vitamin C but did not validate his anecdotal comments or such high doses. In fact, the megadoses Pauling was consuming are believed to cause an increased risk of kidney stones for some people.

The RDA has gone from an often arbitrary number to one that is more scientifically refined. Though RDAs are not yet perfect, doses dramatically higher than the RDA put users at risk for potentially serious problems. See our entry on Vitamin E for a clear example of dose-related increased risk. Proponents of megavitamin therapy, when discussing why they think RDAs should be ignored, stress the early nature of the RDA as an "educated guess" and not the present reality.

Claims

Megavitamin therapy has traditionally been recommended for mental health and psychiatric problems. The first uses of megavitamin therapy in the 1950s were in the treatment of schizophrenia, for which vitamin B_3 (niacin) was recommended. During the 1970s, megavitamin therapy became popular in the treatment of various psychological problems in children, especially those with attention deficit hyperactivity disorder (ADHD). It has also been recommended to treat Down syndrome, autism, and epilepsy and to increase IQ in healthy children. The therapy appears to come and go in popularity, claiming effectiveness in treating a wide range of psychological conditions but also acne, arthritis, and hypertension.

Study Findings

Studies have not found megavitamin therapy to be effective. The vast majority of illnesses for which megavitamin therapy is recommended have not been linked to vitamin deficiencies. A number of controlled studies (✗✗✗) in the 1980s examined megavitamin therapy in ADHD children and consistently found little evidence for any improvements. Some children had poorer behavior when on the therapy. The evidence is just as unconvincing for all alleged benefits of megavitamin therapy in children. The American Academy of Pediatrics and the Canadian Academy of Pediatrics found no evidence to support its use in children and warned of adverse effects. Reviews in the 1990s found many poorly designed studies of megavitamin therapy with children. The only area showing some possible benefit was use of vitamin B_6 and magnesium for autism. A 1995 review of this area found twelve studies, all but one involving the same researcher. Although benefits were found, the studies were poorly designed with no long-term follow-up. The dose of 600 mg of vitamin B_6 is known to cause nerve damage.

The only recent study we located was a 1999 randomized controlled study (✗✗✗) of adults with schizophrenia. Five months of megavitamin therapy showed huge changes in the levels of various vitamins in the patients' blood. No differences were found between the treated and placebo groups in symptoms or behavior.

Cautions

The Dietary Reference Intake recommendations issued in 2000 for antioxidant vitamins included a UL, which is the highest level likely to pose no risk of adverse health effects for almost everyone. Intakes exceeding the UL have increased risks of adverse effects. The UL for vitamin C was set at 2000 mg per day based on the risk of serious diarrhea and other side effects. The UL for vitamin E is 1000 mg per day (equivalent to 1000 IU synthetic, 1500 IU natural) based on the increased risk of hemorrhage due to its anticoagulant properties. Recent studies have found increased risks when only 150 IU (roughly 100 mg) of vitamin E is taken daily.

A number of other vitamins are known to have toxic effects in high doses. Vitamin D in large quantities can lead to muscle weakness, bone pain, and high blood pressure. Chronic overdosing of vitamin A can result in joint pain, cracked skin, bone abnormalities, and anemia. A single overdose can lead to nausea, vomiting, headache, blurred vision, and lack of muscle coordination. Large doses of vitamin A can lead to visual problems in children and are suspected of causing deformities in unborn babies. In January 2001, the UL for vitamin A was set at 3 mg per day.

A number of vitamins, especially the B group, can interfere with one another's absorption. High doses of one can lead to deficiencies in others. The same is true of certain minerals. Use of megavitamin therapy in children is particularly popular, yet unwarranted. The February 2000 issue of *Pediatrics* reported (✗) the death of a two-year-old due to excessive magnesium from megavitamin therapy recommended by a dietitian, but without the child's physician being informed.

As with all dietary supplements, concerns have been raised about the quality and purity of multivitamins in the United States. ConsumerLab.com released the results of tests of multivitamin products in 2001. Among twenty-seven multivitamin products tested, nine (33 percent) failed to contain the amounts of vitamins listed on the label. Another four had amounts of some vitamins that exceeded the Tolerable Upper Intake Level (UL), although the products were made before some new ULs were set. Nonetheless, half the products did not meet accepted standards.

When ConsumerLab.com retested multivitamins in 2004, only 58 percent (fourteen of twenty-four) of multivitamins and fortified waters passed testing. An additional twenty products passed that had been submitted by their manufacturers or distributors through the independent lab's Voluntary Certification Program. Overall, forty-four products were tested, with 32 percent failing the tests. Those taking megadoses of vitamins should be aware of this lack of quality.

Recommendations

Vitamins (the name was derived from the combination of the words *vital* and *amines*) are an essential part of our diet, and adequate amounts are usually available from a healthy, balanced diet. A general, good-quality multivitamin preparation is more than adequate to make up for any shortages most people in developed countries might have. Megavitamin therapy has been tested as a treatment for numerous conditions, ranging from ADHD and mental retardation in children to the flu and cancer in adults, and found to have little or no benefit. The risks of overdosing on some of the vitamins are significant,

warranting avoidance of this therapy. This is especially true with children.

Some of the conditions for which megavitamin therapy is recommended are chronic and difficult to endure. Patients are willing to try anything, especially something "natural" that seems safe. These products are no more natural than pharmaceuticals and are not regulated to ensure their quality. Unfortunately, megavitamin treatments are ineffective and will not provide relief. Anyone who does try this approach should inform his or her physician so that any related developments can be monitored.

Treatment Categories

Scientifically Questionable
For any indication ☹☹

Quackery
As promoted by some practitioners

Risk of Serious Side Effects
From overdoses of various vitamins ⊘⊘

Further Reading

Barrett, Stephen. "Orthomolecular Therapy." Updated August 21, 2003. *QuackWatch: www.quackwatch. org/01QuackeryRelatedTopics/ortho.html.* Accessed December 21, 2005.

Nutrition Committee, Canadian Paediatric Society. "Megavitamin and Megamineral Therapy in Childhood." *Canadian Medical Association Journal* 143, no. 10 (November 1990): 1009–13.

Vaughan, Kevin, and Nathaniel McConaghy. "Megavitamin and Dietary Treatment in Schizophrenia: A Randomised, Controlled Trial." *Australian and New Zealand Journal of Psychiatry* 33, no. 1 (February 1999): 84–88.

MELATONIN

What It Is

With increased air travel for business and pleasure, jet lag has become an issue for more people. This is especially the case with multinational businesses that expect travelers to be alert and efficient as soon as they arrive. Many strategies to avoid or overcome jet lag have been suggested, with recent attention focusing on melatonin. This hormone is involved in the natural sleep-wake cycle under the control of a circadian clock. This "clock" is located in the brain; darkness leads to increased production of melatonin, while light inhibits its production. How melatonin then acts in the body is unclear. While its production in humans is highest at night when most humans sleep, its level is also highest at night in nocturnal mammals. Rather than viewing it as a "sleep hormone," as some do, it might be better viewed as a "darkness hormone." Melatonin is not a natural sleeping tablet.

Flying through several time zones and changing work shifts get the body's melatonin levels out of sync with when a person wants to be awake or asleep, thus disturbing his or her sleep pattern. Supplemental melatonin is taken to help bring the body's melatonin levels back into sync with the person's sleep-wake cycle. This relieves the various symptoms associated with jet lag, such as fatigue, loss of concentration, irritability, and difficulty getting to sleep at night.

Melatonin levels also vary during a person's lifetime. After about age twenty, the body produces less melatonin. Some claim this is connected to increased sleep disturbances that occur with age, but this has not been clearly demonstrated. Melatonin levels are also connected with the levels of several other hormones, such as growth hormone.

Claims

The best-known use of melatonin is for jet lag, but it has also been used to help people with insomnia and people with jobs that involve frequent shift changes. Melatonin has also been recommended for tinnitus (ringing in the ears), headaches, Alzheimer's disease, depression, anxiety, cancer, and many other conditions.

Study Findings

A 2002 Cochrane review (✓✓✓) found ten controlled trials of melatonin for jet lag. The studies varied considerably in design and dosage. All but two of the studies found melatonin significantly better than placebo in reducing jet lag symptoms when the journeys crossed five or more time zones. The optimal dose appeared to be 5 mg daily, with higher doses being no more effective and lower doses failing to improve sleep quality. Two more studies (✓✓✓) were published after this Cochrane review, and both found melatonin better than placebo in helping people overcome symptoms of jet lag.

Melatonin has also been studied as an aid to help people fall asleep faster. While some studies have found benefit, an equal number have found it no more helpful than placebo. The Agency for Healthcare Research and Quality (AHRQ) sponsored a systematic review (✗✗✗✗) that was published by the *British Medical Journal* in 2006. It came to several conclusions based on randomized controlled trials of melatonin. Clinically insignificant benefits were found in the sleep patterns of normal sleepers and those with insomnia. Beneficial effects were noted only for those whose sleep patterns were off-cycle. However, all these studies on sleep were very small and methodologically flawed. Some assumed that people lying still in bed were asleep, yet that may not have been the case. One interesting study pointed to the difficulties of studying sleep agents. This study found statistically significant improvements in people's sleep quality after they had been told they would be given melatonin in a study, but before they actually received any. Such is the power of the placebo effect!

Little evidence supports most of the other uses of melatonin. However, it has a reputation for treating solid tumor cancers. A 2005 systematic review (✓✓✓) found ten controlled studies of its use in a variety of solid tumors. The studies examined survival rates after one year of treatment. However, all the studies were carried out within the same hospital network in Italy and Poland. Independent verification of the results would be important. In addition, none of the studies were blinded. Nonetheless, a statistically significant benefit in survival rate was found for those treated with melatonin.

Cautions

In clinical trials, about one in ten participants experienced hypnotic effects that were relatively mild and quickly went away. Other adverse effects included headaches, disorientation, nausea, and gastrointestinal problems. The 2002 Cochrane review located a number of adverse events involving people with epilepsy and recommended against those people using

it. Melatonin is produced naturally in high levels in children and is involved in sexual development. It has been used safely in studies with children, although the Natural Database rates it as "possibly unsafe" for children and pregnant women. We would not recommend its use while breast-feeding due to insufficient reliable information. The long-term effects of using melatonin are unknown. The Natural Database rates appropriate oral melatonin use for up to two months as "likely safe" and use from two to nine months as "possibly safe."

In 2002, ConsumerLab.com purchased eighteen melatonin-containing supplements — fifteen were quick-release products, and three were time-release. Of the total, twelve were melatonin-only products. The other six were combined with vitamin B_6 or herbs such as valerian. Sixteen of the eighteen products (89 percent) met their label claims and were not contaminated with lead. The two other products were not far from a passing standard.

Recommendations

Melatonin is a hormone involved in sleep-wake cycles. It appears to be most beneficial in helping people adjust to changes in those cycles, as opposed to helping people with sleep problems. As such, it can be recommended to minimize the effects of jet lag, especially with extended flights. When flying westward, best results are reported when melatonin is taken the evening of the departure day and then at normal bedtime at the destination for a few days. When flying eastward, the usual recommendation is to start melatonin after arriving at the destination at the local bedtime. Starting melatonin before departure does not appear to add any benefits. Those experiencing excessive drowsiness should reduce the dosage and be cautious driving or operating machinery.

Dosage

For jet lag, 4 to 5 mg of melatonin is usually recommended at bedtime on the arrival day at the destination and continued for two to five days. Low doses of 0.5 to 3 mg are recommended to avoid the sedative properties of the higher doses. For insomnia, dosages of 0.3 to 5 mg at bedtime are recommended. When treating cancer, 20 to 40 mg daily is recommended.

Treatment Categories

Complementary

To alleviate the symptoms of jet lag ☺☺☺
To facilitate changes in sleep-wake cycles ☺☺
To treat solid tumor-type cancers ☺
To treat insomnia ☺

Scientifically Unproven

For any other indication

Further Reading

Buscemi N., B. Vandermeer, N. Hooton, R. Pandya, L. Tjosvold, L. Hartling, S. Vohra, T. Klassen, and G. Baker. "Efficacy and Safety of Exogenous Melatonin for Secondary Sleep Disorders and Sleep Disorders Accompanying Sleep Restriction: Meta-analysis." *British Medical Journal* 332 (February 2006): 385 – 93.

Mills, E., P. Wu, D. Seely, G. Guyatt. "Melatonin in the Treatment of Cancer: A Systematic Review of Randomized Controlled Trials and Meta-analysis." *Journal of Pineal Research* 39, no. 4 (November 2005): 360 – 66.

Scheer, Frank A. J. L., and Charles A. Czeisler. "Melatonin, Sleep, and Circadian Rhythms." *Sleep Medicine Reviews* 9, no. 1 (February 2005): 5 – 9.

MILK THISTLE

• What It Is

Milk thistle has long been a staple of folk medicine throughout Europe, where it is consistently one of the top-selling herbal supplements. In 2004, it reached the top ten in sales in the United States. For many years, milk thistle was considered valuable for lactating women who needed a boost in their milk production, though studies have now proven that it is ineffective for this purpose. More common these days is its use as a liver tonic and to treat various liver diseases such as hepatitis and cirrhosis.

Milk thistle of the variety called *Silybum marianum* (previously called *Carduus marianus*) is found widely in Europe, eastern Africa, and North America. A member of the aster family, milk thistle grows to a height of up to ten feet. It bears a bright purple brushlike flower, and in the summer it produces black seeds from which the drug is derived.

Milk thistle has been known by a number of other common names, including holy thistle, St. Mary thistle, marian thistle, lady's thistle, and royal thistle. Its spiritual names stem from the belief that the white veins on the plant's leaves carried the milk of the Virgin Mary.

• Claims

For two thousand years, milk thistle has been used as a medicinal herb. The Latin name, *Silybum*, was coined by Dioscorides, an herbalist in ancient Greece who used the term *silybon* to describe thistle-like plants. Pliny the Elder (AD 23 – 79), a Roman writer,

recorded that the plant's juice was excellent for "carrying off bile." Culpepper (1787), an English herbalist, described its use in removing obstructions to the liver and spleen and as a remedy for jaundice. The Eclectics, a late nineteenth-century school of medical herbalists, used milk thistle for congestion in the liver, spleen, and kidney and for varicose veins and menstrual disorders. Milk thistle is widely used in Europe, where it has been commercially available for almost thirty years for such problems as dyspepsia, hepatitis, liver vulnerability, loss of appetite, and diseases of the spleen. It has been used intravenously to treat people poisoned by the *Amanita phalloides* mushroom (also called Death Cap).

• Study Findings

Many studies used a compound isolated from milk thistle called "silymarin," which is not the same as using the plant material itself. Surveys have found that 10 to 15 percent of patients in liver clinics are taking milk thistle products. A 2002 review (✗✗✗) of fifteen studies found that many were of poor quality and few showed any benefit. A 2005 review of seven higher-quality controlled trials was published. Some of the trials used a product called Legalon, which is standardized to contain 70 to 80 percent silymarin. The types of conditions being treated included acute viral hepatitis and chronic liver disease due to alcoholism or other causes. Four of the studies (✓✓✓) found milk thistle more beneficial than placebo, but three (✗✗✗) found no benefit. A 2005 Cochrane review included thirteen studies of milk thistle for liver disease due to alcoholism or hepatitis B or C. While some studies found benefit from milk thistle, when only the highest-quality studies were examined, no overall benefit was found in reducing death rates or any liver complications. The authors concluded that milk thistle was no better than placebo (✗✗✗). This lack of consistency in different studies led the National Institutes of Health to initiate a large study of milk thistle for liver disease in 2005.

Several case studies (✓✓) have reported beneficial effects when intravenous milk thistle was used in people poisoned by the *Amanita phalloides* mushroom (Death Cap). In all cases, conventional therapy had failed, and in some cases people recovered. However, this intravenous formulation of milk thistle is not available in the United States. The German Commission E, an expert committee responsible for evaluating the safety and efficacy of herbal medicines, has recommended milk thistle as supportive treatment for chronic inflammatory liver conditions.

Cautions

No serious adverse effects have been seen with milk thistle. Animals subjected to high doses of milk thistle have shown no toxic effects. Some patients report loose stools. In the largest clinical trial, joint aches, headaches, and hives were rarely reported. There are no reported drug interactions. Milk thistle extracts standardized to contain 70 to 80 percent silymarin seem to be safe when used for up to forty-one months. However, there is insufficient reliable information about the safety of intravenous formulations of milk thistle and its constituents. No reliable information shows whether it is safe for children or women who are pregnant or lactating.

In 2004, ConsumerLab.com published test results for twenty-seven milk thistle supplements. All but one of these passed the company's tests. The one product that failed contained only 18 percent of the claimed silymarin. However, ConsumerLab.com warns, "When choosing a brand, it is important to note that the amount of silymarin will vary considerably among products, largely due to whether the milk thistle used was a concentrated extract or nonconcentrated seed powder/meal."

Recommendations

Milk thistle has become a very popular herbal supplement for hepatitis and cirrhosis. Extensive laboratory and animal data suggest a liver protective benefit with silymarin. However, the clinical studies in humans are mixed. Most European studies used Legalon, available in the United States as Thisylin. The positive studies with alcoholic hepatitis and cirrhosis showing improved liver function tests and longer life must be viewed alongside studies that are equally well done and that show milk thistle to be no better than placebo.

No published controlled trials exist for milk thistle used to treat specific liver diseases, such as chronic hepatitis B or C. For patients with hepatitis or cirrhosis, milk thistle appears to be safe and inexpensive. For patients with alcoholic liver disease, abstinence from alcohol remains the cornerstone of therapy, and for those at risk for hepatitis A and B, vaccines are available. Milk thistle remains unproven for chronic hepatitis C. For patients with acute viral hepatitis, alcoholic hepatitis, and cirrhosis, a modest benefit may exist, but the evidence remains inconclusive.

Dosage

A typical dose is 200 to 400 mg of extract per day, although up to 800 mg daily has been evaluated in studies. German Commission E recommends a formulation standardized to contain at least 70 percent silymarin. Unfortunately, there is no guarantee in the United States that products so labeled actually contain this much silymarin. Recommendations are not given for duration of therapy.

Treatment Categories

Complementary

To treat acute viral hepatitis	☺
To treat cirrhosis of the liver	☺
To treat toxic liver damage	☺
To treat chronic liver disease and hepatitis	☹
Intravenously, if conventional therapy fails, to treat *Amanita phalloides* (Death Cap) poisoning	☺

Scientifically Unproven

For any other indication

Further Reading

Jacobs, Bradly P., Cathi Dennehy, Gilbert Ramirez, Jodi Sapp, and Valerie A. Lawrence. "Milk Thistle for the Treatment of Liver Disease: A Systematic Review and Meta-analysis." *American Journal of Medicine* 113, no. 6 (October 2002): 506–15.

Rainone, Francine. "Milk Thistle." *American Family Physician* 72, no. 7 (October 2005): 1285–88.

Rambaldi, Andrea, Bradly P. Jacobs, Gaetano Iaquinto, and Christian Gluud. "Milk Thistle for Alcoholic and/or Hepatitis B or C Liver Diseases — A Systematic Cochrane Hepatobiliary Group Review with Meta-analyses of Randomized Clinical Trials." *American Journal of Gastroenterology* 100, no. 11 (November 2005): 2583–91.

MSM

What It Is

MSM is one of those products that all of a sudden captures the public imagination. Such remedies pop out of obscurity, become widely popular through some charismatic personality or bestselling book, and leave doctors scratching their heads about what to tell patients. MSM came to prominence in 1999 with the publication of *The Miracle of MSM: The Natural Solution for Pain*. Why this book? No one knows. But some people are reaping the benefits of massive sales of books and products.

MSM stands for "methylsulfonylmethane," but the substance is also called "dimethyl sulfone" or $DMSO_2$. This should not be confused with DMSO (dimethyl sulfoxide), a liquid or gel used topically to treat different forms of pain. After DMSO is taken into the body, it is broken down to form MSM. Some claim that the effects of DMSO are as much the result of MSM as they are of DMSO. (A small number of controlled trials support this use of DMSO, although it is vital that pharmaceutical-grade DMSO be used. DMSO transports many substances through the skin and into the blood, including any impurities in the gel or on the skin.)

MSM is a white crystalline product that occurs widely in nature. It is found in various green plants, vegetables, fruits, and grains and in the adrenal glands, milk, and urine of cows and humans. It is a natural source of organic sulfur, which is needed to make sulfur-containing amino acids (such as cystine) for the body's proteins.

Claims

MSM began as a cure for arthritis. A 1935 study found low cystine levels in people with arthritis, which might be why someone made a connection between MSM and arthritis. From that, MSM was advocated for use in other chronic painful conditions. Sulfur is important in the functioning of insulin, so it was recommended for diabetes. Now it is recommended for all sorts of painful conditions, allergies, premenstrual syndrome, snoring, HIV, cancer, and much more.

Study Findings

Sulfur is widely available in many proteins in the diet. Sulfur deficiency has not been documented, nor has a connection between sulfur and any disease or disorder been established. Some preliminary animal studies suggest MSM may play a role in inflammatory reactions and pain. However, very few studies of MSM have been carried out with humans.

Two studies (✓✓✓) have examined MSM with osteoarthritis. The first, reported in 2004, randomly assigned people to receive either MSM or glucosamine or both — or a placebo. All three treatments significantly reduced pain and swelling. The combination was most effective and acted the fastest. People took 0.5 grams three times daily. The second trial was a 2005 pilot study in which people with knee osteoarthritis received either 3 grams MSM twice a day or placebo. After twelve weeks, those taking MSM had significant improvements in pain

M

relief and physical functioning, but not in degree of stiffness.

One uncontrolled study (✓✓) gave fifty people with hay fever 2.6 grams of MSM daily for thirty days. Improvements were found in the symptoms reported by the participants. However, no changes were found in blood levels of compounds typically released by the body during allergic reactions. The authors noted that these results were preliminary since all participants knew they were receiving MSM and no control group was involved.

Cautions

Clinical trials reported no serious adverse events, even when people took 6 grams per day. The side effects reported by those taking MSM and placebo were similar. No other adverse reports were found, even when 18 grams per day were taken. Most of these studies lasted no more than a month, however. There is insufficient reliable information about using MSM during pregnancy or lactation, so we recommend that women not use it during these times. When ConsumerLab.com reported its testing of MSM products in 2004, nine MSM products and eight glucosamine/chondroitin/MSM products all passed testing.

Recommendations

Very little controlled research has been conducted on MSM. However, preliminary results indicate that MSM may be useful in treating osteoarthritis. Even more benefit was found when MSM was taken along with glucosamine, which has been shown to benefit people with osteoarthritis. The substance apparently is safe to use. However, more research is needed be-fore MSM can be wholeheartedly recommended. Its use for allergies cannot be recommended.

Dosage

No recommended dosage has been established. Capsules with 100 mg of MSM are recommended one to three times a day.

Treatment Categories

Complementary
To relieve pain and swelling in those
with osteoarthritis ☺

Scientifically Unproven
To relieve pain generally ☺
To relieve the symptoms of hay fever ☺

Scientifically Questionable
For any other indication

Quackery or Fraud
In the hands of some who claim it is a cure-all

Further Reading

Kim, L. S., L. J. Axelrod, P. Howard, N. Buratovich, and R. F. Waters. "Efficacy of Methylsulfonylmethane (MSM) in Osteoarthritis Pain of the Knee: A Pilot Clinical Trial." *Osteoarthritis Cartilage* 14, no. 3 (March 2006): 286–94.

"Methylsulfonylmethane (MSM)." *Alternative Medicine Review* 8, no. 4 (November 2003): 438–41.

NONI JUICE

What It Is

Traditional Polynesian medicine has recently contributed two very popular products: kava and noni juice. This juice is made from the fruit of the morinda tree (*Morinda citrifolia*), a small evergreen tree in the Pacific islands, Southeast Asia, Australia, and India that often grows among lava flows. The root of a closely related tree, *Morinda officinalis*, is used to make a different product called "ba ji tian." The two should not be confused, though they are sometimes combined. Morinda fruit is also known as rotten cheese fruit for a very obvious reason: it smells and tastes terrible. In spite of this, *Nutrition Business Journal* reported in 2004 that noni juice topped the list of bestselling natural products in the United States.

Morinda bark contains high concentrations of yellow chemicals called "anthraquinones," which explains its traditional use as a source of yellow dye. Various parts of the morinda tree are used in making many commonly used traditional Polynesian remedies. For the most part, these remedies are used topically to treat wounds and infections. The remedies are believed to "draw out" an infection from a wound.

A 1985 publication by Ralph M. Heinicke in the *Pacific Tropical Botanical Garden Bulletin* changed everything. Using scientific terms, Heinicke explained how noni juice, from the fruit of the morinda tree, contains a chemical called "proxeronine" that is broken down in the body to xeronine. He said that cells throughout the body take up xeronine and become healthy or are cured of diseases. All of a sudden, noni juice became a highly popular health drink. The only problem is that Heinicke did not reference any of the articles he used to support his claims — and no one has ever identified proxeronine or xeronine.

Claims

Heinicke's article claimed that noni juice would benefit those with high blood pressure, arthritis, menstrual cramps, poor digestion, injuries, depression, pain, and many other conditions. He also claimed it had potential for treating cancer. That is one area in which studies are being conducted on the juice. The traditional uses are completely different, with external use recommended for a variety of wounds and infections. Topically, it is also used to treat arthritis and headaches. Morinda bark has been taken orally in traditional settings to induce abortions.

Study Findings

Morinda fruit contains significant amounts of potassium, vitamin C, vitamin A, and fatty acids. No studies were located for the wide variety of indications for which noni juice is used. No controlled studies have been conducted on its external use. A Ph.D. dissertation on noni juice reported the isolation of chemicals with anticancer activity in some laboratory tests. Research funded by the National Institutes of Health is currently investigating the potential of these compounds for treating cancer.

Cautions

ConsumerLab.com lists several concerns about the quality of morinda products:

- Unlike most herbals sold as supplements, quality standards have yet to be defined for noni juice and supplements. Currently, there is no way to judge whether one product is more effective or safer than another.
- Reports have circulated that some companies take the leftover by-products of juicing (the discarded seed, pulp, and fiber material), dry it, grind it up, and deceptively sell it as "100% noni fruit powder." Such a product would not be expected to contain the compounds found in noni juice.
- Distinctive varieties of morinda trees exist, with possibly more than one species being used as the source of fruit. Almost all of the published literature is based on fruit from trees in Hawaii. However, most of the fruit being sold is from trees grown in French Polynesia, Samoa, Fiji, and other South Pacific islands, which may have different chemical constituents.
- Noni fruit is often wild harvested ("wild crafted") and therefore not of consistent quality or origin.
- Noni is also commercially grown and harvested. As with other commercially grown crops, pesticides may be used in its production. Noni fruit is often grown in countries with different laws regulating usage of pesticides and herbicides, including ones that are no longer acceptable in the United States, Canada, or Europe. Some growers, however, do have organic certifications.

- Some, but not all, noni juice is pasteurized. Pasteurization is a heat treatment intended to kill potential pathogens in food products and may prolong shelf life. It has been argued, however, that pasteurization might also inactivate compounds with potential beneficial effect, but this has not been proven.

Noni juice appears to be relatively safe when used orally or topically in appropriate ways, or when the fruit is consumed as food. However, noni juice contains significant amounts of potassium (56 mEq/L, which is similar to orange and tomato juice). Some medications used to treat high blood pressure (such as potassium-sparing diuretics, ACE inhibitors, and angiotensin receptor blockers) can lead to retention of potassium. The two together might lead to very high levels of potassium, which can lead to nausea or potentially lethal cardiac arrhythmias. For the same reasons, noni juice should not be taken by anyone with kidney problems. A small number of case reports (✘✘) of liver toxicity have been connected to noni juice and morinda tea. Anthraquinones, such as those found in noni juice, can negatively affect the liver. Given the traditional use of morinda to cause abortions, it probably should be avoided during pregnancy. There is no evidence that it is safe in breast-feeding women; therefore, we do not recommend its use by lactating women.

Recommendations

As a juice with many vitamins, noni appears to be a healthy food option. It is too early to state if any of its components are effective in treating any particular condition. The claims of any curative properties are highly suspect. In fact, the FDA has issued many warnings to the manufacturers of morinda and noni products about unsubstantiated claims. As we said about mangosteen, enjoy the juice; forget the hype.

Dosage

There is no information on the appropriate dose.

Treatment Categories

Complementary

To add fruit to a more plant-based diet ☺☺☺

Scientifically Unproven

As juice, to treat cancer ☹☹

Scientifically Questionable

For any indication

Quackery or Fraud

In the hands of some practitioners

Further Reading

McClatchey, Will. "From Polynesian Healers to Health Food Stores: Changing Perspectives of *Morinda citrifolia* (Rubiaceae)." *Integrative Cancer Therapies* 1, no. 2 (June 2002): 110–20.

NOPAL

What It Is

Nopal refers to the prickly pear cactus (*Opuntia fuliginosa*). However, there are two hundred to three hundred species of *Opuntia* cacti around the world. Their ability to grow in arid deserts where little else flourishes has made them an important source of food and medicinal agents in those regions. Nopal is one of the most popular natural remedies used in Hispanic regions. It is especially popular in Mexico, where it is the most widely used natural remedy for treating diabetes. In one study of type 2 diabetes patients in Mexico City, almost 62 percent reported using complementary therapies (compared to 20 percent of diabetes patients in the United States). Of the Mexican patients using complementary therapies, almost three-quarters used nopal.

The fleshy stem or pad of the cactus is used, as is the fruit. The fruit is also known as cactus pears or prickly pears. The cactus is believed to be most effective when eaten fresh or broiled. Today, however, dried preparations and extracts are made and marketed as capsules and powders.

Claims

The main claim made for nopal is that it lowers blood glucose and can thus treat diabetes. It is also said to help reduce high cholesterol levels, help with weight loss, relieve hangovers, and treat viral infections. Treatment of benign prostatic hypertrophy (enlargement of the prostate) is a recent addition to its uses.

Study Findings

Much of the nopal stem consists of a fibrous carbohydrate called "pectin." This is believed to combine with other carbohydrates and fats in the diet and slow or prevent their absorption. Animal studies also suggest that nopal may contain substances that either act like insulin or increase the sensitivity of tissues to insulin. This would have the effect of lowering blood glucose levels. Other compounds extracted from nopal interfere with liver production of cholesterol and lower blood cholesterol levels in animals.

A small number of human studies (✓✓) were carried out by one research group in Mexico during the 1980s. Participants were given 500 grams of broiled cactus stem. The studies found consistent reductions in blood glucose levels of between 17 and 46 percent. These changes did not occur when nopal was given to nondiabetic people. The maximal effect occurred a few hours after eating nopal and lasted up to six hours. Most studies involved seven or eight patients who were not blinded to the intervention; control groups were not used to compare results against placebo.

Cautions

Nopal appears to be well tolerated as a food and when used for health purposes for up to eight months. Some people have mild gastrointestinal problems from the food, including nausea, diarrhea, and headache. People with type 2 diabetes whose blood sugar levels are under control should discuss the use of nopal with their health care professionals before making any changes. Nopal could have additive effects with other drugs or dietary approaches being used. Pregnant and lactating women should not use nopal supplements until there is reliable evidence that they are safe and effective for these women.

Recommendations

The stems and fruit of the prickly cactus are a plant food that may provide benefit in the control of type 2 diabetes. Very little research has been conducted in this area, so it is not known whether the effects on blood glucose are maintained with long-term usage. Other long-term effects are not known. The small amount of research was conducted on the cooked cactus, which may not be readily available in many parts of the world. Research on the capsules and dried products available elsewhere has not been done. Whether these products will have the same benefits as the fruit is not known.

Dosage

The usual recommendation for diabetes is 100 to 500 grams of broiled stems a day, divided into three doses. For benign prostatic hypertrophy, dried powdered flowers of prickly pear cactus (500 mg three times daily) were used, although it is not known if this is the best dose.

Treatment Categories

Complementary

To lower blood glucose in type 2 diabetes	☺
To lower blood cholesterol	☺
To treat benign prostatic hyperplasia	☺

Scientifically Unproven

For any other indication

Further Reading

Poss, Jane E., Mary A. Jezewski, and Armando G. Stuart. "Home Remedies for Type 2 Diabetes Used by Mexican Americans in El Paso, Texas." *Clinical Nursing Research* 12, no. 4 (November 2003): 304–23.

Stintzing, Florian C., and Reinhold Carle. "Cactus Stems (Opuntia spp.): A Review on Their Chemistry, Technology, and Uses." *Molecular Nutrition and Food Research* 49, no. 2 (February 2005): 175–94.

OMEGA FATTY ACIDS

What They Are

Interest in this area of nutrition and diet began with the observation of very low death rates from cardiovascular disease in populations that consumed large amounts of fish. The benefit was traced to polyunsaturated omega-3 fatty acids. Hundreds of subsequent studies have been carried out to better understand the role of omega-3 fatty acids in the diet. The main omega-3 fatty acids are eicosapentaenoic acid (EPA), docosahexaenoic acid (DHA), and alpha-linolenic acid (ALA). EPA and DHA are found mainly in fish, while ALA is primarily derived from plants.

Fatty acids are the building blocks of natural fats and oils. Although fat tends to be viewed negatively, all cells of the body require fats to build and maintain healthy membranes. Fatty acids are important sources of energy and are used to make a number of other compounds essential for good health. This is why fatty acids are believed to potentially impact many conditions that affect various parts of the body.

The total amount of fat in the diet is important for body weight. However, the particular type of fatty acid found in dietary fat is also very important for health. The fatty acids found in animal fats tend to have very few double bonds (they are saturated). This gives the molecules a shape that permits them to stack together, which can contribute to various diseases. For example, animal fats more easily contribute to plaque that can clog arteries, leading to atherosclerosis. In contrast, plant and fish oils tend to have fatty acids with several double bonds (they are unsaturated or polyunsaturated). The "omega-3" term identifies where the first double bond is located in the molecule.

The major food sources of EPA and DHA are fish, primarily mackerel, herring, tuna, salmon, sardine, and trout. Commercial fish oils and supplements vary in the relative proportions of these two omega-3 fatty acids. Each fish oil also has other characteristic components. For example, cod liver oil has relatively large amounts of vitamins A and D. Although EPA and DHA can be made from ALA, they all have different effects in the body. ALA comes primarily from vegetable oils such as flaxseed (or linseed) oil, canola (or rapeseed) oil, and soybean oil. ALA is also found in red meat, dairy products, walnuts, vegetables, and chocolate. The impact of ALA appears to be quite different from that of EPA and DHA and much less powerful.

Claims

Omega-3 fatty acids are said to benefit almost every condition a person might ever get. The primary focus has been on preventing cardiovascular diseases, asthma, neurological disorders, cognitive decline, and various mental health problems. The related omega-6 fatty acids are used for reducing the risk of coronary heart disease and cancer. A particular omega-6 fatty acid, arachidonic acid, is used as a supplement in infant formulas.

Study Findings

Many epidemiological studies have demonstrated a connection between omega-3 fatty acid consumption and many diseases. To assess the current research in this area, the Agency for Healthcare Research and Quality (AHRQ) commissioned several reviews. These were published during 2004 and 2005 and form the basis of what is reported here.

Hundreds of studies have examined the impact of dietary fatty acids on cardiovascular health. Most studies have examined the effects on various risk factors for heart disease. The most clear-cut evidence (✓✓✓) is that omega-3 fatty acids reduce total triglyceride levels by between 10 and 33 percent. However, only one of these studies (✗✗✗) involved plant omega-3 fatty acids (rapeseed and linseed oil), and it found increased triglyceride levels. One specific fish oil preparation (Omacor) contains 465 mg of EPA and 375 mg of DHA per 1-gram capsule and is FDA-approved for treating hypertriglyceridemia (triglyceride levels of 500 mg/dL and above) in conjunction with dietary changes.

In cholesterol levels, small but desirable changes were found with fish oils (✓✓✓), but the plant oils produced smaller changes. A few studies (✓✓✓) examined the impact of fish oils on blood pressure and found small reductions (about 2 mm Hg). Other cardiovascular risk factors showed smaller or inconsistent changes. Few studies examined differences among different fatty acids or doses or duration of consumption.

For the 2004 AHRQ review, thirty-nine controlled studies were found that examined the impact of omega-3 fatty acids on heart disease. Of these, twelve were randomized and double-blinded. A clear pattern emerged (✓✓✓) of reduced death rates and reduced cardiovascular disease among those adding omega-3 fatty acids to their diet. The benefit was much more significant for fish oils (EPA and DHA) than for plant oils (ALA). However, the studies were all very different, making generalizations somewhat tentative. More recent studies have shown that fish oils benefit patients who have recently had a heart attack (✓✓✓✓). However, those with chronic heart disease or an implanted cardioverter defibrillator (ICD) had more heart problems when taking fish oil compared to placebo (✗✗✗).

Interest in the impact of omega-3 fatty acids on asthma was stimulated by the observation that the Inuit (the people formerly called "Eskimos") have a very low incidence of asthma. The AHRQ review found twenty-six studies of this issue but concluded that the findings were so inconsistent that nothing firm could be stated. Many studies were very poorly designed, and all were so different that general conclusions could not be made. The intervention did have few adverse effects.

Another review examined the health effects of omega-3 fatty acids on normal cognitive function with aging, dementia, and neurological diseases. Only twelve studies were found in this area. The results varied considerably. For example, one of three studies found a significant reduction in risk of Alzheimer's disease for those consuming more fish. Two of three other studies found reduced disability for those with multiple sclerosis who took an omega-3 fatty acid. The review concluded that much more research is needed in this area. In a similar way, the reviews of omega-3 fatty acids for eye health and mental health found that there was insufficient research to come to any general conclusions.

At least one randomized trial (✗✗✗) has shown that feeding infants a formula containing arachidonic acid (an omega-6 fatty acid) doesn't seem to be effective in improving cognitive and mental development or growth up to eighteen months of age. Other trials have shown that omega-6 fatty acids actually elevate triglyceride levels.

Cautions

The oils containing omega-3 fatty acids tend to be tolerated well. Fish oils leave people with strong fishy tastes, which can lead to belching, nausea, and loose stools. Doses larger than 3 grams of fish oil have been suspected of interfering with blood clotting and suppressing immune function. Because of this, the Natural Database rates omega-3 fatty acids as "likely safe" at doses of 3 grams per day or less and "possibly unsafe" in doses greater than 3 grams per day. There is insufficient reliable information about the safety of omega-6 fatty acids. We therefore recommend that children or women who are pregnant or lactating not use these.

Some very recent studies may indicate that fish oil could increase the risk of irregular and even fatal heart rhythms in people with a history of heart attacks or coronary artery disease. In one study, men with chronic coronary artery disease who took up to 3 grams of fish oil capsules daily had a significantly increased risk of cardiac deaths (29 percent increased risk) and sudden deaths (55 percent increased risk). In another placebo-controlled trial, patients with an implanted cardioverter defibrillator (ICD) had more cardiac arrhythmias if they took fish oil compared to a placebo (olive oil).

In spite of the potential benefits from fish oil, fatty fish can contain toxins such as mercury, polychlorinated biphenyls (PCBs), dioxin, and dioxin-related compounds. A debate erupted in 2004 after publication of an article in a prominent science journal that calculated the *hypothetical* risk of consuming farm-raised salmon that might contain toxins. Much more research is needed to evaluate the best balance between these potential risks from toxins with frequent consumption of shark, swordfish, king mackerel, tilefish, or farm-raised salmon and the potential health benefits from their omega-3 fatty acids. However, caution would suggest limiting the intake of these fish for young children, pregnant and lactating women, and women who may become pregnant. The Natural Database suggests limiting these fish to less than 2 ounces per week for children and less than 12 ounces per week (3 to 4 servings) for women of child-bearing age. Others, such as Walter Willett at Harvard School of Public Health, disagree and lament the drop in fish consumption triggered by the 2004 article.

Because omega-3 fatty acids are obtained from natural sources, levels in supplements can vary, depending on the source and method of processing. The freshness of the oil is also an important consideration, because rancid fish oils have an extremely unpleasant odor and may not be as effective. In 2004, ConsumerLab.com purchased forty-one EPA and DHA dietary supplements sold in the United States. All but two were fresh and contained their claimed amounts of EPA and DHA. None of the products were found to contain detectable levels of mercury, PCBs, or dioxins.

Recommendations

Omega-3 fatty acids are the subject of much current interest. While a lot remains unknown about precisely how these fatty acids can best be used, a number of points can be made. Increasing the amount of omega-3 fatty acids in many diets probably will bring several benefits. However, it cannot be stated at this point precisely what those benefits will be or the extent to which they will be experienced. Much remains to be learned about the optimal amounts of these fatty acids and which sources are best.

Before increasing the amount of omega-3 fatty acids, people should consider a few other points. Fatty acids come in fats and oils that are high in calories. Increasing omega-3 fatty acids should be done by substituting them for other fats or oils you already consume. There are many questions as to whether dietary supplements will provide the same benefits as eating foods high in omega-3 fatty acids. Our general recommendation is that it is better to add more healthy foods to your diet than to add another supplement to your daily intake. The evidence also points to fish sources of omega-3 fatty acids being more beneficial than plant sources.

● Dosage

A wide range of doses have been recommended. A typical dose is 5 grams of fish oil containing EPA and DHA. A typical recommendation of ALA is 1 to 2 grams.

● Treatment Categories

Complementary

To gain overall improvement in
health through a healthier diet ☺☺☺

Omega-3 fatty acids:
to reduce blood triglyceride levels ☺☺☺☺
to reduce the risk of cardiovascular
disease after a recent heart attack ☺☺☺
to reduce the risk of cardiovascular
disease in people with
hypercholesterolemia ☺☺
to reduce the risk of cardiovascular
disease in the general population ☺
to reduce the risk of cardiovascular
disease with chronic coronary
artery disease ☹☹☹
to reduce the risk of age-related
macular disease and cataracts ☺
to prevent restenosis after angioplasty
or graph occlusion after coronary
artery bypass ☺
to treat asthma ☺
to decrease the risk of cancer ☺
to treat dysmenorrhea (painful menses)
in teens ☺
to treat mild hypertension ☺

to reduce the risk of ischemic stroke ☺
to treat ADHD ☹
to treat claudication or peripheral
artery disease ☹
to treat mastalgia (breast pain) ☹
to prevent migraine headaches ☹
to prevent muscle soreness with exercise ☹
to treat diabetes ☹☹

Omega-6 fatty acids:
to improve infant development ☹
to treat hypertriglyceridemia ☹☹☹

Scientifically Unproven
For any other indication

● Further Reading

Agency for Healthcare Research and Quality: *www.ahrq. gov/clinic/epcindex.htm#dietsup.* Accessed December 22, 2005, for the following:

Effects of Omega-3 Fatty Acids on Cardiovascular Risk Factors and Intermediate Markers of Cardiovascular Disease. March 2004.

Effects of Omega-3 Fatty Acids on Cardiovascular Disease. March 2004.

Health Effects of Omega-3 Fatty Acids on Asthma. March 2004.

Effects of Omega-3 Fatty Acids on Cognitive Function with Aging, Dementia, and Neurological Diseases. February 2005.

Effects of Omega-3 Fatty Acids on Mental Health. July 2005.

Effects of Omega-3 Fatty Acids on Eye Health. July 2005.

Effects of Omega-3 Fatty Acids on Child and Maternal Health. August 2005.

Willett, Walter C. "Fish: Balancing Health Risks and Benefits." *American Journal of Preventive Health* 29, no. 4 (2005): 320 – 21.

PEPPERMINT

• What It Is

Peppermint has a long history of use as a mint and flavoring agent and as a medicinal agent. For the latter purpose, peppermint is available as an inhalant, as liquid extracts, as peppermint oil, and as a tea. Topical preparations include such household products as Bengay and Vicks VapoRub.

Peppermint products contain a significant amount of menthol (35 to 70 percent) along with many other closely related compounds. The peppermint plant is *Mentha piperita*, which is a hybrid of *Mentha spicata* (spearmint) and *Mentha aquatica* (water mint). Peppermint and spearmint contain many of the same compounds, but they differ most significantly in that menthol is absent from spearmint oil. Many of the characteristic properties of peppermint are attributed to menthol, and pharmaceutical-grade peppermint oil is usually standardized to contain 44 percent menthol.

• Claims

Claims about peppermint can be divided between those for internal use and those for external use. Internal use is said to help a variety of gastrointestinal disorders. It is said to aid in digestion, treat irritable bowel syndrome, reduce flatulence, treat stomach cancer, and relieve headaches. Peppermint (and menthol) are used externally for headaches, pain, muscle aches, itching, sunburn, and the musculoskeletal pain of arthritis, neuralgia, and rheumatism.

• Study Findings

Animal studies have demonstrated that peppermint oil and menthol relieve intestinal spasms. A small number of controlled studies (✓✓) have shown that peppermint reduces colon spasms that occur when people have barium enemas and endoscopy. Nine controlled trials have examined peppermint oil either applied directly to the colon or taken orally for intestinal spasms. Although most of these studies were not blinded, all but one showed that peppermint oil reduces intestinal spasms more than placebo.

Irritable bowel syndrome (IBS) is experienced by many people and is an uncomfortable condition that is without satisfactory treatments. A 2005 review (✓✓✓) located fifteen randomized double-blind trials of peppermint oil for IBS. Twelve compared peppermint to placebo, and in eight peppermint was found to be more effective. The three others compared peppermint to conventional drugs, and the two treatments were found to be equivalent. These reviewers concluded that peppermint may be the treatment of choice for IBS involving nonserious diarrhea or constipation. One study (✓✓✓) of IBS enrolled children eight to twelve years old and found enteric-coated peppermint capsules significantly better than placebo.

"Dyspepsia" is a medical term for generalized stomach pain of uncertain origin. Peppermint is commonly recommended for such conditions. A 2002 review (✓✓✓) found nine controlled trials of several peppermint products, although all of them contained at least one other herb. Four of the studies used enteric-coated capsules containing a fixed combination of peppermint and caraway available in Germany as a commercial product (Enteroplant). In all these studies, people reported significantly greater relief from the peppermint products compared to placebo. However, some of the studies were poorly designed, and dyspepsia is particularly susceptible to the placebo effect. One study that used only placebos found that 80 percent of people with dyspepsia reported improvements with placebo, with 50 percent reporting marked improvements.

Laboratory studies have shown that the topical actions of peppermint are due to menthol. This stimulates the nerves that detect cold, leading to the typical cooling sensation. The nerves that perceive pain and itching are depressed. This leads to dilation of the blood vessels, which can promote healing. In spite of the widespread use of such preparations, little controlled research has studied peppermint's effectiveness topically.

Cautions

The types of adverse effects reported in studies include heartburn, diarrhea, nausea, and other gastric complaints. These are believed to arise when peppermint relaxes smooth muscles in the upper digestive tract, which allows stomach acid to irritate the esophagus. Enteric-coated capsules have been developed to ensure the active ingredients are released after the capsules pass through the stomach. This allows relaxation of the intestinal smooth muscles and helps to minimize the adverse effects. Some people are allergic to mint, which can manifest as skin irritation or asthmatic symptoms.

Steam distillation of the leaves produces peppermint oil, which contains numerous components, including pugelone. Pugelone does not have any use. While up to 1 percent pugelone is safe, oil with more

than that is toxic to the kidneys and liver. It is therefore important that only high-quality peppermint oil is used to eliminate the chance of getting a toxic level.

Peppermint oil has been found to stimulate menstrual flow and therefore should not be used during pregnancy. Infants and children should not be given peppermint oil or extracts. Topical preparations should not be used on cuts or broken skin.

Recommendations

Peppermint oil has a long tradition of use in food and medicine. Care must be taken to ensure that it is not used on broken skin and that medical attention is sought if the condition does not improve.

Oral use of peppermint oil has been shown to be of benefit in relieving intestinal spasms. The enteric-coated product must be used to ensure effectiveness in the intestines and to minimize adverse effects in the upper gastrointestinal tract. High-quality products are especially important to ensure that the enteric coating has been applied properly and that toxic pugelone levels are minimized.

Dosage

Enteric-coated capsules containing 0.2 ml of peppermint oil are usually taken three times daily in between meals. For dyspepsia, a dose of 90 mg of peppermint oil per day has been used in combination with caraway oil. Topical preparations to relieve pain contain at least 1 percent menthol and are usually applied three or four times daily. For tension headaches, 10 percent peppermint oil in an ethanol solution applied across the forehead and temples and then reapplied after fifteen and thirty minutes is recommended.

Treatment Categories

Complementary

As enteric-coated capsules, to relieve intestinal spasms ☺☺☺

As enteric-coated capsules to relieve the symptoms of irritable bowel syndrome ☺☺

Orally to relieve dyspepsia ☺☺

Topically to relieve pain and itching ☺☺

Topically to treat post-herpetic neuralgia ☺

Inhaled to prevent postoperative nausea ☹

Scientifically Unproven

For any other indication

Further Reading

Grigoleit, H. G., and P. Grigoleit. "Peppermint Oil in Irritable Bowel Syndrome." *Phytomedicine* 12, no. 8 (August 2005): 601–6.

Thompson Coon, J., and E. Ernst. "Systematic Review: Herbal Medicinal Products for Non-Ulcer Dyspepsia." *Alimentary Pharmacology and Therapeutics* 16, no. 10 (October 2002): 1689–99.

PROBIOTICS

What They Are

In the dairy aisle at grocery stores, the word "probiotics" is visible on more and more products, especially yogurts. The term refers to microorganisms or components of microbes that are beneficial to the health and well-being of the consumer. The idea of adding bacteria to our diet may seem counterintuitive given our familiarity with taking antibiotics to eliminate bacteria. However, the idea is catching on and has a reasonable basis.

The human gastrointestinal (GI) tract is home to about four hundred different species of bacteria and yeast. A delicate balance between health-promoting and disease-causing (or pathogenic) microbes is crucial for human health. Probiotics are believed to restrain the growth of pathogenic organisms and promote the growth of healthy microbes.

The general idea behind probiotics was presented in 1908 by the Russian Nobel Prize winner Elie Metchnikoff. He claimed that Bulgarian peasants who regularly consumed yogurt lived longer because of *Lactobacillus* organisms in the yogurt. Various *Lactobacillus* species, especially *Lactobacillus acidophilus*, remain prominent among the organisms used in probiotics. Various fermented dairy products, such as yogurt, cheese, and buttermilk, can contain probiotics, which are also available in tablets, capsules, and powders as dietary supplements.

Claims

Reduced intake of fermented foods in Western diets and increased use of antibiotics are alleged to have tipped the GI microbial balance more in favor of pathogenic organisms. Supplementation with probiotics is proposed as one strategy to restore a healthy balance and prevent disease. They are thus promoted as beneficial for a healthy diet. Probiotics are also said to treat a number of specific diseases. These include diarrhea, inflammatory bowel disease, Crohn's disease, irritable bowel syndrome, and other GI tract disturbances. They are also said to reduce the severity of some allergic reactions and to stimulate the immune system.

• Study Findings

Numerous laboratory and animal studies have demonstrated how *Lactobacillus* and other organisms have beneficial effects. As they grow, they compete with pathogenic organisms for nutrients in the GI tract. As the probiotic organisms grow, they produce chemicals called "bacteriocins." These include lactic acid, acetic acid, and hydrogen peroxide, which can alter the GI environment to make it less suitable for pathogenic microbes. Probiotics also enhance the body's immune reaction and prevent the attachment of pathogenic organisms to the GI tract so they are eliminated more quickly.

Controlled research in humans is furthest along for the use of probiotics in treating diarrhea. A 2003 Cochrane review (✓✓✓✓) found twenty-three controlled trials of various probiotics for diarrhea caused by infectious organisms. This form of diarrhea is especially problematic in developing countries, where it contributes to the deaths of 2 million to 3 million children every year. When adults or children with infectious diarrhea started taking probiotics, the proportion with diarrhea three days later was significantly lower than in the placebo groups. On average, the episodes were thirty hours shorter. Controlled studies have shown that probiotics are effective with some, but not all, types of diarrhea found in developing countries. Diarrhea caused by broad-spectrum antibiotics responds well to probiotics, as do some forms of viral diarrhea.

Irritable bowel syndrome is characterized by abdominal pain, bloating, flatulence, and diarrhea or constipation. One randomized controlled trial (✓✓✓) found that probiotics led to improvements in flatulence only. Another controlled study found improvements in biochemical tests, but not in the symptoms reported (✗✗✗) by patients.

Crohn's disease is one of several conditions arising from inflammation of the bowels. GI discomfort and pain occur in various ways. These conditions have environmental, genetic, and microbial causes. Several case studies (✓✓) have reported relief of symptoms after patients began taking probiotics. A number of small studies (✓✓✓) have similarly shown beneficial effects. However, all these studies had methodological flaws, making it difficult to draw definite conclusions.

People who are lactose intolerant are not able to digest milk products without significant GI discomfort. Reports (✓✓) have documented that some lactose-intolerant people were able to comfortably consume probiotic milk products, presumably because the microbes digest the lactose. However, many other lactose-intolerant people have not been able to digest milk-based probiotics.

Research on probiotics is a relatively new but rapidly growing field. For example, the early 2006 edition of the Cochrane Library contained only one completed review on probiotics (described above). The same edition also listed six other reviews that were being prepared at that time to provide evidence on six other conditions for which probiotics were being used.

Cautions

The most frequently reported adverse effect of probiotics is flatulence. In many people, this normalizes after a number of days of taking probiotics. Although probiotics are naturally occurring microbes, cases (✖✖) have been reported of infections from the products.

An improved microbial environment in the GI tract may lead to better absorption of vitamin K, which will reduce the effectiveness of warfarin, a drug taken to prevent blood clotting.

Product quality is a significant problem with probiotics. Standardization has not yet been developed for the best organisms to use or how to prepare the products. This leaves questions as to whether probiotic foods contain a sufficient number of organisms to have the desired effects. Dietary supplements made from probiotics are of unknown quality.

Recommendations

The use of probiotics is a new and developing area. The rationale for their use is well established. Their effectiveness and safety in treating GI diseases have been demonstrated for a small number of conditions. Signs from preliminary research are positive in other areas. Numerous different organisms are used in probiotics, and each may have different effects. Even different strains of the same species have been found to have different effects, making standardization important but difficult.

The place of probiotics in a generally healthy diet has not been established. Changes to the Western diet have contributed to fewer foods being produced by fermentation, which may have had some detrimental effects. Adding these back into a balanced diet using probiotic foods may have some beneficial health effects. However, much more research is needed before this can be asserted with confidence. Evidence does show that probiotics can be beneficial when used as part of the treatment regimen for a number of GI diseases, especially particular types of diarrhea.

Dosage

Most research reports using doses of 1 to 10 billion organisms per day divided into three or four doses. Products should indicate the amount needed to deliver a particular number of organisms.

Treatment Categories

Complementary

To treat infectious diarrhea, especially viral or caused by antibiotics	☺☺☺☺
To treat bacterial diarrhea	☺☺
To treat Crohn's disease	☺☺
To treat irritable bowel syndrome	☺
To overcome lactose intolerance	☹

Scientifically Unproven

As part of a healthy, balanced diet	☺☺
For any other indication	

Further Reading

Broekaert, Ilse J., and W. Allan Walker. "Probiotics as Flourishing Benefactors for the Human Body." *Gastroenterology Nursing* 29, no. 1 (January/February 2006): 26–34.

Chermesh, Irit, and Rami Eliakim. "Probiotics and the Gastrointestinal Tract: Where Are We in 2005?" *World Journal of Gastroenterology* 12, no. 6 (February 2006): 853–57.

PSYLLIUM

What It Is

Recent interest in psyllium has brought it to twelfth place in *Nutrition Business Journal*'s 2004 order of sales. One particular product, Metamucil, has been on the market for many years as a bulk laxative to relieve constipation. The product is made from the seeds and seed husks of *Plantago psyllium* and *Plantago ovata*. These plants are part of the plantain group and are members of the buckwheat family. The psyllium used here is also called "blond psyllium" to distinguish it from other types of seeds.

The seeds and seed husks can be added to food or are dried and ground into a powder. Most commercial products use only the husk. This contains 10 to 30 percent mucilage, which is a water-soluble fiber. When mixed with water, this forms a viscous gel that moves through the intestine without being absorbed.

Claims

Psyllium is most commonly used to treat digestive problems. As a viscous liquid, it counteracts diarrhea by absorbing water, making the stools more viscous and delaying passage of materials through the intestines. For those with constipation, the gel lubricates the intestines, and substances in psyllium directly stimulate contraction of the intestinal smooth muscles. Psyllium is also said to be beneficial to lower blood glucose and cholesterol levels, to prevent heart disease, and to provide some relief for those with irritable bowel syndrome.

Study Findings

Several randomized double-blind trials have examined psyllium's use as a laxative. Some, but not all, studies showed that psyllium was more effective than placebo in increasing stool frequency. One open trial found psyllium more effective in relieving constipation than a number of other laxatives. One controlled trial found psyllium more effective than senna. A product containing both psyllium and senna (called Agiolax) was found to have better laxative effects than psyllium alone in two studies. Six small controlled trials (✓✓✓) found Agiolax had better results than lactulose, a conventional laxative used as the standard in comparison trials. Overall, studies (✓✓✓) have found psyllium to be effective and relatively well tolerated.

Numerous controlled studies (✓✓✓) have documented that psyllium seed husks or seeds can lead to moderate reductions in total cholesterol of 3 to 14 percent and reductions in low-density lipoprotein (LDL) levels (so-called bad cholesterol) of 5 to 10 percent. Psyllium does not usually lead to increases in high-density lipoprotein (HDL) levels (so-called good cholesterol). However, the LDL to HDL ratio does improve significantly after six months of treatment. Greater benefits can be achieved when psyllium is added to a low-fat diet that is high in fruits and vegetables. When psyllium is taken along with conventional drugs, the same benefit can be achieved with reduced drug doses. The FDA allows foods containing at least 1.7 grams of psyllium per serving to be labeled with the claim that they may reduce the risk of heart disease when consumed as part of a diet low in fat and cholesterol.

A smaller number of studies (✓✓✓) have found that psyllium reduces blood sugar levels in people with diabetes, but not in those who do not have diabetes. The effect is maximal when psyllium is added to a meal, resulting in 14 to 20 percent lower blood glucose levels immediately after the meal. Glucose and cholesterol combine with the psyllium fiber in the intestine, which prevents or slows their absorption. Some claim that fiber similarly combines with carcinogens to prevent cancer. Controlled studies were not found to support this claim.

Cautions

Psyllium can cause flatulence, constipation, diarrhea, dyspepsia, and abdominal pain. Those taking psyllium should begin with a low dose and have their reaction to the product monitored. Plenty of water must be consumed along with psyllium. Some people have allergic reactions to psyllium, and care should be taken with those who have several allergies. Psyllium is also known to combine with iron supplements. Those taking iron supplements, or at risk for low iron, should carefully monitor their intake of psyllium. Those with stable diabetes should consult their physician before adding psyllium to ensure that any changes are detected quickly.

Recommendations

Psyllium and other forms of fiber can be recommended as laxatives that are relatively well tolerated. They sometimes produce side effects, but these are mild and transient. Psyllium appears to be effective in relieving some gastrointestinal disorders. The fiber also produces a moderate but significant reduction in cholesterol and blood glucose levels.

The maximal benefit is obtained when psyllium is included as part of a reduced-calorie diet that is low in cholesterol.

Dosage

Orally, as a laxative, the most common dose is 7.5 grams of psyllium seeds, taken with large amounts of water. The dose is divided up and taken separately, two to four times daily. However, a dose of up to 40 grams has been recommended in some studies.

Treatment Categories

Conventional
As a bulk laxative to relieve
  relatively mild constipation   ☺☺☺☺

Complementary
To reduce cholesterol levels   ☺☺☺
To reduce glucose levels in type 2
  diabetic patients   ☺☺
To relieve the symptoms of irritable
  bowel syndrome   ☺☺
To treat diarrhea   ☺
To treat hemorrhoids   ☺
To treat hypertension as part
  of a low-fat diet   ☺

Scientifically Unproven
For any other indication

Further Reading

Ramkumar, Davendra, and Satish S. C. Rao. "Efficacy and Safety of Traditional Medical Therapies for Chronic Constipation: Systematic Review." *American Journal of Gastroenterology* 100, no. 4 (April 2005): 936–71.

RED YEAST RICE

● What It Is

Lovers of Chinese food have long been familiar with red yeast rice, though they may not realize that fact. A number of Chinese fish and meat dishes have a red color that comes from red yeast. Red yeast rice is the product of rice fermented with the *Monascus purpureus* yeast. It is used as a food preservative and flavor enhancer and for making red rice wine.

Red yeast rice is mentioned in a traditional Chinese medicine book called the *Ben Cao Gang Mu*, written during the Ming Dynasty (1368 – 1644). The medical text states that red yeast rice is helpful in improving blood circulation and reducing blood clotting. Researchers in China published studies in the 1990s showing that animals fed red yeast rice had reduced cholesterol levels. These studies used red yeast rice either as a dried powder called Zhitaior or as an alcohol extract called Xuezhikang.

A company in the United States called Pharmanex began importing the Zhitai form of red yeast rice and marketed it as a proprietary dietary supplement called Cholestin. Then the controversy started. The makers of Mevacor, a prescription cholesterol-lowering drug, claimed Cholestin violated their patent. The active ingredient in Mevacor is lovastatin, a member of the "statin" group of drugs. Cholestin contains naturally occurring lovastatin and other statins.

In 1998, the FDA ruled that Cholestin should not be regulated as a dietary supplement. The 1994 Dietary Supplement Health and Education Act (DSHEA) states that a dietary supplement cannot contain a substance already approved as a drug unless the supplement was commercially available before the drug's approval. The FDA's 1998 ruling was overturned but was later upheld in federal court. Cholestin was ruled to be an unapproved drug and taken off the market in the United States until such time as it provides the required research to support its approval as a new drug. The product remains on the market in Canada, Asia, and Europe and on the Internet.

In a final twist to this saga, Pharmanex announced "a new and improved version" of Cholestin in 2001. The product has the same name and is said to have the same benefits, but it now contains what the company says is policosanol, not lovastatin. The company says its policosanol is an extract of beeswax, but all other sources state it is an extract of sugarcane. The two extracts are mixtures of similar compounds, but the relative proportions of the compounds are completely different. For example, sugarcane policosanol contains 50 to 80 percent octacosanol, while the beeswax extract contains 14 to 22 percent octacosanol. The company states that clinical research supports policosanol having a cholesterol-lowering effect, but that research was carried out on the sugarcane extract, not their product. The company states that "it is expected" that the beeswax and sugarcane extracts will have the same effects. However, a randomized study in 2006 showed that sugar cane policosanol was no better than placebo in lowering cholesterol levels.

Many other red yeast rice products are available on the Internet marketed on the basis of research done on Cholestin when it contained red yeast rice.

Claims

Red yeast rice is sold as a dietary supplement, said to promote healthy blood cholesterol levels. Some say that it both controls high cholesterol levels in patients with elevated levels and maintains desirable levels of cholesterol in those with normal levels. This is important because high cholesterol levels are known to promote the buildup of plaque in the arteries (atherosclerosis). This restricts the flow of blood through the vessels, which can lead to increased blood pressure and a higher chance of heart attack or stroke.

Study Findings

Cholesterol is present in the blood in a number of different forms, including low-density lipoproteins (LDL) and high-density lipoproteins (HDL). Blood tests are reported in terms of total cholesterol, LDL cholesterol, and HDL cholesterol. Studies have found that having low values for the first two measures (total cholesterol and LDL) and a high value for the third (HDL) is most desirable. A small number of studies in China (✓✓✓) showed that both Zhitai and Xuezhikang reduce total cholesterol and LDL cholesterol levels, while simultaneously increasing the HDL cholesterol level.

The first clinical trial of red yeast rice Cholestin (✓✓✓) in the United States was published in February 1999 and reported that it reduced total cholesterol by 16 percent and LDL cholesterol by 22 percent, but left HDL cholesterol levels unchanged. Three other small studies (✓✓✓) have subsequently confirmed these findings. These results were not unexpected.

Conventional medicine has been using a group of drugs called "statins" since 1987 to reduce choles-

terol levels. The first of these was isolated from yeast of the same genus as that used in red yeast rice. That compound was called "lovastatin" and is commercially available as a drug called Mevacor. Analysis of red yeast rice Cholestin revealed that it also contains lovastatin, along with eight other statin-like compounds. Taking the daily recommended dose gives a person the equivalent of about 10 mg of statins. Patients given 10 mg of Mevacor got almost the same amount of lovastatin and had a 17 percent reduction in LDL cholesterol — compared to the 16 percent reduction found with red yeast rice Cholestin. Such data underlies why the FDA sought to have Cholestin regulated as a drug.

While evidence supports the medical use of statins by people with high cholesterol levels, we are not aware of any evidence demonstrating that healthy people with normal cholesterol levels will benefit from taking any red yeast rice product.

Cautions

Studies of red yeast rice have reported no adverse effects other than stomach disturbance in a small number of patients. However, Mevacor has been found to cause liver damage, muscle pain, and kidney damage in a small number of patients. For these reasons, patients taking Mevacor are cautioned to have their livers checked regularly. The same advice would apply to users of red yeast rice.

Because developing fetuses require cholesterol in unique ways, these drugs may harm the unborn. Animal studies have found abnormalities in developing bones. Hence, these products are not recommended for women who might become, or already are, pregnant. The FDA rating for lovastatin is an X rating, meaning that it should never be taken during pregnancy. We can find no studies showing the products are safe in lactating women, and therefore they would best be avoided while breast-feeding. In addition, the safety of red yeast rice (and statins) in children (under eighteen) has not been established, and we therefore recommend against children using these products.

Given that red yeast rice contains the same type of drugs as contained in the pharmaceutical statins, the same cautions and concerns should exist with it. While the presence of other constituents in the preparation may act to prevent some of these side effects, this has not been demonstrated in long-term studies. One of the reasons some drugs are available only by prescription is to ensure adequate monitoring by physicians. Since red yeast rice is available as an unregulated dietary supplement, people will use it to self-medicate without having the blood tests necessary to monitor for any liver damage. While this will not be a problem for the majority of people, it may be for others — and we have no way of predicting whose liver might be damaged by any of the statins. Furthermore, without monitoring of blood cholesterol levels, some people may take it without needing to, and others with very high cholesterol levels may not reduce their cholesterol enough.

Be aware that taking red yeast rice within twenty-four hours of ingesting grapefruit products increases the risk of adverse effects. In 2006, researchers identified the cause of this problem as furanocoumarins in grapefruit. Until grapefruit products free of these compounds are available, do not take red yeast and grapefruit products at the same time.

Before Cholestin was reformulated to remove all red yeast rice, Heber and colleagues examined nine red yeast rice products for their statin-like ingredients (called "monacolins"). None of the other products contained the same ten monacolins as red yeast rice Cholestin. Total monacolin content varied from 0 to 0.58 percent. Total amount of lovastatin ranged from 0.15 to 3.37 mg per capsule. Red yeast rice Cholestin contained 2.46 mg per capsule. Only Cholestin and one other product were found to be free of citrinin, a toxic fermentation by-product that is known to cause genetic changes and kidney damage. Damage has been detected at 0.2 to 1.7 microgram levels. Six of the products had more than that per capsule, and one had 64.7 micrograms per capsule. Because of these many concerns, the American Heart Association has cautioned against using red yeast rice products pending the results of long-term studies.

Recommendations

Red yeast rice appears to be a natural remedy that does what it claims to do — at least for those with elevated cholesterol levels; however, there is no evidence that it helps those with normal levels of cholesterol or triglycerides (a general term for all blood lipids). People with mildly elevated cholesterol levels may benefit from it. It is less expensive than the pharmaceutical products, but then it also comes unmonitored.

The winding history of Cholestin reveals, yet again, the regulatory problems with dietary supplements. A product that appeared to be effective, safe, and manufactured under high-quality conditions has been lost from the market. Its place has been taken by low-quality products being marketed on the coattails of the higher-quality product. Yet the same brand name is being used for a completely different product, probably leading to confusion among those who are aware of the research on red yeast rice. Before using red yeast rice, find a high-quality product and arrange to have regular blood tests for liver function. Cholesterol levels are best kept in check by a combined strategy of diet, exercise, stress reduction, and, in some cases, drug therapy.

Dosage

Most clinical studies used the old form of red yeast rice Cholestin. Nevertheless, most other red yeast rice products claim to contain a similar amount of red yeast rice (600 mg). For hypercholesterolemia, a typical dose of red yeast rice is 1200 mg two times daily with food. A total daily dose of 2400 mg of red yeast rice contains approximately 9.6 mg of total statins, of which 7.2 mg is lovastatin. For products that are not standardized, dosing will be uncertain.

Treatment Categories

Complementary

To lower elevated cholesterol
or triglyceride levels ☺☺☺☺

Scientifically Unproven

To control normal cholesterol
or triglyceride levels ☹☹
For any other indication

Risk of Serious Side Effects

Liver damage is a rare
but serious side effect. ⊘⊘
Many products are contaminated
with the toxin citrinin. ⊘⊘⊘⊘
Do not use during pregnancy. ⊘⊘⊘⊘

Further Reading

Heber, David, Audra Lembertas, Qing-Yi Lu, Susan Bowerman, and Vay L. W. Go. "An Analysis of Nine Proprietary Chinese Red Yeast Rice Dietary Supplements: Implications of Variability in Chemical Profile and Contents." *Journal of Alternative and Complementary Medicine* 7, no. 2 (2001): 133 – 39.

Journoud, Mélanie, and Peter J. H. Jones. "Red Yeast Rice: A New Hypolipidemic Drug." *Life Sciences* 74, no. 22 (April 2004): 2675 – 83.

SAM-e

• What It Is

SAM-e (S-adenosyl-L-methionine) is a naturally occurring compound found throughout the human body, but in particularly high concentrations in the liver and brain. It is required for the normal production of many hormones and membranes. Since 1975, commercial SAM-e preparations have been available by prescription in different European countries for depression and other conditions. These entered the United States market in 1999 and rapidly became popular.

• Claims

The most widespread claims for SAM-e are to treat depression, osteoarthritis, and liver disease. Many other uses are promoted based on claims that supplementation can restore youthful levels of SAM-e and overcome conditions said to be related to deficiencies.

• Study Findings

Initial interest in SAM-e arose after depressed patients were noticed to have reduced levels of SAM-e. Other compounds involved in SAM-e activities were also found to be outside normal ranges in people with major depression. This led to the use of SAM-e as a treatment for depression. Over forty-five controlled clinical trials have been conducted in this area. However, SAM-e is poorly absorbed from the intestinal tract and rapidly broken down in the body. For this reason, in Europe SAM-e is usually administered by injection, and much of the research has been conducted there. Both intravenous and intramuscular injections are used. In contrast, SAM-e is available in the United States as a dietary supplement with all the usual concern about quality.

Starting in the 1970s, several unblinded studies (✓✓) showed that injected SAM-e produced significant improvements in depressed patients. These results were confirmed in randomized double-blind studies (✓✓✓). Injected SAM-e has been shown to have similar effectiveness to conventional antidepressants. Early studies with oral SAM-e did not show greater effectiveness than placebo. In the early 1990s, the FDA required a number of trials of oral SAM-e to stop because of problems found with poor release of SAM-e from tablets. A number of later studies (✓✓✓) found oral SAM-e to be more effective than placebo and as effective as conventional antidepressants. A 2002 review sponsored by the Agency for Health Research and Quality (AHRQ) found twenty-eight studies of injection and oral formulations and combined their results in a meta-analysis (✓✓✓). This calculated that SAM-e could be expected to bring about a roughly 25 percent improvement in symptoms of depression compared to placebo. It found no statistically significant differences between SAM-e and conventional antidepressants. However, combining the results of injection and oral formulations is questionable.

SAM-e is naturally involved in reactions that lead to the production of cartilage. This has led to interest in its use in treating osteoarthritis. The 2002 AHRQ review found few studies of SAM-e for osteoarthritis compared to the number of studies conducted for depression. However, twelve studies (✓✓) were reported during the 1980s, but these were all unblinded studies that did not include a control group. Positive effects on pain were found in many. Since that time, one large randomized controlled trial (✓✓✓) found SAM-e more beneficial than placebo for relief of osteoarthritic pain. The AHRQ found a number of studies (✓✓✓✓) that found SAM-e as effective as conventional painkillers used with osteoarthritis. A 2004 controlled study (✓✓✓) found SAM-e as effective as Celebrex in relieving pain. SAM-e in all cases took longer to have its effect, but after a few weeks, the treatments were similar in pain relief effectiveness. There is no evidence that SAM-e reverses or prevents the damage caused by osteoarthritis.

The high level of SAM-e in the liver, along with results of animal studies, has suggested that SAM-e may protect the liver from damage. One study (✓✓✓) with alcoholic patients found that cirrhosis of the liver progressed more slowly in those given SAM-e. The AHRQ review (✓✓✓✓) found a small number of studies in which SAM-e was preferable to placebo in treating pruritus (itching). However, it was not as effective as conventional medications.

At least seven studies (✓✓) have examined SAM-e in treating fibromyalgia. This condition is characterized by general and chronic pain and often leads to depression. Many of these studies found benefits, but the trials did not include placebo controls and the results were based mostly on subjective evaluations. However, the evidence from depression studies would support a role for SAM-e in treating fibromyalgia.

Cautions

Common side effects of SAM-e include gastrointestinal problems, jitteriness, insomnia, and exacerbation of underlying manic symptoms. When compared to conventional drugs used for the same conditions, SAM-e in many cases appeared preferable. The number and severity of the adverse effects increase as the dose of SAM-e is increased.

Since SAM-e is expensive, many have been concerned about the quality and quantity of SAM-e in supplements. Another concern is that SAM-e can break down under certain circumstances resulting in less ingredient than what is stated on the label. In 2004, ConsumerLab.com purchased and tested ten SAM-e products. One product failed the tests, containing only 30 percent of the labeled amount of SAM-e.

Recommendations

SAM-e is a naturally occurring substance known to play an important role in many processes throughout the body. Clinical studies have clearly demonstrated beneficial effects for those with depression. Positive effects have also been seen with pain related to osteoarthritis. The evidence with other conditions is not so clear. However, product quality is a major concern with SAM-e. Even with the best of products, the active ingredient is poorly absorbed and quickly broken down in the body. There is much debate over what type of formulation will lead to the best results. SAM-e is an expensive supplement, and much of an oral dose will not survive digestion. This is why injected formulations are commonly used in Europe.

● Dosage

The usual dose given by injection is 200 to 400 mg daily. Oral doses are significantly higher, usually 800 to 1600 mg per day in divided doses. For depression, an oral dose of 1600 mg per day is most commonly used in clinical trials. For osteoarthritis, an oral dose of 200 mg three times daily is typical. For fibromyalgia, 800 mg per day is a typical dose.

● Treatment Categories

Complementary

To treat depression	☺☺☺
To relieve pain due to osteoarthritis	☺☺
To protect the liver from various types of damage	☺☺
To relieve fibromyalgia	☺☺

Scientifically Unproven

For any other indication

Risk of Serious Side Effects

If conventional drugs are stopped without medical supervision	⊘⊘⊘⊘

● Further Reading

Fetrow, C. W., and Juan R. Avila. "Efficacy of the Dietary Supplement S-Adenosyl-L-Methionine." *Annals of Pharmacotherapy* 35, no. 11 (November 2001): 1414–25.

Hardy, Mary, Ian Coulter, Sally C. Morton, Joya Favreau, Swamy Venuturupalli, Francesco Chiappelli, Frederico Rossi, Greg Orshansky, Lara K. Jungvig, Elizabeth A. Roth, Marika J. Suttorp, and Paul Shekelle. *S-Adenosyl-L-Methionine for Treatment of Depression, Osteoarthritis, and Liver Disease.* Evidence Report/Technology Assessment No. 64. AHRQ Publication No. 02-E034. Rockville, Md.: Agency for Healthcare Research and Quality, 2002. *AHRQ: www.ncbi.nlm.nih.gov/books/bv.fcgi?rid=hstat1a. chapter.2159.* Accessed December 23, 2005.

Papakostas, George I., Jonathan E. Alpert, and Maurizio Fava. "S-Adenosyl-Methionine in Depression: A Comprehensive Review of the Literature." *Current Psychiatry Reports* 5, no. 6 (December 2003): 460–66.

S

SAW PALMETTO

What It Is

Saw palmetto might be called the "great berry hope" of the aging male population. Rumored to at least maintain and possibly improve a man's sex life (some herbalists consider it to be an aphrodisiac), it has a history of use for genital and urinary tract problems. This was especially true with Native Americans, who also used the berries to create a tonic that was believed to improve nutritional health. In the first half of the twentieth century, saw palmetto tea was included in *The United States Pharmacopeia* and *The National Formulary*. In 2004, it was the third most purchased herbal remedy in the United States, according to *HerbalGram*.

Saw palmetto is a small palm tree found along the southeastern coasts of the United States and in the West Indies. It is also called the American dwarf palm tree, the palmetto shrub, or the cabbage palm. Its most common scientific name is *Serenoa repens*; however, other scientific names include *Sabal serrulata* and *Serenoa serrulata*. It produces blue-black berries early in the winter, and the herbal remedy is extracted from these.

Claims

Saw palmetto extract has been used traditionally as an aphrodisiac, a tonic for the male reproductive system, and a remedy for respiratory complaints, urinary conditions, migraine headaches, genital problems, and cancer. It has also been promoted to restore hair growth and to increase breast size. It is currently used most commonly for problems related to enlargement of the prostate gland. Benign prostatic hyperplasia (BPH) is the most common non-malignant tumor in men (which means it does not spread and thus is usually less serious than metastatic cancers).

Most men over sixty years of age have BPH, resulting in numerous urinary problems, which are irritating, frustrating, and embarrassing. While conventional pharmaceuticals are available, most commonly drugs called "finasteride" (Proscar) or "alpha blockers" (Hytrin, Cardura, Flomax), these have the potential to cause serious side effects such as impotence and dizziness. Recently the alpha blockers have been associated with increased death rates in patients with hypertension or heart disease. A natural, safe treatment available without a prescription is a very attractive option for many patients.

Study Findings

Most of the studies on saw palmetto extract have been done in Europe with standardized preparations called Prostagutt and Permixon. Many of these used small numbers of patients, but recent studies have been larger and better controlled. A 2002 Cochrane review found twenty-one controlled trials, eleven of which were evaluated as well controlled. Overall, these studies (✓✓✓✓) found saw palmetto extract close to twice as effective as placebo in improving urinary flow and relieving the symptoms of BPH.

When studies (✓✓✓✓) compared the extract to finasteride, they were equally effective, and people taking the berry preparation reported fewer problems with impotence. However, these studies used numerous types of saw palmetto preparations and were of relatively short duration (only two lasted six months or more). Another limitation is that finasteride has the advantage that its effects can be monitored by reduced size of the prostate and reduced blood levels of PSA (prostate specific antigen). Neither of these changes occurs when patients take saw palmetto, raising questions about whether and how saw palmetto makes physiological changes.

Some experts feel that saw palmetto may be most useful in stages I and II (early stage) BPH. Stage I is characterized by increased frequency of urination during the day and night, delayed onset of urination, and a weak stream. Stage II is characterized by the symptoms of stage I accompanied by failure to completely empty the bladder.

How saw palmetto might affect BPH is not precisely known. A significant proportion of the extract is made up of "free fatty acids," which may be responsible for its activities. How these would act is not clear. The extract also contains a number of steroids that act somewhat like estrogen, the female sex hormone. The most active of these, beta-sitosterol, was found (✓✓✓✓) to be as effective as pharmaceutical drugs used for BPH.

There is no convincing evidence that saw palmetto is effective in the treatment or prevention of prostate cancer.

Cautions

Side effects reported in clinical trials have been relatively mild, including headache, nausea, and dizziness. The compounds in saw palmetto that are most likely to be beneficial for BPH are water insoluble — not water soluble — so teas made from the plant material are not likely to be beneficial. Concerns that saw palmetto might falsely raise the PSA (prostate specific antigen) level in men have not proven to be warranted. Because of the steroids found in saw palmetto, it should not be used during pregnancy or breast-feeding.

Almost all the clinical research was done on standardized European extracts, which may differ from products available in the United States. Therefore, caution is needed in choosing reliable products. Free fatty acids are regarded as important active ingredients, with debate over the contribution from other compounds. The percent of plant material made up of free fatty acids is a standard way to determine the quality of saw palmetto products. The free fatty acid content of fourteen European brands was analyzed in 2004 and found to vary considerably. It was highest in Permixon (81 percent); the lowest was 41 percent. Such variation in free fatty acid content is likely to give different effects and may explain the variability seen in clinical trials.

ConsumerLab.com purchased fourteen saw palmetto products in 2002 and 2003 to determine their quality. Eight additional products were tested at the request of their manufacturers or distributors through the company's Voluntary Certification Program. Of the twenty-two products, seventeen passed testing and five failed (a 23 percent failure rate). A full list of the products is available at *www.consumerlab.com*. Interestingly, prices ranged from $4 to $20 for a one-month supply, with the $4 product passing the tests and the $20 product failing.

Recommendations

Saw palmetto appears to bring relief to many men who have an enlarged prostate gland. However, the evidence for this is based primarily on German products. Some of these are now available in the United States. Even European products vary considerably, as found in the 2004 study discussed above.

BPH is a condition for which treatment may be needed for many years. No studies have been done on people taking saw palmetto for extended periods of time. Caution is therefore needed, along with monitoring of vital functions. Before using saw palmetto, check with a health care professional for a proper diagnosis, as symptoms of BPH may signal other more serious conditions that require conventional treatment. Given its lower cost and fewer side effects, saw palmetto extract may be a helpful alternative for people with mild to moderate BPH.

Dosage

An extract containing 80 to 90 percent free fatty acids is recommended at a dose of 160 mg twice daily or 320 mg once daily.

Treatment Categories

Complementary

To relieve the symptoms of benign
prostatic hyperplasia (BPH)   ☺☺☺☺

Scientifically Unproven

To treat prostate cancer   ☹☹☹
To treat chronic (nonbacterial)
prostatitis   ☹
For any other indication

Risk of Serious Side Effects

If saw palmetto is used to treat
prostate cancer   ⊘⊘⊘⊘

Further Reading

Gong, Edward M., and Glenn S. Gerber. "Saw Palmetto and Benign Prostatic Hyperplasia." *American Journal of Chinese Medicine* 32, no. 3 (2004): 331 – 38.

Habib, F. K., and M. G. Wyllie. "Not All Brands Are Created Equal: A Comparison of Selected Components of Different Brands of *Serenoa repens* Extract." *Prostate Cancer and Prostatic Diseases* 7, no. 3 (2004): 195 – 200.

SELENIUM

What It Is

Selenium is a naturally occurring mineral with some remarkable properties. While we may think of other minerals as more familiar, such as copper, or more precious, such as silver, selenium has a unique property. Recent discoveries have found that it is the only trace element specified in our genetic code and that it forms its own amino acid. Biochemistry books have long noted that all the proteins of the body are built from twenty amino acids. Selenium is now known to make up the twenty-first amino acid.

The most abundant sources of organic selenium (that which is chemically bonded to amino acids and proteins) are seafood, cereal grains, liver, and Brazil nuts. The nuts are the richest source. Selenium is attached to a number of enzymes (which are proteins) that play crucial roles in protecting the body from oxidative damage. This may be how selenium impacts health.

Selenium also occurs in inorganic forms (as salt) and is in many ways similar to sulfur. Selenium is required in the diet, with a deficiency leading to specific forms of heart and osteoarthritic diseases. Deficiencies are more common in China, New Zealand, and most of Europe, where little selenium is found in the soil. Plants grown in these countries are selenium-deficient. Plants extract inorganic selenium from the soil and convert it into organic selenium.

Claims

The main claim regarding selenium is that it helps prevent cancer. This has made it one of the best-selling dietary supplements. It is also reported to protect against heart disease, infertility, muscular dystrophy, rheumatoid arthritis, depression, and aging. Some alternative practitioners recommend selenium to treat AIDS and to prevent heart disease, atherosclerosis, macular degeneration of the eye, and premature graying of hair. Selenium is also said to protect the skin from the damaging effects of ultraviolet light. Large amounts of selenium are found in human liver, spleen, and lymph, suggesting that it may play a role in immunity.

Study Findings

For a long time, people have believed that selenium protects against cancer, heart ailments, and other diseases and that it improves immunity. But studies report conflicting conclusions. Animal studies have clearly demonstrated that selenium reduces the risk of cancer. Uncontrolled studies (✓✓) have found that those who have lower blood levels of selenium have higher incidences of cancer. However, in controlled studies, the results have been less positive, although some lowering of cancer rates has been found compared to placebo.

HERBAL REMEDIES, VITAMINS, AND DIETARY SUPPLEMENTS

A 1996 study of selenium called the Nutritional Prevention of Cancer (NPC) trial caused quite a stir. Numerous reports have subsequently emanated from this large study. The NPC trial started as a randomized study to examine the possibility that selenium supplements protect people against basal-cell and squamous-cell skin cancers. The researchers recruited 1,312 patients from the eastern United States, where selenium levels in the soil and crops are low and skin cancer rates are high. All the patients had a history of skin cancer. Half the group received a placebo pill every day for an average of 4.5 years, and the other half took pills with 200 micrograms of selenium each day.

The NPC trial (✗✗✗) found that selenium supplements had no effect on skin cancers; however, halfway through the study, the researchers decided to look at other types of cancers and cancer mortality. They found some surprising results (✓✓✓). The people who had taken selenium had 63 percent fewer prostate cancers, 58 percent fewer colorectal cancers, and 46 percent fewer lung cancers than the placebo-treated group.

Overall, there were 39 percent fewer new cancers among those taking selenium, and half as many people in that group died from cancer. Since the selenium seemed to be so beneficial, the researchers stopped the placebo phase of the trial early so that everyone could benefit.

Weaknesses have been pointed out in the NPC trial. For example, few women were included. Furthermore, the results are not consistent with those of other studies — although some of those studies used lower doses of selenium. Therefore, the researchers and other cancer specialists are calling for further trials before any national recommendations are made about selenium supplementation to prevent cancer.

Another study in China (✓✓✓) found significantly lower cancer rates in people given supplements of selenium, beta-carotene, and vitamin E. However, China has selenium-deficient soil and it was not possible to determine which of the supplements may have led to the effects seen. A 2004 review (✓✓✓✓) of such trials showed that selenium supplementation significantly reduced the risk of some cancers. However, much remains to be understood about the best dose for selenium supplementation. A large randomized double-blind trial is under way that will hopefully provide many of the answers needed. This Selenium and Vitamin E Cancer Prevention Trial (SELECT) has recruited more than thirty thousand volunteers, but its results will not be available until 2013.

Regarding other uses of selenium, a 2003 Cochrane review (✗✗✗) of selenium supplement for preterm infants found three relevant trials. One found (✓✓✓) reduced incidence of sepsis (widespread infection) in preterm infants given selenium supplements. No differences were found (✗✗✗) in overall survival or in the reduction of neonatal chronic lung disease or eye problems related to prematurity. Observational studies have suggested a role for selenium in treating asthma. A 2004 Cochrane review (✓✓) was able to locate only one relevant study, which involved twenty-four patients. While subjective benefits were noted, objective improvements were not visible. Another 2004 Cochrane review (✗✗✗✗) examined the role of selenium in helping critically ill adults. A benefit has been proposed on the assumption that selenium improves the immune system and helps combat infection. Seven trials were found that supplemented seriously ill adults with selenium. No statistically significant improvements were found in any aspect of the health of these people.

Cautions

A condition called "selenosis" occurs (✖✖) when people take more than 1 mg (1000 micrograms [mcg] = 1 mg) of selenium daily. The effects range from a garlic-like odor on the breath to loss of hair and nails, diarrhea, skin lesions, nausea, vomiting, fatigue, irritability, muscle tenderness, tremor, light-headedness, facial flushing, liver and kidney dysfunction, and, in the extreme, death. Those with thyroid problems are particularly prone to these side effects. Even daily doses above 400 mcg may cause significant toxicity and should not be used.

For children, selenium is safe when used in doses below the Tolerable Upper Intake Level (UL) of 45 mcg per day for infants up to age six months, 60 mcg per day for infants seven to twelve months, 90 mcg per day for children one to three years, 150 mcg per day for children four to eight years, 280 mcg per day for children nine to thirteen years, and 400 mcg per day for children age fourteen years and older.

Selenium interacts with many drugs and vitamins, such as vitamins E and C. Most dietary selenium occurs in its organic form, but commercial supplements often use inorganic selenium. The two do not act in the same way, with organic selenium being preferable.

It is particularly important that women who are pregnant or lactating not exceed their RDA (65 mcg for pregnancy, 75 mcg for lactation). In the case of pregnancy, higher doses may cause birth defects or miscarriage.

Recommendations

Sufficient evidence exists to warrant supplemental selenium in the diet. Selenium is already being added to some foods and fertilizers, and selenium-rich crops are being developed. Selenium is readily available in some foods: you can get 120 mcg of selenium in just one Brazil nut grown in the region of Brazil that has soil rich in selenium. Other good sources are seafood (especially tuna), wheat germ, and bran.

Although more studies are needed, especially into the long-term effects of supplementation, selenium does appear to protect people against some types of cancers. However, caution should be exercised as this mineral produces toxicity at a relatively low level. If you take selenium and notice any changes in the strength or appearance of your fingernails, especially your thumbnails, you should immediately stop taking the selenium and discuss the matter with your primary health care provider.

Dosage

The 2000 Institute of Medicine (IOM) report on antioxidants set the daily recommended intake level for selenium at 55 mcg per day (65 mcg for pregnancy and 75 mcg for lactation). Food sources include seafood, liver, meat, grains, and Brazil nuts. The average daily intake is 106 mcg per day in the United States and 155 mcg in Canada, thus making supplementation unnecessary for most in North America. The IOM report set the selenium upper intake level for adults at 400 mcg per day. This maximum level is based on nutrients from all sources. More than this amount could cause selenosis, the toxic reaction described under Cautions.

• Treatment Categories

Conventional

In doses up to 75 mcg per day
as an antioxidant ☺☺☺☺

Complementary

In doses up to 200 mcg per day
to protect against cancer, in
particular the incidence of lung,
colon, rectal, and prostate cancers ☺☺☺

To protect against cardiovascular
disease ☹

To treat rheumatoid arthritis ☹

To treat osteoarthritis ☹

To treat HIV/AIDS ☹

To treat hypothyroidism ☹

Scientifically Unproven

For any other indication

Risk of Serious Side Effects

When taken in large doses ⊘⊘

• Further Reading

Clark, Larry C., Gerald F. Combs Jr., Bruce W. Turnbull, Elizabeth H. Slate, Dan K. Chalker, James Chow, Loretta S. Davis, Renee A. Glover, Gloria F. Graham, Earl G. Gross, Arnon Krongrad, Jack L. Lesher Jr., H. Kim Park, Beverly B. Sanders Jr., Cameron L. Smith, and J. Richard Taylor. "Effects of Selenium Supplementation for Cancer Prevention in Patients with Carcinoma of the Skin: A Randomized Controlled Trial." *Journal of the American Medical Association* 276, no. 24 (December 1996): 1957–63.

Rayman, Margaret P. "Selenium in Cancer Prevention: A Review of the Evidence and Mechanism of Action." *Proceedings of the Nutrition Society* 64, no. 4 (November 2005): 527–42.

Ryan-Harshman, Milly, and Walid Aldoori. "The Relevance of Selenium to Immunity, Cancer, and Infectious/Inflammatory Diseases." *Canadian Journal of Dietetic Practice and Research* 66, no. 2 (Summer 2005): 98–102.

SENNA

What It Is

The senna shrub, known technically as *Cassia senna* (other names include *Senna alexandrina* and *Cassia acutifolia*), has long been a part of medicine in the Middle East and northern Africa. The plant grew along the Nile River, where the leaves and berries were found to be a gentle laxative. Another form of senna, *Cassia angustifolia*, is found in India, where its properties are said to be similar.

The Arab nations introduced senna throughout Europe around the ninth or tenth century. Since then it has remained a popular natural laxative and is available in many over-the-counter pharmaceutical products (e.g., Senokot).

Claims

Senna has long been used to treat constipation and remains a popular laxative. In addition, senna has traditionally been used as a cathartic to clear toxins from the bowels. Native Americans used a senna species (*Cassia marilandica*) indigenous to eastern North America to reduce fevers. In a few cultures, senna also has been used to kill intestinal worms, alleviate indigestion, and treat ringworm and hemorrhoids. Traditional healers in northern Africa used it to heal various types of stomach pain. An unlikely traditional use, given that senna tastes awful, was as a mouthwash to freshen the breath.

Today senna is used almost exclusively to treat constipation and constipation-related disorders such as hemorrhoids and anal fissures. Senna is considered more potent than another widely used stimulant laxative, cascara sagrada bark (from the bush *Frangula purshiana*). Senna is sometimes combined with herbs such as ginger or coriander to avoid intestinal cramps. Senna is included for its laxative properties in some diet teas; however, the use of laxatives for weight loss is highly questionable and can be dangerous.

Study Findings

Compounds in senna called "anthraquinones" stimulate the colon to contract more frequently, moving material through the intestines faster. These compounds also cause secretion of electrolytes and water into the intestines to facilitate movement. A small number of randomized controlled trials (✓✓✓✓) support the use of senna as an effective, relatively safe laxative when used occasionally.

Senna has been compared with other conventional and herbal laxatives in controlled trials. A Spanish study (✓✓✓) found that senna had similar efficacy and adverse effects when used to treat constipation caused by opioid drugs in patients with advanced cancer. Senna was viewed as preferable because of its lower cost. However, another trial for constipation (✗✗✗) found lactulose more effective than senna. Another study in India (✗✗✗) found that senna worked as well as a liquid Ayurvedic herbal preparation, but recommended the latter because of its better taste and fewer side effects. Senna was compared to polyethylene glycol to clear the bowels prior to surgery of the colon or rectum in a randomized controlled trial. The colons of the patients who took senna were cleaner, and those patients reported it was easier to take compared to those taking the polyethylene glycol (✓✓✓). Senna has also been found to be as effective (✓✓✓) as another conventional laxative, sodium picosulfate. It was also found to relieve general constipation as effectively (✓✓✓) as adding 10 grams of bran to the diet.

Another herbal remedy used to treat constipation is psyllium. One controlled trial found psyllium more effective than senna. However, a combination of psyllium with senna (called Agiolax) was found to give better results than psyllium alone. Six small controlled trials (✓✓✓✓) have found Agiolax to have better results than lactulose, a conventional laxative.

• Cautions

Potential side effects (✗✗) of senna include diarrhea, nausea, and abdominal cramps or pain. Because of these side effects, most practitioners recommend trying milder laxatives before resorting to senna.

Pregnant or lactating women should avoid senna, as should persons with acute or chronic intestinal diseases and persons taking diuretics, steroids, or licorice, because senna interferes with their intestinal absorption. The Natural Database rates senna "possibly unsafe" during pregnancy, primarily because pregnant women should not self-medicate when constipated. The active ingredients pass into breast milk, so senna should not be used during lactation. Senna was reported as the second most commonly prescribed laxative by family physicians and pediatricians (after milk of magnesia). However, parents should be cautious about giving senna to children without medical consultation.

Extended use can also lead to more serious adverse effects from dehydration, potassium loss, and electrolyte imbalance, including muscle and heart ailments. For years there have been concerns that chronic (daily) use of senna can lead to a "laxative-dependency syndrome." This disorder leads to a poorly functioning colon, poor gastric motility, and laxative-induced diarrhea. We found little research evidence to support this concern, but authorities commonly recommend that laxatives such as senna not be taken for more than seven days in a row. Chronic use of senna can lead to a disorder called "pseudomelanosis coli," in which pigment is deposited in the lining of the intestine. This appears to be a harmless feature that usually goes away when people stop using senna. There are several case reports (✗✗) in the medical literature of long-term use or high doses of senna causing liver toxicity.

In 1996, California became the first state to require warning labels for products containing senna and other stimulant laxatives. Chronic use is also suspected of increasing the chances of getting colon cancer. This concern led the FDA in 2002 to reclassify senna from Category I (Generally Regarded as Safe) to Category III (More Data Needed). Manufacturers are now being required to produce evidence of the safety of senna products. The American Herbal Products Association recommends that senna leaf products contain this notice: "Do not use this product if you have abdominal pain or diarrhea. Consult a health care provider prior to use if you are pregnant or nursing. Discontinue use in the event of diarrhea or watery stools. Do not exceed recommended dose. Not for long-term use."

Senna teas are best avoided, as they deliver highly variable doses of active ingredients.

Recommendations

Senna is a readily available and inexpensive laxative. However, its effects may not occur for a number of hours and then can be rather dramatic! The ingredients in senna must be chemically broken down in the intestines before becoming active, which can take eight to twelve hours. It is important that additional tablets not be taken during this lag time. Less drastic products to treat constipation are commonly available. As with any laxative, senna should not be used for more than a week and is not a safe way to lose weight.

Dosage

The usual dose is 187 mg extract taken at bedtime. Standardized over-the-counter preparations should be used.

Treatment Categories

Conventional

To treat constipation
in the short term ☺☺☺☺

Complementary

To evacuate the bowel
for medical indications
and procedures ☺☺☺☺

Scientifically Unproven

For any other indication

Further Reading

Foster, Steven, and Varro E. Tyler. *Tyler's Honest Herbal: A Sensible Guide to the Use of Herbs and Related Remedies.* 4th ed. New York: Haworth Herbal, 1999, 355–57.

Ramkumar, Davendra, and Satish S. C. Rao. "Efficacy and Safety of Traditional Medical Therapies for Chronic Constipation: Systematic Review." *American Journal of Gastroenterology* 100, no. 4 (April 2005): 936–71.

Vanderperren, Bénédicte, Michela Rizzo, Luc Angenot, Vincent Haufroid, Michel Jadoul, and Philippe Hantson. "Acute Liver Failure with Renal Impairment Related to the Abuse of Senna Anthraquinone Glycosides." *Annals of Pharmacotherapy* 39, nos. 7–8 (July–August 2005): 1353–57.

S

SHARK CARTILAGE

• What It Is

Shark cartilage is a cancer therapy made popular by Dr. William Lane in his books *Sharks Don't Get Cancer* (1992) and *Sharks Still Don't Get Cancer* (1996). Lane believed that sharks do not get cancer. He noted that their skeletons don't contain bones but instead are made of cartilage that contains no blood vessels. Other research has shown that cancers require extensive blood supplies to grow. This occurs through a process called "angiogenesis." If cartilage contains something that prevents the growth of blood vessels, this might be able to stop cancers from growing by cutting off their blood supply. The search for effective "antiangiogenic" agents is a significant area of cancer research.

• Claims

Shark cartilage is sold in the United States as a dietary supplement and therefore does not have to be tested or regulated by the FDA. For this reason, it is advertised as beneficial for the health of bones and joints. However, its most popular reputation is as a treatment for cancer, especially breast, colon, intracranial, and spinal cancers. It is estimated that about 50,000 Americans use it every year for this purpose. One study found that shark cartilage was the most popular cancer remedy recommended in health food stores. Among Dutch cancer patients, 60 percent reported they had used the Houtsmuller Diet, named after a Dutch physician who claimed a diet rich in shark cartilage and other vitamins cured his cancer; the doctor has since admitted he never had cancer.

Shark cartilage is also used to treat psoriasis, intestinal inflammation and retina problems related to diabetes and to help in wound healing.

• Study Findings

Although Dr. Lane states he has research support for his claims about shark cartilage, the results of these studies are not very convincing. Research on animals has shown that cartilage from a variety of animals does slow the growth of blood vessels. Lane extracted shark cartilage and tested the product on humans in cancer clinics in Cuba and Mexico. This research led to three publications used to support shark cartilage's effectiveness against cancer. One study (✓✓) involved only eight patients and no control group. The second reported only differences in microscope slides made of tumors in treated and untreated animals. The third (✓✓) reported interviews with twenty-one cancer patients who contacted Lane to express their appreciation for his product. Taken together, these constitute extremely weak evidence for effectiveness.

One review of shark cartilage found five reports of studies, but all were small and poorly designed. Also, the reviewers were only able to locate brief summaries of the studies. Of these, three found no benefit from shark cartilage in patients with breast, prostate, or brain cancers, one found a "positive trend" among cancer patients, and the fifth found improved quality of life in half of the patients enrolled. A 1998 study published by Denis Miller and colleagues (✗✗✗) tested the safety and efficacy of shark cartilage in sixty patients with advanced forms of cancer. They found that shark cartilage was inactive with all forms of cancer studied, primarily breast, colon, and lung cancer. A small proportion of patients became stable during the study, but this was about the same percent as respond to placebos in other studies.

In response to popular usage, the National Cancer Institute sponsored the first randomized double-blind trial of shark cartilage, published in 2005. The study (✘✘✘) was designed to involve six hundred patients with advanced breast or colorectal cancer. After two years, only eighty-three patients had enrolled in the study when it was closed down by its oversight body. Such groups oversee clinical trials to ensure studies are conducted properly and do not continue any longer than necessary. The shark cartilage study was closed because there was clearly no benefit from the supplement compared to placebo. Also, half the people taking shark cartilage (according to the manufacturer's recommendations) had dropped out of the study within one month primarily because of gastrointestinal problems.

The search for effective antiangiogenic agents continues, and promising agents appear to be on the horizon. One of these (called AE-941, or Neovastat) has been isolated from an extract of shark cartilage and has shown promising results in early studies. The product is now being tested in a large controlled trial involving patients with lung cancer. Also, there is some evidence that AE-941 may improve the appearance of and decrease the itching caused by psoriasis. In addition, taking AE-941 orally seems to increase survival in patients with advanced renal cell carcinoma (the most common form of kidney cancer in adults). Because of these data, the FDA granted AE-941 orphan-drug status for renal cell carcinoma. This gives producers of drugs for relatively rare diseases tax breaks in the United States and a seven-year marketing monopoly if the drug is eventually approved for human use.

These approaches, however, are very different from the current way that shark cartilage is used as a dietary supplement. People are said to need 60 to 90 grams of shark cartilage per day to treat cancer. A dose of less than 0.1 gram of AE-941 is taken daily. The product is being made and tested according to the highest pharmaceutical standards. Its manufacturers are seeking approval for AE-941 as a regulated drug, not a dietary supplement. The results of studies with AE-941 do not provide evidence regarding shark cartilage supplements.

Cautions

No serious adverse effects have been reported in the trials conducted on shark cartilage. However, the huge doses recommended to treat cancer cause many gastrointestinal problems. It also has a strong fishy smell and taste, which makes it very unpalatable. The most common side effects are nausea, vomiting, a bad taste in the mouth, dyspepsia, dizziness, elevated blood sugar and calcium levels, decreased strength and performance, weakness and fatigue, altered consciousness, and constipation. Half the patients in both of the controlled studies (✘✘✘) reported significant problems of this type.

Another serious concern with shark cartilage, and other alternative cancer treatments, is that people may avoid effective treatments while taking these ineffective ones.

Recommendations

Shark cartilage costs about $700 to $1,000 per month. This is a high price to pay for a therapy with no evidence of effectiveness. While cancer remains a devastating disease, conventional medicine has developed reliable and effective treatments for some types of cancer. If the cancer progresses to the point where no effective treatments remain, studies show that shark cartilage used as recommended will negatively affect a patient's quality of life and provide no benefit. As difficult as this time can be, people should use the time to pursue spiritual and relational blessings rather than elusive "cures" such as shark cartilage.

Dosage

Doses recommended to prevent cancer range from 0.5 to 4.5 grams daily, divided into smaller doses taken thirty minutes before meals. To treat cancer, manufacturers recommend starting with 24 grams per day, increasing toward a goal of 96 grams per day.

Treatment Categories

Complementary

To treat cancer	☹☹☹☹
To prevent cancer	☹☹☹☹
To treat osteoarthritis	☹☹☹

Scientifically Unproven

For any indication

Quackery or Fraud

In the hands of some practitioners

Risk of Serious Side Effects

If used instead of effective
cancer treatment   ⊘⊘⊘⊘

Further Reading

Loprinzi, Charles L., Ralph Levitt, Debra L. Barton, Jeff A. Sloan, Pam J. Atherton, Denise J. Smith, Shaker R. Dakhil, Dennis F. Moore Jr., James E. Krook, Kendrith M. Rowland Jr., Miroslaw A. Mazurczak, Alan R. Berg, and George P. Kim. "Evaluation of Shark Cartilage in Patients with Advanced Cancer: A North Central Cancer Treatment Group Trial." *Cancer* 104, no. 1 (July 2005): 176–82.

Miller, Denis R., Gary T. Anderson, James J. Stark, Joel L. Granick, and DeJuran Richardson. "Phase I/II Trial of the Safety and Efficacy of Shark Cartilage in the Treatment of Advanced Cancer." *Journal of Clinical Oncology* 16, no. 11 (November 1998): 3649–55.

SOY

What It Is

During the 1980s, Westerners were confronted with the idea of small white cubes, called "tofu," replacing meat in their food. For some, tofu was another interesting way to change and improve their diet. For others, the tasteless, almost textureless cubes were an example of taking health foods too far. The blandness of soy tofu contrasted with soy sauce, which gained wider popularity. Then came tempeh (fermented soybeans), soy flours, and soy milk. Then recipe books claimed soy could be used to prepare tasty meals. Reports regularly appeared about additional health benefits of replacing animal protein with soy. Yet even among Americans convinced that soy consumption is healthy, only a small proportion eat soy products at least once a week. Almost all the health claims are based on daily consumption of soy.

In October 1999, the FDA approved the use of a health claim on foods containing soy. The labels were permitted to state that a daily diet of 25 grams of soy protein, as part of a diet low in saturated fat and cholesterol, may reduce the risk of heart disease.

This claim does not apply to soy dietary supplements. Interest in soy supplements increased after studies on hormone replacement therapy for menopausal women reported high levels of adverse effects.

Broadly speaking, soy can be divided into soy foods and soy supplements. Soybeans contain soy proteins and are used to make soy flour, soy milk, vegetable protein, tofu, and tempeh. Soybeans also contain a variety of compounds called "isoflavones," which are isolated and used to make soy supplements. These polyphenolic compounds are antioxidants but also have some of the same actions as the female hormone estrogen, though at a much weaker level. Because of these effects, they belong to a group of compounds called "phytoestrogens" (*phyto* means "having to do with plants"). The most abundant isoflavones in soy are called "genistein" and "daidzein." Soy sauce and soybean oil are made from soy, but they contain very small quantities of soy protein or isoflavones.

Claims

Addition of soy to the diet is said to have many beneficial health effects. These benefits are best achieved when animal proteins are replaced by soy. The 1999 FDA designation was based on hundreds of studies showing changes in blood lipids compatible with protection against heart disease. Soy is recommended as a healthy food that protects against many other diseases. The most commonly cited ones are kidney and gastrointestinal diseases, cancer, osteoporosis, menopausal symptoms, and reproductive problems.

Study Findings

Soy and its isoflavones have been shown in laboratory experiments to impact the body in different ways. Genistein both mimics and counteracts the effects of estrogen. It can stimulate the growth of some cancer cells and inhibits the growth of others. These properties give rise to the possibility of soy being useful in treatment of menopausal symptoms, but also to concerns that it might stimulate the growth of estrogen-dependent cancers, such as some breast cancers. Isoflavones also act as antioxidants, which may underlie their potential benefit in reducing the risk of heart disease.

A comprehensive review of the clinical evidence on soy was published by Ethan Balk and colleagues in August 2005. Their report for the Agency for Healthcare Research and Quality provides a comprehensive review of the controlled studies conducted on soy. Cardiovascular disease was the area with the most research. However, no controlled studies were found that examined the effectiveness of soy consumption in reducing cardiovascular disease or any related clinical events. Numerous epidemiological studies (✓✓) have shown that cultures with high soy consumption have reduced incidence of cardiovascular disease. All the controlled studies of soy consumption measured changes in various risk factors for cardiovascular disease.

Sixty-eight studies were found that measured various lipid levels, such as total cholesterol, high-density lipoprotein (HDL, or "good" cholesterol), or low-density lipoprotein (LDL, or "bad" cholesterol). The amount of soy consumed varied considerably, with an average of 36 grams of soy protein or 80 mg of isoflavones. Very few studies were rated as of good quality, about half were of fair quality, and another considerable number were of poor quality.

The results varied from study to study, but overall beneficial effects were found (✓✓✓). A relatively consistent benefit was found in the majority of studies, although the size of the benefit was only a few mg/dL.

The blood levels of several other substances are correlated with risk of various cardiac diseases. These substances include lipoprotein(a), C-reactive protein, and homocysteine. Twenty studies (✗✗✗✗) have examined the impact of soy on lipoprotein(a) levels, with almost all studies finding no benefit.

Three studies (✗✗✗✗) found no benefits in C-reactive protein levels from soy consumption. Five poorly designed studies (✓✓✓) found small beneficial changes in homocysteine levels.

Nine studies (✗✗✗) have examined the functioning of arteries or the flow of blood through them and found either no changes or small, insignificant changes. Twenty-five studies examined blood pressure changes related to soy consumption. A meta-analysis (✗✗✗✗) found no statistically significant benefit, although one study (✓✓✓) did find large reductions in blood pressure. The results of that one study have not been repeated in other studies. Overall, then, soy consumption, either as soy protein or purified isoflavones, has small beneficial effects on blood lipid levels. Other risk factors associated with heart disease have not been changed by soy consumption.

Surveys (✓✓) have found that countries where soy consumption is high have reduced incidences of various cancers. As with cardiovascular disease, though, no controlled studies have examined the impact of increasing soy consumption on the occurrence of cancer. Most have measured only risk factors for different cancers. The results have been inconsistent and inconclusive (✗✗✗✗). Three studies raised concerns that soy may stimulate some types of estrogen-dependent breast cancers. Although the overall data are inconclusive, women with breast cancer are usually cautioned against increasing soy consumption.

In countries where soy consumption is relatively high, only 10 to 20 percent of women have menopausal hot flashes, compared to 60 to 90 percent of women in Western countries. With heightened concern about the adverse effects of hormone replacement therapy, many women have turned to soy during menopause. Twenty-one studies measured soy's impact on menopausal symptoms, most commonly hot flashes. All studies found that the frequency and severity of hot flashes were reduced in both those who increased soy consumption and in the control or placebo groups. In half the studies, the soy group improved more than the placebo group, but in the other half there was no difference between the two groups. The two most recent controlled trials, one lasting two years, found no beneficial effects (✗✗✗). The significantly reduced incidence of menopausal symptoms in countries where soy consumption is high may result from many years of consuming soy.

Bone mineral density is an important factor in monitoring development of osteoporosis. Studies shorter than one year (✗✗✗) found no benefit from soy consumption. A few studies lasted longer than one year and found inconsistent results.

The impact of increased soy consumption has been studied for numerous other conditions. However, even fewer studies are available for these conditions, and the results are generally inconclusive.

A 2004 Cochrane review (✗✗✗) examined the effectiveness of soy infant formula for the prevention of generalized allergic reactions such as eczema and hay fever. The children in the five studies reviewed did not have milk allergies but did have a family history of allergies. There was no evidence that children fed soy formula had fewer allergic reactions compared to those fed cow's milk formula, whereas those fed soy had significantly greater allergic reactions compared to those fed a hydrolyzed protein formula. The review recommended against using soy formula when children do not have evidence of a milk allergy.

• Cautions

Soy is generally well tolerated by most people. However, a very small number of people can be allergic to it. Some people also get gastrointestinal problems after eating it. Those with cancers that are sensitive to estrogen (some breast cancers) should avoid soy. While eating soy is unlikely to cause any problems, high doses of isoflavone supplements may have adverse effects. One study of women taking 150 mg of soy isoflavones per day for five years found that they had higher levels of endometrial hyperplasia.

Concerns have also been raised about the long-terms effects on infants if they consume large amounts of soy instead of breast milk or dairy products. In 2005, Israel's health ministry warned that soy products should be limited in children and avoided in infants — although there may be no alternative for some infants (those with a milk allergy). The concern is based on the estrogen-like effects of soy and phytoestrogens and the unknown long-term effects of these compounds. Similar concerns have been expressed by health agencies in New Zealand, Australia, and the United Kingdom.

Labeling of isoflavone supplements is very confusing. In nature, most isoflavones are found connected to sugar molecules (called "glucosides"). A manufacturer may therefore choose to include the weight of the sugar in the stated amount of isoflavones in the product. In such products, as much as 40 to 50 percent of the claimed "isoflavones" may really be sugar. A more precise label will state just the weight of the isoflavone. The potency of two products claiming to contain the same amount of isoflavones can differ significantly, depending on how the isoflavone concentration is calculated.

In July 2005, ConsumerLab.com tested a number of isoflavone supplements. Most contained their claimed amounts of isoflavones and properly released their contents, but three did not. Two contained only roughly half of what their labels claimed, while a third failed to break apart and release its ingredients properly. ConsumerLab.com also warned that "even among products that passed testing, the amount of isoflavones varied."

Recommendations

Most people could benefit from replacing some animal protein with soy protein. This would be one way to increase the proportion of plant products in a healthy diet. There are many ways to increase soy in the diet through food and supplements. Many more resources are now available to plan tastier foods that contain soy. The benefits that can be expected are more likely to be those of a healthier diet rather than the prevention or treatment of any specific diseases. However, in general, infants should not be fed soy formula unless there is a medical reason to avoid milk-based formula.

Dosage

The usual recommendations are to include about 25 grams of soy protein in the daily diet, or about 50 mg of isoflavones. These could be obtained from four glasses of soy milk, one-third of a brick of tofu, or one serving of soy protein powder.

Treatment Categories

Complementary

As part of a plant-rich diet	☺☺☺
To reduce total and LDL cholesterol levels	☺☺☺
To reduce the risk of cardiovascular disease	☺

Scientifically Unproven

To prevent cardiovascular disease	☺
To treat cyclical breast pain (mastalgia)	☺
To reduce the risk of breast, endometrial, lung, or thyroid cancer	☺
To treat or prevent diabetic neuropathy	☺
To treat type 2 diabetes in postmenopausal women	☺
To reduce the severity or frequency of hot flashes	☺
To treat cardiovascular disease	☹☹☹
To prevent other cancers	☹☹
To reduce the severity or frequency of hot flashes in breast cancer survivors	☹☹☹
To prevent the development of osteoporosis	☹☹

Risk of Serious Side Effects

In infants who are not medically required to use soy formula	⊘⊘
In women at risk of estrogen-sensitive cancers	⊘⊘

Further Reading

Balk, Ethan, Mei Chung, Priscilla Chew, Stanley Ip, Gowri Raman, Bruce Kupelnick, Athina Tatsioni, Yannan Sun, Brian Wolk, Deirdre DeVine, and Joseph Lau. *Effects of Soy on Health Outcomes.* Evidence Report/Technology Assessment No. 126. AHRQ Publication No. 05-E024-2. Rockville, Md.: Agency for Healthcare Research and Quality, 2005. *AHRQ: www.ahrq.gov/downloads/pub/evidence/pdf/soyeffects/soy.pdf.* Accessed December 10, 2005.

Haimov-Kochman, Ronit, and Drorith Hochner-Celnikier. "Hot Flashes Revisited: Pharmacological and Herbal Options for Hot Flashes Management. What Does the Evidence Tell Us?" *Acta Obstetricia et Gynecologica Scandinavica* 84, no. 10 (October 2005): 972–79.

Siegel-Itzkovich, Judy. "Health Committee Warns of Potential Dangers of Soya." *British Medical Journal* 331 (July 2005): 254.

ST. JOHN'S WORT

What It Is

For centuries, many people plagued by emotions that led them to despair turned to St. John's wort (*Hypericum perforatum*) for relief. "St. John's" derives from the way the flower blooms around St. John's Day (June 24). Also, when the buds and flowers are squeezed, they exude a red pigment that was associated with the blood of John the Baptist.

Today depression has become a global concern. The World Health Organization estimates that depression will be the second leading cause of disability in the world by the year 2020. Some estimates claim that one in five people will become depressed at some point in their lives. Fifty years ago, the estimate was one in a thousand. Has life become harder, resulting in many more people suffering from depression? Or have people recognized that depression is something that should be talked about and that medicine should treat? Do more people now look for something to take to get rid of their depression?

Debate rages over all these issues. Prescriptions for antidepressants have skyrocketed. Some of the bestselling drugs in the world are the newer SSRI drugs such as Prozac and Zoloft. (SSRI stands for selective serotonin reuptake inhibitors, which describes the presumed way these drugs work.) At the same time, many turn to St. John's wort as the preferred way to treat mild depression. The remedy, made from an extract of the flowers of *Hypericum perforatum*, is the most widely prescribed antidepressant in Germany, used even more than Prozac. Over the last several years, it has been one of the bestselling herbal remedies in the United States.

Claims

St. John's wort is used primarily for mild to moderate forms of depression and anxiety. Some also recommend it for people with insomnia and generalized chronic fatigue. More recently, St. John's wort has been postulated as a treatment for viruses. Testing is in the very earliest stages to see if it — in particular, one of its active ingredients, hypericin — will have an impact against HIV infections. However, pending the outcome of the research that is just beginning, this remains conjecture.

Study Findings

Numerous clinical studies (✓✓✓✓) were conducted in Germany on St. John's wort during the 1990s. In 1996, Klaus Linde and colleagues published a review of prior research that was very influential in bringing St. John's wort to people's attention outside of Germany. This review concluded that St. John's wort was better than placebo, although it could not be determined if it worked better for one type of depression over another.

Linde published an updated review in 2005 that had stricter criteria for the studies it would consider. This review included thirty-seven different studies, reflecting the extensive research conducted on this herbal remedy. Twenty-six of these studies compared St. John's wort with placebos, and fourteen compared it with other conventional antidepressants. Both mild to moderate forms of depression and more severe depression were examined. The results of the review were complex but can be summarized as follows:

- Studies (✓✓✓) involving people with mild to moderate depression found that St. John's wort is more effective than placebo and of similar effectiveness to conventional antidepressants.
- The six most recent trials (✗✗✗) had the highest quality ratings and all involved people with major depression. St. John's wort was only minimally beneficial compared to placebo.
- The effectiveness of St. John's wort for depression was called into question based on two studies performed in psychiatric care clinics (✗✗). However, the overwhelming majority of evidence in primary care clinics shows that St. John's wort is effective for patients with mild depression. This discrepancy may be due to the fact that most patients in primary care settings have less severe depression than patients seeking psychiatric care.
- Clinical guidelines from the American College of Physicians/American Society of Internal Medicine suggest that St. John's wort can be considered an option (instead of conventional antidepressants) for short-term treatment of mild depression.
- The adverse effects reported (✓✓✓) with St. John's wort were less severe compared to older antidepressants (e.g., imipramine) and slightly less severe compared to newer antidepressant drugs (e.g., the SSRIs).

Overall, then, St. John's wort appears to have clear benefits for mild to moderate depression, minimal benefit for major depression, and similar benefits to conventional antidepressants.

However, some are still cautious about recommending St. John's wort. To date it is still unclear which chemicals in St. John's wort are the active ingredients. This creates uncertainty over how to standardize the products. Some manufacturers ensure their products contain a set amount of hypericin, but others use a different compound, hyperflorin. Both are present in St. John's wort, but no one knows which one ensures the product will have the correct effect when people take it. Until this is known, evaluation and standardization of products will be difficult.

Furthermore, because of the lack of regulation of dietary supplements in the United States, there is significant variation in the available products. The amount of hyperflorin has been shown to vary one-hundred-fold among different brands. Significant variation has also been found among different batches of the same brand. Even in Germany, where herbal remedies are more stringently regulated, the potency of products sold in pharmacies was found to be significantly greater than those sold in supermarkets. Such inconsistency in quality may explain much of the inconsistency found in people's responses to St. John's wort.

In addition, since St. John's wort has not been shown to be more effective or significantly better tolerated than conventional antidepressants, and since St. John's wort causes many drug interactions, it might not be the best choice for many patients, especially those who are taking other conventional drugs.

Although St. John's wort is also used to treat anxiety and other psychological disorders, few if any studies have examined its use with these conditions. A few studies (✗✗✗) examined its use in treating viral infections, but these did not find it to be effective.

● Cautions

Side effects of St. John's wort itself are infrequent and relatively mild. The most common symptoms were intestinal discomfort, fatigue, dry mouth, dizziness, skin rash, and (with very high doses) hypersensitivity to sunlight. Most studies lasted only a few months, so the long-term effects of taking the herb are not known.

The major concern about St John's wort relates to the way it interacts with other drugs. About 40 percent of prescription drugs are broken down in the body by the cytochrome P450 metabolic pathway. Now, before you turn the page (after all, who cares about a P450 pathway?), let us explain how important this is.

This P450 pathway is an important way for the body to eliminate foreign compounds. If it is induced (a form of stimulation suspected to occur with St. John's wort), it will cause many drugs to be broken down more quickly than usual, possibly even before they can have their proper effect. This means St. John's wort could have a potentially dangerous impact on many prescription medications. Some of these drugs include oral contraceptives, warfarin (a drug used to prevent blood clotting), digoxin (used to treat congestive heart failure), simvastatin (used to lower cholesterol levels), a number of drugs used to treat HIV (including most of the reverse transcriptase inhibitors and protease inhibitors), cyclosporine (which all tissue transplant recipients must take), the triptans (used to treat migraine headaches), alprazolam (Xanax), antidepressant drugs, clopidogrel (Plavix), dextromethorphan (Robitussin DM and many others), fexofenadine (Allegra), and many others.

More recent research has noted that the interactions with other drugs may be more complicated. Some drugs are broken down more slowly when people take St. John's wort, leading to higher blood levels than normal. Interactions with other antidepressants are also possible. How St. John's wort combats depression is not known, but it is highly likely to interact with other antidepressants. Therefore, people on prescription antidepressants should alert their physicians before starting St. John's wort or any other herbal remedy. You should not suddenly stop antidepressants you are currently taking without medical supervision. There is a risk of adverse withdrawal effects from abruptly discontinuing St. John's wort or prescription antidepressants.

To lessen the risk of these drug interactions, you should not take St. John's wort and prescription medications without first discussing the situation with your doctor and pharmacist.

As usual, concerns must be raised about product quality. The most recent evaluation of St. John's wort by ConsumerLab.com was published in 2004. Among the ten products purchased for evaluation, two were dropped from testing because they lacked information about which part of the plant was used to make the product (which should be the flowers and leaves of St. John's wort). It is an FDA requirement to put this information on dietary supplement labels. Among the eight that were analyzed, half failed the testing, some for more than one reason. Three were contaminated with the heavy metal cadmium, one was contaminated with excessive lead, three contained less hypericin than their labels claimed, and one recommended a dose much lower than what is known to be effective. Subsequent to this review, an additional four products were tested at the request of their manufacturers or distributors and all four passed.

The Natural Database rates St. John's wort as "possibly safe" for children and "possibly unsafe" for women who are pregnant or lactating.

● Recommendations

St. John's wort appears to be a relatively safe treatment for mild forms of depression. The evidence regarding anxiety or insomnia is much weaker. Milder forms of depression respond better than more severe forms, and there may be other variations in people's responses. However, no information is available on the long-term effects of taking this herb, so it should be used only as a short-term option. Given the complicated nature of depression and anxiety, taking St. John's wort, or any other pill, alone should not be viewed as an adequate way to deal with these conditions. The psychological, relational, and spiritual issues should also be addressed.

Furthermore, St. John's wort should never be taken with any prescription medication without a doctor or pharmacist first checking for possible interactions. When deciding on a product, remember that most studies have been conducted with German formulations, some of which are available in the United States.

● Dosage

For mild to moderate depression, most clinical trials have used St. John's wort extract standardized to contain 0.3 percent hypericin. Doses are most commonly 300 mg three times daily, with up to 1200 mg daily used. Other studies used a 0.2 percent hypericin extract with people taking 250 mg twice daily. An extract standardized to contain 5 percent hyperforin has been used at 300 mg three times daily. For children under twelve years of age with depression, the 0.3 percent hypericin extract of St. John's wort has been used at 300 mg per day.

● Treatment Categories

Complementary

To treat mild depression	☺☺☺☺
To treat mild anxiety	☺☺
To treat PMS	☺
To treat Seasonal Affective Disorder (SAD)	☺
To treat major depression	☹

Scientifically Unproven

To treat obsessive-compulsive disorder	☺
To treat viral infections	☹☹☹
To treat Hepatitis C	☹
To treat HIV-AIDS	☹
To treat polyneuropathy	☹
For any other indication	

Risk of Serious Side Effects

When taken along with other prescription drugs without medical supervision	⊘⊘⊘
If conventional drugs are stopped without medical supervision	⊘⊘⊘⊘

● Further Reading

Linde, Klaus, Gilbert Ramirez, Cynthia D. Mulrow, Andrej Pauls, Wolfgang Weidenhammer, and Dieter Melchart. "St. John's Wort for Depression — An Overview and Meta-Analysis of Randomised Clinical Trials." *British Medical Journal* 313 (August 1996): 253 – 58.

Linde, Klaus, Michael Berner, Matthias Egger, and Cynthia Mulrow. "St John's Wort for Depression: Meta-analysis of Randomised Controlled Trials." *British Journal of Psychiatry* 186 (February 2005): 99 – 107.

Mills, Edward, Victor M. Montori, Ping Wu, Keith Gallicano, Mike Clarke, and Gordon Guyatt. "Interaction of St John's Wort with Conventional Drugs: Systematic Review of Clinical Trials." *British Medical Journal* 329 (July 2004): 27 – 30.

Williams John W., Jr., and Tracey Holsinger. "St. John's for Depression, Worts and All." *British Medical Journal* 330 (March 2005): 154 – 55.

TEA TREE OIL

What It Is

The tea tree is native to Australia and got its name from British sailors under Captain James Cook, the first to report its use (and that of kava) to Westerners. Cook and his crew used it to make a hot tea. Captain Cook did not realize that the native tribes had used the tea tree for its antiseptic properties.

The tea tree has the official name *Melaleuca alternifolia*, and the oil is obtained from its leaves. The oil is sometimes sold as Melaleuca oil, a substance that should not be purchased without a careful check. There are several species of tea trees, and the oils from species other than *Melaleuca alternifolia* contain high concentrations of skin irritants.

Tea tree oil has a faint lemon color and a nutmeg-like odor. The oil is a complex mixture of almost one hundred compounds called "terpenes."

Claims

Tea tree oil is used as a general antimicrobial agent. It became known outside of Australia during World War I because of its widespread use by Australian troops for burns, wounds, and infections. Based on this history, tea tree oil remains popular as a natural antiseptic and is added to many "natural" cosmetics, toothpaste, and hair products.

Tea tree oil is believed to be effective in treating a wide range of bacterial, viral, and fungal conditions, including athlete's foot, ringworm, respiratory infections, and vaginitis. As a first-aid remedy, it readily penetrates the skin and is believed useful for treating burns, scrapes, bites, stings, and various skin irritations. Some people feel it is an effective insect repellent. Tea tree oil is used to help prevent or treat acne, cold and flu, yeast infections, warts, nasal congestion, and sore throat.

Tea tree oil is used in aromatherapy, whether by inhalation or in various body care products. Tea tree oil also has been used in dental care. Diluted in water, it is used as a mouthwash and gargle. In more concentrated forms, it is used to relieve canker sores, cold sores, and gum disease.

Study Findings

Tea tree oil has been shown in laboratory tests to kill a variety of microorganisms. A 2000 review found four controlled studies (✓✓✓) of tea tree oil for a variety of skin conditions. Newer studies were not found. Fungal infections of the feet and nails are relatively difficult to control, even with conventional prescription drugs. However, 10 percent tea tree oil has been shown in one study (✓✓✓) to be as effective as 1 percent tolnaftate cream in reducing the symptoms of athlete's foot (tinea pedis). In another study (✓✓✓), 100 percent tea tree oil was as effective as 1 percent clotrimazole in improving nail appearance and symptoms. However, both conditions are known to have high rates of recurrence. Furthermore, there is at least one study (✗✗✗) showing that tea tree oil was no better than placebo against fungal foot infections. A few clinical studies (✓✓✓) have shown it to be somewhat effective against acne. In one study (✗✗✗), comparing 5 percent tea tree oil to benzoyl peroxide lotion, the tea tree oil was better tolerated but was less effective and had a slower onset of action. Case reports (✓) of tea tree oil pessaries relieving vaginal yeast infections have been reported. There are no demonstrated benefits (✗✗) from adding tea tree oil to toothpaste.

Cautions

Tea tree oil should never be taken internally and should always be diluted when applied to broken skin. Research on how it kills microbes has revealed that it also kills certain types of human cells. This may result in slower healing and increased scarring when used for burns. All of these findings should caution against its use in toothpaste, mouthwashes, and lozenges, all of which can easily be ingested. A relatively small number of allergic reactions have been reported, and long-term use can lead to dermatitis. The Natural Database rates tea tree oil as "likely unsafe" for anyone to use orally — adults and children.

For topical use, tea tree oil is possibly safe for all people, including children and women who are pregnant or lactating. Since tea tree oil may irritate the skin, test it first by applying a tiny amount on a small patch of skin. Tea tree oil can safely be applied full strength in drops to fingernails or toenails (to treat fungal infections, for example). It should not be applied to broken skin or near the eyes.

Recommendations

This natural oil is effective against a number of microorganisms and may be a helpful agent for minor skin infections. However, it should be used cautiously, if at all, with open wounds, more serious infections, and burns. Tea tree oil should never be ingested.

Dosage

The oil should be applied to the affected areas twice a day. It should not be taken internally.

Treatment Categories

Complementary

Topically to treat fungal nail infections or athlete's foot	☺☺
Topically to treat mild acne	☺☺
Topically to treat bacterial vaginosis	☺
With care, as a mouthwash to treat oropharyngeal candidiasis in HIV/AIDS patients	☺
As a mouthwash to treat other mouth or throat infections	☹☹

Scientifically Unproven

For any other indication, especially orally

Risk of Serious Side Effects

When used orally	⊘⊘⊘

Further Reading

Ernst, E., and A. Huntley. "Tea Tree Oil: A Systematic Review of Randomized Clinical Trials." *Forschende Komplementarmedizin und Klassische Naturheilkunde* 7, no. 1 (2000): 17–20.

Foster, Steven, and Varro E. Tyler. *Tyler's Honest Herbal: A Sensible Guide to the Use of Herbs and Related Remedies.* 4th ed. New York: Haworth Herbal, 1999, 369–70.

VALERIAN

What It Is

Both cats and their humans have long delighted in the use of valerian. The roots and rhizomes of common valerian (*Valeriana officinalis*) form the number one over-the-counter sedative in Germany, with a chemical similar to catnip. Humans use valerian for a gentle sleep. Some Native American tribes also used it to treat cuts and wounds, while ancient Greeks used it to treat urinary tract and digestive disorders. The cats simply like to "get high."

The pink-flowered perennial valerian grows wild in temperate areas of the Americas and Eurasia. The root, which is politely described as "pungent" or "malodorous," smells terrible — unless you're a cat. Its odor comes close to that of well-worn, long-unwashed socks or a sharp cheese even starving mice might avoid. It may be used as a tea, tincture (alcohol-based solution), or extract in capsules.

Claims

Valerian has been used as a sedative and to treat anxiety. It is said to act as a central nervous system depressant, binding to benzodiazepine receptors. Benzodiazepine is the active ingredient in the prescription drug Valium, once the most commonly prescribed tranquilizer in the United States. However, unlike Valium-like prescription drugs, valerian is said to be nontoxic and does not interact with alcohol.

In the eighteenth and nineteenth centuries, valerian was indispensable for treating various types of nervous conditions, not only insomnia, but also anxiety, nervous headache, exhaustion, and hysteria. Doctors often recommended it to women who suffered from emotionally induced exhaustion of the nervous system. The association among women, nervous conditions, and valerian was so strong that valerian has been called the "Valium of the nineteenth century."

Valerian is now the most prominent herbal remedy for insomnia as well as nervous conditions related to anxiety, tension, and stress. It is believed to work well as a nerve tonic for people who suffer from nervous exhaustion, panic attacks, and emotional disturbances. It is used as a pain-relieving agent for conditions such as tension-related headache, nerve pain, and menstrual cramps. Valerian is felt by some to soothe the digestive system and relieve indigestion, constipation, irritable bowel syndrome, and stomach cramps, especially those that may be due to excessive nervousness.

Valerian is used by some herbalists to prevent or treat high blood pressure, cough (often in combination with other herbs such as licorice), attention deficit disorder (ADD and ADHD), and altitude sickness.

Study Findings

Over one hundred different substances have been identified in valerian, of which valeric and isovalerenic acid are thought to be most active. Valerian has been studied in several small, double-blind clinical trials (✓✓✓✓) that showed improvement of sleep quality. However, some of the studies (✗✗✗)

457

have found the effect on sleep to be no different than that from a placebo. A number of studies (✓✓✓✓) revealed an important pattern to the way valerian affects sleep patterns. A single dose does not put people to sleep, but beneficial effects usually develop after about two weeks. Valerian seems to improve slow-wave sleep (SWS) more than rapid eye movement (REM) sleep. SWS is the most restorative sleep, whereas REM sleep is lighter. Another pattern observed was that people with insomnia tended to experience sleep improvement, whereas those without sleep problems were largely unaffected by valerian.

Herbal products combining valerian and other herbs have been studied in a small number of trials. A few studies (✓✓✓✓) have found valerian beneficial when used in combination with regular brewing hops (*Humulus lupulus*). In one controlled clinical trial, an herbal formula containing hops and valerian was just as effective as a benzodiazepine (the class of tranquilizers that includes Valium and Xanax) for patients suffering from nonchronic and nonpsychiatric sleep disorders. Valerian seems to work similarly to benzodiazepines, though with weaker effects. Valerian combined with St. John's wort or kava has been found to be helpful.

German health officials have approved valerian for use as a mild sedative and sleep aid, based on several European clinical trials (✓✓✓✓). In contrast, the U.S. Pharmacopeia in 1998 decided there was too much conflicting data to recommend the use of valerian as a short-term treatment for insomnia. A preliminary 2002 study (✓✓✓) involving five children with intellectual deficits found that valerian significantly improved sleep patterns, especially with children with hyperactivity issues. No adverse effects were reported.

Cautions

In the United States, valerian is approved for use in flavoring foods and beverages such as root beer. No serious side effects have been reported. However, when valerian is taken in medicinal doses (✗✗), unusual side effects include morning sleepiness, headache, cardiac disturbances, and trouble walking. One of the consistent findings in clinical trials (✓✓✓) is that people report fewer side effects with valerian than pharmaceutical drugs, with less residual sedation in the morning. For unknown reasons, a small minority of people may find valerian stimulating instead of calming, causing insomnia, restlessness, or uneasiness. These people become restless and get palpitations, particularly with long-term use. Addiction has not been reported, but rare cases of liver toxicity and withdrawal symptoms have been reported.

Whether or not valerian interacts with alcohol is disputed. Most experts recommend against taking valerian and alcohol together. Valerian has been reported to slow the metabolism of barbiturates and should not be used with these medications. A few people experience stomach complaints from taking valerian.

Some components display cancer-causing activity in the laboratory; however, these effects have not been reproduced in laboratory animals, even at extremely high doses. Nevertheless, most experts warn that valerian probably should not be used by pregnant or lactating women. The Natural Database rates valerian as "possibly safe" for use in children. The safety of using valerian daily for longer than a month is unknown.

In July 2004, ConsumerLab.com tested thirteen valerian products. Eight were selected by ConsumerLab.com, and five were tested at the request of their manufacturers or distributors. Five products (39 percent) failed the tests. Four products did not contain the labeled amount of valerenic acids, and two were contaminated with cadmium or lead (one product failed both tests).

In 2006, ConsumerLab.com retested valerian products and found that over 70 percent of the nineteen products tested lacked key ingredients or were contaminated. Overall, ten products failed to meet quality standards, with most containing lower amounts of the active ingredients used in clinical trials. One product had less than 1 percent of the usual dose of these compounds. Three supplements were contaminated with cadmium or lead. Of the nineteen products tested, only six met quality standards.

Recommendations

Valerian has very few reported side effects and may be an effective over-the-counter treatment for sleep problems or anxiety, as it appears to have mild sedating and tranquilizing effects. It appears to take a week or two before most people notice its effect, so it will not work as well for those with occasional sleep problems as it will for those with chronic insomnia. No studies have examined the side effects of taking valerian long-term. Valerian should not be taken with other sedatives or before driving or in other situations when alertness is required.

Dosage

The studies have used a variety of doses, ranging from 60 mg to over 1200 mg (which is a problem in assessing overall effect). A 300 to 900 mg dose of valerian one to two hours before bedtime for up to twenty-eight days is most commonly used.

Treatment Categories

Complementary

To improve sleep duration and quality
after being taken for at least a week   ☺☺☺☺
To accelerate the onset of sleep
when taken occasionally   ☹☹☹
To relieve restlessness and sleep
disorders caused by anxiety   ☺☺
To relieve anxiety   ☺

Scientifically Unproven

For any other indication

Further Reading

Hadley, Susan, and Judith J. Petry. "Valerian." *American Family Physician* 67, no. 8 (April 2003): 1755 – 58.

Wheatley, David. "Medicinal Plants for Insomnia: A Review of Their Pharmacology, Efficacy and Tolerability." *Journal of Psychopharmacology* 19, no. 4 (July 2005): 414 – 21.

V

VITAMIN C

What It Is

Vitamin C, also called "ascorbic acid," is most commonly found in citrus fruits, but large quantities also exist in strawberries, kiwi fruit, and tomatoes. A certain amount of vitamin C is required in everyone's diet to maintain health. A lack of vitamin C in the diet leads to scurvy. Vitamin C is required for many functions in the body, including tissue repair, metabolism of carbohydrates, and synthesis of proteins.

Vitamin C can be extracted from natural sources (rose hips, acerola), but no research has proved any nutritional difference between synthetic and "natural" forms of vitamin C. Vitamin C is often combined with plant bioflavonoids (e.g., rutin, hesperdin, quercetin) to enhance absorption or activity, but studies have not examined whether this actually occurs.

Vitamin C comes in a wide variety of forms, including tablets, capsules, powders, liquids, and chewable wafers. Buffered vitamin C provides added calcium and magnesium, which help to reduce irritation from stomach acid, and buffered chewable tablets protect teeth from ascorbic acid — an especially important feature for children and anyone with soft enamel. "Corn-free" vitamin C is designed for those who are sensitive to corn (unlike most vitamin C, it is derived from sago palm rather than corn). There is no proof that sublingual vitamin C sprays or tablets (which are much more expensive) have any additional benefit.

Claims

The importance of vitamin C in the diet is well understood and scientifically proven. The only controversy is the amount we need, both from day to day and when our bodies are exposed to unusual stress. Some people claim high daily doses prevent colds. Linus Pauling, a dual Nobel Prize winner for chemistry and for peace, was the most outspoken proponent of this view, recommending that everyone take 1 gram of vitamin C daily and increase the dose to 2 grams a day as soon as they feel a cold coming on. Pauling himself claimed that by the end of his life he was taking 18 grams of vitamin C daily, which he increased to 40 grams when he felt a cold starting. He also claimed vitamin C could treat everything from cancer to schizophrenia.

Some advocates believe that large amounts of vitamin C improve athletic performance, mood, and cardiovascular health. Vitamin C is believed by some to prevent cancer, increase longevity, prevent cataracts, and enhance brain function.

Study Findings

In 1992, researchers at the University of California, Los Angeles (UCLA), reported that among 11,000 participants surveyed over a ten-year period (✓✓), those getting the most vitamin C (300 mg per day) had the lowest rates of heart disease and cancer and lived the longest. These findings took into account differences in exercise, diet, and lifestyle.

VITAMIN C

Optimal levels of vitamin C have been suggested in a number of studies (✓✓) to benefit a wide range of health conditions, including cataracts, diabetes, eczema, periodontal disease, glaucoma, gout, high cholesterol, menopause, heavy menstruation, minor injuries, morning sickness, recurrent ear infections, and urinary tract infections. Vitamin C enhances vitamin E's antioxidant properties and promotes the absorption of other nutrients (such as iron).

Confirming earlier epidemiological studies, a study of 247 older women (✓✓) determined that vitamin C supplementation over a ten- to twelve-year period was associated with a dramatically reduced prevalence of age-related cataracts. Another human study (✓✓) confirmed earlier animal research in finding that eight days of combined vitamin C (2000 mg per day) and vitamin E (1000 IU per day) protect the skin from sunburn. Another recent epidemiological study (✓✓) conducted in a retirement community in Australia found that consumption of vitamin C supplements was associated with a lower percentage of severe cognitive impairment, although not with any effects on tests of verbal fluency.

The use of vitamin C as a treatment has focused on the common cold. Linus Pauling made his original claims about vitamin C and the common cold in a book published in 1970. He based his conclusion on four studies (✓✓✓✓). (See p. 47 for a detailed discussion of problems with his review.) Since then, dozens of other high-quality clinical studies have been conducted on vitamin C. A 2004 Cochrane review came to the following conclusions based on the results of fifty-five controlled trials:

- Taking up to 2 grams vitamin C daily on an ongoing basis does not in general reduce someone's chances of getting a cold (✗✗✗).

- Six studies with people regularly exposed to physical stress and cold (marathon runners, skiers, and soldiers) who took up to 2 grams vitamin C daily halved their risk of getting a cold (✓✓✓✓).
- Taking up to 2 grams vitamin C daily on an ongoing basis does slightly reduce the length of a cold when someone gets one. The average reduction was 8 percent for adults and 14 percent for children (✓✓✓✓).
- Taking 1 to 2 grams vitamin C daily as soon as someone gets a cold does not alter the length or severity of the symptoms (✗✗✗). However, one large trial that used 8 grams did find that the duration of the cold was shortened slightly.
- Megadoses of vitamin C (more than 2 grams daily) do not have any beneficial effects (✗✗✗).

Vitamin C has also been tested as a treatment for a small number of other conditions. Another 2004 Cochrane review (✗✗✗) examined its use in treating asthma. Eight controlled trials were found, with the reviewers concluding that there was insufficient evidence to recommend its use in asthmatic patients. A 2005 Cochrane review (✗✗✗) found that there was not enough evidence to recommend using vitamin C to reduce complications during pregnancy. Vitamin C's antioxidant properties have led to its use in preventing Alzheimer's disease, but this has not been examined in controlled studies. The most recent epidemiological studies (✗✗) found no connection between vitamin C intake and Alzheimer's disease.

The Agency for Healthcare Research and Quality (AHRQ) sponsored a systematic review of vitamin C for the prevention and treatment of cancer

V

and another for cardiovascular disease. Both were published in 2003 and found little evidence of benefit. With cancer, some individual studies showed benefit, but the overall pattern (✗✗✗✗) was not beneficial. With cardiovascular disease, all studies (✗✗✗✗) found no benefit from vitamin C.

The body's cells routinely transform dietary vitamin C into other substances called "metabolites." Some research indicates that supplements that combine vitamin C with its metabolites may permit it to be absorbed better and faster into the blood and immune cells and last longer in body tissues. A patented supplement called Ester-C is composed of esters of vitamin C and its metabolites (an ester is a slightly modified form of any acid group, one of which is in vitamin C, or ascorbic acid). However, we are aware of no proven clinical benefit of this more expensive form of vitamin C.

Regarding the debate over how much vitamin C to take, several studies (✗✗) have demonstrated that it is very unlikely that high doses of vitamin C could benefit people. A dose of up to 200 mg is absorbed well from the digestive tract. At higher doses, some of the vitamin C is not absorbed. Taking any more than 500 mg of vitamin C per day will result in hardly any of the additional vitamin C making it to your cells. All the rest will get flushed down the drain.

Cautions

Vitamin C does not cause serious adverse effects, even when taken in very high doses. However, some people report (✗) nausea, heartburn, diarrhea, and other intestinal problems. People who are prone to get kidney stones should be cautious about how much vitamin C they take, as high doses (2000 mg per day or more) may cause kidney stones and may be associated with deep vein blood clots (thromboses).

Some researchers believe that vitamin C exceeding 1000 mg per day may cause oxidation rather than have an antioxidant effect. At least one study (✗✗) has shown an increase in atherosclerosis in people taking 500 mg of vitamin C per day.

Although there has been great variability in the quality of vitamin C products in the past, the situation appears to be improving. For example, in March 2005, ConsumerLab.com purchased twenty-nine brands of vitamin C – containing products: twenty-seven for adults and two for children. All twenty-nine products met their claims for vitamin C content, and all disintegrated properly as needed for absorption. Similar results were obtained in 2003. In 2001, several products were found to contain somewhat less vitamin C than claimed, and one product would not disintegrate properly.

Recommendations

Everyone needs a certain amount of vitamin C in the diet. Western diets often are deficient, and therefore many people may benefit from some supplementation. Taking 1 to 2 grams of vitamin C per day may lead to a small benefit when someone catches a cold, but it won't prevent getting a cold. However, those exposed to rigorous exercise in cold temperatures do seem to benefit significantly from taking regular vitamin C. Such patterns have only recently been noticed and will presumably be researched further. The use of vitamin C to prevent or treat any other illness is not supported by the evidence.

Dosage

The recommended daily allowance of vitamin C was increased somewhat in 2000 by the Institute of Medicine (IOM). The institute, a private nonprofit organization that advises federal health officials, is part of the National Academy of Sciences, which has set the nation's Recommended Dietary Allowances, or RDAs, for nutrients since 1941. The Food and Drug Administration (FDA) uses these recommendations to set "daily values" that appear on food labels.

The IOM recommended that women should consume 75 mg per day, and men 90 mg. Because smokers are more likely to suffer from biological processes that damage cells and deplete vitamin C, they need an additional 35 mg per day. The RDA for children increases gradually from 15 mg per day for one- to three-year-olds to 45 mg per day for nine- to thirteen-year-olds, up to adult levels by eighteen years of age.

The IOM states that these levels can easily be met without taking supplements by eating citrus fruits, potatoes, strawberries, broccoli, and leafy green vegetables. An 8-ounce glass of orange juice provides about 100 mg of vitamin C.

The report also set the upper intake level for vitamin C, from both food and supplements, at 2000 mg per day for adults. Intakes above this amount may cause a number of medical problems. Those who recommend vitamin C to treat the common cold usually suggest 1 to 3 grams a day.

Treatment Categories

Conventional

To prevent vitamin C deficiency or scurvy	☺☺☺☺
To achieve recommended dietary allowances	☺☺☺☺

Complementary

As an antioxidant supplement	☺☺☺☺
To increase iron absorption	☺☺☺
To prevent colds in the general population	☹☹☹☹
To prevent colds among those who exercise vigorously in the cold	☺☺☺
To treat the common cold once symptoms appear	☹☹☹
In doses of up to 2000 mg (2 g) per day to reduce the severity of colds	☺
To prevent some forms of cancer	☹
To prevent cardiovascular disease	☹☹

Scientifically Unproven

Megadoses (greater than 2000 mg [2 g] per day) for any indication	☹☹☹☹
To treat asthma	☹☹☹
To treat ADHD	☹☹
To prevent complications during pregnancy	☹☹☹
To treat or prevent Alzheimer's disease	☹☹☹
For any other indication	

Further Reading

Boothby, Linda A., and Paul L. Doering. "Vitamin C and Vitamin E for Alzheimer's Disease." *Annals of Pharmacotherapy* 39, no. 12 (December 2005): 2073–79.

Douglas, Robert M., and Harri Hemilä. "Vitamin C for Preventing and Treating the Common Cold." *PLoS Medicine* 2, no. 6 (June 2005): e168. *PLoS Medicine: www.plosmedicine.org.* Accessed October 3, 2005.

Levine, Mark, Steven C. Rumsey, Rushad Daruwala, Jae B. Park, and Yaohui Wang. "Criteria and Recommendations for Vitamin C Intake." *Journal of the American Medical Association* 281, no. 15 (April 1999): 1415–23.

V

VITAMIN E

What It Is

Vitamin E is a mixture of eight different, but very similar, compounds called "tocopherols." They make up the fat-soluble vitamin that is found in vegetable oils, nuts, whole grains, and greens. Wheat-germ oil is the single richest source of the vitamin. However, the amount present naturally in foods is much lower than what is needed to get the health benefits reported from those who take a supplement of at least 100 IU per day (IU stands for International Units; 100 IU of vitamin E = 67 mg). Much of the absorbed vitamin ends up in low-density lipoprotein particles (LDL, or "bad" cholesterol). LDL plays a central role in transporting cholesterol around the body. The rest forms part of the cell membranes throughout the body.

Claims

Vitamin E is an antioxidant. The oxidation of LDL is an important step in the development of atherosclerosis, or hardening of the arteries. Vitamin E is said to prevent this chemical reaction and thus to play a role in the prevention of heart disease. The vitamin is also said to help the user resist infections, to treat hepatitis B, to reverse early memory loss problems due to dementia, and to prevent some cancers. There have also been anecdotal stories of vitamin E used to restore sexual drive in former psychiatric patients believed to have temporary drug-damaged libido.

Study Findings

Laboratory studies have shown that vitamin E prevents the oxidation of LDL. Based on questionnaires (✓✓) given to tens of thousands of people, those who took the most vitamin E had lower levels of heart disease; those who took the least vitamin E had the most heart problems. However, results from more controlled studies have not been completely positive, leading to some hesitation about vitamin E's benefits. In the area of resistance to infections, one controlled study (✓✓✓) found that elderly patients taking 200 mg of vitamin E per day had about one-third of the infections experienced by those taking a placebo.

In early 2000, the Institute of Medicine (IOM) released a report on vitamins E and C and other antioxidants. This report, and the research on which it was based, is a good example of how confusing medical research can sometimes be. It also demonstrates the importance of patience before making broad recommendations about dietary supplements. The report concluded that it was too early to make firm statements about the ability of vitamin E, or any other dietary antioxidant, to prevent or treat any disease. This caution has been borne out by subsequent research.

The results from major trials with cardiovascular disease came in a roller-coaster pattern. A 1993 study in China (✓✓✓) found that healthy volunteers taking vitamin E (30 mg), beta-carotene, and selenium for five years had 9 percent fewer deaths from heart disease compared to those taking placebo. A

1994 study in Finland (✗✗✗) found no effect on coronary heart disease for smokers given 50 mg of vitamin E daily for five to eight years. A 1996 British study (✓✓✓) found an impressive 77 percent drop in nonfatal heart attacks for those taking 400 or 800 IU of vitamin E daily for a little over a year, though deaths from all cardiovascular causes remained unchanged. A 1999 Italian study (✗✗✗) found no cardiac benefit for patients given 300 mg of vitamin E for three to five years. The first major United States study (✗✗✗), published in 2000, found no significant benefit for those taking 400 IU (267 mg) of vitamin E for four to six years. In fact, among the 10,000 participants at high risk for cardiovascular events, those taking conventional drugs did so much better (20 to 25 percent improvement in all areas) that the journal in which the study was published took the unusual step of pre-publishing the results on its website so physicians could make changes in their recommendations as soon as possible.

Then followed five more trials, some with huge numbers of participants (approaching 30,000). Two found some cardiovascular benefit (✓✓✓) from vitamin E (though only among certain subgroups of participants), while three found no benefit (✗✗✗). While the studies have conflicting results, their similar design allows them to be combined into a meta-analysis. One published in 2004 (✗✗✗) reported no statistically significant or clinically important benefits from vitamin E supplementation for any important cardiovascular event: heart attack, stroke, or death from cardiovascular diseases. Another meta-analysis (✗✗✗), published by Miller and colleagues in 2005, focused on the risk of death among those taking vitamin E supplements. This risk was increased by vitamin E, especially at higher doses (400 IU per day or greater), but was still higher among those taking 150 IU per day.

Two more randomized controlled studies (✗✗✗) published in 2005 added strength to the growing concern about vitamin E supplements. The HOPE-TOO trial found no cardiac benefit and an increased risk of heart failure and hospitalization for heart failure among those taking vitamin E for seven years. Then a study with almost 40,000 women from the Women's Health Study found no cardiac benefit and a 4 percent increase in mortality among those taking 600 IU of vitamin E every other day. All of a sudden, experts recommend that people *not* take vitamin E to prevent heart disease.

Another area in which vitamin E was thought to be beneficial was with cancer. Epidemiological studies (✓✓) again suggested that those consuming more vitamin E got cancer less frequently. Four of the above cardiac studies (✗✗✗) also examined incidence of cancer. Only one examined vitamin E supplementation alone, and it found no benefit in occurrence of cancer or deaths from cancer. The others found no overall benefit but did show some beneficial effects for some subgroups. The HOPE-TOO and Women's Health Study found no beneficial effects from vitamin E in preventing cancer or reducing deaths from cancer.

As an antioxidant, vitamin E has been recommended to prevent or retard other diseases thought to be connected with oxidative stress. These include Parkinson's disease, Alzheimer's disease, tardive dyskinesia, and cataracts. The evidence examining vitamin E supplements for these diseases is sparse and conflicting. Given the risks found with the cardiac studies and the lack of clear benefit with any of these diseases, vitamin E supplements cannot be recommended here either.

According to the IOM, the vitamin E consumed should be "alpha-tocopherol," the only type that human blood can maintain and transfer to cells when needed. Other experts contend that it is preferable to consume "mixed tocopherols," including *d*-beta, *d*-gamma, *d*-delta-tocopherols, tocotrienols, and others. They maintain that each form of vitamin E offers different antioxidant effects, and vitamin E occurs in foods as mixed tocopherols. There is no clear evidence to make a definite recommendation.

Another controversial area is whether you should take "synthetic" vitamin E (which contains all-racemic alpha-tocopherol, containing equal amounts of all eight stereoisomers, and is the form of vitamin E in fortified foods and most vitamin E supplements) or "natural" vitamin E (which contains only one specific isomer of alpha-tocopherol and occurs naturally in foods such as nuts, eggs, meats, and oils). Natural vitamin E supplements seem to be better absorbed and may therefore be more potent than synthetic forms. But there's no evidence that natural is more effective or safer than synthetic when equally potent doses are used. There is not enough evidence that one form of vitamin E, or any combination, is better or safer than any other.

Cautions

Direct adverse effects from vitamin E are rare. However, it may interfere with the blood's clotting mechanisms, so it should not be taken by those already taking blood thinners (such as aspirin or warfarin). This is believed to be the source of the higher risk of cardiac problems in the long-term studies. The increased risk was dose-related and first noticeable at 150 IU per day. The RDA (Recommended Dietary Allowance) is 22 IU (15 mg).

The Tolerable Upper Intake Level of vitamin E, based only on intake from vitamin supplements, was set at 1000 mg of alpha-tocopherol per day for adults. This amount is equivalent to roughly 1500 IU of "*d*-alpha-tocopherol," sometimes labeled as "natural source" vitamin E, or 1100 IU of "*dl*-alpha-tocopherol," a synthetic version of vitamin E. The Natural Database rates vitamin E as "likely safe" for women who are pregnant or lactating when taken in amounts that do not exceed the RDA. People consuming more than the tolerable upper limit face an even greater risk of stroke and uncontrolled bleeding because the vitamin can prevent blood clotting.

In August 2004, ConsumerLab.com reported on its testing of the leading vitamin E products sold in the United States. Thirty-four products were purchased, including capsules, creams, and topical oils. All but four products passed the tests. Three had less vitamin E than their labels claimed, and two contained synthetic forms when their labels claimed to be natural (with one product failing on both counts).

Recommendations

The evidence concerning vitamin E's role in protecting people from heart disease or cancer is now clearer. There is no benefit, and beyond 150 IU per day, there is some increased risk. While the percent risk is very small, any risk is too much when there is clear evidence of no benefit. The evidence regarding vitamin E's benefit with other diseases is less substantial. However, in no condition is there clear evidence of benefit.

Everyone needs to consume some vitamin E. Once again, the benefit seems to come from a healthy, balanced diet in which vitamin E is obtained as part of a plant-rich diet. Problems arise when large doses of a single antioxidant are taken in the hope of obtaining what a balanced diet provides through a diverse selection of antioxidants.

Dosage

The 2000 IOM recommended intake level (RDA) of vitamin E for both women and men is 15 mg (22 IU). Food sources include nuts, seeds, liver, and leafy green vegetables. Daily multivitamins will usually provide about 30 IU. A healthy, balanced diet should also provide approximately 20 to 30 IU of mixed tocopherols.

Treatment Categories

Conventional

As part of a balanced diet,
up to 22 IU per day ☺☺☺☺

Complementary

To prevent or treat any
cardiac disease ☹☹☹☹

To prevent or treat high
blood pressure ☹☹☹☹

To prevent or treat colds ☹☹

To treat Alzheimer's disease ☹☹

To prevent or treat osteoarthritis ☹☹

To prevent or treat cataracts ☹

To prevent or treat cancer ☹☹☹☹

To treat diabetes ☹

To prevent or treat any chronic
disease related to antioxidants ☹☹☹☹

Scientifically Unproven

For any other indication

Risk of Serious Side Effects

When more than 150 IU per day is taken ⊘

Further Reading

Pham, David Q., and Roda Plakogiannis. "Vitamin E Supplementation in Cardiovascular Disease and Cancer Prevention: Part 1." *Annals of Pharmacotherapy* 39, no. 11 (November 2005): 1870–78.

_____. "Vitamin E Supplementation in Alzheimer's Disease, Parkinson's Disease, Tardive Dyskinesia, and Cataract: Part 2." *Annals of Pharmacotherapy* 39, no. 12 (December 2005): 2065–71.

Miller, Edgar R., III., Roberto Pastor-Barriuso, Darshan Dalal, Rudolph A. Riemersma, Lawrence J. Appel, and Eliseo Guallar. "Meta-analysis: High-Dosage Vitamin E Supplementation May Increase All-Cause Mortality." *Annals of Internal Medicine* 142, no. 1 (January 2005): 37–46.

WILD YAM

What It Is

Wild yam (*Dioscorea villosa*) is a climbing vine that grows in the wet woodlands of North and Central America. Historically, it was very important as the sole source of steroids used to make contraceptive hormones, cortisone, and anabolic hormones. These pharmaceutical drugs are now made from other starting materials, but wild yam remains of interest as a natural source of steroids. Other species of wild yam are also used, including *Dioscorea floribunda*, *Dioscorea composita*, and *Dioscorea mexicana* (also called *Dioscorea macrostachya*).

Claims

Hundreds of yam species exist worldwide, and a number of cultures have discovered medicinal applications. The Chinese, for example, have long used a yam species as a liver tonic, digestive aid, and muscle relaxant. Ayurvedic practitioners in India have used a yam species as a remedy for impotence and infertility. Wild yam is also known as colic root because of its antispasmodic action. In some cultures it is a folk remedy for diverticulitis, nausea during pregnancy, and flatulence.

With revelations of the problems with hormone replacement therapy, wild yam creams were among the alternatives recommended to reduce menopausal symptoms. They were also recommended to relieve menstrual or uterine cramps. Wild yam is said to promote the secretion of bile and may help

to alleviate liver ailments. The herb is believed by some to have anti-inflammatory properties that make it useful in treating rheumatoid arthritis and other conditions. Others use it to prevent or treat indigestion.

Wild yam contains DHEA (see the DHEA entry), which is the source of much publicity and controversy of its own. Wild yam is recommended for many of the same conditions as DHEA, such as AIDS, cancer, chronic fatigue syndrome, fibromyalgia, multiple sclerosis, and various psychological disorders.

Study Findings

Wild yam contains compounds that, in purified form, are being researched for their role in treating some conditions. These include DHEA and dioscin, shown to have anti-inflammatory activity. However, wild yam preparations will not necessarily produce the same effects as the pure compounds. Studies with an extract of wild yam taken orally have not found increased blood levels of DHEA. While the diosgenin in wild yam can be converted into human steroids in the laboratory, there is no known biochemical pathway within humans to carry out this conversion. This makes it unlikely that wild yam can act as a source of human hormones such as estrogen or progesterone.

Wild yam cream was tested in one small trial (✗✗✗) involving menopausal women. The randomized double-blind trial lasted three months and found no differences in menopausal symptoms between women using wild yam cream and women

using a placebo. No changes in estrogen or progesterone levels, nor in any other health measurement,
were found.

Cautions

Preparations made from wild yam show all the natural variability of any herbal remedy and have the
same lack of standardization as other dietary supplements. Given that steroids are very active in the
body, often at very low concentrations, taking them
in herbal remedies is risky because of the variability
in dosages. These products have produced numerous
side effects, all typical of steroids: acne, hair loss,
headache, menstrual irregularities, and (in women)
development of male voice and hair patterns.

A number of cancers have been shown to be stimulated by steroid hormones, so wild yam should be
completely avoided by anyone with a family history
of breast, ovarian, uterine, or prostate cancer. Wild
yam should not be taken orally during pregnancy, as
the steroids may adversely affect fetal development.

There is insufficient information to determine if
wild yam is safe when applied topically during pregnancy or lactation; therefore, it should be avoided by
women during these times.

Recommendations

Wild yam has played an important role in the development of steroid pharmaceuticals. Steroids are
powerful drugs, actively involved in many different
bodily functions. They are also active in very small
quantities. There is much uncertainty about how
much of any particular steroid may be found in any
particular wild yam product. Given that these wild
yam products have not been shown to be effective for
any particular disease, their potential side effects do
not warrant their use.

When appropriate and necessary, standardized
pharmaceutical steroid products (or DHEA) should
be used since they are readily available and not
overly expensive.

Dosage

Some products recommend 2 to 4 grams three times
a day, although recommendations vary widely.

Treatment Categories

Complementary
To treat menopausal symptoms   ☹☹☹☹

Scientifically Unproven
For any other indication

Risk of Serious Side Effects
Because wild yam contains steroids   ⊘

Further Reading

Komesaroff, P. A., C. V. Black, V. Cable, and K. Sudhir.
"Effects of Wild Yam Extract on Menopausal Symptoms, Lipids and Sex Hormones in Healthy Menopausal Women." *Climacteric* 4 (2001): 144–50.

WILLOW BARK

What It Is

Willow bark tea was once the drink of choice for those who overindulged in wines and beer as well as those suffering from arthritis. Although the ancients didn't know they were getting salicylic acid from the tea, that ingredient probably was the reason for the early popularity of willow bark tea. We now know it was the forerunner of aspirin (*acetylsalicylic acid*).

Willow bark has been used as an anti-inflammatory at least since the time of ancient Egypt. Both the white willow (*Salix alba*), native to Europe but now growing widely in the United States, and the black willow (*Salix nigra*), native to North America, have bark used in powdered form or extracted with alcohol to make a tincture. Other *Salix* species are also used.

Willow bark contains a compound called "salicin" in low levels (1 to 2 percent). The liver and intestines convert salicin into salicylic acid. Salicin, salicylic acid, and aspirin belong to the group of compounds called "salicylates." Early in the nineteenth century, pure samples of salicylates were isolated from willow bark. In 1852, salicylic acid was chemically manufactured from other, more readily available compounds, thus eliminating the need to use plant material. In 1899, the German company Bayer chemically modified salicylic acid to make a form less irritating to the stomach: aspirin. This represented one of the first successes for pharmacognosy, the science of taking an herbal remedy, identifying the active ingredient, and chemically producing a form that was better tolerated and more readily available. Aspirin has been studied extensively in human trials, with the results validating some traditional uses of willow bark.

Claims

Various cultures around the world have been known to use willow bark medicinally, not only for its pain-relieving and fever-reducing properties but also as a digestive tonic. Native American tribes were using willow species for pain and fever in the seventeenth century and probably knew of these medicinal effects before the arrival of Europeans.

Willow bark was a popular remedy among Colonial Americans to reduce inflammation and fever and to treat ailments ranging from gout to food poisoning. Willow leaves were also sometimes used in remedies for colic and other conditions. Ointments with willow bark were used topically for cuts and burns.

Modern uses for willow bark still rely on its aspirin-like effects, though it is considered milder and slower acting than aspirin. As a pain reliever, willow bark is said to alleviate muscle aches, tension headaches, and arthritis.

Because studies have found that aspirin works as a thermogenic (heat-creating and calorie-burning) agent synergistically with caffeine and ephedrine, willow bark is sometimes included in weight-loss formulas. Willow bark is also believed to help prevent or treat bursitis, rheumatism, nerve pain, and many other diseases involving tissue inflammation.

Study Findings

Two studies were conducted using willow bark to treat acute back pain. One randomly assigned people to receive either 120 or 240 mg of salicin or a placebo. Those taking willow bark (✓✓✓) had significantly less pain than those taking a placebo. One person (✗✗) had a severe allergic reaction to the lower dose of willow bark. Another trial (✓✓✓) randomly assigned people with acute back pain to either willow bark extract or a conventional COX-2 inhibitor anti-inflammatory drug. After four weeks, pain reduction did not differ between the two groups, nor did adverse effects.

Two controlled studies have also examined willow bark extract to treat osteoarthritis. One study (✓✓✓) gave patients an extract containing 240 mg of salicin or placebo. After two weeks, patients taking willow bark had significantly less pain than the placebo group, although the reduction was only 14 percent. No differences existed in physical function or stiffness. However, a 2004 trial (✗✗✗) with osteoarthritis found willow bark extract (240 mg of salicin) no more effective in reducing pain than placebo. A third group taking the conventional pain reliever diclofenac had a significant reduction in pain. Another trial (✗✗✗) with rheumatoid arthritis patients showed no difference in pain relief between willow bark and placebo.

Cautions

All salicylates can have some adverse effects and drug interactions. This includes willow bark products. They can be irritating to the stomach, and a condition known as salicylate toxicity (characterized by nausea, vomiting, diarrhea, dizziness, and lethargy) can develop. Some people are hypersensitive to salicylates, and people with a history of allergies or asthma should avoid using willow bark products. In clinical trials, 1 to 3 percent of participants had allergic reactions.

Willow bark shouldn't be given to children who have a fever that may be due to certain viral illnesses, including chicken pox or influenza, because of the risk of Reye's syndrome. Although the connection between Reye's syndrome and willow bark is not as well defined as with aspirin, this is due mostly to a lack of research. Willow bark should also be avoided by pregnant women and anyone with ulcers. In addition, willow bark should not be taken by lactating women, as its salicylates can be excreted in breast milk and have been linked to adverse effects in breast-fed infants. Side effects are infrequent but may include nausea, diarrhea, and digestive upset. Excessive long-term use could cause stomach ulcers.

Aspirin slows blood clotting and is recommended for some people at risk of stroke (caused by blood clots). However, if someone is already taking anticoagulant medication, using willow bark products may increase the risk of bleeding.

Recommendations

While modern research has validated the traditional uses of willow bark, this doesn't mean that taking willow bark instead of aspirin is the best thing to do. Willow bark, like all other herbs and plants, varies in the concentrations of active ingredients, depending on when and how it is harvested, stored, and processed. Since aspirin is widely available, inexpensive, and standardized, it should always be used by those taking these products for extended periods. For occasional use in relieving headaches or other aches and pains, willow bark appears effective and safe.

● Dosage

Usually 60 to 120 mg of salicin is recommended per day. Up to 240 mg can be taken, which may be the most effective dose. People vary in how well they can tolerate salicylates.

● Treatment Categories

Complementary

To relieve pain in adults	☺☺☺
To relieve headaches in adults	☺☺
To treat back pain in adults	☺☺
To reduce fever in adults	☺
To treat osteoarthritis	☹
To treat rheumatoid arthritis	☹☹
To relieve arthritic stiffness	☹☹

Risk of Serious Side Effects

When taken by children under seventeen years of age	⊘⊘⊘

● Further Reading

Biegert, Claudia, Irmela Wagner, Rainer Lüdtke, Ina Kötter, Claudia Lohmüller, Ilhan Günaydin, Katja Taxis, and Lutz Heide. "Efficacy and Safety of Willow Bark Extract in the Treatment of Osteoarthritis and Rheumatoid Arthritis: Results of Two Randomized Double-Blind Controlled Trials." *Journal of Rheumatology* 31, no. 11 (November 2004): 2121 – 30.

Clauson, Kevin A., Marile L. Santamarina, Christian M. Buettner, and Jacintha S. Cauffield. "Evaluation of Presence of Aspirin-Related Warnings with Willow Bark." *Annals of Pharmacotherapy* 39, no. 7 – 8 (July – August 2005): 1234 – 37.

WITCH HAZEL

What It Is

Witch hazel, or *Hamamelis virginiana*, is a small tree native to North America. It forms distinctive yellow treadlike flowers in the fall while other trees are losing their leaves. Hamamelis water, a witch hazel extract used medicinally, is made by passing steam through the plant parts and adding alcohol to keep the cooled material soluble.

Claims

An extract of witch hazel was used by Native Americans to reduce inflammation and as an astringent for the treatment of diarrhea, hemorrhoids, and a variety of skin conditions. All astringents contract tissues and thus reduce fluid secretions. A tea would be drunk or gargled for relief of cold, flu, or sore throat. Witch hazel was also taken internally for diarrhea, internal bleeding, and menstrual pain. Topical remedies were used to stop minor bleeding; to soothe insect bites, sunburn, and poison ivy; and to relieve the pain and inflammation of sore backs and muscle pain. The herb became a common ingredient in patent medicines of the nineteenth century and was the active ingredient in the popular Pond's Extract.

Many of witch hazel's topical uses remain popular today. Astringent compounds in witch hazel are believed to stem bleeding, whether from abrasions or from minor cuts such as shaving nicks. Witch hazel is said to reduce the pain and swelling of hemorrhoids and bruises. Many people use witch hazel pads, small pieces of thin cloth packaged in a witch hazel solution, to cool sunburn and other minor burns, to help relieve the itching of insect bites and poison ivy, and to dry out cold sores. Witch hazel is used as a remedy for varicose veins and other venous conditions. Hospital personnel use witch hazel pads to soothe the itching and burning of rectal or vaginal surgical stitches.

Some companies sell witch hazel in teething preparations. Witch hazel is also said to help prevent or treat inflammation of the mouth, eczema, skin ulcers, and bedsores.

Study Findings

Some studies have been done on the compounds extracted from witch hazel. The astringent compounds are called "tannins." Alcohol extracts of witch hazel leaves contain the highest concentration of tannins. However, the most commonly available preparations are made by steam distillation to which alcohol is added later. These contain no tannins. Since alcohol is an astringent, this may account for any observed astringent activity of these preparations.

German scientists determined that a witch hazel bark extract exhibited significant antiviral activity against herpes simplex type 1. Witch hazel was also shown to have antioxidant and anti-inflammatory properties. Japanese researchers tested sixty-five plant extracts (✓) for antioxidant activity. Witch hazel was one of two herbs (the other being horse chestnut) found to have strong free-radical scavenging activity. The researchers concluded that these herbs were likely candidates for use in antiaging or antiwrinkle products for protecting the skin — although no clinical trials have been completed.

Lab tests have shown that witch hazel extracts have weak antimicrobial activity. In one of the few controlled human trials (✓✓✓) of witch hazel's anti-inflammatory properties, an after-sun lotion containing witch hazel was shown to protect the skin from ultraviolet-induced inflammation and redness. A later study (✓✓✓) confirmed these findings, but the improvements were significantly less than those seen with a 0.25 percent hydrocortisone lotion. However, another study (✗✗✗) did not find any benefit beyond a placebo effect.

Cautions

Topical use of witch hazel is very safe, although it may on rare occasions cause minor skin irritations. "Witch hazel water" and other commercial products are often for external use only. Drinking witch hazel tea is thought to be relatively safe, with one drawback being the possibility that when taken internally, the high level of tannins may cause nausea, vomiting, or constipation (✗✗). There is some concern they may also cause liver damage.

According to the Natural Database, there is insufficient reliable information to evaluate the use of witch hazel during pregnancy and lactation; therefore, we recommend women avoid using it during these times.

Recommendations

Alcohol extracts of witch hazel may have some value as astringents, but this is not a readily available form of the remedy. Varro Tyler quotes from a 1947 pharmacy manual: "Hamamelis [witch hazel] is so nearly destitute of medicinal virtues that it scarcely deserves official recognition." He claims it would be better to use red wine as an astringent since it also contains tannins and about as much alcohol as witch hazel extract. Witch hazel preparations appear to bring relief for different skin injuries, though we question whether this relief is the result of witch hazel or of the other ingredients in the preparations — or even the pads themselves. Regardless, when used externally, these are safe. Conventional therapies should be pursued if the irritation persists or worsens in any way.

Dosage

The extract is used to make creams and various preparations and pads for topical application.

Treatment Categories

Conventional

Topically to relieve itching and
burning of anorectal disorders
and external hemorrhoids ☺☺
Topically to reduce minor bleeding ☺☺
Topically as an antiseptic for mild
skin injuries ☺☺

Complementary

To treat fever blisters, sunburn, or varicose veins ☺

Scientifically Unproven

For any internal use

Further Reading

Foster, Steven, and Varro E. Tyler. *Tyler's Honest Herbal: A Sensible Guide to the Use of Herbs and Related Remedies.* 4th ed. New York: Haworth Herbal, 1999, 383–85.

Hughes-Formella, B. J., A. Filbry, J. Gassmueller, and F. Rippke. "Anti-inflammatory Efficacy of Topical Preparations with 10% Hamamelis Distillate in a UV Erythema Test." *Skin Pharmacology and Applied Skin Physiology* 15, no. 2 (March–April 2002): 125–32.

ZINC

What It Is

Zinc is a naturally occurring mineral that is required in the diet. In the body, it is incorporated into a number of enzymes involved in various reactions throughout the body. Zinc deficiencies are rare and occur primarily when other problems prevent the absorption of zinc from the intestines. Deficiencies lead to skin problems, diarrhea, problems with the immune system, and failure to thrive in babies. Zinc is present in legumes, grains, peanuts, and many meats. Both meat eaters and vegetarians generally get enough of the mineral in their diet.

Claims

Zinc supplements have been recommended to treat acne, diarrhea, diabetes, high blood pressure, ulcers, and enlarged prostates and to fight off infections.

Popular interest in zinc has focused on lozenges to cure the common cold, treat recurrent ear infections, and prevent acute lower respiratory infections. Zinc supplements have been promoted to benefit those who are HIV positive. Zinc is also recommended for a huge range of other conditions.

Study Findings

Zinc lozenges are popularly advertised as an effective way to treat the common cold. In 1984, the first clinic trial on this topic reported a dramatic average seven-day reduction in the duration of cold symptoms. Further clinical trials reported beneficial effects, but none as great as the 1984 study. A 2004 review found twelve clinical trials, seven of which (✓✓✓✓) found that zinc lozenges shortened the duration of cold symptoms, while five (✗✗✗) found them no better than placebo. Meta-analyses in 1997 and again in 2000 concluded that while beneficial effects had been reported from randomized controlled trials, the results were very weak and did not warrant recommending zinc lozenges for the common cold.

However, the 2004 review carried out a detailed analysis of the amount of zinc ions released by the lozenges. Zinc is believed to work when zinc ions (Zn^{2+}) combine with charged particles on the surfaces of cold viruses and nasal passageways to interfere with the life-cycle of the virus. This means that the amount of Zn^{2+} released from lozenges is very important. The review found that little or no Zn^{2+} was released in the studies that found no benefit from the lozenges. These primarily used a popular brand (Cold-Eeze) that used zinc acetate to mask the bad taste of zinc but released little Zn^{2+} into the body. Some are therefore recommending that only the form of zinc used in the 1984 trial, called "zinc gluconate," be used. Another recommendation is that higher-dose lozenges be used. In those studies with positive effects, the zinc lozenges contained 13.3 to 23 mg of zinc, whereas some of the negative studies used lozenges containing about 5 mg each. Although the evidence is still unclear, the higher-dose lozenges do appear to somewhat reduce the duration of cold symptoms.

Another change has been to use zinc nasal gel to apply zinc directly to where the cold viruses replicate. A small number of trials (✓✓✓) have shown that the gel can reduce the duration of symptoms. It should be noted that in all these cases, zinc is taken within twenty-four hours of initially feeling the cold symptoms. There is no evidence that regular intake of zinc supplements will prevent the common cold.

Zinc has also been recommended in the treatment of wounds for thousands of years. Applying zinc topically to skin wounds is mentioned in three-thousand-year-old Egyptian papyri. More recently, oral zinc supplements have been recommended to promote healing of many different types of wounds, including surgical ones. Zinc does play an important role in normal wound healing. Zinc deficiencies can thus delay wound healing. However, evidence of benefit from zinc supplementation is not clear-cut. Both a 1998 Cochrane review (✗✗✗) and another 2003 review (✗✗✗) found no evidence to support routine use of zinc supplements when people have leg ulcers.

Some studies (✓✓✓) have found faster recovery time and reduced incidence of postoperative complications with zinc supplementation. Zinc may be helpful in speeding healing after burns or injury. The results seem to be particularly pronounced when there is zinc deficiency prior to the treatment. An easy, reliable method of determining adequate zinc levels is not available. However, when people with poor or inadequate diets have wounds, zinc supplementation should be considered.

Zinc deficiency is more likely to occur in developing countries, where diarrhea is often another serious and widespread problem. Zinc supplements have been recommended to treat diarrhea. A 2000 systematic review (✓✓✓✓) found ten studies carried out with children in developing countries. The studies examined the impact both on the day zinc supplements were given and after seven days of supplementation. Half the studies examined acute diarrhea and half examined chronic diarrhea. On average, the number of children with acute diarrhea was 15 percent lower on the first day and 22 percent lower after seven days. For those with chronic diarrhea, 24 percent fewer had diarrhea on the first day and 39 percent fewer seven days later. All children were also given adequate water and nutrition. Since that review, positive effects have been noted in other studies in Nepal and India, though a 2005 study in Turkey found no benefits from zinc supplements.

Use of zinc by people infected with HIV became popular after it was noticed that many infected people had lower than normal zinc levels. Since zinc deficiency is known to adversely affect the immune system, it was logical to conclude that supplements might help those with HIV. However, studies have now shown (✖✖✖) that HIV patients taking zinc supplements were twice as likely to develop AIDS and more likely to die sooner. The reasons for these connections are not known.

Cautions

Zinc lozenges have a very bad taste, yet they are to be taken every two hours or so. The taste is so bad that about one-third of the research subjects in studies had nausea, and about 10 percent had diarrhea. This has also created problems for blinding of trials since the zinc is easily distinguishable from placebo.

High doses of zinc have been found to negatively impact the immune system and to lower HDL levels (which can lead to higher overall cholesterol levels) and hinder the absorption of copper (another essential element). The Tolerable Upper Intake Limit is 40 mg per day for adults, which would quickly be exceeded taking high-dose lozenges every two hours. The upper limit for children ranges from 4 mg per day during the first six months to 23 mg for nine- to thirteen-year-olds and 34 mg for adolescents.

High levels of zinc can prevent absorption of copper, another mineral required in small amounts. Copper deficiency leads to anemia. Zinc effectively treats Wilson's disease, a hereditary disease in which the body retains too much copper, thus damaging the brain, eyes, and kidneys.

In April 2004, ConsumerLab.com reported testing on zinc lozenges, pills, and liquids. All seven lozenges tested contained their claimed amount of zinc. However, there was significant variation in the amount of zinc per lozenge and the suggested doses. These ranged from as little as 5 mg per day to as much as 80 mg. Of the nine pills and liquids, two contained less zinc than claimed, ranging from 73 to 85 percent of the label amounts. Ironically, the product with the greatest shortfall indicated that it was made under "good manufacturing practices." No products were contaminated with unacceptable amounts of lead.

Recommendations

The evidence regarding zinc supplements and cold symptoms is complicated. Some benefit has been found for certain formulations that deliver the correct form and dose of zinc. However, the most popular brand of lozenge (Cold-Eeze) has not fared well in controlled studies. Other brands containing higher doses of zinc gluconate appear to be more effective, though they also have the bad taste. Zinc nasal gel may overcome some of these problems.

The use of zinc supplements for other conditions has even less support. However, people can have zinc deficiency, especially in developing countries. Supplementation there can be a simple and effective means of treating various disorders, including diarrhea and impaired wound healing.

Dosage

Different forms of zinc provide different amounts of elemental zinc. Most lozenges contain 9 to 24 mg of zinc, with one lozenge being recommended every two hours. For treating or preventing the common cold with intranasal zinc, 2.1 mg of zinc per day has been used.

The RDA recommended by the Institute of Medicine in 2001 is 11 mg per day for men and 8 mg per day for women. Vegetarians require an additional 50 percent because chemicals commonly found in plants hinder the absorption of zinc. Pregnant and breast-feeding women should increase their consumption of zinc by a few milligrams per day but should discuss dosage with a physician.

Treatment Categories

Conventional

To overcome zinc deficiency	☺☺☺☺
To treat Wilson's disease	☺☺☺☺

Complementary

To treat diarrhea in zinc-deficient children	☺☺☺
With the appropriate formulation, to reduce the duration of common cold symptoms	☺☺

To prevent the common cold	☹☹☹
To prevent or treat the flu (influenza)	☹☹
To enhance wound healing in zinc-deficient people	☺
To enhance wound healing in general	☹
To treat hypogeusia (taste dysfunction)	☺☺
To treat psoriasis	☹☹

Scientifically Unproven

For any other indication

Further Reading

Eby, George A. "Zinc Lozenges: Cold Cure or Candy? Solution Chemistry Determinations." *Bioscience Reports* 24, no. 1 (February 2004): 23 – 39.

Gray, Mikel. "Does Oral Zinc Supplementation Promote Healing of Chronic Wounds?" *Journal of Wound Ostomy and Continence Nursing* 30, no. 6 (November 2003): 295 – 99.

Hulisz, Darrell. "Efficacy of Zinc Against Common Cold Viruses: An Overview." *Journal of the American Pharmacists Association* 44, no. 5 (September – October 2004): 594 – 603.

INDEXES

EFFECTIVENESS OF THERAPIES

LISTED BY DISEASE OR SYMPTOM

This index shows the authors' rating for the effectiveness of each therapy, herb, vitamin, and supplement, listed alphabetically by disease, condition, or symptom. For more information on any of the author-rated therapies, see the listing for that therapy. Therapies or remedies for which insufficient evidence exists for a reliable recommendation are not included in this section. Before acting on these recommendations, please read the complete entry. The index is intended to guide you to the evidence discussed in each entry.

Since the evidence for any particular therapy can not only support its benefits but also show its potential for harm, we have compiled a single guide that we hope will be useful. The rating is our "best estimate" of the benefit or harm for any particular indication. Others could (and often do) look at the same evidence and derive different conclusions.

Overall Recommendation	Criteria
☺☺☺☺	75% – 100% confidence that the therapy is potentially beneficial
☺☺☺	50% – 74% confidence that the therapy is potentially beneficial
☺☺	25% – 49% confidence that the therapy is potentially beneficial
☺	0% – 24% confidence that the therapy is potentially beneficial
☹	0% – 24% confidence that the therapy is of no benefit or potentially harmful
☹☹	25% – 49% confidence that the therapy is of no benefit or potentially harmful
☹☹☹	50% – 74% confidence that the therapy is of no benefit or potentially harmful
☹☹☹☹	75% – 100% confidence that the therapy is of no benefit or potentially harmful

EFFECTIVENESS OF THERAPIES: LISTED BY DISEASE OR SYMPTOM

Abrasions

☹☹ comfrey

Acid Reflux

☹☹ licorice

Acne

☹☹☹☹ aloe
☺☺ tea tree oil

Addictions

☹☹☹☹ acupuncture

ADHD

☹ omega fatty acids
☹☹ vitamin C

Adrenal Insufficiency

☺☺☺ DHEA

AIDS

☹ St. John's wort
☹ selenium

Alertness. Mental

☺☺☺ green tea

Allergies

☺☺☺☺ bee products

Alzheimer's Disease

☺ DHEA
☺☺☺ ginkgo biloba
☹☹☹ vitamin C
☹☹ vitamin E

Amyotrophic Lateral Sclerosis (ALS)

☹☹☹ antioxidants
☹☹ creatine

Angina

☹☹☹☹ chelation therapy
☺ Coenzyme Q$_{10}$

Anti-Aging

☹☹☹ Coenzyme Q$_{10}$
☺☺ DHEA

Antioxidant Source

☺☺☺ grape seed extract
☺☺☺ green tea
☺☺☺☺ lutein
☺☺☺☺ mangosteen
☺☺☺☺ selenium
☺☺☺☺ vitamin C

Anxiety

☺☺☺ aromatherapy
☺☺☺☺ biofeedback
☺☺☺ breathing techniques
☺☺☺ kava
☺☺☺☺ meditation
☺☺☺ reflexology
☺☺ St. John's wort
☺☺ tai chi
☺ valerian

Arthritis

☺☺☺ capsaicin
☺☺☺☺ chondroitin sulfate
☹☹☹ creatine
☹☹☹ feverfew
☺ ginger
☺☺☺☺ glucosamine
☺ MSM
☺☺ SAM-e
☹ selenium
☹☹☹ shark cartilage
☹☹ vitamin E
☹ willow bark

ALTERNATIVE MEDICINE

Asthma

- ☹☹☹☹ acupuncture
- ☺☺☺☺ breathing techniques
- ☺ omega fatty acids
- ☹☹☹ vitamin C
- ☺☺ yoga

Atherosclerosis

- ☹ garlic

Athlete's Foot

- ☺☺ tea tree oil

Athletic Performance Enhancement

- ☹☹☹☹ androstenedione
- ☹☹☹☹ chromium
- ☹☹ Coenzyme Q$_{10}$
- ☺☺☺☺ creatine
- ☹☹☹☹ DHEA
- ☹☹☹☹ ginseng
- ☹☹☹☹ guarana

Back Pain

- ☺☺ biofeedback
- ☺☺ willow bark

Back Pain (Acute)

- ☹☹ acupuncture
- ☺☺☺☺ chiropractic

Back Pain (Chronic)

- ☺ acupuncture
- ☺☺☺☺ chiropractic

Balance Development

- ☺☺☺☺ tai chi

Benign Prostatic Hyperplasia (BPH)

- ☺☺☺☺ saw palmetto

Bleeding

- ☺☺ witch hazel

Blood Glucose

- ☺ bilberry
- ☺ ginseng
- ☺ nopal

Blood Pressure Reduction

- ☺☺☺☺ biofeedback
- ☺☺ Coenzyme Q$_{10}$
- ☺☺☺☺ meditation

Bruises

- ☹ comfrey

Burns (Mild)

- ☺☺☺ bee products

Cancer

- ☺☺☺☺ diet and nutrition
- ☺ green tea
- ☺ lutein
- ☺ melatonin
- ☹☹ noni juice
- ☺ omega fatty acids
- ☺☺☺ selenium
- ☹☹☹☹ shark cartilage
- ☺ soy
- ☹ vitamin C
- ☹☹☹☹ vitamin E

Cancer (Breast)

- ☹☹ garlic
-   green tea
-   soy

Cancer (Colorectal)

- ☺ garlic

Cancer (Gastrointestinal)

- ☹☹☹☹ antioxidants

Cancer (Lung)

- ☹☹ garlic

Cancer (Prostate)

- ☺ garlic
- ☹☹☹ saw palmetto

Cancer (Stomach)

- ☺ garlic

EFFECTIVENESS OF THERAPIES: LISTED BY DISEASE OR SYMPTOM

Cardiovascular Disease

☹☹☹☹ antioxidants
☺☺☺☺ diet and nutrition
☺ grape seed extract
☺☺ lutein
☺☺☺ omega fatty acids
☹ selenium
☺ soy
☹☹ vitamin C
☹☹☹☹ vitamin E

Cataracts

☺☺☺☺ chondroitin sulfate
☺☺ lutein
☺ omega fatty acids
☹ vitamin E

Chemotherapy-Induced Nausea

☺☺☺ acupuncture
☹ ginger

Cholesterol (High)

☺ bee products
☺ chromium
☺☺ Coenzyme Q$_{10}$
☺☺ garlic
☹ ginseng
☺ green tea
☺ nopal
☺☺☺ psyllium
☺☺☺☺ red yeast rice
☺☺☺ soy

Chronic Disease Prevention

☺☺☺ antioxidants
☺☺☺☺ diet and nutrition
☹☹☹☹ vitamin E

Chronic Fatigue Syndrome

☹ DHEA

Circulatory Problems

☺ bilberry

Cirrhosis

☺ milk thistle

Claudication

☺☺☺ ginkgo biloba
☹ omega fatty acids

Cognitive Function

☺☺☺ ginkgo biloba
☺ ginseng

Colds

☺☺☺ echinacea
☹☹ goldenseal
☹☹☹☹ vitamin C
☹☹ vitamin E
☺☺ zinc

Congestive Heart Failure

☺☺☺ Coenzyme Q$_{10}$
☺ creatine
☹ ginseng

Constipation

☺☺ cascara
☺☺☺☺ colonics
☺☺☺☺ psyllium
☺☺☺☺ senna

Cough

☺☺ licorice

Cramps (Intestinal)

☺ chamomile

Crohn's Disease

☺☺ probiotics

Cuts

☹☹ comfrey

ALTERNATIVE MEDICINE

Dementia

☺☺ ginkgo biloba

Dental Pain

☺☺☺ acupuncture

Depression

☹☹☹ ginkgo biloba
☺ light therapy
☺☺☺ SAM-e
☺☺☺☺ St. John's wort
☺☺ tai chi

Detoxification

☹☹☹☹ colonics

Diabetes

☺☺☺ chromium
☺ Coenzyme Q$_{10}$
☹☹☹☹ cranberry
☺☺☺☺ diet and nutrition
☹☹ garlic
☺ nopal
☹☹ omega fatty acids
☺☺ psyllium
☺ soy
☹ vitamin E

Diarrhea

☺☺ bilberry
☺☺☺☺ probiotics
☺ psyllium
☺☺☺ zinc

Digestive System Stimulation

☺☺ capsaicin

Disease Prevention

☹☹☹ aromatherapy

Dizziness

☺☺ ginkgo biloba

Dry Eyes

☺☺ chondroitin sulfate

Dyspepsia

☺ capsaicin
☺☺ chamomile
☹☹ licorice
☺☺ peppermint

Eczema

☹☹☹☹ aloe
☹☹☹☹ evening primrose

Energy Improvement

☹☹ chromium
☺ ginseng

Erectile Dysfunction

☺ DHEA

Exercise Tolerance

☺ creatine

Eye Health

☹☹ bilberry
☺☺☺ lutein
☺ omega fatty acids

Fatigue

☺ ginseng

Fever

☺ willow bark

Fever Blisters

☺ witch hazel

Fibromyalgia Syndrome

☺☺ SAM-e

EFFECTIVENESS OF THERAPIES: LISTED BY DISEASE OR SYMPTOM

Flexibility Development

☺☺☺☺ tai chi
☺☺☺☺ yoga

Flu

☹☹ echinacea
☺☺ elderberry
☹☹ goldenseal
☹☹ zinc

Fungal Infections

☺☺ tea tree oil

Glucose Intolerance

☹☹☹ chromium

Hay Fever

☹☹☹☹ grape seed extract
☺ MSM

Headache (Various)

☺☺ acupressure
☺ acupuncture
☺☺ chiropractic
☺☺ ginkgo biloba
☺☺☺ hypnosis
☺ reflexology
☺☺ willow bark

Healing Promotion

☹☹ comfrey

Heart Disease

☹☹☹☹ chelation therapy
☹☹☹ green tea
☺☺ hawthorn

Heavy Metal Poisoning

☺☺☺☺ chelation therapy

Hemorrhoids

☺☺ horse chestnut
☺ psyllium
☺☺ witch hazel

Hepatitis

☺☺ licorice
☺ milk thistle
☹ St. John's wort

High Blood Pressure

☺ garlic
☹☹ grape seed extract
☺☺ green tea
☹☹☹☹ vitamin E

HIV/AIDS. *See also* AIDS

☹ St. John's wort
☹ selenium

Hot Flashes

☺☺☺ black cohosh
☹☹☹ ginseng
☺ soy

Huntington's Disease

☺ Coenzyme Q_{10}

Hypertension

☺ omega fatty acids
☺ psyllium

Hypertriglyceridemia

☹☹☹☹ omega fatty acids

Hypogeusia

☺☺ zinc

Hypoglycemia

☺☺ chromium

ALTERNATIVE MEDICINE

Hypothyroidism

☹ selenium

Immune System

☹ ginseng

Incontinence

☺☺☺☺ biofeedback

Indigestion

☹☹ licorice

Infections

☺☺ bee products
☺ chamomile
☺☺ tea tree oil

Insomnia

☺ ginseng
☺ melatonin

Intestinal Spasms

☺☺☺ peppermint

Irritable Bowel Syndrome (IBS)

☹ capsaicin
☺☺ peppermint
☺ probiotics
☺☺ psyllium

Itching

☺☺ peppermint

Jaundice

☺☺☺☺ light therapy

Jet Lag

☺☺☺ melatonin

Labor Pains

☹☹☹☹ evening primrose
☺☺☺ hypnosis

Lactose Intolerance

☹ probiotics

Laxative

☺☺☺☺ aloe

Liver Problems

☹☹☹☹ kava
☺ milk thistle
☺☺ SAM-e

Macular Degeneration

☺ ginkgo biloba
☺☺☺☺ lutein

Mastalgia

☺☺ evening primrose
☹ omega fatty acids
☺ soy

Memory Loss

☺☺ ginkgo biloba
☺ ginseng

Memory Loss (Age-Related)

☺☺ ginkgo biloba

Menopause Symptoms

☺☺☺ black cohosh
☺☺ DHEA
☹☹☹☹ dong quai
☺ ginseng
☺ kava
☹☹☹☹ wild yam

Menstrual Problems

☹☹☹ evening primrose
☺ omega fatty acids

Mental Performance

☹☹☹ DHEA
☺ ginseng

EFFECTIVENESS OF THERAPIES: LISTED BY DISEASE OR SYMPTOM

Migraine Headache

- ☺☺☺☺ biofeedback
- ☺☺ breathing techniques
- ☺☺ chiropractic
- ☺☺☺ Coenzyme Q_{10}
- ☺☺ feverfew
- ☺ omega fatty acids

Mood Enhancer

- ☹☹☹ ginkgo biloba
- ☺ ginseng
- ☺☺ tai chi

Morning Sickness

- ☺ acupressure
- ☺ ginger

Motion Sickness

- ☺ ginger

Muscle Aches

- ☹ omega fatty acids

Muscular Dystrophy

- ☺ creatine

Nail Infections (Fungal)

- ☺☺ tea tree oil

Nausea

- ☺☺☺☺ acupressure
- ☺ ginger
- ☹ peppermint
- ☺☺☺ progressive muscle relaxation

Neck Pain

- ☹ chiropractic

Neuralgia

- ☺ peppermint

Neuropathy

- ☺☺☺☺ capsaicin
- ☺ soy

Night Vision

- ☹☹☹ bilberry
- ☺ grape seed extract

Obsessive-Compulsive Disorder

- ☺ St. John's wort

Osteoarthritis (*See* Arthritis)

Osteoporosis

- ☺ DHEA
- ☺ evening primrose
- ☹☹ soy

Pain (Acute or Chronic)

- ☺☺ aromatherapy
- ☺☺☺☺ capsaicin
- ☺ ginger
- ☺☺☺ glucosamine
- ☺☺☺☺ hypnosis
- ☺ MSM
- ☺ magnet therapy
- ☺☺ massage therapy
- ☺☺☺ meditation
- ☺☺ peppermint
- ☺☺☺ progressive muscle relaxation
- ☺ reflexology
- ☹☹☹☹ reiki
- ☺☺ SAM-e
- ☺☺☺☺ visualization or guided imagery
- ☺☺☺ willow bark
- ☺☺ yoga

Parkinson's Disease

- ☺ Coenzyme Q_{10}

Periodontal Disease

- ☹☹☹ comfrey

ALTERNATIVE MEDICINE

Peripheral Arterial Disease

☹☹☹☹ chelation therapy
☺☺☺ ginkgo biloba
☹ omega fatty acids

Physical Fitness

☺☺☺ yoga

Polyneuropathy

☹ St. John's wort

Preeclampsia

☺☺ antioxidants
☹☹☹☹ evening primrose

Pregnancy Complications

☹☹☹ vitamin C

Premature Ejaculation

☹ dong quai

Premenstrual Syndrome (PMS)

☹☹☹ evening primrose
☺ St. John's wort

Preventive Medicine

☹☹☹☹ chiropractic

Prostate Problems

☺ nopal
☹ saw palmetto

Psoriasis

☺☺☺ aloe
☹☹ zinc

Quality of Life Improvement

☺ aromatherapy

Relaxation

☺☺☺ aromatherapy
☺☺☺☺ massage therapy
☺☺ naturopathic medicine
☺☺☺☺ progressive muscle relaxation
☺☺☺ reflexology
☹☹☹☹ reiki
☺☺☺☺ visualization or guided imagery

Respiratory Problems

☺☺ massage therapy

Restenosis

☺ omega fatty acids

Restlessness

☺☺ kava
☺☺ valerian

Retinitis Pigmentosa

☺ lutein

Retinopathy

☺☺ bilberry

Rheumatoid Arthritis (See Arthritis)

Scurvy

☺☺☺☺ vitamin C

Seasickness

☺☺ ginger

Seasonal Affective Disorder (SAD)

☹☹☹ ginkgo biloba
☺☺☺☺ light therapy
☺ St. John's wort

Sexual Arousal

☹☹☹☹ androstenedione

EFFECTIVENESS OF THERAPIES: LISTED BY DISEASE OR SYMPTOM

Sexual Dysfunction

☹ DHEA
☹☹ ginkgo biloba
☹☹☹ horny goat weed

Sexual Performance

☹☹☹☹ androstenedione
☹☹☹☹ horny goat weed

Shoulder Pain

☹ chiropractic

Skin Disorders

☺☺☺ aloe
☺☺ chamomile
☺☺ DHEA
☺☺☺☺ light therapy
☺☺ lutein

Sleep Inducement

☺☺☺ chamomile
☺☺ melatonin
☺☺☺☺ valerian

Smoking Cessation

☹☹ acupressure
☹☹☹☹ acupuncture
☹☹☹ hypnosis

Sore Throat

☹☹☹ comfrey

Sprains

☹ comfrey

Strength Development

☺☺☺☺ tai chi

Stress Relief

☺☺☺ aromatherapy
☺☺ kava
☺☺☺☺ massage therapy
☺☺☺☺ meditation
☺☺ progressive muscle relaxation
☺☺☺ yoga

Stroke

☺ omega fatty acids

Sunburn

☺ witch hazel

Systemic Lupus Erythematosis

☺☺ DHEA

Tension

☺☺☺☺ biofeedback
☺☺☺ reflexology
☺☺☺☺ visualization or guided imagery

Tinnitus

☹☹☹ ginkgo biloba

Triglycerides (High)

☺ chromium
☺☺☺☺ omega fatty acids
☺☺☺☺ red yeast rice

Ulcers

☺☺☺ bee products
☺ capsaicin
☺ horse chestnut
☺ licorice

Urinary Tract Infection (UTI)

☺☺☺ cranberry

ALTERNATIVE MEDICINE

Vaginosis

☺ tea tree oil

Varicose Veins

☺☺ grape seed extract
☺☺☺ horse chestnut
☺ witch hazel

Vertigo

☺ ginger

Viral Infections

☹☹☹ St. John's wort

Vomiting

☺☺☺☺ acupressure
☺☺☺ progressive muscle relaxation

Weight Loss

☹☹☹☹ acupuncture
☹☹☹☹ cascara
☹☹☹ chromium
☹☹☹☹ guarana
☹☹ hypnosis

Well-Being

☺ DHEA
☺☺☺☺ diet and nutrition
☺ ginseng
☺☺ meditation

Wilson's Disease

☺☺☺☺ zinc

Wounds (Minor Skin)

☺☺☺ aloe
☺ zinc

SCRIPTURE INDEX

SCRIPTURE INDEX

ALTERNATIVE MEDICINE

SUBJECT INDEX

SUBJECT INDEX

SUBJECT INDEX

SUBJECT INDEX

Christian
Medical
Association
Resources

Medically reliable ... biblically sound. That is the promise of Christian Medical Association *Resources* and our publishing partnership with Zondervan. Because your health is at stake, you cannot settle for anything less than the whole truth.

From these resources, people's faith can draw from both the knowledge of medical science and the wisdom of God's word. You will benefit from the cutting-edge knowledge of experienced, trusted, and respected doctors. These persons of faith and science can help you gain new insights into the vital link between health and spirituality. A sound biblical analysis of treatments and technologies is essential to protecting yourself from seemingly harmless — yet spiritually, ethically, or medically unsound — options.

Founded in 1931, the Christian Medical Association helps thousands of doctors minister to their patients by imitating the Great Physician, Jesus Christ. The Christian Medical Association provides a voice on the important bioethical issues of our time to the public, the media, and our policy makers. We minister to needy patients around the world through medical missions. We evangelize and disciple the next generation of Christian doctors via campus ministries on nearly every medical and dental school. And, we provide educational and inspirational resources to the church.

To learn more about the Christian Medical Association and its sister organization, the Christian Dental Association, browse the website at *www.cmda.org* or call Christian Medical & Dental Associations' Life & Health Resources at 888-231-2637.

> *"Dear friend, I pray that you may enjoy good health and that all may go well with you, even as your soul is getting along well."*
>
> 3 John 2

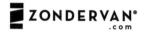